CW00954330

Stell and Maran's

Head and Neck Surgery

Stell and Maran's

Head and Neck Surgery

Third Edition

A. G. D. Maran
MD, FRCS(Ed), FRCS, FACS, FRCP(Ed)
Professor of Otolaryngology, University of Edinburgh, UK

M. Gaze
MRCP, FRCR
Consultant Radiation Oncologist,
University College London Hospitals and
Hospitals for Sick Children, Great Ormond Street, London, UK

J. A. Wilson
MD, FRCS(Ed), FRCS
Consultant Otolaryngologist, Royal Infirmary,
Glasgow, UK

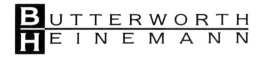

Butterworth-Heinemann Ltd
Linacre House, Jordan Hill, Oxford OX2 8DP

A member of the Reed Elsevier group

OXFORD   LONDON   BOSTON
MUNICH   NEW DELHI   SINGAPORE   SYDNEY
TOKYO   TORONTO   WELLINGTON

First published 1972
Second edition 1978
Third edition 1993

British Library Cataloguing in Publication Data
Stell, P. M.
  Stell and Maran's Head and Neck Surgery.
  – 3 Rev. ed
  I. Title II. Maran, A. G. D.
  III. Gaze, M.   IV. Wilson, J. A.
  617.51059

ISBN 0 7506 0916 8

Photoset by Wilmaset Ltd., Birkenhead, Wirral.
Printed and bound in Great Britain by The Bath Press Ltd, Avon.

Contents

Preface

It is now almost 25 years since the first edition of this book was begun. At that time, head and neck surgery in most European countries was in its infancy. Linear accelerators had only just become available, reconstructive surgery was in its infancy: axial flaps, musculocutaneous flaps and free flaps were scarcely thought of, let alone in general use. On the diagnostic front, CT scans and MRI were luxuries of the future. Much of the painstaking pathological work which has done so much to improve our understanding of these diseases had not yet been undertaken. Furthermore, many otolaryngologists had a poor basic surgical training and were, therefore, unsuited and untrained to embark upon major soft tissue surgery. We started a head and neck surgery course in 1968 and have now held 27 such courses which have attracted 500 applicants from all over the world. This small textbook encompasses what is now taught on that course.

In the succeeding quarter of a century, the field has changed enormously and a comprehensive textbook of head and neck surgery which included technical details would run to several volumes. By our trainees we have been encouraged to believe that there is still a place for a simple text describing the techniques of head and neck surgery for the trainee in otolaryngology, plastic, oral and general surgery, for the occasional surgeon who is required to carry out one of these procedures without skilled assistance and for oncologists wishing to have an understanding of the surgery their patients may require.

Head and neck surgery has not found its identity. In the UK there is no Specialist Advisory Committee to oversee it, there is no American board of head and neck surgery and it is not an EEC listed speciality. It has, however, come through the confrontational interdisciplinary minefield to become a very much better integrated combined subject.

Many things have changed. The frightful disasters have passed into history and our sympathies are with the brave patients who were part of the learning curve of the specialty. The damaging irradiation, the poorly placed incisions, the wrongly designed flaps but, most importantly, the lack of understanding of the disease process and the often unrealistic expectations of the surgeon of his results.

The main change as far as this book is concerned, however, is the early retirement of Professor Philip Stell. Without his initial enthusiasm and clarity of thought the first edition would never have been created. His place has been ably taken by Dr Mark Gaze and Miss Janet A. Wilson. Their talents have allowed us to enlarge the scope of the book into a multidisciplinary text. As well as a complete rewrite, attention has been directed at new diseases and surgical procedures, there are sections on biology, controversies, imaging and, most importantly, radiotherapy. We still feel that a referenced book of necessity is dated and we hope that readers will find the topic-based reading lists of greater value.

AGDM
JAW
1993

1

Nature of head and neck cancer

Introduction

A variety of different tumour types may arise at a host of anatomical sites within the head and neck. Head and neck cancer when otherwise unqualified is generally taken to mean squamous carcinoma arising in the upper aerodigestive tract. This is often characterized by similar behaviour irrespective of site. The tumour is usually confined to the primary site and perhaps the regional lymph nodes and haematogenous metastases are rare. For this reason, locoregional treatment by either surgery, radiotherapy or a combination of the two techniques is frequently curative. This chapter describes the aetiology, immunology, genetics and prognosis of head and neck cancer.

Aetiology

The larynx and hypopharynx are much the commonest sites of squamous cell carcinoma of the head and neck in the wesetern world. Although both are clearly related to cigarette smoking and, to a lesser extent, alcohol consumption, the widely varying incidence in different regions of Europe and North America remains unexplained. The highest mortality rates in Europe occur in France, Spain and Italy. Other areas of high incidence include Poland and Ohio, USA. The peak incidence of northern Thailand had been linked to the smoking of a particular cigarette. The usual sex ratio of laryngeal carcinoma is around 10:1 male:female, but there is an abnormally high incidence in Scottish women, which is also unexplained. Laryngeal tumours are twice as common in heavily industrialized areas, and their incidence shows a slow but steady increase over the last few decades. The different penetration of blond and black tobaccos may be one reason for the observation that smoking appears to increase lung cancer rates rather than larynx cancer rates, as in south-west Europe. Alternatively, as alcohol and tobacco seem to have a synergistic role in carcino-

genesis in the oral cavity, oesophagus, hypopharynx and epilarynx, alcohol may be the key factor. This is supported by the finding that the average mortality rates for cancer of the larynx correlate more closely with alcohol consumption than with cigarette smoking, although the risk of developing carcinoma of the larynx increases directly in proportion to the amount smoked.

The burning of tar gives off a variety of substances, including methyl cholanthrine, benzopyrene and benzanthracene, which are broken down by arylhydrocarbon hydroxylase into carcinogenic epoxides which bind to DNA. Smoking filtered cigarettes seems to be associated with a slightly lower risk than smoking untipped cigarettes. A large autopsy study showed that the incidence of histological changes such as cells with atypical nuclei, carcinoma-*in-situ* and invasive carcinoma in the larynx was directly related to the number of cigarettes smoked. One European study showed an increase in incidence risk over non-smokers from 2.4 for smokers of up to 7 cigarettes per day to 16.4 for smokers of over 25 a day. For ex-smokers, the risk declines by 70% after 10 years. In some areas up to 30% of laryngeal cancer patients have had asbestos exposure – but the vast majority are also smokers. Asbestos has been found in tumour-free larynges at postmortem in former asbestos workers. Nickel and chromate dust are principal inorganic chemicals which can cause lesions in the nose, larynx, lung and paranasal sinuses. Further site-specific carcinogens, such as dietary factors in Chinese nasopharyngeal carcinoma and wood dust exposure in nasal adenocarcinoma, are considered in later chapters. Radiation exposure is another potential risk factor but the 9% incidence of second primary malignancies has been shown not to be affected by a history of external beam irradiation of the initial tumour. Vitamin A deficiency is known to cause epithelial metaplasia, and trials are currently under way to assess the effect of retinoid therapy in the prevention of second neoplasms.

The relatively high incidence of postcricoid carcinoma in the UK and Scandinavia may be due to an association with Paterson-Brown Kelly syndrome (iron deficiency, glossitis, koilonychia and an upper oesophageal web), as originally suggested by Paterson in 1919 on the basis of his observations in Wales, and later documented by others in rural North Sweden. In Sweden as a whole, the fall in incidence of postcricoid carcinoma has been attributed to a fall in the prevalence of Paterson–Brown Kelly syndrome. One retrospective study from Wales suggested that up to 9% of women with postcricoid carcinoma had a previous web, compared with less than 1% of the surrounding population. Conversely, in patients with a web, the reported incidence of subsequent postcricoid cancer ranges from 4 to 16%. Dietary analysis in Scandinavian countries with a high prevalence of the disease has indicated that a deficiency of ascorbic acid (vitamin C), with secondary reduced iron absorption, may be important, particularly in days before the fortification of flour with iron and vitamins.

There are somewhat conflicting reports of the importance of human papillomavirus (HPV) subtypes in the aetiology of head and neck neoplasms. A study of HPV-6 and HPV-11 using polymerase chain reaction found no greater prevalence of either subtype in laryngopharyngeal tumours than in histologically normal biopsies from the nasopharynx. Similar techniques were used with gene amplification to study the E6 region of HPV-16 and the E1 region of HPV-6b, which were detected in 17.6% and 2.9% of tumours respectively. There is also anecdotal evidence for the presence of HPV-16 DNA in carcinoma of the antrum and tonsil.

Tumour immunology

The immune system operates as a continuous surveillance mechanism for the recognition of non-self antigens, and is also an important determinant of tumour behaviour in established disease. Head and neck cancer is remarkable for its ability to cause extensive local tissue destruction and regional nodal involvement, in the absence of distant metastatic spread, which is usually a very late event. This has led many workers to believe that there may be some distinctive immunological characteristics and that these might be amenable to diagnostic and/or therapeutic exploitation.

Cell-mediated immunity is thought to account for most of the host response to tumours, although it is known that serum immunoglobulin A (IgA) levels are elevated in head and neck cancer. There is, however, little correlation between the degree of elevation and the clinical course, except in nasopharyngeal cancer where specific levels to the early and viral capsid antigens of Epstein–Barr virus correlate with tumour load. The level of secretory IgA in saliva is also increased in nasopharyngeal tumours. Histologically, lymphoid infiltration of the primary tumour appears to improve prognosis only in well-differentiated tumours. Patients with squamous cell carcinoma of the head and neck have lower levels of CD4 (helper) cells than controls. The reduction of helper:suppressor T cell ratio bears some relationship to the stage of the disease in nasopharyngeal cancer, but is of inconsistent prognostic value at other sites. Tumour-infiltrating lymphocytes have low levels of antitumour cytotoxicity, which can be boosted by *in vitro* incubation with interleukin-2. Radiotherapy may selectively affect helper cells, while suppressor cells seem relatively radioresistant. A rebound increase in T cells in responsive tumours has also been described.

Head and neck cancer is unusual in that it is associated with low peripheral blood T cell counts, but there are conflicting reports of the clinical importance of the extent of the depletion. One of the most significant nodal factors is the presence of extracapsular spread, which has been shown to affect 65% of nodes under 3 cm. If absent, the patient's prognosis is similar to that of an N0 patient. During immune reactions, lymphocytes and monocytes produce soluble substances such as lymphokines, including interleukin-2, which promotes interferon-γ production. Prostaglandins are also produced (by suppressor monocytes) in head and neck cancer. Prostaglandin has a variety of immunosuppressive mechanisms, including reduction of interleukin-2 production.

Genetic aspects of head and neck cancer

In 1911 Rous described the ability of a cell-free extract, taken from a tumour, to induce the development of a sarcoma in chickens. The aetiological agent was later identified as a retrovirus, known also to cause cancer in primates, and a single gene was found to be responsible for initiating this malignant change. It was not until 1969 that the oncogene hypothesis of cancer was proposed. The genome of an RNA virus encodes three genes, but those causing tumours have a fourth gene, the v-*onc* or oncogene. The 30 different types identified are each known by the name of the relevant virus, e.g. v-*erb* is the avian erythroblastosis virus. The two types of RNA virus are the rapidly transforming type which carries oncogenes capable of causing tumours directly, and the slowly transforming type which induces tumours by inserting into the host genome and altering the transcription of cellular genes. In cell culture, cell transformation is indicated by the loss of contact inhibition and a disorderly heaping-up of cells. The relevance of viral oncogenes to human tumours was indicated by the discovery of almost identical DNA sequences in the genome of higher animals. These cellular or proto-oncogenes occur in most normal tissues.

The *myc* gene is associated with four distinct strains of viruses known to cause cancer in chickens. Thus, a common set of genes may hold the key to many types of cancer. Up to 25% of human tumours have oncogenes which have been activated by one of three mechanisms. Activation follows single point mutation of an oncogene, e.g. the mutation of the gene encoding the protein p53. This protein is usually a tumour suppressor, but mutation can turn the gene into one which transforms cells. Secondly, activation follows translocation of a proto-oncogene, e.g. in Burkitt's lymphoma where there is translocation of the c-*myc* oncogene from its usual position on chromosome 8 to a location on chromosome 14 adjacent to an immunoglobulin-producing gene. This juxtaposition seems to increase transcription of the *myc* gene which becomes an activated oncogene. Finally, there is gene amplification which results in an increase in production of the oncogene product or oncoprotein.

The products of proto-oncogenes (oncoproteins) also include certain soluble growth factors and their receptors, but the normal function of proto-oncogenes is still under investigation. Indeed the term 'oncogene' can be somewhat misleading as it covers a wide variety of different genes which participate in growth control, including nuclear proteins, signal transducers and kinases. The nuclear oncogenes are DNA-binding genes whose products can activate other genes and can stimulate DNA replication, either directly or indirectly. An example is the c-*myc* gene which is implicated in the spontaneous development of such a wide range of tumours that it appears to be activated by purely regulatory changes, in the absence of any structural alteration. The *ras* family comprises signal transducer genes. Normal, inactive *ras* proteins bind guanosine diphosphate (GDP) until stimulated, e.g. by a transmembrane receptor, to synthesize GTP and activate the protein. Mutation of the gene may cause abnormal stabilization of the *ras* protein in the active state. Like the receptor group of oncogenes discussed below, the proto-oncogenes of the non-receptor kinase category can be turned into active oncogenes by structural changes which increase the kinase activity of their products.

There are also tumour suppressor genes or anti-oncogenes whose range of gene products includes growth inhibitory factors and their receptors and DNA repair enzymes. The loss of heterozygous expression of such suppressor genes has been associated with tumour development. Homozygous expression of the long arm of chromosome 22 (22q) is associated with the development of acoustic neuroma. Markers for the short arm of chromosome 17

(17p) have loss of heterozygous expression in a large number of tumours, e.g. the p53 gene is lost in colon cancer and osteosarcoma. Tumours rarely develop as the result of a single genetic event and the concept of oncogenes and suppressor genes should remain fluid, because factors which promote growth at one stage may inhibit it at another.

There is still no widely accepted genetic explanation for the differences between benign and malignant tumours. The errors produced by genetic instability viruses and probably also by mutation appear to be more or less random. Multiple errors, such as those which follow repeated exposure to carcinogens, may accumulate and give rise to later tumour formation when one of the variants develops a growth advantage. Five classes of gene contribute to normal stability of the genome, including those responsible for DNA repair and nuclear division. Metastatic tumour cells may be formed by misexpression of an oncogene, or loss of genetic stability, or both. Misexpression of stability genes may be of more importance in tumour progression. In other words, physiological genetic events can be altered to contribute to the development of cancer, and thus cancer research is now intimately related to cellular biology.

Growth factors and markers

Growth factor research was stimulated by observations on cell cultures, which suggested that neoplastic cells have reduced requirements for the usual essential substances, and that often the cultures produce substances which stimulate growth of normal cells. The finding that many oncoproteins (oncogene products) transpired to be abnormal or supernumerary copies of growth factors or their receptors has strengthened the concept that disordered growth regulation is not an epiphenomenon, but is causally related to the development of neoplasia. The most extensively studied substance is epidermal growth factor (EGF). It is a 53 amino acid polypeptide, derived from a 1217 residue precursor (pre-pro-EGF) whose short hydrophilic segment may play a role in intercalation through cell membranes. EGF is present in most mammalian fluids, with high concentrations being found in prostatic fluid and precolostrum from mammary glands. The EGF receptor (EGFr) has extracellular, intracellular and transmembrane components. The intracellular domain has strong homology with v-*erbB* which was isolated from an avian erythroleukaemia virus. When EGF binds to the EGFr, various biochemical processes are stimulated which culminate in cell division 6–8 h later. Several qualitative studies have shown the presence of EGFr in head and neck squamous cancer. A minority of head and neck squamous cancers also appear to have EGFr gene amplification. A recent quantitative analysis has indicated that the levels of EGFr expression in head and neck tumours are intermediate between those of breast cancer and the high levels found in brain tumours. EGFr levels were found to be higher in laryngeal tumours than in normal laryngeal mucosa, but not directly related to T stage. A study of oesophageal tumours indicated a correlation between the level of EGFr expression and poor prognosis, but an immunohistochemical study of EGFr and transferrin receptors found neither to be a useful marker of cell growth. Radiolabelled EGF has been used in lymphoscintigraphy to detect recurrence of carcinoma of the uterine cervix, but this methodology has not yet been applied to the head and neck. Receptors for the intracellular messenger cyclic adenosine monophosphate have been detected in a wide variety of normal and neoplastic tissues of the head and neck, but with no clear relationship to malignant potential.

In breast cancers, EGFr expression appears to be inversely related to the level of oestrogen receptor (ER), and thus to be a poor prognostic indicator. The growth of a cell line derived from human salivary gland adenocarcinoma has none the less been shown to be inhibited by a glucocorticoid-induced stimulation of EGFr production which results in a fall in EGF secretion. The presence of ER has been demonstrated in low concentration in a wide variety of head and neck normal and neoplastic tissues. Some laryngeal tumours have also been shown to contain androgen receptors. In cell lines ER expression seems much more common in tumours of laryngeal than non-laryngeal origin. Furthermore, in ER-positive human laryngeal cell lines, the anti-oestrogen tamoxifen appears to have a synergistic antiproliferative effect with cisplatinum.

Transforming growth factor-α (TGF-α) is also present in many tumours and may represent a fetal form of EGF, but its role in the induction of neoplastic phenotype is debated. TGF has been consistently detected in human oral cancer, both *in vitro* and *in vivo*, and there is some evidence that TGF-α is responsible for many cases of hypercalcaemia in malignancy. Platelet-derived growth factor (PDGF) is responsible for most of the stimulation of growth of cells in culture by serum. The gene which codes for one of its two polypeptide chains is identical to the *sis* oncogene. Normally PDGF is released by platelets which disintegrate after bleeding, thus stimulating fibroblasts to participate in wound healing. Abnormal (e.g. retrovirus-induced) activation can lead the fibroblast to produce its own growth factor. When cells in culture develop the ability to produce their own growth factor, they become immortal, although the relevance of this autocrine mechanism to human tumour growth is not known. Other growth factors include fibroblast growth factor which stimulates angiogenesis; insulin-like growth

factors, which are produced by several tumour lines; nerve growth factor which is produced by melanoma, neuroblastoma and gliomas; and interleukin-2 which has a role in T cell transformation by human T lymphotropic viruses (HTLV).

Various groups have attempted to identify a serum marker for squamous carcinoma which could be used to assess the response to therapy and to detect subclinical recurrence. A radioimmune assay of squamous cell carcinoma antigen in patients with head and neck cancer showed that 44% had abnormally elevated levels, but that only half of the disease-free patients had post-treatment levels within normal limits. Others have studied carcinoembryonic antigen, ferritin and circulating immune complexes, but no serum marker of clinical benefit has so far been identified.

Prognostic indicators

It was reported in 1987 that in solid tumours, including those at head and neck sites, where surgery was the primary therapy, survival rates over the past 20 years were substantially unchanged. Data from Iowa, on the other hand, indicate a gradual increase in 5-year survival from 39% in 1960 to 47% in 1984, largely due to increased survival in patients with 'regional stage' disease. Untreated, the median survival in advanced head and neck cancer is 88 days. Surviving squamous cell carcinoma has been shown to be significantly related to sex (less good prognosis in females), T stage and general condition. Age is not a significant predictor of survival when allowance is made for untreated patients, those with second primary malignancies and deaths from intercurrent disease. General health performance status does, however, significantly affect outcome. Pathological features, with the exception of extracapsular nodal disease alluded to, rarely contribute much prognostic information.

In a study of end-stage disease, significant predictors of survival were found to be Karnofsky status, response to chemotherapy and ploidy. When a normal, diploid cell divides, if there is abnormal separation of the chromosomes during mitosis, then an aneuploid cell results. The degree of DNA aneuploidy reflects the frequency of cell division and, therefore, tumour chemosensitivity. Several studies have, however since failed to show that ploidy is of clinical significance in head and neck tumours.

There has been considerable recent interest in the possible association of blood transfusion during therapy and long-term outcome of head and neck cancer. No prospective, randomized study has addressed this issue, and indeed there would be clear ethical problems associated with such a study, particularly in view of the risk of transmitting hepatitis or human immunodeficiency virus during transfusion. One retrospective study of 16 possible prognostic factors showed that tumour stage, surgical margin status, the number of pathologically positive nodes, type of therapy and blood transfusion status were the only five factors which correlated significantly with prognosis. Using multivariate analysis, these were reduced to just two useful prognostic factors – surgical margin status and blood transfusion. At least one other study has also suggested that, stage for stage, recurrence rates are higher following transfusion, perhaps because of its known immunosuppressive effects.

References and further reading

Epidemiology/aetiology

Auerbach O, Hammond E C, Garfinkel L (1970) Histologic changes in the larynx in relation to smoking habits. *Cancer* 25:92–104.

Friedman M, Toriumi D M, Strorigl T, Grybauskas V T, Skolnik E (1988) Effects of therapeutic radiation on the development of multiple primary tumors of the head and neck. *Head Neck Surg* Suppl:S48–51.

Kleinsasser O (1988) Epidemiology, etiology and pathogenesis. In: *Tumours of the Larynx and Hypopharynx* Stell P M (Tr). Stuttgart, Thieme Verlag, pp. 2–24.

Krajina Z, Kulcar Z, Konic-Carnelutti V (1975) Epidemiology of laryngeal cancer. *Laryngoscope* 85:1155–61.

Kuylenstierna R, Munck-Wikland E (1985). Esophagitis and cancer of the esophagus. *Cancer* 56:837–9.

Moore C (1971) Cigarette smoking and cancer of the mouth, pharynx and larynx: a continuing study. *JAMA* 218:553–8.

Parnes S M (1990) Asbestos and cancer of the larynx: is there a relationship? *Laryngoscope* 100:254–61.

Ramadan M F, Morton R P, Stell P M, Pharoah P O D (1982) Epidemiology of laryngeal cancer. *Clin Otolaryngol* 7:417–28.

Vaughan C W, Homburger F, Shapshay S M, Soto E, Bernfield P (1980) Carcinogenesis of the upper aerodigestive tract. *Otolaryngol Clin North Am* 13:405–12.

Ward P H, Harrison D G (1988) Reflux as an etiological factor of carcinoma of the laryngopharynx. *Laryngoscope* 98:1195–9.

Wynder E L, Covey L S, Mabuchi K, Mushinski M (1976) Environmental factors in cancer of the larynx: a second look. *Cancer* 38:1591–601.

Prognostic indicators and tumour markers

Cooke L D, Cooke T G, Bootz F *et al.* (1990) Ploidy as a prognostic indicator in end stage squamous cell carcinoma of the head and neck region treated with cisplatinum. *Br J Cancer* 61:759–62.

Eibling D E, Johnson J T, Wagner R L, Su S (1989) SCC-RIA in the diagnosis of squamous cell carcinoma of the head and neck. *Laryngoscope* 99:117–24.

Goldsmith M M, Cresson D H, Arnold L A, Postma D S, Askin F B, Pillsbury H C (1987) Pt I DNA flow cytometry as a prognostic indicator in head and neck cancer. *Otolaryngol Head Neck Surg* 96:307–18.

Goldsmith M M, Cresson D H, Askin F B (1987) Part II.

The prognostic significance of stromal eosinophilia in head and neck cancer. *Otolaryngol Head Neck Surg* 96:319–24.

Holm L E (1982) Cellular DNA amounts of squamous cell carcinomas of the head and neck region in relation to prognosis. *Laryngoscope* 92:1064–9.

Hsu H-C, Chen C-L, Hsu M-M, Lynn T-C, Tu S-M, Huang S-C (1987) Pathology of nasopharyngeal carcinoma; proposal of a new histologic classification correlated with prognosis. *Cancer* 59:945–51.

Jackson R M, Rice D H (1989) Blood transfusions and recurrence in head and neck cancer. *Ann Otol Rhinol Laryngol* 98:171–3.

Jones K R, Weissler M C (1990) Blood transfusions and other risk factors for recurrence of cancer of the head and neck. *Arch Otolaryngol Head Neck Surg* 116:304–9.

Kearsley J H, Furlong K L, Cooke R A, Waters M J (1990) An immunohistochemical assessment of cellular proliferation markers in head and neck squamous cell cancers. *Br J Cancer* 61:821–7.

Kurniawan A N, Susworo R, Sumanto (1985) Nasopharyngeal carcinoma: correlation of histopathology with radiation response. *Southeast Asian J Trop Med Pub Hlth* 16:613–19.

Stell P M (1990) Prognosis in laryngeal carcinoma: tumour factors. *Clin Otolaryngol* 15:69–81.

Stell P M (1990) Prognosis in laryngeal carcinoma: host factors. *Clin Otolaryngol* 15:111–19.

Urba S G, Carey T E, Kudla-Hatch V, Wolf G T, Forastiere A A (1990) Tamoxifen therapy in patients with recurrent laryngeal squamous carcinoma. *Laryngoscope* 100:76–8.

Watson D M A, Wilson J A (1990) Cyclic-AMP binding proteins in the head and neck. *Clin Otolaryngol* 15:427–30.

Genetic aspects of head and neck cancer

Bryan R L, Bevan I S, Crocker J, Young L S (1990) Detection of HPV 6 and 11 in tumours of the upper respiratory tract using the polymerase chain reaction. *Clin Otolaryngol* 15:177–80.

Dimery I W, Jones L A, Verjan R P, Raymond A K, Goepfert H, Hong W K (1987) Estrogen receptors in normal salivary gland and salivary gland carcinoma. *Arch Otolaryngol Head Neck Surg* 113:1082–5.

Ferguson B J, Hudson W R, McCarty K S (1987) Sex steroid receptor distribution in the human larynx and laryngeal carcinoma. *Arch Otolaryngol Head Neck Surg* 113:1311–15.

Hoshikawa T, Nakajima T, Uhara H *et al.* (1990) Detection of human papillomavirus DNA in laryngeal squamous cell carcinomas by polymerase chain reaction. *Laryngoscope* 100:647–50.

Ishibashi T, Matsushima S, Tsunokawa Y *et al.* (1990) Human papillomavirus DNA in squamous cell carcinoma of the upper aerodigestive tract. *Arch Otolaryngol Head Neck Surg* 116:294–8.

Kashima H, Mounts P, Kuhajda F, Loury M (1986) Demonstration of human papilloma-virus capsid antigen in carcinoma-in-situ of the larynx. *Ann Otol Rhinol Laryngol* 95:603–7.

Kiyabu M T, Shibata D, Arnheim N, Martin W J, Fitzgibbons P L (1989) Detection of human papillomavirus in formalin-fixed, invasive squamous carcinomas using the polymerase chain reaction. *Am J Surg Pathol* **13**:221–4.

Michalopoulos G K (1989) Growth factors in neoplasia. In: Sirica A E (ed) *The Pathology of Neoplasia*. New York, Plenum Press, pp. 345–70.

Minden M D (1987) Oncogenes. In: Tannock, I F, Hill R P (eds) *The Basic Science of Oncology*. New York, Pergamon Press, pp. 72–88.

Miyaguchi M, Olofsson J, Hellquist H B (1990) Expression of epidermal growth factor receptor in laryngeal dysplasia and carcinoma. *Acta Otolaryngol* **110**:309–13.

Reiner Z, Cvrtila D, Petric V (1988) Cytoplasmic steroid receptors in cancer of the larynx. *Arch Otorhinolaryngol* **245**:47–9.

Scambia G, Panici P B, Battaglia F *et al.* (1991) Receptors for epidermal growth factor and steroid hormones in primary laryngeal tumours. *Cancer* **67**:1347–51.

Steel C M (1989) Oncogenes and anti-oncogenes in human cancer. *Proc R Coll Phys Edinb* **19**:413–29.

Todd R, Donoff B R, Gertz R *et al.* (1989) TGF-α and EGF-receptor mRNAs in human oral cancers. *Carcinogenesis* **10**:1553–6.

Volpe J. (1990) Genetic stability and instability in tumours. In: Shyser M (ed) *Molecular Biology of Cancer Genes*. Chichester, Ellis Horwood, pp. 9–23.

Wilson J A, Hawkins R A, Rogers M J, Gilmour H M, Maran A G D (1991) Estimation of oestrogen receptors (ER) and epidermal growth factor receptors (EGFR) in normal and neoplastic tissues of the head and neck. *Clin Otolaryngol* **16**:523–4.

Yamahara M, Fujito T, Ishikawa T *et al.* (1988) Phenotypic expression of human epidermal growth factor in foetal submandibular gland and pleomorphic adenoma of the salivary gland. *Virchows Arch A Pathol Anat Histopathol* **412**:301–6.

Tumour behaviour

Cooper J S, Pajak T F, Rubin P *et al.* (1989) Second malignancies in patients who have head and neck cancer: incidence, effect on survival and implications based on the RTOG experience. *Int J Radiat Oncol Biol Phys* **17**:449–56.

Gluckman J L (1979) Synchronous, multiple primary lesions of the upper aerodigestive system. *Arch Otolaryngol* **105**:597–8.

Incze J, Vaughan C W, Lui P, Strong M S, Kulapaditharou B (1982) Premalignant changes in normal appearing epithelium in patients with squamous cell carcinoma of the upper aerodigestive tract. *Am J Surg* **144**:401–5.

Stell P M, Morton R P, Singh S D (1983) Squamous carcinoma of the head and neck: the untreated patient. *Clin Otolaryngol* **8**:7–13.

Immunology

Gaze M N, Wilson J A (1988) Head and neck tumour immunology. *Clin Otolaryngol* **13**:495–9.

Johnson J T, Barnes L, Myers E N, Schramms V L, Borochovitz D, Sigler B A (1981) The extracapsular spread of tumours in cervical node metastasis. *Arch Otolaryngol* **107**:725–9.

Katz A E (1983) Immunobiologic staging of patients with carcinoma of the head and neck. *Laryngoscope* **93**:445–63.

Medina J E (1983) The controversial role of BCG in the treatment of squamous cell carcinoma of the head and neck. *Arch Otolaryngol* **109**:543.

Ortega I S, Nieto C S, Forcelledo M F F, Gomis J E (1987) Lymph node response and its relationship to prognosis in carcinomas of the head and neck. *Clin Otolaryngol* **12**:241–7.

Watanabe T, Iglehart J D, Bolognesi D P (1983) Secretory immune response in patients with oropharyngeal carcinoma. *Ann Otol Rhinol Laryngol* **92**:295–9.

Wolf G T, Schmaltz S, Hudson J *et al.* (1987) Alterations in T lymphocyte populations in patients with head and neck cancer. *Arch Otolaryngol Head Neck Surg* **113**:1200–6.

Wolf G T, Hudson J, Peterson K A, Poore J A, McClatchey K D (1989) Interleukin 2 receptor expression in patients with head and neck squamous carcinoma. Effects of thymosin-a, in vitro. *Arch Otolaryngol Head Neck Surg* **115**:1345–9.

2

Assessment

Clinical examination

Some patients with head and neck cancer are untreatable and some who are treatable are better left alone; deciding who shall be treated however is more difficult than in most other fields because there are seldom any objective signs to show that the patient is beyond treatment. When the patient is first seen, the tumour is virtually always confined to the head and neck with no distant metastasis; furthermore head and neck tumour is very rarely irremovable–virtually every structure to which a tumour may be fixed can be removed in continuity with the tumour and repaired. Thus the vast majority of patients with head and neck cancer are potentially treatable but some of them should not be treated, usually due to a combination of advanced stage, poor general condition and advanced local disease, making the mutilating effects of surgery not worthwhile. Generally speaking the first decision to be made is *whether* to treat before deciding *how* – if a patient is unfit for surgery because of age or poor general health it will usually be unwise to treat him or her by radiotherapy or chemotherapy. Therefore the final decision on treatment hinges on a full assessment of the patient including age and general condition.

There are four possible end-points of the initial assessment exercise:

1 that the patient is potentially curable;
2 that the patient is curable of the primary tumour but is likely to succumb to another illness within a few months;
3 that the patient is incurable of the tumour but ought to be treated;
4 that the patient is incurable and should not be treated.

Much of the following shows how we reach these end-points.

History

Taking the history from a patient with a head and neck tumour is no different from taking a history from a patient with any other medical or surgical condition. Three items, however, are of particular significance in making the ultimate decision on treatment policy.

The first is age. Head and neck tumours generally occur in people over the age of 45. If somebody has a head and neck tumour under the age of 45 then they are not liable to do as well as someone over 45 and something odd has gone on in their immunological make-up to have caused the tumour to develop. Most head and neck tumours are epithelial carcinomas and are due to years of abuse of the epithelium by cigarettes and tobacco. For a young person to develop such a tumour, therefore, there is a more sinister significance. Similarly, while it can be expected that a smoker may develop a cancer of the larynx it would be unexpected, unusual and of a more sinister significance if a non-smoker developed a cancer of the larynx.

The next important issue is social circumstance. Most of the head and neck operations interfere with anatomy, physiology and/or psychology of the patient. Every patient who has a head and neck operation requires some moral and physical support afterwards. If there is nobody to look after them when they leave hospital then this should play a part in deciding whether or not the patient has surgery or radiotherapy as the primary treatment.

Finally, tumour biology must be assessed. Poorly differentiated tumours have a worse prognosis than well-differentiated tumours. Tumours in the young have a worse significance than tumours in the old and the growth pattern of tumours has to be assessed. John Conley used to have a useful teaching aphorism, namely: 'listen to what the tumour tells you – sometimes it says "I am going to kill you".' A tumour that is growing very quickly may not be amenable to treatment by any modality and the treatment indeed may be worse than the end-point of the disease.

Table 2.1 Eastern Co-operative Oncology Group (ECOG) scale

Grade	
0	Fully active, able to carry on all predisease activities without restriction (Karnofsky 90–100)
1	Restricted in physically strenuous activity but ambulatory and able to carry out work of a light or sedentary nature; for example, light housework, office work (Karnofsky 70–80)
2	Ambulatory and capable of self-care but unable to carry out any work activities. Up and about more than 50% of waking hours (Karnofsky 50–60)
3	Capable of only limited self-care, confined to bed or chair 50% or more of waking hours (Karnofsky 30–40)
4	Completely disabled. Cannot carry on any self-care. Totally confined to bed or chair (Karnofsky 10–20)

Similarly the tumours that develop in immuno-compromised individuals seldom to do well by any modality.

The patient's general condition should always be classified using one of the methods of measuring the performance status, such as the Eastern Co-operative Oncology Group (ECOG) scheme or the Karnofsky status (Table 2.1).

Examination

Examination of the primary site

When you are examining a patient with a head and neck tumour always think in terms of T staging. When you are examining the local lesion being considered for treatment, delineate its borders exactly both by inspection and by a palpation and make a permanent record of your finding in the case chart. Acquire the habit of drawing every region from different angles and giving an idea of size by using normal landmarks. Although not as important as previously, the status of the teeth is important if radiation is to be considered and the head and neck surgeon should acquire some expertise in assessing dental health.

Examination of the neck

You should develop a routine for examination of the lymphatic fields on both sides of the neck. We suggest the following.

Stand behind the patient and flex his or her head slightly. Have all clothing removed until the points of the shoulders can be seen. Begin by placing the index fingers in both mastoid processes and work down the trapezius muscle until the fingers meet at the clavicle.

There are nodes under the trapezius muscle and for this reason fingers should be inserted under the anterior border of the muscle with the thumb pressing down on top with the shoulder blades forward. When the clavicle is reached the posterior triangle is palpated. Here the nodes lie between the skin and the muscles of the floor of the triangle and thus can be rolled between these surfaces. Now take the tension off the sternomastoid muscle by lateral movement of the head to one side. Place your fingers in front of and medial to the sternomastoid and your thumb behind it. Move down the muscle carefully because this is where 80% of the nodes are. One common reason for a palpable lump here is a normal but tortuous carotid artery but this is pulsatile.

Continue this examination down to the clavicle and then palpate the trachea and at this point assess the size of the thyroid gland. Then working upwards to the neck assess the mobility of the larynx and examine the submental triangle on the submandibular gland from anterior to posterior using the mandible as a strut. At the posterior border of the submandibular gland continue upwards over the face to assess the state of the nodes in and around the parotid gland.

General examination

The patient's general health should be assessed with the usual investigations. A decision as to whether the patient is operable or not should be shared with the anaesthetist who takes the final responsibilities for the patient's health during any procedure. The anaesthetist will therefore order any further investigations which will decide the patient's operability.

The staging of cancer

Cancer is a very heterogeneous disease, or rather group of diseases, and the natural history and response to treatment can be very varied. There are obvious advantages in subdividing cases of cancer into groups in which the behaviour is similar. This process is called staging, and is done for the following reasons:

Firstly, it acts as a guide to the appropriate treatment. The question, 'how should a patient with carcinoma of the larynx be treated?' cannot be answered without reference to stage. A patient with a small tumour confined to the true cord which remains mobile can be treated successfully by irradiation with voice preservation, but a man with an advanced transglottic carcinoma, causing airway obstruction and invading the thyroid cartilage with nodal metastases requires laryngectomy and neck dissection.

Secondly, the stage of a tumour acts as a guide to

prognosis. Multivariate analysis of one large recent study showed stage, anatomical site and age, in that order, to be the most significant predictors of survival. Accurate prognosis is important, not just to satisfy a patient who wants to know the likelihood of successful treatment, but also to ensure equivalence of groups in clinical trials. For example, suppose a new form of treatment is being compared with standard practice in the treatment of oropharyngeal carcinoma. If there arises by chance a preponderance of more advanced cases in the conventional treatment arm, the survival rate in the experimental arm may be greater, even if in reality there is no difference between the treatments, stage for stage. Pre-randomization stratification by stage will prevent this source of error.

Staging permits more reliable comparison of results between centres. For example, if one hospital, A, publishes better survival figures for laryngeal cancer, it may be assumed that it is a better hospital offering better treatment. Yet different hospitals serve different populations and consequently the pattern of cancer cases they see may be different. The observed discrepancy may therefore result from the fact that hospital B serves a large population of socially disadvantaged men who present late with advanced disease. If survival figures are published separately for each stage, it may be found that there is no difference between hospital A and hospital B, or even that truly better results from hospital B have been masked by the large proportion of poor prognosis cases treated there.

Finally, staging permits a more reliable examination of reasons behind time trends. For example, the incidence of both malignant melanoma and testicular cancer are increasing in Scotland, yet the proportion of patients dying from these diseases is diminishing. It might be assumed that the improved survival from melanoma has been caused by the development of effective systemic therapy, as is the case for testicular tumours. In fact, examination of the distribution of stages at presentation shows that more cases of melanoma are now being diagnosed early as a result of a public education campaign, but the prognosis of advanced cases has not changed.

It will be seen that most of the reasons for staging are of no benefit to the individual patient, and so it must be tempting for a busy surgeon to make no attempt at staging beyond a brief assessment for the purposes of choosing treatment, or worse still for him hurriedly to assign an inaccurate stage. Yet if the biology of cancer is to be more fully understood, and if treatments are to be improved, it is imperative that staging is carried out fully and accurately on all patients.

So how do we stage cancer? The basic requirement is to define in each patient all the factors relevant to the natural history and outcome of his cancer, thereby enabling a patient with cancer to be grouped with other similar cases. The first subdivision of cancer is of course by primary site, as no one would contemplate applying generalizations about, say lung cancer, to skin cancer. However, this grouping is still inadequate, and mention of histological type is necessary to distinguish basal cell carcinoma of the skin from malignant melanoma, and small cell from squamous carcinoma of the lung.

Even amongst tumours of one histological type arising at one primary site, there are still variations in prognosis. The most important factor determining this is usually the size and extent of the primary tumour, and whether or not lymphatic or haematogenous metastases are present. Together these constitute the stage of the tumour. While assessment of the tumour, nodes and metastases is usually sufficient for staging purposes, other factors which are sometimes taken into account include the histological differentiation or grade in the case of soft tissue sarcoma, and the patient's age in the case of differentiated thyroid carcinoma of follicular cell origin. For tumours such as lymphoma, which do not follow an orderly progression from primary tumour to nodal involvement then distant metastases, special staging systems have been devised.

Even for epidermoid cancer there is a variety of different staging classifications, which although they have similar aims and use similar data, differ in important regards and therefore lead to groupings which may not be directly comparable. Fortunately, over the years, the two principal staging classifications for head and neck cancer, those of the American Joint Committee on Cancer (AJCC) and the Union Internationale Contre le Cancer (UICC), have undergone a convergent evolution, and are now identical. Details can be found in the *Manual for Staging of Cancer*, third edition, 1988, published by the AJCC, and in the UICC handbook, *TNM Classification of Malignant Tumours*, fourth edition, 1987. For each primary site in the head and neck, the factors taken into account in the stage classification are described in the appropriate chapter in this book, but the following general definitions are applied to all sites.

The primary tumour is indicated by the letter T, the status of regional lymph nodes by N and distant metastases by M. In each case the letter is followed by a suffix, usually an Arabic numeral, to indicate the extent of disease in each category.

The extent of primary tumour is indicated by the suffixes 1, 2, 3, or 4, representing progressively more advanced disease. Increasing size is usually the sole criterion for categories 1, 2, and 3, while 4 often indicates direct extension outwith the primary area, or invasion of underlying bone or cartilage. Other criteria are applied in special circumstances, such as fixation of the cord in laryngeal carcinoma, and the number of subsites involved in nasopharyngeal carcinoma. T0 is used when there is no evidence of a primary tumour. Tis is used when the primary is non-invasive or carcinoma *in situ*, and TX is used when for some reason the extent of the primary tumour cannot be assessed.

Three categories are used to describe progressive involvement of the regional lymph nodes, which for all head and neck sites, except the thyroid gland, are as follows. N1 indicates metastasis in a single ipsilateral lymph node, 3 cm or less in its greatest dimension. The N2 category is subdivided into three sections. N2a indicates metastasis in a single ipsilateral lymph node, more than 3 cm but not more than 6 cm in greatest dimension. N2b indicates metastasis in multiple ipsilateral lymph nodes, none more than 6 cm in greatest dimension. N2c indicates metastasis in bilateral or contralateral lymph nodes, none more than 6 cm in greatest dimension. N3 disease is any lymphatic spread more than 6 cm in greatest dimension. As in the case of T staging, the suffix 0 means no evidence of regional lymph node involvement, and the suffix X means that the nodes cannot be assessed.

The presence or absence of distant metastases are indicated by M1 or M0, respectively. If the presence of metastases cannot be assessed, the X suffix is used.

TNM staging can be performed on data obtained in various ways. At the simplest level, it is a clinical system based on examination findings and investigations such as radiology. If definitive surgery has been performed, a post surgical pathological assessment is used. A prefix can be used to designate the source of the information, c for clinical staging, p for pathological staging, but often the prefix is omitted, and the classification is assumed to be clinical.

With five principal options for the T stage, four for the N stage and two for metastases, there are 40 possible TNM options, more if the various subcategories are included. This is clearly too many for easy use. Even in the largest reported patient series, there would be some combinations with too few patients for meaningful comparison. Therefore different TNM categories are aggregated into *Stage Groupings*, designated by Roman numerals. In general terms, Stage 0 disease is carcinoma *in situ*. Stage I disease comprises a node negative operable primary.

Stage II is an operable primary with operable nodes, Stage III is disease considered inoperable by virtue of either an advanced primary tumour or advanced nodal involvement, and in Stage IV disease, distant metastases are present.

Despite the obvious value of staging, both in the management of individual patients, and for the grouping of patients in trials and reports of treatment, it does have its limitations. The most insidious of these is that attempts to increase the accuracy of staging lead to greater complexity, and hence paradoxically to more errors, and an increased likelihood of non-compliance by the person responsible for staging.

Secondly, recognising that current staging systems do not discriminate perfectly between good and poor prognosis categories, investigators often create their own staging system to report their own results. When reading the literature, it is wise to make sure you know which system is being used. It is perhaps in the case of nasopharyngeal carcinoma (NPC) that the greatest number of staging systems is currently in operation. One recent study, for example, reported superior prognostic prediction in NPC by the use not only of disease extent but also various parameters such as the presence of cranial nerve involvement and the duration and number of other associated symptoms. Unless results are reported using also an internationally recognized staging classification, it is virtually impossible to compare series meaningfully. Thirdly, although the anatomical site classification is for the most part satisfactory, showing a significant difference in observed survival between laryngeal and pharyngeal tumours, the dual listing of the aryepiglottic fold in both categories and the occurrence of large tumours involving both sites present problems. It appears to be better to classify these large tumours as being of pharyngeal origin.

Finally, in recent years the advent of sophisticated imaging technology has made assessment more accurate. Cases are now often demonstrated to be more extensive than is clinically apparent, and are accordingly put into higher stages. Table 2.2 shows the results of treatment for a form of cancer, as staged by an older, less accurate clinical method and using modern sophisticated imaging techniques. The

Table 2.2 Comparison of results of treatment for cancer using an old and new staging system

Stage	Old staging system			New staging system		
	Number of patients	Percentage cured	Number cured	Number of patients	Percentage cured	Number cured
I	30	80%	24	25	84%	21
II	30	50%	15	25	60%	15
III	30	20%	6	25	28%	7
IV	10	10%	1	25	12%	3
All	100	46%	46	100	46%	46

cure rate for each stage of the disease is higher in those staged with the more modern technique. Yet the overall cure rate for the entire cohort of patients, at 46%, is identical whichever staging system is used. This illustrates the phenomenon of stage migration, where apparently superior results are produced by the downstaging of patients. While it would be inadvisable to contemplate major surgery before excluding the presence of distant metastases, in practice very few patients with squamous carcinoma have disease outwith the head and neck at presentation. The converse situation, of a secondary lesion in the head and neck should be considered when adenocarcinoma occurs in cervical lymph nodes, or in the salivary glands, and a primary lesion in breast, bowel etc., excluded.

Radiology

It is now almost 20 years since the introduction of computerized tomography (CT) scanning and the generation of the first magnetic resonance images (MRI). Recent refinements have greatly increased the usefulness of both systems in the assessment of head and neck tumours. MR scanning appears likely to overtake CT scanning as the investigative method of choice in the larynx, where it yields greater cartilage detail, and in the parotid and nasopharynx, where it offers better soft tissue contrast. MR imaging has the advantages of lack of bony/dental amalgam artefacts, direct multiplanar imaging, infrequent need for contrast and the potential for MR angiography to visualize vasculature non-invasively.

The production of MRI depends on the absorption of radiowaves by hydrogen nuclei and, therefore, on the distribution and chemical environment of the hydrogen atoms in the tissue studied. Hydrogen nuclei behave as small bar magnets, spinning on their axes. The 'wobble' of the spin (precession) allows transfer of the energy of radiowaves to the nuclei, if the radiowave frequency is resonant with the frequency of the precessing nuclei. The energy absorption moves the atom through an angle, generating a measurable oscillating current in the receiver coils. The resonant frequency is proportional to the strength of the surrounding magnetic field. A T_1 relaxation curve is determined by the rate at which the excited protons realign with the field. T_2 relaxation time reflects signal decay, as the spinning protons lose phase with one another. Alteration of the timing and frequency of the radiofrequency pulses will 'weight' the resulting MRI to reflect primarily T_1 or T_2 relaxation times. Images can be enhanced by the use of paramagnetic substances like gadolinium diethylenetriaminepenta-acetic acid (Gd-DTPA) which readily passes from the blood-stream, e.g. into acoustic neuromas, shortening the

T_1 relaxation time and causing the lesion to appear bright on T_1 weighted images. Where available, Gd-DTPA has supplanted air CT cisternography in visualization of cerebellopontine angle tumours.

Errors of clinical staging of tumours of the laryngopharynx are reduced by imaging technology, although where used in isolation, like clinical staging, CT tends to understage disease. One series comparing operative specimens with clinical and CT findings showed that the accuracy of clinical staging was 59% and that of CT staging 71%, rising to 88% when both results were combined. Other series confirm CT understaging of laryngeal disease, largely attributable to the under-recording of invasion of the thyroid and arytenoid cartilages. Although CT is known to be accurate in diagnosing laryngeal muscle involvement, this is in any case readily assessed by direct inspection. MR is superior to CT in assessing tumour extension into ossified hyaline cartilage (because of loss of the marrow space signal). MR imaging of the larynx is improved by the use of surface coils, which reduce the signal-to-noise ratio by almost 50% compared with the use of head/body coils alone. The method is particularly helpful in determining the limits of the disease, especially the subglottic extent, which is harder to assess than the supraglottic limit at direct laryngoscopy.

As at other sites, CT gives more detail about bony invasion by tumours of the nasopharynx than MR, but the latter's superior soft tissue definition gives useful information about tumour extension along the V, VII, IX and X cranial nerves, and detects infiltration of the carotid sheath. The pharyngobasilar fascia, which separates the pharynx from the parapharyngeal space, is also well delineated on MR, yet is not seen on CT. T_2 weighted images are also helpful in distinguishing nasopharyngeal tumour from inflammation but mucosal spread is hard to detect by either method. Within the nasal cavity, as elsewhere, cancer presents a lower intensity signal than inflammatory processes on T_2 weighted images. Again, although Gd-DTPA causes tumour enhancement, the substance also enhances normal nasal mucosa. A T_1 weighted sequence without enhancement is, therefore, also always needed for correct assessment of the contrast between tumour and adipose tissue, which decreases after Gd-DTPA. MR is superior in the distinction of tumour from dura or CSF but CT is required to define the cribriform plate in detail. Both techniques are, therefore, very helpful in planning craniofacial resection. On T_2 images nasopharyngeal angiofibroma is particularly difficult to differentiate from mucosa of the nasopharynx and its adjacent musculature. The use of Gd-DTPA greatly enhances the contrast between muscles and tumour. Similarly, in the orbit, MR is emerging as superior to the evaluation of intraocular disease including lesions of the orbital apex in adults, while CT is useful for the assessment of intraorbital calcifications and orbital fractures.

Clinical staging of tumours of the oral cavity and oropharynx has an accuracy of 90% for T1 and T2 lesions, but 70% of larger tumours are understaged – a finding which clearly has grave consequences for planning adequate therapy. Because of the beam-hardening artefacts caused by dense bones, teeth and fillings, the accuracy of CT in the oral cavity is only 60%, compared with 80–90% in the floor of mouth or oropharynx. The cardinal CT sign of early floor of mouth lesions is the loss of the sublingual space between the mylohyoid and geniohyoid muscles. Tumours of the tongue or floor of mouth are readily seen on MRI due to their dark contrast with the surrounding fat. Gd-DTPA enhanced images are better overall and quick to obtain but give less good imaging of tumour infiltration of fat than plain images. CT takes only about 10 min to image the whole area from the base of skull to the clavicles, i.e. including a search for cervical nodes, while MR takes 40 min to image the oral cavity and oropharynx alone. The slower MR scanning is also, therefore, more open to motion artefact, and yields a relatively large number of non-diagnostic scans in elderly subjects, although with increasing refinement, scanning time is gradually being reduced. In summary, then, the particular indications for MR imaging of oral tumours are if CT has excess artefact, if there is insufficient contrast with normal tissues on CT, or if problems are encountered in determining the cranio-caudal extent, when the sagittal cuts of MR may be useful.

Particularly since the advent of fine needle aspiration cytology, it is easy to be nihilistic about the role of the radiologist in the investigation of salivary gland swellings, most of which will ultimately undergo surgical excision. It can, however, be useful to assess radiologically whether a small lesion is intra- or extraglandular, or to determine the parapharyngeal extent of parotid tumours, which are usually larger at operation than they appear clinically. Such information may spare a patient with a benign lesion an unnecessary superficial parotidectomy, or a patient with deep lobe extension inadequate primary surgery. With modern CT scanners, sialography is felt now not to be necessary, and indeed parenchymal staining may actually make a tumour harder to assess. MR is probably preferable to CT, and attempts have been made to identify CT features of malignant tumours, which have a high nuclear-to-cytoplasm ratio, relatively little free water, and thus low signal intensity on all imaging frequencies.

Radionuclide ^{123}I scanning remains very important in the investigation of thyroid nodules – a cold nodule has a 10% chance of being malignant. CT is useful in thyroid lymphoma, as the scan can be combined with a chest examination, while MR is good at demonstrating anatomical abnormalities such as the extent of a large goitre or the degree of muscle invasion (but not benign from malignant tumours). Ultrasonography still plays a major role: in this superficial gland, the examination is straight-forward, and it is also safe and cheap. Ultrasound has also been shown to be a sensitive method for the detection of cervical lymph nodes. In one series of 62 patients, a third were found to have enlarged neck nodes which had been missed on palpation, half of which contained tumour. Ultrasound of the parotid gland is also useful in children to support a diagnosis of sialectasis or to follow the regression of parotid lymphadenopathy.

It is sometimes also important to assess the patency of the arterial supply in the management of head and neck cancer. Formerly, this committed the patient to undergo arteriography, which carried an appreciable risk of inducing a cerebrovascular accident, sometimes fatal. The technique of digital venous subtraction angiography, introduced in the 1980's was associated with a much lower complication rate in the definition of vessel patency or the nature of a pulsatile mass. The next development in vascular imaging was Doppler ultrasound. The method is based on a phenomenon described by Doppler in 1872, in fact in relation to the behaviour of light. The compressions and rarefactions of sound waves pass through a given medium at a predicted interval (frequency) and at a constant speed. If the transmitter and receiver are stationary, the received frequency = the transmitted frequency. If, however, the receiver is moving towards the transmitter, it will encounter more compression beats per second and will, therefore, register a higher frequency (positive Doppler shift). If the receiver is moving away from the transmitter, it will receive fewer compressions per second (negative Doppler shift).

In clinical ultrasound, the phenomenon is produced by the movement of blood cells in a vessel. Colour Doppler machines incorporate powerful computers for simultaneous sampling of multiple tiny volumes. The resultant colour graphics allow assessment of the actual pattern of flow in a vessel or area of tissue. The method may ultimately be of value in the investigation of thyroid swellings, as it can distinguish the characteristic pulsatile pattern of Graves' disease, the 'thyroid inferno', from those of autonomous adenomas or carcinomas. Another refinement is the use of Duplex Doppler ultrasound, which combines a Doppler probe with real-time ultrasound, allowing the operator to define both vessel orientation in relation to the Doppler beam and to locate precisely the portion of tissue from which the beam originates. Whether the advent of MR angiography will render some of these methods obsolete remains to be seen.

Endoscopy

The patient with a head and neck tumour undergoes endoscopy for three reasons: to define the tumour accurately, to exclude a second tumour and to take a biopsy. It has been suggested that outpatient video-laryngoscopic examination can, in some hands, be adequate, but most otolaryngologists require rigid endoscopy under general anaesthesia to allow the necessary biopsies to be taken. Try to define the limits of the tumour in all directions, and relate them to anatomical landmarks. Make a drawing of the findings. Next, take a biopsy from the viable part of the tumour, i.e. not from its centre, which may be necrotic, and not from its edge, which may show dysplasia only. Take a big piece with cutting forceps that do not crush the tissue, and place it directly in formalin – do not poke it with needles or put it on a swab, as these manoeuvres can distort the tissue. A biopsy of a tumour in the mouth is best taken with a knife if this is feasible. If a lymphoma is suspected the pathologist will prefer a specimen that has not been put in formalin and is fresh (see Chapter 7).

The presence of a synchronous primary tumour is in general more likely than the presence of distant metastases. The cumulative incidence of second lesions following primary lesions at any head and neck site is up to 15%. Fewer than half will have a detectable synchronous primary lesion, almost half of which will be detected by a thorough ear, nose and throat examination. The pick-up rate of routine endoscopy at the time of primary diagnosis of an upper aerodigestive tract carcinoma is thus likely to be of the order of 2–3%. While detection of a second primary may modify the therapy of the original tumour, there is no substantial evidence about the effect on survival. Certainly, every patient must have a chest X-ray, as most head cancer patients are also high-risk candidates for lung cancer.

The reported incidence of synchronous oesophageal primaries ranges from 0.7 to 1.7%. In some series, radiology is as accurate as endoscopy in detecting these lesions, while others find oesophagoscopy to be superior. There are few, if any data, on the later development of oesophageal neoplasia in patients with negative screening at the time of presentation, perhaps because in that situation there is no way to distinguish a missed synchronous lesion from a metachronous lesion. One small study of laryngopharyngo-oesophagectomy with gastric pull-up had a 17% incidence of oesophageal primaries detected at endoscopy, rising to 25% when the resected specimens were examined pathologically. All were small (and, by inference, potentially curable) lesions whose development was associated with a 33% incidence of Barrett's oesophagus. In another study, only 4 of 69 patients were asymptomatic and had a normal chest X-ray when their synchronous or metachronous oesophageal or bronchial neoplasms were diagnosed. In fact all 4 died from a variety of causes soon after therapy and the 5-year survival of 43 similar patients (0.7% of those endoscoped) was just 7%. It is perhaps the generally poor status and outcome in patients with multiple primaries, as much as the cost ($1000 in the USA), or potential morbidity, which leads surgeons to question the value of triple endoscopy at presentation.

Fine-needle aspiration cytology

Incisional biopsy of a lymph node is rarely justified: a squamous carcinoma may be implanted into the tissues; if the tumour is a lymphoma, the specimen will not give node architecture information – and in vascular tumours the procedure can even be fatal! The former practice of Tru-cut needle core biopsy has now been superseded by fine-needle aspiration cytology (FNAC).

FNAC of head and neck lesions increased *pari passu* with the development of skills in exfoliative cervical cytology and in FNAC at other sites, particularly breast. In the head and neck it is of great value because of the multiplicity of accessible organs and the heterogeneous pathology encountered. An early clue as to the tissue or tumour of origin may thus greatly influence the early management of a patient with head and neck swelling, reducing dramatically both patient anxiety and resource consumption. The early detection of, for example, a goitre, lymphoma or adenocarcinoma will lead to a very different clinical approach from the detection of a pleomorphic adenoma or a squamous cell carcinoma. It is this very plethora, however, which makes head and neck FNAC particularly challenging. The involved cytologist needs to be skilled and committed. Under these circumstances the accuracy is at least in excess of 90%. Although not every open biopsy is conclusive either, FNAC is clearly no substitute for histology, especially in the determination of nodal architecture in lymphoma, the malignant potential of a follicular thyroid tumour or of extracapsular spread in squamous carcinoma, or in the distinction of a pleomorphic from a monomorphic adenoma. Conversely, open biopsy is contraindicated in pleomorphic adenoma or nodal deposits of squamous carcinoma. All series report a small but appreciable false-negative rate (2%) and any suspicious lump should, therefore, be explored or otherwise investigated as appropriate.

The technique is simple and cheap, as the only specialist input is that of the cytologist. (Although ultrasound or CT-guided aspiration may be required in postnasal or parapharyngeal space lesions, most lumps are readily accessible.) The cost saving compared with excisional biopsy in the USA is estimated to be between $1000 (outpatient) and $2000 (in-patient). One of the commonest reasons for failure is the submission of inadequate material for diagnosis, in which case often the best course is simply to repeat the aspirate.

The necessary equipment should be kept in a small box ready for use and comprises a 20 ml syringe, 21 G needles, microscope slides, slide carriers, fixative spray and skin swabs. Air is expelled from a syringe and a needle attached. The lump is stabilized with the left hand as the needle enters. Apply suction, and while this is maintained, make several radial passes within the substance of the swelling. Release the suction. Withdraw the needle through the skin. The tissue core should thus be retained within the needle itself, rather than transferred to the syringe. Disconnect the needle and aspirate 10 ml of air into the syringe. Reconnect it to the needle and expel the specimen on to a slide. Use a second slide to smear the specimen and repeat this with further slides until the smear is of the right thickness. This can be judged only with experience, and feedback from the cytologist. The slides should be sprayed at once with alcohol fixative, if Papanicolaou or similar stains are to be used. Alternatively, they may be air-dried if May Grunwald Giemsa is to be used. Blood in the specimen will cause drying artefact but may not render it useless. If fluid is aspirated, this should be sent in a clean universal container so that a cytospin preparation can be obtained.

Several clinical and animal experiments have been performed to assess the safety of FNAC. Some report no cell seeding at all; others have detected spillage of 10^2–10^4 cells but have also shown that the number of cells required to cause a seeded growth in humans is about twice that observed. Transperitoneal implantation of advanced retroperitoneal lesions has been reported in a small number cases to have been followed by seeding but there are no reports of seeding of head and neck tumours, including parotid tumours. One fatality has, however, been reported, following aspiration of a carotid body tumour. Suspicion of this lesion is variously regarded as a contraindication, or as an indication for the use of a finer (23 G) needle.

References and further reading

Staging

American Joint Committee on Cancer (1988) *Manual for staging of cancer*, 3rd edn. Philadelphia, J B Lippincott.

Hermanek P, Sobin L H (eds) (1987) *Union Internationale Contre le Cancer*, 4th edn. Berlin, Springer-Verlag.

Neel H B, Taylor W F (1989) New staging system for nasopharyngeal carcinoma. *Arch Otolaryngol Head Neck Surg* 15:1293–303.

Sulfaro S, Barzan L, Querin F *et al.* (1989) T staging of the laryngopharyngeal carcinoma: a 7 year multidisciplinary experience. *Arch Otolaryngol Head Neck Surg* 115:613–20.

Wiernik G, Alcock C J, Fowler J F, Haybittle J L, Hopewell J W, Rezvani M (1990) The predictive value of tumor classification compared with results of the British Institute of Radiology fractionation trial in the treatment of laryngopharyngeal carcinoma. *Laryngoscope* 100:863–72.

Radiology

Atlas S W (1988) MR of the orbit: current imaging applications. *Semin Ultrasound* 9:31–40.

Dillon W P (1986) Magnetic resonance imaging of head and neck tumours. *Cardiovasc Intervent Radiol* 8:275–82.

Feinmesser R, Freeman J L, Noyek A M, Birt B D (1987) Metastatic disease. A clinical/radiologic/pathologic correlative study. *Arch Otolaryngol Head Neck Surg* 113:1307–10.

Hasso A N (1984) CT of tumours and tumour-like conditions of the paranasal sinuses. *Radiol Clin North Am* 22:119–30.

Havas T E, Motbey J A, Gullane P J (1988) Prevalence of incidental abnormalities on computed tomographic scans of the paranasal sinuses. *Arch Otolaryngol Head Neck Surg* 114:856–9.

Hirano M, Kurita S, Cho J S, Tanaka H (1988) Computed tomography in determining laryngeal involvement of hypopharyngeal carcinoma. *Ann Otol Rhinol Laryngol* 97:476–82.

Holliday R A, Reede D L (1989) MRI of mastoid and middle ear disease. *Radiol Clin North Am* 27:283–99.

Jacobson H G (1988) Magnetic resonance imaging of the head and neck region. Present status and future potential. *JAMA* 260:3313–26.

Jong R J B de, Rongen R J, Jong P C de, Lameris J S, Knegt P (1988) Screening for lymph nodes in the neck with ultrasound *Clin Otolaryngol* 13: 5–9.

Kondo M, Ando Y, Inuyama Y, Shiga H, Hashimoto S (1986) Maxillary squamous cell carcinomas staged by computed tomography. *Int J Radiat Oncol Biol Phys* 12:111–16.

Lloyd G A S (1989) Magnetic resonance imaging of the nose and paranasal sinuses. *J R Soc Med* 82:84–7.

Mikulis D J, Chisin R, Wismer G L *et al.* (1989) Phase contrast imaging of the parotid region. *Am J Neuroradiol* 10:157–64.

Noyek A M, Shulman H S (1987) Diagnostic imaging of the larynx. In: Tucker H M (ed) *The Larynx*. New York, Thieme Medical, pp. 79–133

Platts A D, Valentine A R (1986) The use of intravenous digital subtraction angiography in the evaluation of neck masses. *Ann R Coll Surg Engl* 68:249–51.

Rafto S E, Gefter W B (1988) MRI of the upper aerodigestive tract and neck. *Radiol Clin North Am* 26:547–71.

Som P M (1987) Lymph nodes of the neck. *Radiology* 165:593–600.

Teresi L M, Lufkin R B, Hanafee W N (1989) Magnetic resonance imaging of the larynx. *Radiol Clin North Am* 27:393–406.

Voorman G S, Petti G H, Schulz E, Chonkich G D, Kirk G A (1988) The pitfalls of technetium Tc^{99m}/thallium 201 parathyroid scanning. *Arch Otolaryngol Head Neck Surg* 114: 993–5.

Yuh W T C, Sato Y, Loes D T *et al.* Magnetic resonance

imaging and computed tomography in pediatric head and neck masses. *Ann Otol Rhinol Laryngol* **100**:54–62.

Endoscopy

Atkinson D, Fleming S, Weaver A. (1982) Triple endoscopy: a valuable procedure in head and neck surgery. *Am J Surg* **144**:416–19.

Bastian R W, Collins S L, Kaniff T, Matz G J (1989) Indirect videolaryngoscopy versus direct endoscopy for larynx and pharynx cancer staging. *Ann Otol Rhinol Laryngol* **98**:693–8.

Grossman T W (1989) The incidence and diagnosis of secondary esophageal carcinoma in the head and neck cancer patient. *Laryngoscope* **99**:1052–6.

Grossman T W, Kita M S, Toohill R J (1987) The diagnostic accuracy of pharyngoesophagram compared to esophagoscopy in patients with head and neck cancer. *Laryngoscope* **97**:1030–2.

Leipzig B, Zellmer J E, Klug D (1985) The role of endoscopy in evaluating patients with head and neck cancer. *Arch Otolaryngol* **111**:589–94.

Neel H B (1984) Routine panendoscopy – is it necessary every time? *Arch Otolaryngol* **110**:531–2.

Nino-Murcia M, Vincent M E, Vaughan C *et al.* (1990) Esophagography and esophagoscopy: comparison in the examination of patients with head and neck carcinoma. *Arch Otolaryngol Head Neck Surg* (1990) **116**:917–19.

Price J C, Jansen C J, Johns M E (1990) Esophageal reflux and secondary malignant neoplasia at laryngoesophagectomy. *Arch Otolaryngol Head Neck Surg* **116**:163–4.

Shons A R, McQuarrie D G (1985) Multiple primary epidermoid carcinomas of the upper aerodigestive tract. *Arch Surg* **120**:1007–9.

Tucker H M (1987) Laryngoscopy, endoscopic surgery and special techniques. In: *The Larynx*. New York, Thieme Medical, pp. 163–79.

Fine-needle aspiration cytology

Peters B R, Schnadig V J, Quinn F B *et al.* (1989) Interobserver variability in the interpretation of fine-needle aspiration biopsy of head and neck masses. *Arch Otolaryngol Head Neck Surg* **115**:1438–42.

Schneider K L, Schreiber K, Silver C E (1984) The initial evaluation of masses of the neck by needle aspiration biopsy. *Surg Gynecol Obstet* **159**:450–2.

Trapp T, Lufkin R, Abermayor E, Layfield L, Hanafee W, Ward P (1989) A new needle and technique for MRI-guided aspiration cytology of the head and neck. *Laryngoscope* **99**:105–8.

Weymuller E A, Kiviat N B, Duckert L G (1983) Aspiration cytology: an efficient and cost-effective modality. *Laryngoscope* **93**:561–4.

Wilson J A, McIntyre M A, Haacke N P, Maran A G D (1987) Fine needle aspiration biopsy and the otolaryngologist. *J Laryngol Otol* **101**:595–600.

Zajicek J (1979) The aspiration biopsy smear. In: Koss L G (ed) *Diagnostic Cytology and its Histopathologic Bases*, vol. 2. Philadelphia, J B Lippincott, pp. 1001–47.

Zajicek J, Eneroth C-M (1970) Cytological diagnosis of salivary gland carcinomas from aspiration biopsy smears. *Acta Otolaryngol* **263**:183–5.

Treatability

Aaronson N K (1988) Quality of life: what is it? How should it be measured? *Oncology* **2**:69–74.

Gardine R L, Kokal W A, Beatty J D, Riihimaki D U, Wagman L D, Terz J J (1988) Predicting the need for prolonged enteral supplementation in the patient with head and neck cancer. *Am J Surg* **156**:63–5.

Hussey D H, Latourette H B, Panje W R (1991) Head and neck cancer: an analysis of the incidence, patterns of treatment, and survial at the University of Iowa. *Ann Otol Rhinol Laryngol* **100** (Suppl) **152**:2–16.

Olson M L, Shedd D P (1978) Disability and rehabilitation in head and neck cancer patients after treatment. *Head Neck Surg* **1**:52–8.

Padilla G V, Grant M M, Martin L (1988) Rehabilitation and quality of life measurement issues. *Head Neck Surg* **10** (Suppl 11):S156–60.

Schag C C, Heinrich R L, Ganz P A (1984) Karnofsky performance status revisited: reliability, validity and guidelines. *J Clin Oncol* **2**:187–93.

Stell P M (1987) Can we afford to treat head and neck cancer? *Clin Otolaryngol* **12**:321–5.

3

Treatment options

Surgery

Preparation

The patient

It is vital to prepare both the patient and relatives psychologically before major treatment options are undertaken for a fatal disease, possibly with a fatal outcome. The statements made here are the opinions of the authors and are not intended to be dogmatic.

One of the ever-present problems of cancer therapy is what to tell the patient about the disease. An abdominal or thoracic malignancy can usually be treated without the patient being aware of extensive resection and thus it is possible to treat the patient without telling him or her precisely what has been done, if this is the preferred option. In head and neck cancer this is not so. All operations mutilate the patient to some extent and deprive him or her temporarily or permanently of an important function such as speech and swallowing. Therefore it is essential that the patient should be given an accurate account of the facts.

Many patients now use the words 'malignancy' and 'cancer' with greater ease than was once the case. These words can therefore now be used more freely by the medical profession. At the first interview the authors usually confine themselves to telling the patients and relatives that he or she has a malignancy or a growth (or indeed a cancer if the patient volunteers that word). Further explanations at this stage are usually useless because the news has induced a massive mental block in most patients and to talk further at this stage is a waste of time. Some degree of optimism should however be expressed at this first interview but the full explanation of the details of the treatment is better left for a few days until the patient is a bit more receptive.

Informed consent

The doctrine of informed consent has not yet been enshrined in English or Scottish law but may well be soon. It is essential to explain what is involved in the patient's illness, both to the patient and to the relatives. It is better to carry out this part of the interview with the relatives and the patient together at the same time. Talking to the patient and relatives separately can easily lead to suspicion and to misinterpretations in a situation which is fraught with opportunity of misunderstanding.

Informed consent consists of four items:

1 Your advice on the alternatives.
2 The effects of not taking your advice.
3 The specific risks of the operation.
4 The risks of surgery in general.

Your advice on the alternatives

In the management of cancer of the head and neck the alternatives of surgery or radiotherapy always exist and therefore both must be discussed. It is best to indicate to the patient the results you get in your institution because the patient will be treated by you and not some prince of surgery who has just written up his lifetime's work. His conclusions will not usually be transferable to your practice and this applies both to surgery and to radiotherapy. To talk about one therapy to the exclusion of the other would be entirely wrong but at this point you must indicate to the patient which modality you think is preferable for this particular tumour.

The effects of not taking your advice

If the patient opts for surgery when radiotherapy has been suggested or vice versa then the explanation of the effects has been taken care of in the previous part of the interview. If however the patient opts for no treatment then no term of life should ever be given to patient and relatives for two reasons. Firstly, you cannot begin to be accurate in estimating somebody's lifespan with an untreated carcinoma, and secondly anything that you will say will be taken as definitive and quoted back at you.

16

The specific risks of the operation

Strictly speaking, in English law, according to the Sidaway case, all you need to tell the patient about are serious risks such as paralysis, death and blindness. Most courts however would judge that the prudent doctor would expect the prudent patient to be told of any complications and effect of surgery that would materially alter his or her life quality. It is not enough just to use words, but you must also explain the effects of things like aphonia, dysarthria, dysphagia and the problems of prosthesis.

The risks of surgery in general

The risks of surgery in general are the problems of the anaesthetist and should form part of the interview that the anaesthetist has with a patient before any surgery is undertaken.

Finally, all of the above should be recorded in the case record. The permission form which is available in most British hospitals is insufficient to take care of all of the above and while it is not yet necessary to have statements signed and countersigned, this may well come to pass in the UK within the next decade.

Opinions are divided about whether or not to let a patient see a successful patient prior to operation. The authors feel that it is not always helpful for a patient who is to undergo a total laryngectomy to talk to one who has undergone the same operation and has been fully rehabilitated. Firstly, even the very best rehabilitation from a laryngectomy is ill-considered by the normal population and by no means every laryngectomee gets fully rehabilitated. Secondly, a target may be set that can never be reached by the patient in question.

The surgeon and team

Smooth performance of the operation is greatly enhanced if you discuss the operation beforehand with all of the surgical team and discuss policy issues and individual duties. You need to warn the anaesthetist of any difficult intubation and you need to ask about any special requirements such as hypertension, omission of long-acting relaxants etc. The nursing team needs to be warned about the major steps of the operation and their order. For example, many head and neck procedures begin with a tracheostomy, often followed by endoscopy for a final check on the findings. Both of these steps require separate trays, which must be arranged. If microvascular surgery is to be done the nurses skilled in this technique need to arrange their duty rota so that they are available in the latter part of the day.

Skin preparation

If the patient is shaved the day before operation this increases the bacterial count on the skin. Therefore the patient should be shaved immediately before the procedure.

Before preparing the skin in theatre, adjust the position of the patient exactly, either yourself before scrubbing up, or have it done by trained theatre staff under supervision. Extend the patient's neck by putting a small sandbag underneath the shoulders. If the patient is to have a radical neck dissection, extend the neck and also turn it to the other side, by placing the sandbag mainly under the ipsilateral shoulder.

Make sure that there is a plastic sheet under the patient's head and shoulders, because wet towels allow bacteria from the theatre table to pass through.

Use a separate trolley to clean the patient's skin and also put on a larger size of gloves, which you discard after cleaning the skin and putting on the towels.

The only important point about sterilizing solutions in head and neck surgery is that the particular preparation should not be coloured, so that any changes in colour in the skin flap can be seen at an early stage. Use whatever is the fashion in your hospital at the time.

After the skin has been prepared, spray the edges of the operative field with Nobecutaine so that the towels stick to the skin. This eliminates spaces between the towels and the skin through which infection can gain access. Towel clips get in the way in a long operation and tend to slip, so stitch the towels to skin with 3/0 silk.

The incision

Principles of incisions

Incisions for operations in the head and neck must conform to the basic requirements of any incision, as follows. An incision must provide adequate access. To achieve this, those made in neck surgery are fundamentally different from those in abdominal or thoracic surgery, where access is obtained to the appropriate cavity by a cut that is deepened through overlying structures, and by retraction of the edges of the incision, so that skin flaps are not raised. In neck surgery, large skin flaps must be developed to provide adequate access; these flaps must sometimes be so large that their blood supply becomes tenuous, particularly in a patient who has been irradiated. This is best illustrated by the operation of radical neck dissection in which the operative field extends from the clavicle below to the mandible above, from the border of the trapezius laterally to the midline medially; thus the entire skin of the neck must be elevated.

There is a well-known surgical aphorism that a wound heals from side to side and not from end to end, implying that a large wound heals as well as a small wound. Doubtless this is true of incisions used for abdominal or thoracic surgery in which flaps are not developed. But in neck surgery, where extensive flaps must be elevated, this aphorism is untrue; blind adherence to this principle will lead, on occasion, to avoidable disasters.

Any incision must be capable of extension, during the operation or later, so that any present or future eventuality can be dealt with. It is particularly important when operating on the neck for the first time to bear in mind that a further operation may be required at some future date, so that the incision used must be capable of being reopened to deal with a further problem. An obvious example of this is a laryngectomy in which a neck dissection may later be needed. In this instance if the laryngectomy is done through an apron type of flap, it is subsequently difficult to fashion a satisfactory incision through which to do a neck dissection.

An incision must not damage vital structures in or beneath the skin. The most important structures running in the skin are the cutaneous blood vessels. Cadaver studies have shown that the blood supply of the neck is taken largely from two pedicles, one anterosuperior derived from the carotid artery, and one inferomedial derived from the branches of the subclavian artery. There is thus a watershed running in an inferomedial direction in the neck and it is said that incisions which take advantage of this are particularly safe (Fig. 3.1). This may not be the whole story, because in the live patient a flap delineated by horizontal incisions is very safe and very rarely undergoes necrosis, which is not true of those delineated by vertical incisions.

The most important structures beneath the skin are the branches of the facial nerve, and elevation of the flap in the upper part of the neck must proceed in such a manner as to preserve these. This will be dealt with in Chapter 10.

An incision must always heal well, producing a scar which is cosmetically acceptable. To achieve this it is well-known that an incision should always, if possible, be placed in the lines of election for scars in the neck or in relaxed skin tension lines. These run in a horizontal direction and coincide with the skin creases, which should always be used for siting a scar (Fig. 3.2). (It should be noted that the lines of election for scars do not coincide with Langer's lines, which indeed run vertically on the neck.) A further factor which may mitigate against healing is the use of a three-point junction. It is a well-known surgical principle that the use of such a junction increases the incidence of wound breakdown, and wherever possible such a junction should not be used.

To summarize these principles, an incision in the neck should lie in a horizontal plane, if possible; it should be so designed that it can be extended if complications are encountered; and the flaps raised should be as small as possible, compatible with the extent of the operation envisaged.

Marking the skin incision

Mark the site of the incision with methylene blue and a mapping pen. The technique of traction and counteraction causes distortion of the skin so that sewing up the cut edges in correct apposition may be difficult. Therefore, before making the incision, make marks on each side of the incision line at opposing points with a needle dipped in methylene blue (Fig. 3.3).

At this stage infiltrate the site of the incision in the skin with not more than 6 ml of Xylocaine in 1:80000 adrenaline. Also infiltrate the underlying soft tissue of the entire area of the neck widely with up to 200 ml of 1:250000 adrenaline. The local anaesthetic in the skin prevents the wheal-and-flare reflex when the skin is cut, and the infiltration of the soft tissues markedly reduces the bleeding during operation. With preparation of the operative site in this way, coupled with careful operative technique, the blood loss should be minimal. For example, the blood loss of a radical neck dissection, or a total laryngectomy, should be less than 200 ml. In view of the increasing difficulty of obtaining blood, and of increasing anxiety about diseases transmitted via transfused blood, the advantages of low blood loss are obvious.

Making the incision

The knife should be held at right angles to the skin, which in some parts of the body is difficult to achieve. Where the skin is very loose, the pressure of the knife will distort it, causing the resulting cut to be slanted and untidy, which makes suturing difficult. Also, skin edges cut on the bevel may undergo necrosis (Fig. 3.4). The answer is to provide external tension. In most cases, this can be achieved by spreading the skin with the other hand. Occasionally, it is necessary to have tension in all directions, and it is a useful trick also to have an assistant stretch the skin in the line of the cut with a pair of skin hooks.

Make the cut with sufficient boldness to part the skin with one clean stroke rather than a process of erosion, but not so bold as to damage underlying structures. Hold the knife blade at right angles to the skin using the belly of the blade. Where a small cut is required, a small blade, such as a no. 15, is easiest. Larger cuts, for example when developing chest flaps, need larger blades, such as no. 10 or no. 22.

The assistant now retracts the flaps vertically

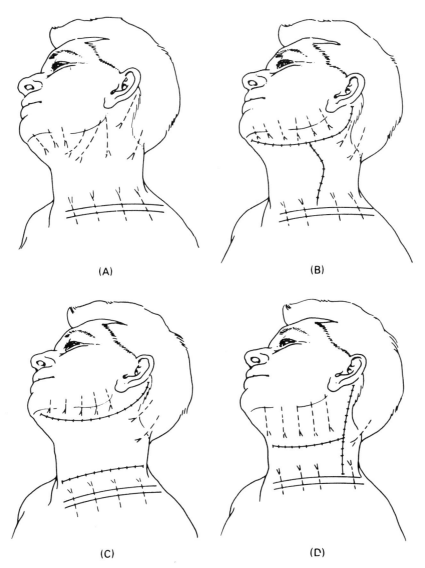

(A)

(B)

(C)

(D)

Fig. 3.1 Blood supply of the skin of the neck in relation to various incision lines.

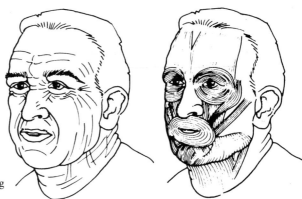

Fig. 3.2 Lines of election for scars related to wrinkling and the underlying musculature.

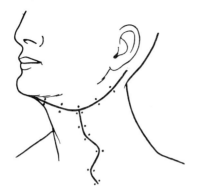

Fig. 3.3 Skin incision marked.

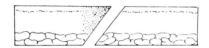

Fig. 3.4 Bevelled skin edges.

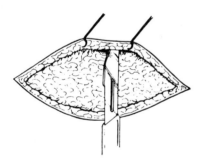

Fig. 3.5 Skin edges retracted.

upwards with double skin hooks in the subcutaneous tissues (Fig. 3.5). This demonstrates a clear plane deep to the platysma: sharp dissection in this plane is bloodless. Never apply Allis forceps to the skin and do not let the assistant fold the flap upon itself – this leads to buttonholing.

After elevating the flaps, the skin surface must be excluded completely from the wound, either by stitching the flaps back to the towels or by retracting them with a Joll's clamp and side towels. If the skin flaps are stitched to the towels, never pass the needle through the skin, only through the subcutaneous tissues. On no account should an upper skin flap be stretched over the chin to hold it out of place.

Dissection

Use a limited range of instruments, know each instrument by name, and become thoroughly familiar with each. Remember one of the basic rules of surgery: pick it up, use it, put it down. Do no wave it about, and 'keep your eye on the ball'.

Another of the secrets of good surgery is space: each individual step of surgery is easy, but access to allow that manoeuvre to be executed can be difficult. Access requires space, and the creation of space demands the ability to think in three dimensions.

Dissect with a knife with a sharp blade. Only use scissors exceptionally because these separate the tissues and do not cut them.

As regards bleeding points, a good rule is to use coagulation diathermy on the specimen only, and to tie with chromic catgut any large vessel that is left in the patient. Any vessel that has a name should be tied with 3/0 silk.

Do not leave long-ended ligatures, do not tie a large mass of tissue, and do not coagulate a large area – these are all causes of abscess formation.

Bone excision

The most obvious reason for excising bone in head and neck cancer surgery is because it is invaded by cancer. Also, it is often necessary to excise bone to close the defect resulting from excision of a tumour of the tonsil, and sometimes bone must be cut to provide access – the common example of this is mandibulotomy for access to a tumour of the tongue or of the floor of the mouth. In mandibulotomy, the bone will be put back together again, and so it has to be cut with the edges planned for good immobilization. The safest way to do this is to mark a step in the mandible with methylene blue and to drill holes for the immobilization wires before cutting the bone – if the bone is cut first it is very difficult to drill decent holes in its loose ends. Mark the step as shown (Fig. 3.6): the shape of the fragments is such that pull on the proximal fragment by the pterygoid muscles will impact the fragments after they are

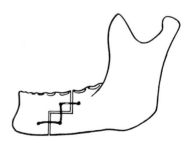

Fig. 3.6 Mandibulotomy.

replaced. Once the holes have been drilled it is easy to cut along the line, separate the parts of the mandible, excise the tumour, replace the mandible and wire it. Remember that heavily irradiated bone often becomes infected if it is divided and then exposed to saliva.

The best instruments for cutting bone is a Stryker saw, but if this is not available then a fissure burr on a dental drill is adequate. A Gigli saw can also be used: keep it taut, and do not pause because the wire curls up and sticks in the bone if it is not kept taut, resulting in a broken wire; also keep the handles as far apart as possible, cutting with the wire almost straight.

Excision drill

After excising the specimen, in continuity, leave the table with the specimen and examine the edges. In oral or pharyngeal cancer the margin around the tumour often appears narrow – this may be due to the fact that mucosa retracts after it has been cut.

However, if there is no margin at one edge go back and excise another strip of mucosa at this point. Also send specimens from the edges nearest the tumour for frozen section to ensure that excision has been complete.

After examining the specimen make sure that the theatre sister takes away all the instruments used in the removal of the tumour, because they are all contaminated. Take off your gown and gloves, put on new ones and make sure everybody else does the same.

In times past, didactic recommendations were made for safe margins. However, pathological studies have refined our knowledge of this area, and it is now known that the margin must be dictated by the tumour. Lip cancers require a margin of not more than 1 cm, and the excellent results from supraglottic laryngectomy have shown that only millimetres of clearance are needed near the vocal cords. Conversely, some tumours require more than 2 cm margin; the most notorious of these are tumours of the tongue and hypopharynx. Each case will have to be treated on its merits but one should always strive to perform as wide a removal as possible within the limits of possible reconstruction and cosmetic deformity.

If preoperative radiotherapy has been used in the treatment of a head and neck cancer, it is important not to be fooled by the subsequent reduction in the size of the tumour. The margin to be excised is the same as would have been taken had the patient not had radiotherapy; this is also true of induction chemotherapy.

Tissues become distorted during excision, so tattoo a line of clearance around the tumour before starting to remove it. If preoperative radiotherapy is to be used, tattoo the selected line of excision before irradiation. This is best done at the time of biopsy under general anaesthetic.

Wound irrigation

Before beginning to close the wound, wash it out well. Many different solutions are advised – sterile water, cytotoxic solutions, Cetavlon, etc., but the important part of this process appears to be the mechanical action of the washing, rather than any lytic action on the cells. Wash all areas thoroughly with at least 1 l of solution. The washout will almost certainly restart bleeding from several points – now is the time to secure final and absolute haemostasis.

Drains

Suction drainage must be used: a wick type of drain is as likely to allow bacteria into the wound as serum to come out.

Methods
Polythene tubes

These are the simplest and easiest method of establishing suction drainage. Cut holes in thin polythene tubing and connect the tubing to a suction machine, or wall suction. The disadvantage of this method is that the patient cannot walk about.

Vacuum systems

Various closed suction systems are available but are more expensive. The tubes are already perforated and sterilized, and drain into bottles or canisters which are evacuated of air. In accordance with the 'laws' of technology, the best and cheapest of these is no longer made. These systems have the advantage that the patient is mobile. The disadvantage is that a close watch is needed to detect exhaustion of the vacuum.

Fixation of the drainage tube

Hold each drain in place within the wound by two 3/0 chromic catguts sutured to the underlying muscles. Take care that no holes are within about 2.5 cm of the skin puncture or else air will leak; stitch the drains to the skin by a Roman garter stitch of 3/0 silk. Additional fixation is supplied by laying the drains parallel to each other 2.5 cm apart on the chest and holding them down with a 15 cm piece of 7.5 cm elastic adhesive. Nobecutaine acts as an additional seal at the pucture holes, but apply it with suction off, in case an air leak sucks Nobecutaine under the skin flaps.

Closing the skin

It is very important to produce a good scar after a head and neck operation: the scar is the only sign available to the patient and relatives for assessing your workmanship. The principles of sewing the skin are to have no tension on it; to avoid dead spaces; to have no haematomas; and to get perfect apposition of the skin edge. Achieve these by using suction drainage, and stitching up in two layers.

Instruments

Healthy tissues should not be pinched, crushed or otherwise abused. There is no doubt that having the right instrument for the right job makes the procedure less of a trial for surgeon and patient alike. For example, closing a wound with a fine suture using a pair of heavy forceps and a pair of Kilner needle holders (which have a particularly strong ratchet) irritates the experienced and is likely to make the inexperienced feel unnecessarily clumsy. Fine work requires fine instruments.

Do not grasp skin with forceps – non-toothed forceps crush it, and toothed forceps produce puncture marks. To overcome this, grasp the wound edges by the subcutaneous tissues, or use the toothed forceps as a hook and lever. This means using the forceps with the tips open, hooking the subcutaneous tissues with one tip and exerting gentle pressure with the tip to lever the skin backwards to facilitate the passage of the needle (Fig. 3.7). This is a habit that is worth acquiring early, as the novice's frustration at trying to place a suture with one hand is directly

proportional to the force applied to the forceps held in the other, with consequent damage to the skin edges.

An excellent alternative is to hold the skin edges with a skin hook, but this can be harder than it looks. The purpose of forceps is to evert the skin while the suture is being placed. This aim can often be achieved by pressing the open forceps down on either side of the wound, which has the effect of pushing the skin edges up (Fig. 3.8), and then passing the needle through both sides with one movement. The same effect can be produced by using fingers instead of forceps.

Sutures

There is an increasing number of sutures available on the market and a list of those most frequently used is given in Table 3.1. Absorbables are used where a suture is expected to be removed or where removal may be difficult, for example, in subcutaneous closure and suturing mucosa. They are absorbed at different rates, and this is reflected in their ability to take the tension of a sutured wound. Plain catgut loses its tensile strength fastest (after about 5 days) and polydioxanone (PDS) lasts longest, about 60 days. These sutures are all absorbed by varying degrees of inflammatory response, except PDS, which is absorbed by hydrolysis, although what practical difference this makes has yet to be determined.

From the above, two points emerge:

1 Do not put absorbables too close to the skin if possible, because of the inflammatory response.

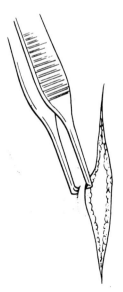

Fig. 3.7 One tip of a toothed forceps used as a hook and the other as a lever.

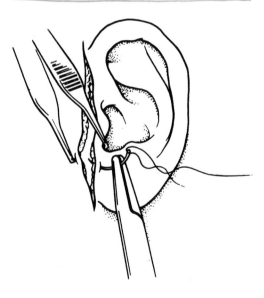

Fig. 3.8 Open forceps used for simultaneous counterpressure and eversion.

Table 3.1 Suture materials

	Non-absorbable	Absorbable
Monofilament	Polyamides (nylon)	Polydioxanone (PDS)
	Polypropylene (Prolene)	Catgut
	Polybutester (Novafil)	
	Steel	
Multifilament	Silk	Polyglycolic (Dexon)
	Linen	
	Polyamide (Nurolon)	Polyglactin (Vicryl)
	Polyester (Ethibond, Mersilene)	

2 Use longer-lasting absorbables where there is tight skin closure or the skin tension is naturally high, to take the weight of the wound.

Catgut is easy to work with and ties a good knot. Dexon and Vicryl are easy to work with but require very careful multiple knots, and PDS is hard to work with but ties an excellent knot.

Non-absorbables are used as skin sutures or permanent subcutaneous sutures. Silk is the easiest of any suture to handle and ties the best knot: best, meaning the most secure knot with the least number of throws. However, there is some evidence that because it is a multifilament and therefore has some capillary action, it is more likely to cause hatch marks (suture marks) than an equivalent monofilament. Nurolon is very similar to silk, but ties a less secure knot. Monofilaments in general are harder to handle, and require more care in tying a knot. Prolene and Novafil are more slippery than nylon, and are therefore better for subcuticular closure of wounds and tie better knots. Clips are quicker but more expensive. They do however give an excellent end-result.

Suturing

An indication of choice of sutures has been given above. It remains to decide on the type of suture for any given situation. Use the finest suture that will hold the wound, and consider how long the sutures will need to remain in place. Subcutaneous sutures are used to close the dead space and take the weight of the wound, while skin sutures should do no more than provide fine edge approximation of a wound that already has a 'kissing fit' from the subcutaneous closure.

The incidence of hatch marks is directly related to the length of time the suture is left in and its tightness. Therefore, if a suture needs to be left in for any length of time, consider using a subcuticular one.

Most sutures are now atraumatic, that is to say, the needle is swaged on to the suture. All needles discussed in this chapter, except the one used for subcuticular sutures, are meant to be used with needle holders, which means that they are curved. They may be round-bodied or cutting. Round-bodied needles have a simple tapering tip and are used where minimal tissue trauma is obligatory, such as in bowel or vascular surgery. However, they are extremely difficult to pass through tough tissues such as skin. Always use a cutting needle for suturing skin or subcutaneous tissues. As the name implies, cutting needles have a cutting tip, in a variety of types, which permits them to be passed easily through most tissues. Taper cutting or reverse cutting needles are a compromise between cutting and round-bodied needles.

Curved needles should be mounted in the needle holder in their flattened mid-section at the tip of the holder (Fig. 3.9a). If they are mounted at the swaged section, which is round, there is a tendency for the needle to twist in the holder and bend or break off (Fig. 3.9b).

Subcutaneous sutures are used to obliterate dead spaces and approximate the wound edges. Use an absorbable material on a cutting needle. Close the platysma with a continuous suture, and invert the final knot. This layer must produce an airtight closure: it also provides the strength of the wound. Skin sutures are used to provide accurate edge approximation with skin eversion. To achieve eversion, the deep tissues should push the edges upward when the knot is tied (Fig. 3.10), which is the reason for turning the skin back with forceps or a skin hook

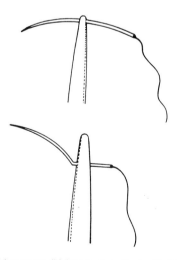

Fig. 3.9 (a) correct; (b) incorrect method of holding a needle.

as the needle is passed. Eversion of the wound edges is mandatory for primary healing with a good scar – an inverted wound may look fine until the sutures are removed, and then the edges gape and heal by secondary intention.

There are many different methods of skin closure. The commonest is the simple interrupted stitch. However, continuous sutures have some advantages over interrupted sutures. They are faster and easier to remove for the patients and doctor or nurse, and of course have fewer knots to accumulate blood clots, making them easier to keep clean. Continuous sutures have to be placed with proper regard to edge eversion and tightness; they are unsuitable where a suture might need to be removed prematurely, unless it is a locked suture, for once one side is cut, the whole wound is at risk of separating.

A continuous blanket stitch, using a non-absorbable material, is probably the most satisfactory suture for the curving incision of a major neck procedure (Fig. 3.11). Put the needle in at more than right angle to the skin edge to get a bigger bit of dermis and fat than skin. Put the needle in 2 mm from the skin edge and place the sutures 6 mm apart in order to distribute tension evenly. Take equal bites because unequal ones lead to poor apposition of the skin edges. This stitch should evert the skin edges.

Where sutures are to be left in for over 10 days, and where a good scar is of overriding importance and the wound is relatively short and straight (for

example, after surgery for a pharyngeal pouch), a subcuticular suture should be used. A non-absorbable suture must be a monofilament; Prolene and Novafil are easiest to remove. Either a straight or curved needle may be used, depending on personal preference.

Satisfactory and rapid skin closure can now be achieved using staples in a disposable handpiece. A three-point junction must be sewn up first if staples are to be used. Prevent necrosis of the corners and bunching of the tip of the flap as follows: put the needle in 1 cm from the edge of the reception side of the wound, take a subcutaneous bite of the tip, and then bring the needle out again 1 cm from the skin edge on the reception side, and tie the knot, making sure that the suture enters and leaves the reception side at the same level as it does in a V flap (Fig. 3.12).

Postoperative care

Tracheostomy care

Nursing

A trained nurse should be in attendance at all times for the first 24–48 h after a tracheostomy. The nurse should be acquainted with all complications of the operation and the principles of sterile suction and humidification, and also be able to replace the tube if necessary.

Tell the patient before the operation that he or she will not be able to speak until the tracheostomy is closed. He or she should have a 'magic slate' on which to write, and a bell with which to summon assistance.

Fixation of the tracheostomy tube

A tracheostomy tube can be very difficult to replace if it is dislodged within the first 48 h. Therefore stitch the tube to the skin. These stitches must be cut out when the tube is changed for the first time: tapes are then applied to the second tracheostomy tube. Tie the tapes so that they are doubled over, with the head in the neutral position; if they are tied to the extended position they will be too loose when the head is in the neutral position. Always use a reef knot and always place the knots so that there is one on each side of the neck. The tapes should not be tied so tightly that they obstruct the lymphatic drainage, causing oedema of the skin flaps above the ties. Never take the tapes across a pedicled skin flap from the chest.

Removal of secretions

Excess secretions are inevitable after a newly created tracheostomy because the tube acts as a foreign body and stimulates secretions, and the trachea has never

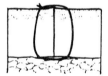

Fig. 3.10 Correct position of skin suture.

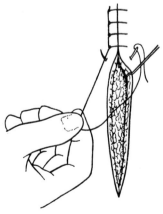

Fig. 3.11 Blanket suture.

CORRECT METHOD   INCORRECT METHOD

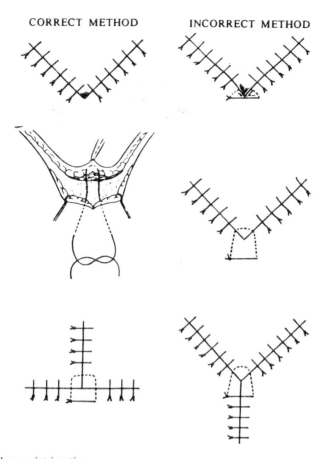

Fig. 3.12 Suturing of a three-point junction.

before been exposed to cold dry air; there may also be some oozing of blood from the operation site. Secretions should be removed by suction every half hour, or more often if indicated. After the first 48 h this period may be lengthened but suction will always be required at least every 4 h. The nurse should wear sterile gloves, and use the special suction tubes that minimize tracheal and bronchial trauma.

Humidification

The normal channels for warming and humidifying the air have been bypassed so artificial humidification is required to prevent crusting of secretions. Humidification is provided by hot water bath humidifiers or by nebulizers delivering cold droplets. An alternative is the heat and humidity exchangers. The humidified air is delivered by a mask or a T-tube applied to the tracheostomy tube. A satisfactory alternative to prevent crusting is the instillation of slaine into the trachea. If secretions (and therefore crusting) are particularly severe it is useful to administer nebulized mucolytics for a few days. This problem is common as many patients have chronic obstructive airways disease.

Changing the tracheostomy tube

Normally for the first 48 h a cuffed plastic tube is used, or occasionally a silver tube, in which case the inner tube is cleaned at hourly intervals. Change the tracheostomy tube after 48 h and insert a smaller one. Thereafter change it every 2–3 days in order to avoid wound infection or crusting. After a tube is inserted into the trachea, establish with absolute certainty that it is actually in the tracheal lumen, as it is easy to place the tube in the mediastinum anterior to the trachea. Ask the patient to take deep breaths, and feel the air coming out of the tube. The safest method of changing the tube at 48 h is to insert a sterile catheter into the old tube, which is then withdrawn over the catheter. The new tube is then threaded over the catheter into the trachea. There is always a risk of failure of reintubation and this can result in unnecessary death. A pair of tracheal dilators should always be taped to the head of the bed, and a tracheostomy set, a battery laryngoscope and bronchoscope should be available on the ward in case of dire emergencies.

Care of the inflatable cuff

When a cuff is blown up to occlude an airway its pressure can exceed that of the systolic blood pressure, so that the area of the tracheal wall with which it is in contact is in danger of ischaemic necrosis. Leave the tube inflated for the first 12 h after operation, deflating the cuff for 5 min every hour, and then let it down. New low-pressure cuffs on most makes of tubes minimize the risk of tracheal damage but the above is still good practice.

Breathing exercises

The patient almost always needs postoperative breathing exercises from the physiotherapist. If secretions are excessive, more vigorous treatment by intermittent positive-pressure breathing triggered by the patient is used. If this is not available the patient's lungs can be inflated with an Ambu bag after suction has been performed. This gives greater ventilation than deep breathing exercises and can be done more often. After sucking out the trachea the Ambu bag is fitted on to the tracheostomy connection, the cuff of the tracheostomy tube is blown up, and the patient ventilated for 3 min. The Ambu bag is then taken off and the cuff let down.

Removal of a temporary tracheostomy tube

About the fifth day after operation place a spigot in the tracheostomy tube during the day. The next day, block the tracheostomy tube overnight as well. If the patient can sleep with the tube closed then withdraw the tracheostomy tube the next day, dress the wound, and allow it to close. It is important to block only a small tube because a no. 36 or 39 tube may cause total respiratory obstruction when blocked, even if the patient's upper airway is patent.

Dressings

Waterproof squares are used in the care of tracheostomies: they have a slit on their top surface that is passed around the edges of the tube and secured above it with a safety pin.

Drains

A suction type of drainage tube will have been inserted in the operating theatre. Continuous suction must be maintained on the drainage tube for bacteria are as likely to go up a drainage tube as serum is to come down it, unless a vacuum is maintained. Whenever suction is taken off the tube it should be clamped. It is important also not to allow the patient to wander around the ward with the drainage tube dangling free; the canister or the bottle should be fixed to the patient's dressing gown.

Leaking drains

All the advantages of suction drainage are lost if air is allowed to leak into the drainage tube from the anastomosis, from the skin incision, or from the tracheostomy. This in turn means that saliva, air or infected secretions are drawn underneath the skin flaps, almost certainly leading to wound infection and skin breakdown. The leak must be stopped immediately to prevent this. Examine the wound to ascertain whether the leak comes from the tracheostomy, the skin incision or the internal suture line.

The best method of preventing an air leak from the tracheostomy is to keep the tracheostomy wound separate from the main wound. This is possible if the tracheostomy is temporary. If the two incisions are joined by accident then the junction should be closed carefully to provide an airtight seal. A permanent tracheostomy should be fashioned with great care in layers, as described in Chapter 9.

If air is heard leaking around the tracheostomy, local packing with cotton wool soaked in Hibitane will usually stop it. This is the easiest site of an air leak to diagnose, and the site of the leak can often be seen if the tracheostomy tube is moved around.

If the *incision* has been stitched properly in two layers it cannot leak. If it does leak, however, a useful manoeuvre is to go along the suture line pulling the edges apart slightly. When the site of the leak has been found there will be a large gush of air into the suction tube. Apply Nobecutaine and local pressure to the leak after stopping the suction, and 5 min later start the suction again; alternatively insert another stitch under local anaesthetic.

Air leaks can also occur at the skin exits of the *drains*, if the holes have been made with anything other than the special needle introducer, or if a drain has slipped and a perforation lies outside the skin. It is often quite difficult to push a tube back to stop a leak here, but Nobecutaine together with adhesive tape is usually successful.

After stitching up the mucosa the *suture line* should be watertight: if you are not sure that it is, the easiest way to find out is to pour water into the pharynx to test it. If the closure is watertight it will also be airtight. If the suture line is leaking, this is particularly bad, because the air will be mixed with saliva, and the flaps will very rapidly become lifted and infected. If this is the leaking site – and usually the diagnosis is made by exclusion of the previous two sites – stop the suction for at least 24 h and apply a pressure dressing. Then, 24 h later, move the tubes a little and restart gentle suction; if the original leak was small, it will usually have sealed.

Type of drainage

Within the first 24–48 h, the drainage from a radical neck dissection consists entirely of blood, and measures about 200 ml/day. After 48 h it becomes serous, and after 6 days only 25 ml drains in 24 h. A lot can be learnt from the character of the drainage and its smell. Air, saliva or a bad smell is often the first sign of an internal fistula: if this happens, localize the fistula with the finger, make a small hole in the skin over it, and apply suction directly to it. This converts a long fistulous tract into a small fistula that will usually heal on its own.

Milky fluid coming into the drainage tube is not milk but chyle. This complication is dealt with in Chapter 8.

Removal of drains

If there are problems with drainage tubes, particularly intractable failure or blockage, it is better to remove them early rather than risk ascending infection under the flaps. The drainage tubes should not be removed until the daily drainage is less than 25 ml. However, as a drain cannot be left *in situ* indefinitely and as in itself it causes some secretion, it should be removed on the sixth day if the daily drainage has been consistent for 48 h.

Intravenous fluids

Most head and neck patients can be fed within 48 h of operation. In the first 48 h the worst mistakes that can be made are to give the patient too much water and salt, resulting in pulmonary oedema. Between the end of the operation and the next morning give the patient 1 l of half-strength Hartmann's solution or dextrose subsequently. This can usually be given via the central intravenous line left in by the anaesthetist at the end of the procedure. This line can be removed the next day provided that the haemoglobin and electrolyte levels are satisfactory, that nasogastric feeds are tolerated, and that the line is not needed for administration of other solutions. Examples of other fluids to be given include dextran 40, 500 ml of which is often given during the first 12 h to patients undergoing microvascular surgery, followed by 500 ml the next day; mannitol to patients undergoing a second neck dissection; calcium replacement after total thyroidectomy; and intravenous hyperalimentation.

Oral feeding

In contrast to most major abdominal operations, when the gut does not function properly for several days postoperatively, gastrointestinal function after most forms of major head and neck surgery is normal. Provided bowel sounds have returned, most patients can be fed via the gastrointestinal tract from day 1. In view of the fact that many patients having major head and neck surgery are already malnourished this is generally desirable. There are many commercial enteral feeding preparations now available that provide a balanced intake and usually contain about 1 kcal (4.2 kJ)/ml. In the absence of gastrointestinal disease the more expensive elemental feeds are unnecessary.

A nasogastric tube is placed during the operation and feeding can normally be started the following day. The best way of ensuring an adequate intake is to give the feed continuously throughout the 24 h using gravity feed or a special pump. Intermittent bolus feeding is associated with abdominal discomfort and it is often not possible to maintain an adequate intake this way. The day after operation a graduated regimen such as that in Table 3.2 is begun. Full-strength feeds, providing about 2400 kcal (10 MJ) in 24 h, can be achieved on the second day, which is adequate for most adult patients. Before feeding starts, care should be taken to ensure the feeding tube is in the stomach by aspirating the stomach contents or listening over the epigastrium while air is injected.

Although narrow-bore feeding tubes are often used for feeding as they are more comfortable, they are less than ideal after head and neck surgery as they are more likely to get displaced if the patient vomits, and also more likely to get blocked. Displacement of a feeding tube after some forms of head and neck surgery is undesirable as it may be impossible to replace it until after the pharyngeal wound has healed.

In patients who are particularly malnourished and who have had surgery involving the gastrointestinal tract (ileal loop etc.), it may be judged desirable to feed intravenously for several days after operation until full gastrointestinal function returns.

Table 3.2 Post-head and neck surgery feeding regimen

1st hour	30 ml warm sterile water
2nd hour	60 ml warm water with glucose
3rd hour	30 ml water and 30 ml warm milk with glucose
4th hour	60 ml water and 30 ml warm milk with glucose
5th hour	30 ml water and 60 ml warm milk with glucose
6th hour	60 ml water and 60 ml warm milk with glucose
7th hour	30 ml water and 90 ml warm milk with glucose
8th hour	120 ml warm milk with glucose
9th hour	200 ml milk feed
11th hour	Full feed

Medications

Antibiotics

Prophylactic antibiotic cover is only needed if the pharynx or mouth has been opened. It is *not* needed for operations such as radical neck dissection and parotidectomy. Before surgery, Gram-negative organisms are rarely present. However, to be absolutely sure, perhaps a swab should be taken from the mouth and throat in clinic, so that culture and sensitivity tests are available at the time of surgery. Other swabs, e.g. from the nose, axilla, groin, are of little value and are no longer taken.

The mouth and pharynx normally contain Gram-positive cocci and anaerobes – Gram-negative cocci are seldom present, but do colonize the mouth within 2–3 days of the passing of a nasogastric tube, which allows the ascent of intestinal organisms. Provided that the patient has no nasogastric tube any antibiotic needed must cover only the Gram-positive cocci and anaerobes. Preferably an antibiotic should be used that is not in frequent use for other purposes. Erythromycin fulfils these criteria admirably. Cover is only needed during, and for a brief period after, opening the pharynx. Therefore give one dose of 1 g erythromycin intravenously during the operation just before the pharynx is opened and 8-hourly for the first 24 h. This regimen has been shown to be highly effective. Many surgeons would also add metronidazole to this but it is not strictly necessary. If postoperative infection becomes established despite this regimen take a swab for culture in the usual way and use the appropriate antibiotic. Augmentin is a broad-spectrum antibiotic covering Gram-negative bacteria (which erythromycin does not), and is therefore a very useful agent. However, generalized use may result in proliferation of resistant bacterial strains, which could limit its usefulness.

Chest infection should be prevented as far as possible by dental hygiene, preoperative treatment of chronic bronchitis and sinusitis, and sterile precautions during tracheostomy care. If it becomes established, treat it with the appropriate antibiotics after having the sputum cultured.

If the patient has a tracheostomy before the operation, take a swab from it a few days before the operation, and start the appropriate antibiotic immediately.

Thyroid and parathyroid replacement

Total thyroidectomy, carried out either for thyroid carcinoma or in continuity with a pharyngolaryngectomy for a carcinoma of the pharynx, may include removal of the parathyroid glands. Some of the problems of postoperative management are calcium balance and thyroid replacement.

Thyroid replacement need not begin for at least a week after the operation, after which time the patient is almost always swallowing or being fed by a nasogastric tube. Begin with thyroxine 0.2 mg/day in a man, and 0.15 mg/day in a woman. Assess the correct dosage by monthly estimates of total thyroxine, which should be kept within the normal limits of 54–166 nmol/l, or of free thyroxine between 8.8 and 23 pmol/l.

Parathyroid replacement is more difficult. Parathormone maintains the serum calcium by releasing it from bone into the blood stream, and by controlling urinary excretion. The natural hormone is replaced with vitamin D_2; calcium supplements must also be given.

Immediately after operation add 120 ml 10% calcium gluconate per day to any intravenous regime. As soon as possible go on to 1.6 g calcium a day given in the form of Calcium-Sandoz tablets. Vitamin D_2 is given as calciferol forte tablets (BP) 50 000 units; one tablet a day is usually enough.

The dose of calcium is adjusted according to the serum calcium level and the serum albumin. For every 1 g of albumin below 40 g/l an allowance of 0.02 mmol/l in the calcium level should be made. For example, if a patient has a serum albumin of 30 g/l and a serum calcium of 2.05 mmol/l, the latter figure should be corrected to 2.25 mmol/l. After these corrections have been made the serum calcium should be maintained between 2.2 and 2.7 mmol/l. The dose of vitamin D_2 is adjusted according to the urinary calcium level because the urinary level fluctuates more rapidly than the serum level. A urinary calcium based on a 24-h collection of urine is therefore needed and this usually requires admission to a metabolic unit. The urinary calcium should be maintained between 3.0 and 7.5 mmol/24 h in men and 2.5–6.25 mmol/24 h in women. Great care is needed with patients in chronic renal failure in whom the serum calcium levels can fluctuate more rapidly than the urinary levels. For some unknown reason the patient's requirements for vitamin D_2 gradually becomes less over the years. To prevent a fluctuation beyond acceptable limits these patients must, therefore, be assessed at monthly intervals. An accurate assessment cannot be carried out without an estimation of the serum calcium, the urinary calcium, the serum pH, the electrolytes and the serum albumin: it should usually be done by a physician interested in this problem.

Dressings and sutures

Wound dressings

Wound dressings have several 'functions': they make the wound warm, macerated and liable to infection; they successfully conceal impending complications, such as haematoma; and they encourage the inquisitive to draw them aside with a dirty fingernail to inspect the wound. If all the bleeding points have been secured, and the incision properly closed, dressings have no other contribution to make to the care of the patient. However, a pressure dressing should be applied for 24 h after the drainage tubes have been removed, to prevent a seroma.

Never put a bandage around the neck after bilateral neck dissection or a second neck dissection as it occludes the remaining venous return via the vertebral veins.

If flaps have been elevated by saliva tracking out of a fistula they can be encouraged to reseat by fenestrating the fistula, and applying a pressure dressing to the flaps.

Necrotic areas should be cleaned twice daily and dressed. Surgical debridement is performed on the ward – no analgesia is needed as dead tissue has no nerve supply.

Sutures

If an adequate subcutaneous layer has been used, skin sutures may be removed after 7 days if the wound appears normal. Stomal sutures after laryngectomy are usually left for up to 12 days as the mucocutaneous junction is often under greater traction.

Monofilament synthetic sutures can be left in place longer than silk, which because it is braided has a wick action, causing microabscesses within 72 h. For this reason silk stitches must be removed early.

Intraoral sutures may be of silk (these can be removed through the mouth 7 days later) or of Dexon that does not need to be removed.

Before removing the stitches, clean the wound edge of all crusts. Cut the material flush with the skin on the opposite side to the knot and then pull the knot over the wound to remove the stitch. Never pull the loose ends away from the skin edges as this can cause wound disruption. When removing a blanket suture take great care not to disrupt the wound edges – cut the free end when it becomes more than about 4 cm long.

Getting up

After operation the patient is supported in bed, sitting up at 45°, in order to avoid lymphatic stasis in the head and neck. Never allow a patient who has had a bilateral neck dissection to lie flat, because of the danger of cerebral oedema.

If the common or internal carotid artery has been ligated, for example after a carotid blow-out, the patient must be nursed flat for 48 h. Thereafter the patient's head may be raised by one pillow a day.

There are very few head and neck procedures that stop the patient getting out of bed the next day; the patient should be walking freely around the ward within 72 h, with the drainage canister attached to his or her dressing gown. This helps to prevent postoperative chest infection and deep venous thrombosis.

Follow-up

Any patient who has had a head and neck cancer procedure should be followed up monthly for the first year, then 2-monthly for the second and third year, then 6-monthly for the fourth and fifth years; after this he or she should be seen yearly for another 5 years.

At each follow-up visit examine both the primary site for recurrence, and neck for enlarged lymph nodes. A primary recurrence may be treated by further surgery, and an enlarged lymph node is certainly treatable, and often curable, by radical neck dissection. A further lymph node metastasis is most likely to present within the first 2 years but remember that a node can grow rapidly, and within 6 weeks be irremovable without heroic surgery. After 2 years a 2 monthly follow-up will be satisfactory, because a node will almost certainly be slow-growing if it appears after this period of time.

The above follow-up principles also apply if radiotherapy has been used as the prime form of treatment.

Radiotherapy

General principles

The rationale for radiotherapy

Radiotherapy, that is, treatment with ionizing radiation, has been recognized as a valuable modality in the management of cancer for nearly a century. Over this period, radiotherapeutic technology has evolved *parri passu* with advances in surgery, and disease that some years ago was best treated with one modality may now be better treated with the other or with both. It can be misleading to base judgements of the value of current treatment practices on reports published decades ago about the outcome of patients treated in the preceding quarter-century. As far as head and neck cancer is concerned, radiotherapy, like surgery, is a local treatment. Its purpose is to eradicate tumour at the primary site, and in some cases the regional lymph nodes. Its principal advantage is that it can often do so while sparing normal tissue function. For example, radiotherapy is certainly no better, and perhaps slightly worse, at curing advanced laryngeal cancer than surgery, yet it offers the chance of voice preservation, which is not possible with laryngectomy.

How radiotherapy works

Radiation causes damage to DNA in both normal and malignant cells. If cells are unable to repair this damage by the time of their next division, then they die in mitosis. The response of both normal and malignant cells to radiation is qualitatively similar, but in general malignant cells have a lower repair capacity than normal ones, and have a shorter cell cycle. Thus the chances of a dose of radiation killing a malignant cell are greater than those of killing a normal cell. It is on these quantitative differences in the response to radiation of normal and malignant cells that radiotherapy depends.

The relationship between cure and complications

The basic principle of radiotherapy is to get as high a radiation dose into the tumour and any occult extensions as possible to ensure a cure, while minimizing the dose to surrounding normal tissue, in order to avoid complications as far as possible. In the head and neck the situation is more complex for several reasons. Firstly, squamous cancer is less radiosensitive than some other tumours such as lymphoma and requires a high dose for cure which is at the level of radiation tolerance of much normal tissue, and exceeds the tolerance of the more sensitive normal structures. Secondly, radiotherapy in the head and neck requires greater technical precision than at other anatomical sites, because of the close juxtaposition of critically radiosensitive organs such as the eye and brainstem to the tumours requiring treatment. In addition there are also other structures such as the salivary glands and mucosa which, while not as critically susceptible to radiation damage as the brainstem, should none the less be spared unnecessary irradiation in order to minimize both acute and long-term sequelae.

For these reasons, the *therapeutic ratio,* that is the relationship between the dose that is required for cure and the dose which causes unacceptable damage, is low. In general terms, a tumour is more likely to be cured if a higher dose is given. Similarly, complications are more likely if a higher dose is used. This relationship is shown graphically in Figure 3.13. It is a matter of philosophy and judgement what incidence of serious complications can be justified in pursuit of cure, although 5% is generally accepted as reasonable. It can be seen that the likelihood of an uncomplicated cure diminishes beyond a certain critical dose level. Another factor to be noted from this graph is that the central part of both curves is quite steep. This means that a relatively small increment in dose may greatly increase the likelihood of cure, or greatly increase the risk of complications. Conversely, a small dose reduction, as may occur if the last one or two treatments in a fractionated course are omitted because of acute side-effects, may greatly diminish the likelihood of cure. The aim of any modification in treatment technique is to enhance the therapeutic ratio. This enables a

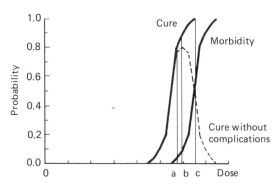

Fig. 3.13 The relationship between radiation dose and the probability of tumour cure, severe late normal tissue morbidity and uncomplicated cure, with a particular treatment regimen.

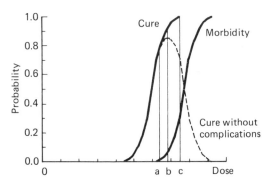

Fig. 3.14 Using an alternative treatment schedule the therapeutic ratio is enhanced.

higher dose to be given, achieving a greater cure rate for a given complication rate (Fig. 3.14).

Treatment intent

Radical and palliative treatment

In general, cancer treatment may be considered radical or palliative. In radical treatment the aim is to cure the patient, even though the chances of achieving this end may be recognized to be slim. Complex, time-consuming and unpleasant treatments can be justified if cure is a possible outcome. On the other hand, when the disease is recognized to be incurable, palliative treatment aimed solely to alleviate symptoms is recommended. This should be simple, quick and should not produce side-effects worse than the symptoms it aims to treat.

Radical treatment with palliative intent

In head and neck cancer the division between radical and palliative treatment is less clear-cut. There are many occasions where a radical style of treatment is rightly used in an attempt to achieve local tumour control, despite the fact that the disease is considered to be incurable. This may be justified by the particularly horrible nature of uncontrolled cancer in some head and neck situations. In addition, unlike many forms of advanced malignancy such as lung cancer or bone metastases, where a short course of low-dose radiotherapy, or even a single treatment, may greatly improve symptoms, this is rarely the case for head and neck cancer. Here a full course of radiotherapy – radical radiotherapy with palliative intent – usually needs to be given to achieve adequate palliation, and conventional palliative radiotherapy is rarely used.

Combined treatment

Types of combination

Although radiotherapy is often used as the sole modality, it is frequently used in combination with surgery or chemotherapy, and sometimes both. It may be decided at the initial assessment to use radiotherapy in combination with surgery either preoperatively or postoperatively as definitive management or as an adjuvant. Alternatively, while surgery may originally have been intended as the sole treatment, radiotherapy is sometimes subsequently indicated in the light of operative findings because of residual disease, or at a later date because of the development of recurrence. Similarly, surgery is sometimes required to salvage recurrent or residual disease following primary radiotherapy.

Preoperative and postoperative radiotherapy

The patterns of failure of surgery and radiotherapy are different. Surgery is good at removing the central bulk of disease, but residual viable tumour, often microscopic, can be left at the resection margins. Radiotherapy is best at eradicating small volumes of disease, and is more likely to fail if there is a large bulky tumour. The two modalities can therefore be combined usefully, the advantages of each overcoming the shortcomings of the other. Preoperative radiotherapy was once advocated on the grounds that the tumour will shrink prior to surgery, making the operation easier, and that by sterilizing the majority of viable cells, the risk of tumour dissemination at the time of operation was reduced. In most circumstances, however, postoperative irradiation is now considered preferable for several reasons. Firstly, proper pathological staging of the tumour and nodes is now possible, and is a better guide to the extent of irradiation required. Secondly, the recent introduction of free as opposed to pedicled flaps in reconstructive surgery has meant that postoperative radiotherapy can commence sooner than was previously the case. In addition, tumour dissemination

at the time of operation is now considered more of a theoretical problem than a real one. Finally, following surgery, only microscopic, well-vascularized tumour should be left behind, which should be relatively easy to cure with radiation.

Adjuvant radiotherapy

Adjuvant radiotherapy is given following the definitive treatment which has apparently removed the malignancy, in order to reduce chances of recurrence. In the radiotherapy of head and neck cancer this includes elective postoperative irradiation following complete surgical excision of a tumour, and prophylactic irradiation of a clinically negative neck. The irradiation of known residual disease following incomplete surgery is not considered to be adjuvant. Adjuvant radiotherapy entails giving a high-dose fractionated course, similar to that used in radical treatment.

Types of radiation treatment

There are three ways of administering ionizing radiation to a tumour, of which by far and away the most important is external beam radiotherapy, or teletherapy. Interstitial radiotherapy and unsealed sources have a small part to play in the treatment of head and neck cancer.

External beam radiotherapy

In this form of treatment, a beam of radiation is directed by a machine to the tumour-bearing part of the patient who is some distance away, usually lying on a couch. A variety of different types of radiation are in current use. Others have been tried in the past, and have now been superseded. In general terms ionizing radiation is either particulate or high-energy electromagnetic radiation, called photons, similar to radiowaves or visible light, but with a much shorter wavelength. These photons are either X-rays or gamma rays. The only particulate radiation in common use is the electron beam. The X-rays used in therapy are classified by their energy level which is measured in electron volts (eV). The least energetic have an energy up to about 100 000 eV, or 100 keV. This type of radiation, called superficial, is poorly penetrating, treating an effective depth of only about 1 cm, and is used exclusively for treating small skin tumours. In the first half of this century, the most penetrating beams generally available came from orthovoltage equipment. They had an energy of about 300 kV, and were also called deep X-rays, a name which still lingers on although this type of equipment is virtually obsolete. Supervoltage or megavoltage machines such as linear accelerators are now universally available. They operate at 4–20 million volts (MV), and produce much more penetrating beams than was possible in the orthovoltage era. Although increased penetration is the principal advantage of megavoltage irradiation, there are also other benefits. With orthovoltage beams, the maximum dose was delivered to the skin, with progressively lower doses to underlying tissues. As a consequence, damage to the skin limited the amount that could be given to deep-seated tumours. With 4 MV beams, the skin is relatively spared, with the maximum dose at a depth of 1 cm, and a much more gradual fall-off of dose at depth. In addition, the edges of linear accelerator beams are much more precisely defined – in technical terms there is less penumbra – meaning that narrower margins can safely be used around a tumour than was possible with orthovoltage. A final important benefit for megavoltage irradiation is that its absorption in different tissues is quite homogeneous. Orthovoltage beams had a much greater absorption in dense materials such as bone and calcified cartilage, and so complications such as osteoradionecrosis and laryngeal cartilage necrosis, which are now only rarely seen, were a considerable problem.

In addition to X-rays, the gamma rays emitted by some radioactive isotopes are of megavoltage quality and can be used for teletherapy. The beam from a radium 'bomb' was the earliest form of high-energy external beam treatment available. Radium was superseded as a source after the Second World War when artificially radioactive isotopes of caesium and cobalt became available. Cobalt, which produced more penetrating radiation, was preferred in most circumstances. The physical characteristics, especially the penetration and penumbra, of the beams from linear accelerators are in many respects preferable to those of cobalt units. However the latter are by comparison low-technology equipment which is cheaper and requires less maintenance by skilled staff, and so cobalt units are still used fairly widely throughout the world for economic and logistic reasons.

Some linear accelerators are dedicated to X-ray production; others are dual-purpose, and can also be used to produce electron beams. While the bulk of radiotherapy is carried out using photons, there are some circumstances in which electrons are preferable. They give a relatively uniform dose up to a certain depth of penetration, and then the dose falls off very rapidly. They are, therefore, used to treat superficial parts, where it is desired to spare an underlying structure from excess irradiation. For example, they can be used to boost the dose to a node mass overlying the spinal cord, following initial photon treatment to a cord tolerance dose. Orthovoltage treatment also has limited penetration but electrons are superior as the fall-off of dose at depth is more rapid, they show some skin-sparing and they are not preferentially absorbed by bone or cartilage. For this last reason they are also the radiotherapeutic treatment of choice for lesions of the pinna and nose.

Neutron beam therapy is the only other form of particle radiation to have been widely used. Despite radiobiological predictions that neutrons would be advantageous, a large number of clinical trials conducted in various centres throughout the world on many different tumour types including head and neck cancer have failed to demonstrate the anticipated benefit. It remains possible that neutrons may have a role in a few circumstances, but most neutron therapy facilities have closed and are not being replaced.

Interstitial radiotherapy

In interstitial radiotherapy or brachytherapy, sealed sources of radioactive isotopes are either implanted into the tumour or placed in a natural body cavity, for example the maxillary antrum or nasopharynx (intracavitary therapy). Implants of long half-life materials which require removal after about 1 week are most commonly used. As an alternative, short half-life elements may be permanently implanted. Originally, radium needles were used for removable implants, and radon for permanent implants. The former were superseded initially by caesium, later by iridium, and radon has been replaced by gold or iodine. Thick, rigid needles were previously the principal type of implant but over the last few years, more versatile, flexible systems have become more widely used. This form of treatment is obviously more easily used in anatomically accessible parts of the body such as the oral cavity, and a detailed description of the use of iridium implants is given in Chapter 16. The main reason for using interstitial therapy is that it enables a very high radiation dose to be given to a very limited volume. Because of the inverse square law, there is a very rapid fall-off of dose from the surface of the source. Interstitial therapy can either be used on its own to treat small tumours, or to give a boost to a residual mass after initial external beam therapy.

Use of unsealed sources

Radioactive isotopes can be used in the form of drugs given orally or intravenously. These drugs are then concentrated by metabolic pathways in malignant tissue, enabling large radiation doses to be given to the tumour, with relative sparing of the normal tissue. There is only one example in the treatment of head and neck malignancy, and that is the treatment of differentiated thyroid carcinoma of follicular cell origin with radioactive iodine. This is fully discussed in Chapter 20.

Volume to be treated

It might reasonably be thought that the volume to be treated by radiotherapy is self-evident. Surely it should be enough to cover the bulk of the tumour as defined by clinical examination and imaging, allowing a reasonable margin for microscopic infiltration. In fact the volume which should be treated remains a matter of some controversy, and practice varies. None the less, despite the fact that the size of the margin treated around tumours varies, and that in some centres clinically uninvolved nodes are irradiated prophylactically, reported survival rates are remarkably constant. The need for salvage treatment may be greater if elective neck irradiation is withheld in tumours which have a high incidence of occult nodal involvement, but this does not appear to compromise overall survival. It becomes a matter of philosophy whether you choose, despite the increased morbidity, to overtreat a proportion of patients to ensure that the maximum number of patients are cured first time around, or whether you prefer to minimize initial treatment so as to spare side-effects, recognizing that more patients will require salvage treatment. Another factor to be considered is that when a smaller volume is treated, the dose which may be given is higher. This might enable more tumours to be cured. One way to combine the treatment of a large volume, so as to treat some part prophylactically, with giving the highest possible dose to a small volume, is to use a shrinking field technique. Initially a large volume is covered, and taken to a modest dose deemed to be adequate to treat subclinical disease, then the volume is reduced to cover only bulk disease which is then boosted to a high dose. Alternatively, a boost may be given by interstitial therapy.

Fractionation of radiotherapy

Conventional fractionation

The maximum amount of radiation which can be given as a single dose is limited by normal tissue tolerance and, with the exception of a small skin tumour, is inadequate to cure cancer. If the total dose is divided up into a number of small doses (fractions) given for example daily, the maximum dose tolerated by normal tissues increases, and cure becomes more likely. For this reason radical radiotherapy is given as a fractionated course over a number of weeks. As the practice of radiotherapy has to a large extent developed empirically, the precise fractionation schedule varies considerably from centre to centre. Despite the variation in total dose, number of fractions per week, total number of fractions and overall time, each institution reports broadly similar results. At one end of the spectrum, a patient might be treated in 16 fractions over 3 weeks; at the other a patient might receive 35 treatments in 7 weeks. A higher total dose, say 65 Gy, will be given for the protracted treatment, compared with perhaps 50 Gy for the shorter regimen. A number of clinical

trials have addressed the question of fractionation. One of the largest, organized by the British Institute of Radiology, showed no significant differences in outcome comparing three with five fractions per week, or a short with a long overall treatment time in the management of laryngeal and hypopharyngeal carcinoma. As the acute mucosal reaction is more severe when the overall treatment time is short, more protracted fractionation is recommended when a large area of mucosa requires irradiation. As brain tissue is more likely to be damaged if large doses per fraction are used, a protracted schedule is preferred if any of the central nervous system is included within the treated volume. Except in these circumstances, there is probably no reason to opt for longer treatment courses.

Experimental fractionation

Hyperfractionation is when the number of fractions is increased beyond conventional levels, and the dose per fraction is reduced correspondingly. Acceleration is when the overall treatment time is reduced. These two modifications are combined in the treatment regimen known as CHART (continuous, hyperfractionated, accelerated radiation therapy) which is currently undergoing clinical trials. This gives a radical course of treatment in just 12 days, using three fractions per day, 7 days per week. The short overall time is designed to overcome the repopulation of malignant cells which is believed to occur during long courses of treatment, and the reduced fraction size is used to prevent increased late tissue damage. Uncontrolled studies have supported the theoretical advantages of such scheduling, but whether the anticipated benefit will be confirmed in a proper trial remains to be seen.

Split courses

It has already been mentioned that the acute mucosal reaction may be dose-limiting. In an attempt to overcome this problem, some workers have divided the radiotherapy course into two halves, separated by a gap of about 2 weeks, allowing the mucosal reaction to settle. However, this gap gives time for the remaining tumour cells, stimulated by the first phase of treatment, to divide rapidly and repopulate the tumour. Studies have shown that split-course regimens produce inferior results to continuous schedules, and this practice is mentioned only to be condemned.

Formulae of equivalence

In physical terms, radiation dose is prescribed using the SI units of absorbed dose, the Gray (Gy). Some people prefer to talk in terms of the centigray (cGy), which is one-hundredth of a Gray. This unit has replaced the previous unit of radiation absorbed dose, the rad, which is equivalent to 0.01 Gy. However in biological terms it is not adequate to describe the dose to a tumour in terms of the physical dose alone. Other factors which must be mentioned are the number of fractions, fraction size, interval between fractions, overall time, volume treated, radiation quality (e.g. photons or neutrons) and beam energy. Over the years, a variety of complex mathematical formulae have been invented by which time, dose and fractionation factors can be rolled into one number to describe a course of treatment. However the biological factors which affect probability of tumour cure and risk of complications are different. Thus a time–dose–fractionation formula may say that two different treatment schedules are equivalent. While this may be the case as far as likelihood of tumour cure is concerned, the two regimens may be very different in terms of complications. For this reason, such formulae are best avoided, and treatment schedules should be fully described in terms of all the relevant factors.

The planning and quality control of radiation therapy

Selecting the treatment volume

When it has been decided to treat a patient with radiation, the precise technical details of the treatment must be decided upon before it is commenced. The extent of the tumour will be known from clinical examination and radiological studies. This information, combined with a knowledge of the natural history of that tumour type and its usual patterns of spread, determines the volume which needs to be treated. In the head and neck it is important to confine the treatment to this volume, in order to protect vulnerable structures such as the eye, lacrimal and salivary glands, the brainstem and spinal cord.

Preparation of a shell

For accurate treatment of the target volume with sparing of adjacent structures to be possible, the patient needs to lie still during treatment, in a constant position from day to day. To ensure this, the patient's head is immobilized in a plastic shell. Such shells, sometimes called masks, moulds or casts, are prepared individually for each patient. This process takes about 3 working days, and requires skilled technical staff, working in a well-equipped mould room. Firstly, with the patient lying in the intended treatment position, strips of plaster of Paris bandages are applied like a mask to the head and neck. When these have set, the mask, which has an impression exactly the same shape and size as the patient, is removed. This impression is filled with

liquid plaster, and a cast is formed. A thermoplastic vacuum-forming machine is used to shape a piece of plastic over the cast. The shaped plastic is then trimmed, holes are cut for the eyes and nostrils, and it is fitted to a neck rest and base board. The shell is then checked on the patient, to ensure that it fits snugly and comfortably.

Simulation

The treatment simulator is a diagnostic X-ray machine with image intensification facilities. It can rotate around the patient, like the treatment unit with exactly matching geometry. The screen shows a pair of parallel wires perpendicular to another pair. The distance between the wires in each pair can be adjusted to make rectangles of any size, indicating the treatment field. The patient lies in the shell in the treatment position on the simulator couch. Using the image intensifier, a treatment field of appropriate size is chosen. Blocks can be introduced into the beam to produce an irregularly shaped field to shield any vulnerable structures. The position of the beam and any blocked areas are marked on to the shell to guide radiographers during treatment. The shell is also used to ensure that the beam alignment, as well as beam position, is correct. A radiograph is taken as a permanent record of treatment intent, showing the position of the selected field and any blocks, in relation to the tumour and normal structures. As in most cases more than one field is used to cover the tumour, this process is repeated for the other fields.

Wedges and compensators

The aim of treatment planning is to ensure that the target volume which contains the tumour gets a high and uniform dose, and the surrounding areas, particularly if they are prone to radiation damage, get a minimal dose. Beyond the depth where the absorbed dose is maximum (about 1 cm for 4 MV photons), the dose received from one beam gets less as it penetrates further into the patient. Two or more beams are thus often used. These are fired from different angles and intersect at the tumour, which therefore receives the highest dose. Because of the oblique incidence of a beam on the surface of the patient, or because two beams from the same side of the patient converge, the dose received by the tumour can vary across its depth. In order to achieve a uniform dose distribution, therefore, metal wedges may be inserted in the head of the treatment unit into the beam to attenuate the dose differentially across its width. In certain circumstances it may be necessary to use individually prepared devices to achieve dose homogeneity. These are called compensators as they compensate for the variations in dose which would otherwise exist.

Isodose plans

A computer is used to create a map or plan of the radiation dose distribution within the patient. Usually this plan is of one cross-section through the middle of the tumour, although in complicated cases several sections at different levels are required. The plan shows the outline of the patient and the position of the tumour and any adjacent vulnerable structures. The position of treatment fields is indicated, and contour lines are drawn joining points which receive the same dose (isodose lines). The isodose plan is checked to ensure that the tumour is contained within the high dose volume and therefore receives an adequate and uniform dose, and that the dose received by any critical structure is within its limits of tolerance.

Treatment verification

During the first treatment session, radiographs may be taken using the beam from the treatment unit. These verification or check films are compared with the simulator films to ensure that the treatment field is positioned as planned, and that any blocks are correctly located.

Lasers

Laser (light amplification by stimulated emission of radiation) is used increasingly in the head and neck region. The emitted wavelengths of a laser light source are usually only of one frequency and comprise an intense, narrow beam of uninterrupted waves. This is generated by the controlled, stimulated emission of photons from excited atoms by using mirrors to reflect atoms along the long axis of a tube. One of the end mirrors is made partially transmitting and emits a parallel laser beam of light. A red-emitting laser is used as a visible, aligning beam. One of the most powerful surgical lasers is the solid-state neodymium-doped yttrium-aluminium garnet (Nd-YAG) laser, a crystal laser whose photon beam is in the near infrared (wavelength 1064 nm) and has a power output of up to 100 W. The 60×100 mm YAG crystal is excited by a krypton arc lamp. Its beam is poorly absorbed by water but heavily scattered by tissue inhomogeneities, resulting in deep tissue penetration, which can be used to coagulate vessels up to 4 mm diameter. Although the wavelength is infrared, it is short enough to be transmitted down an optical fibre, e.g. in the biopsy channel of a fibreoptic bronchoscope. It is thus used to coagulate and necrose obstructing lesions of the trachea and bronchial tree. A modification of the YAG laser incorporates a crystal of potassium titanyl phosphate to produce a 532 nm wavelength visible green light.

This KTP laser is readily transmitted down a flexible quartz fibre and can be manipulated precisely, even down a paediatric bronchoscope.

The CO_2 laser discharge tube contains a mixture of CO_2, helium and nitrogen. The beam has a wavelength 10 times greater than that of the YAG laser (10600 nm), and its power is around 20–60 W. The beam is very strongly absorbed by water, resulting in vaporization of successive layers of tissue. The temperature does not exceed 100°C, limiting the subsurface thermal damage, especially if the beam is highly focused. In the oral cavity, the CO_2 laser allows precise tissue dissection, sealing vessels and lymphatics under 0.5 mm diameter with minimal postoperative pain, inflammation and oedema. It is very useful for the removal of leukoplakia of the floor of the mouth, avoiding damage to the submandibular duct and apparently with a lower recurrence rate than conventional therapy. It can also be used to remove benign lesions – haemangiomas, papillomas, minor salivary gland tumours or even small tumours of the mobile tongue, with no requirement for a skin graft or flap. The CO_2 laser can be incorporated into a rigid bronchoscope system for the palliation of obstructing tracheobronchial malignancy (sometimes after prior coagulation with the YAG laser). Endoscopic laser resection of early laryngeal carcinoma is now being advocated as an alternative to radiotherapy. A recent review of 22 patients following laser resection of T_1 lesions showed good preservation of voice function, but the results were not compared with a radiotherapy cohort. A German group has attempted to use the technique for larger lesions, showing that T_3 tumours cannot be resected by the CO_2 laser but that the method may be feasible for T_2 lesions, if combined with radiotherapy and neck dissection in selected patients. CO_2 laser cordectomy or arytenoidectomy has been used to relieve the airway obstruction associated with bilateral vocal cord paralysis.

The twin dangers of laser are the destruction of human tissue, especially the cornea, and the ignition of combustible material. Corneal exposure is limited to the maximum permitted exposure (MPE) by the wearing of protective eyewear which incorporates filters. General aspects of laser safety are usually coordinated by a physicist, under the auspices of the local laser protection adviser. Performance of microlaryngeal surgery with a laser requires special instruments, including finger-control suction, a cricoid protector for anterior commissure work and saline soaks to guard the endotracheal cuff. Use of a laser in the upper airway requires special anaesthetic techniques to prevent laser ignition of the oxygen–anaesthetic gas mixture; fire will severely damage the patient's airway. Available methods include a standard tube protected by aluminium tape; a stainless steel or silicon tube, and jet ventilation with a Saunders injector with intravenous anaesthesia such as propofol. None of these is ideal. A wrapped tube can cause postintubation oedema, while the specially designed tubes continue to be refined, e.g. to incorporate a double cuff to be filled with saline to protect the distal cuff from the laser. Jet ventilation requires particular care in children because of the risk of surgical emphysema.

Photodynamic therapy

It has long been known that certain dyes, when activated by light, have antineoplastic properties. Modern photodynamic therapy entails injecting a patient with a photosensitizing agent which is activated about 48 h later by the application of laser light. The most commonly used agent is haematoporphyrin derivative (HPD) or its purified form, photofrin. HPD is given by slow intravenous infusion, at a dose of 3 mg/kg body weight. The process by which HPD is absorbed into tumours is not fully understood but its concentration in the stroma is five times greater than that in the cells. Photoactivation of HPD results in the release of cytotoxic singlet oxygen, which also affects the tumour circulation. The laser light used is usually 630 nm red light which clearly has limited penetration, and thus the depth of necrosis is only 5–10 mm. It is therefore curative only for small, superficial skin or mucosal lesions, but it does appear successful in the palliation of more bulky disease. Patients become photosensitized and must avoid strong sunlight for 8 weeks after therapy. Current studies are in progress to compare photodynamic therapy with Nd-YAG laser therapy in oesophageal and lung tumours. Although the method has yet to be evaluated fully, it retains obvious appeal for potential therapy of head and neck tumours, many of which are relatively small, localized and easily accessible.

Chemotherapy

Chemotherapy may be used alone as a palliative treatment for advanced or recurrent disease, or in combination with surgery or radiotherapy as an adjuvant.

Adjuvant chemotherapy

This may be given after, during or prior to definitive treatment, in which case it is termed neoadjuvant therapy. The chemotherapy may be given as a single agent, or as a combination of drugs. The most widely used drugs are antifolate antimetabolites such as methotrexate, antitumour antibiotics like bleomycin, pyrimidine antimetabolites such as 5-fluorouracil and also vincristine and cisplatin. These drugs undoubtedly have biological activity against squamous carcinoma, as objective response rates up to 40% are reported, rising to 75% if combinations (e.g. methotrexate, bleomycin and vinblastine) are used. However, despite the fact that over the last two decades dozens of trials have examined its use, the place of adjuvant chemotherapy remains uncertain. Many of these trials have been too small to detect a modest improvement in survival but it is unlikely that they would have overlooked a major beneficial effect. Such beneficial effects as have been seen relate principally to improved local control rather than increased survival. Local control is improved in oropharyngeal carcinoma by the use of synchronous chemotherapy and radiotherapy, although sometimes at the expense of a fierce mucosal reaction. Indeed in some studies the potential benefit of adjuvant chemotherapy is offset by treatment-related deaths. Induction therapy, unlike synchronous therapy, has never been shown to confer a survival advantage overall, and although patients who achieve a complete remission have improved survival times, this may be because response to induction chemotherapy is a predictor of radiotherapy response. The results of further, large-scale studies are awaited. In the meantime, adjuvant chemotherapy should be used only in a trial setting, and not considered for the routine management of squamous carcinoma of the head and neck.

Palliative chemotherapy

If other options have been exhausted, chemotherapy should be considered in patients with significant symptoms caused by advanced or recurrent tumour considered to be incurable. This can often produce considerable improvement, but the benefit is usually short-lived. Chemotherapy is toxic. Its safe administration is expensive, requiring considerable expertise and, in a palliative context, frequent hospitalization of a patient whose life expectancy is very limited. It is also difficult to determine whether a patient has benefited in terms of survival and/or symptom relief. Any costly treatment of questionable benefit must be administered only after careful consideration, as its use inevitably means a reduction in available resources elsewhere. Savings made by stopping inappropriate chemotherapy in the terminally ill would increase funds available for consultation time, and supportive care.

How chemotherapy works

All chemotherapeutic agents are toxic to both malignant and normal tissue. Normal tissue toxicity is described on page 30. To be useful in humans, the agent must be more toxic to the tumour than to its host. All tumour cells have a resting phase and then, at varying time intervals, pass through the cell cycle

(Fig. 3.15). Many cytotoxic agents are active only at one particular point in this cycle. Others are toxic throughout the cycle. Vincristine, for example, is known to arrest cells in metaphase. Drugs may also be classified according to their type into alkylating agents, antimetabolites, natural products and miscellaneous agents. These two areas of knowledge are more of theoretical than practical importance.

As the effectiveness of chemotherapy within a class of tumours is variable many attempts have been made to find *sensitivity tests,* which would predict response of an individual tumour to chemotherapy. Sadly, all have failed and treatment of individual patients therefore remains empirical.

Assessment of new drugs

Because of the limited efficacy and significant toxicity of all presently available cytotoxics, new drugs and analogues of existing chemotherapeutic agents are being developed with the hope of improving efficacy or diminishing toxicity. Following initial assessment in *in vitro* and *in vivo* laboratory models, the place of a particular agent is assessed by passing it through a series of clinical trials called phase I, II and III.

Phase I studies are usually carried out by or in close collaboration with a drug company to assess dosage levels and toxicity. Heavily pretreated patients with recurrent untreatable disease are used. Three patients are treated at one dosage level, and the toxicity and response, if any, are assessed. The dose is then increased by increments on further groups of 3 patients each, until intolerable toxicity is reached. If the drug shows any signs of activity it then passes to a phase II study.

Patients with previously untreated end-stage disease are the usual subjects for *phase II* studies. The maximum tolerated dose established in a phase I study is used. The main end-points of interest in a phase II study are toxicity and response. The toxicity in various organs is assessed on a five-point scale laid down by the World Health Organization for each course of treatment. The size of the tumour is measured before treatment (not always an easy or possible task) and after each course of treatment. If the tumour disappears completely this is counted as a complete response. If the product of two perpendicular diameters decreases by more than 50% of the original, this is counted as a partial response. For head and neck cancer median survival in a study of this sort is usually around 6 months.

The disadvantages of this type of trial are, firstly, that an untreated control arm is virtually never included. Secondly, the value of response of the tumour in terms of palliation of the patients' symptoms is unmeasured. Thirdly, about one-third of all patients eligible for such a study do not receive treatment for a variety of reasons. They are rarely reported, so that the results of the treatment are artificially inflated because only favourable patients are included. Finally, many reports of studies of this type compare the survival of responders with non-responders. Most authors then make the completely illogical and unjustified conclusion that the responders have benefited. Unless treated responders are compared to an untreated group no such conclusions can be drawn.

These phase II studies usually contain about 20 patients and can be completed in a year or less. Recently, very high response rates have been claimed by some authors for the combination of cisplatin and 5-fluorouracil. Some American authors claim response rates as high as 95% – for some unexplained reason this is about three times the response rate for similar regimens on similar patients

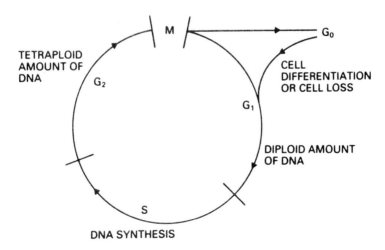

Fig. 3.15 The cell cycle and its phases.

reported from Europe. It is also difficult to explain why response rates as high as this – better even than in the lymphomas – have not produced any effect whatever on survival. It is difficult to escape the conclusion that many of these reports are untrue.

A *phase III* trial has two or more arms and the main end-point is survival of the patient. This type of trial requires several hundred patients and several years to complete. In this type of trial, toxicity and response are recorded, but the main criterion is survival. Furthermore, all patients, once randomized, are included in the analysis whether they were treated or not. This type of trial therefore provides a much more objective answer. It is important when designing such a trial to estimate the number of patients likely to be required in order to judge whether the trial is feasible; most clinicians have a very optimistic view of the size of the trial. There are various formulae for calculating the trial size but all are approximations.

Planning the size must take into account the chances of a type I and type II error. A type I error is the chance of rejecting a hypothesis when it should be accepted – usually because the trial contains too few patients to have the required power to detect a difference between the two arms. A type II error is the chance of accepting a result as significant when it should be rejected. The minimal acceptance level for power is 80%, and for significance the minimum is 5%. The calculation must also take into account the survival rates which are already known from past experience, and any likely improvement. Again, clinicians are usually optimistic in guessing the latter – a true improvement in survival of 5% would be an enormous advance in current circumstances: a true improvement of 10% is exceedingly unlikely, and an improvement of more than this would demand an entirely new form of treatment. The appropriate numbers required for a trial are shown in Table 3.3.

Principles of terminal care

It has been pointed out earlier that while the treatment of patients with cancer is traditionally divided into radical or palliative categories according to the likelihood of cure, this distinction is not infrequently difficult to make. Initial treatment is most often

radical in intent, and even following relapse salvage treatment usually is performed in the hope of cure but with the realization that this goal is less likely to be achieved. As the disease progresses it may become apparent that further attempts at potentially curative therapy are not possible, yet active anti-cancer therapy may still be appropriate in carefully selected cases if this might relieve distressing symptoms or prolong useful life. There usually comes a time, however, when further active palliation is not possible and symptom control measures become paramount.

As the patient progresses along this spectrum from radical primary treatment through salvage procedures to palliative treatment and onwards to terminal care, it can be difficult to decide at just which point the transition in therapeutic aim should be made. Continuity of care is important, and while it may be necessary for the surgeon or oncologist to seek the aid of a palliative medicine physician it is also essential for the patient and family to realize that he or she has not been abandoned, and that care will be continued. The proper management of the patient with advanced malignant disease is one of the most demanding aspects of medical practice, requiring experienced clinical judgement, compassion and common sense in equal measure. A display of insensitivity or indifference in this field is never forgotten and rarely forgiven by the bereaved.

The location of terminal care

The aim of terminal care should be to make the patient free of pain, mobile and sufficiently alert so that he or she can spend time in comfort at home with his or her family if possible. Domiciliary care of the terminally ill patient requires a close liaison between the hospital services which have provided care earlier in the course of the illness and the community health service. The latter comprises the general practitioner, nursing support and ancillary help. The care provided by district nurses is often supplemented with help from those with special experience and training in terminal care, such as Macmillan or Marie Curie nurses. Advice may also be sought from palliative medicine physicians who are often hospice-based. Attendance at a day hospice may enable patients to stay longer at home. Admission to a hospice is not necessarily permanent. It is common practice for patients to be admitted for short periods for convalescence following hospital treatment or to obtain symptom control before returning home. Sometimes hospices will admit patients for a period of respite care to allow their domiciliary carers to take a holiday. If domestic circumstances are not suitable for terminal care, for example patients without immediate family or the socially disadvantaged head and neck cancer patients who live in hostels, institutional care is necessary. Similarly,

Table 3.3 Numbers required in a phase III trial

Known 5-year survival	Improvement in survival	
	5%	*10%*
30%	1124	300
40%	1248	325
50%	1273	325

some patients are well-managed at home during the early part of their terminal illness, but require institutional care later on. The options here are either continued care in the hospitals which have looked after the patient earlier, or hospices. The former is particularly appropriate if a strong relationship has developed between the patient and the staff on the ward where the patient has been previously treated and where the staff have the necessary time and skills to provide appropriate care, or if specialized nursing is required, say for a laryngectomee. The appropriate location for terminal care should be decided jointly between the patient, family and medical attendants.

Pain relief

In the minds of many patients and their families, death from cancer is synonymous with pain and anguish. In the past, this fear was well-founded, but with modern analgesic techniques intractable pain should be very rare. Unfortunately, many patients with pain which could be alleviated are still left to suffer unnecessarily. For adequate analgesia, more than analgesics are required: the prerequisite of successful pain control is careful assessment of the patient's symptoms.

As pain in the patient with far advanced cancer can affect several areas, and may be completely unrelated to the cancer itself, or be caused by its treatment, the site or sites, nature, severity and causes of the patient's discomfort need to be elucidated. In the majority of cases when the pain is rightly attributed to the cancer, it is also important to determine the mechanism underlying it, as the treatment may depend on the cause. For example, the pain of constipation caused by opiates will not be relieved by increasing the dose, but requires the use of laxatives or enemas. It is important to record the details of the pain, and to review the patient regularly to monitor the response to changes in therapy, to evaluate any new symptoms and to provide explanations of the pain and the necessary medication to the patient and relatives. As attention to detail is an important ingredient in the recipe for success, and polypharmacy is often unavoidable, it is helpful if to write out the medication schedule for the patient.

Persistent pain caused by tumour infiltration requires regular therapy to abolish the pain and prevent its recurrence. The pain should not be allowed to recrudesce before the next analgesic dose is due. For this reason, 'as required' or p.r.n. medication is inappropriate as the sole treatment. It is the doctor's responsibility to ensure not only that adequate analgesia is prescribed, but that the patient and carers understand the need for its regular administration. If pain does break through before the next dose, it is better to increase the regular dose rather than to increase the frequency of administration or to prescribe small supplementary doses.

Analgesics may be classified according to the severity of pain that they can treat effectively. For mild pain, simple analgesics such as paracetamol may be all that is required. Simple analgesics with some anti-inflammatory effects such as aspirin or ibuprofen may be more effective than paracetamol, especially in the case of bone pain. As a second simple analgesic is unlikely to succeed where a first has failed, the prescriber should use a more powerful analgesic in this case. Moderate pain may call for a simple analgesic – mild opiate combination such as paracetamol and codeine. If this is inadequate, the pain is by definition severe and strong opiates such as morphine or diamorphine are required. Analgesic regimens should be kept as simple as possible, and there is no sense in using more than one analgesic of any class, although there is logic in combining analgesics which act through different mechanisms, such as aspirin and morphine. Short-acting analgesics such as pethidine should be avoided. Buprenorphine (Temgesic) is also best avoided, despite its longer duration of action and potential for sublingual administration, as being a partial antagonist it can precipitate withdrawal symptoms including pain in patients who have been using other opiates. If possible, oral medication should be used. For patients unable to swallow tablets, liquid preparations are available. For patients who are vomiting, parenteral administration may be required temporarily until effective antiemetic therapy has been instituted. For patients in whom oral therapy is impossible, subcutaneous injections are far preferable to intramuscular injections, especially in those with cachexia. If a patient comfortable with oral morphine becomes unable to swallow, the appropriate parenteral dose is half the oral. Alternatively, suppositories may be used. Syringe drivers giving a continuous subcutaneous infusion are especially valuable in the dying patient who is bed-bound and semicomatose, as sedatives and antiemetics such as haloperidol may be given simultaneously, but may also be used in ambulant patients. Syringe drivers are not without their own problems, and should not be used prematurely in a patient who is quite able to take drugs by mouth. Oral medication is often erroneously deemed inadequate when in reality it is the prescribed dose which is inadequate rather than the oral route which is inappropriate. When injections are necessary, diamorphine is generally preferred to morphine as it is much more soluble, and the volume to be injected is therefore less.

Two fears, drug dependence and respiratory depression, sometimes limit the proper use of strong opiates in the terminal care setting. It is often the patient rather than the doctor who is unwilling to commence opiates as they are concerned about becoming addicted. This possibility is however of no significance in the patient who is destined to die from malignancy within weeks. On the other hand, in this day and age it is increasingly common for unscrupulous drug misusers to steal opiates from their dying relatives for either their own use or for resale, and the prescriber should be alert to this crime. Pain is a powerful respiratory stimulant, and respiratory depression as a result of opiate use is uncommon in terminally ill patients. None the less it may occur, and antagonists should be available for use if necessary.

When strong opiate therapy is initiated, it is best to use oral morphine solution regularly every 4 h. The dose given can be rapidly titrated to the level required to control the pain. Thereafter the patient can continue on this schedule, or an equivalent dose as slow-release tablets which are given only twice a day may be preferred by the patient. As all opiates cause constipation which can be very troublesome, it is essential that a laxative is given concurrently. When the patient is reviewed, it is important to enquire if bowel function is satisfactory and adjust the laxative if necessary.

As well as laxatives, other drugs may be required in combination with opiates. Nausea or vomiting is often a problem following the initiation of opiate therapy, and a wide variety of effective antiemetics is now available. These should be prescribed separately from the opiate, so that the dose of each can be adjusted independently. Tablets which contain combinations of opiates and antiemetics such as dipipanone and cyclizine are available but should not be prescribed, as the fixed ratio of the combination makes it impossible to increase the analgesic level without increasing the antiemetic also. Antiemetics are generally needed only for the first few days after the start of opiate treatment, and may then be discontinued. Care should be taken to distinguish vomiting due to opiates from that due to other causes, for example intestinal obstruction or raised intracranial pressure. There is no place for cocaine in dying patients, although this drug was once popular as an ingredient of 'the Brompton cocktail'. Pain caused by raised intracranial pressure or by nerve compression may be helped by the coadministration of corticosteroids. Superficial dysaesthetic pain which is caused by nerve infiltration or compression may be alleviated by amitriptyline. Sodium valproate or carbamazepine may help sudden lancinating pain which occurs intermittently. Bone metastases are not common in patients with head and neck cancer, but radiotherapy should be considered if painful osseous deposits become manifest, and, as mentioned above, non-steroidal anti-inflammatory agents may also be of value.

Other symptoms

While psychotropics should not be used routinely, anxiety and depression frequently occur in the patient with pain due to advanced malignant disease. These symptoms may abate when pain control is achieved, but if no improvement is seen despite good analgesia, anxiolytics or antidepressants may be indicated. Insomnia is a frequent problem. Once obvious precipitating factors such as pain have been dealt with on their own merits, benzodiazepines such as temazepam may be used. Restlessness and confusion may occur, especially in the dying patient. Major tranquillizers such as haloperidol are then indicated. Chlorpromazine is an alternative, but causes a greater degree of sedation. Methotrimeprazine is also occasionally useful. Patients complaining of a dry mouth or dysphagia should be examined for signs of oropharyngeal candidiasis, which can be treated with nystatin suspension, amphoteracin lozenges or miconazole gel. A dry mouth can also be caused by morphine, amitriptyline or prior radiotherapy to the parotid salivary glands. Patients with intracranial disease or metabolic disturbance may develop epileptic fits. If intermittent these may be controlled by oral anticonvulsants. A prolonged fit may be terminated by intravenous administration of diazepam emulsion. Diazepam may also be administered rectally.

One symptom, generally more distressing for the attending relatives than the sufferer, is the death rattle due to accumulation of excessive respiratory secretions in the moribund patient. This may be reduced by the use of an anticholinergic agent such as atropine or hyoscine.

Summary

Terminal care, like most other aspects of medicine, requires experience, careful assessment of the patient's needs and meticulous attention to therapeutic detail, if it is to be practised successfully. Emotional and social factors, as well as physical ones, need to be taken into consideration in tailoring treatment to an individual patient's requirements. Good terminal care requires a large investment by the doctor of both time and effort, and should, therefore, not be undertaken lightly or unwillingly.

References and further reading

Radiotherapy

Emami B, Bignardi M, Spector G J, Devineni V K, Hederman M A (1987) Reirradiation of recurrent head and neck cancers. *Laryngoscope* 97:85–8.
Henk J M, James K W (1978) Comparative trial of large

and small fractions in the radiotherapy of head and neck cancer. *Clin Radiol* **29**:611–16.

Hong A, Saunders M I, Dische S *et al.* (1990) An audit of head and neck cancer treatment in a regional centre for radiotherapy and oncology. *Clin Oncol* **2**:130–7.

Kramer S, Gelber R D, Snow J B *et al.* (1987) Combined radiation therapy and surgery in the management of advanced head and neck cancer: final report of study 73–03 of the radiation therapy oncology group. *Head Neck Surg* **10**:19–30.

Kumar P P, Good R R, Epstein B E, Yonkers A J, Ogren F P, Moore G F (1987) Outcome of locally advanced stage III and IV head and neck cancer treated by surgery and postoperative external beam radiotherapy. *Laryngoscope* **97**:615–20.

Chemotherapy

Campbell J B, Dorman E B, Helliwell T R *et al* (1987) Factors predicting response of end stage squamous cell carcinoma of the head and the neck to cisplatinum. *Clin Otolaryngol* **12**:167–76.

Eisenberger M (1990) Chemotherapy in head and neck cancer. In: Myers E N, Suen J Y (eds) *Cancer of the Head and Neck*, 2nd edn. New York, Churchill Livingstone, pp. 979–1004.

Ervin T J, Clark J R, Weichselbaum R R *et al.* (1987) An analysis of induction and adjuvant chemotherapy in the multidisciplinary treatment of squamous cell carcinoma of the head and neck. *J Clin Oncol* **5**:10–20.

Hill B T, Price L A (1990) The role of adjuvant chemotherapy in the treatment of advanced head and neck cancer. *Acta Oncol* **29**:695–703.

Morton R P, Stell P M (1984) Cytotoxic chemotherapy for patients with terminal squamous carcinoma – does it influence survival? *Clin Otolaryngol* **9**:175–80.

O'Connor D, Clifford P, Edwards W G *et al.* (1982) Long-term results of VBM and radiotherapy in advanced head and neck cancer. *Int J Radiat Oncol Biol Phys* **8**:1525–31.

Rees G J G (1991) Cancer treatment: deciding what we can afford. *Br Med J* **302**:799–800.

Snow G B, Vermorken J B (1988) Neo-adjuvant chemotherapy in head and neck cancer: state of the art, 1988. *Clin Otolaryngol* **14**:371–5.

Stell P M, Rawson N S B (1990) Adjuvant chemotherapy in head and neck cancer. *Br J Cancer* **61**:779–87.

Tobias J S (1990) Has chemotherapy proved itself in head and neck cancer? *Br J Cancer* **61**:649–51.

Surgery

Friedman M, Mafee M F, Pacella B L, Strorigl T L, Dew L L, Toriumi D M (1990) Rationale for elective neck dissection in 1990. *Laryngoscope* **100**:54–9.

Wickham M H, Narula A A, Barton R P, Bradley P J (1990) Emergency laryngectomy. *Clin Otolaryngol* **15**:35–8.

Yuen A, Medina J E, Goepfert H, Fletcher G (1984) Management of stage T3 and T4 glottic carcinomas. *Am J Surg* **148**:467–72.

Lasers

Borland L M, Reilly J S (1987) Jet ventilation for laser laryngeal surgery in children. *Int J Pediatr Otorhinolaryngol* **14**:65–71.

Carruth J A S, Simpson G T (eds) *Lasers in Otolaryngology*. London, Chapman & Hall.

Castro D J, Saxton R E, Ward P H *et al.* (1990) Flexible Nd:YAG laser palliation of obstructive tracheal metastatic malignancies. *Laryngoscope* **100**:1208–14.

Davis R K, Jako G J, Hyams V J, Shapshay S M (1982) The anatomic limitations of CO_2 laser cordectomy. *Laryngoscope* **92**:980–4.

Hawkins D B, Joseph M M (1990) Avoiding a wrapped endotracheal tube in laser laryngeal surgery: experiences with apneic anesthesia and metal laser-flex endotracheal tubes. *Laryngoscope* **100**:1283–7.

Krespi Y P, Meltzer C J (1989) Laser Surgery for vocal cord carcinoma involving the anterior commissure. *Ann Otol Rhinol Laryngol* **98**:105–9.

Krespi Y P, Weiss M H, Bhatia P (1990) Laser de-epithelialization of muscle-based flaps. *Laryngoscope* **100**:661–2.

Ossoff R H (1989) Laser safety in otolaryngology – head and neck surgery: anesthetic and educational considerations for laryngeal surgery. *Laryngoscope* **99** (Suppl 48):1–26.

Oswal V H, Kashima H K, Flood L M (1988) *The CO_2 Laser in Otolaryngology Head and Neck Surgery*. London, Wright.

Shapshay S M, Davis R K, Vaughan C W, Norton M, Strong M S, Simpson G T (1983) Palliation of airway obstruction for tracheobronchial malignancy: use of the CO_2 laser bronchoscope. *Otolaryngol Head Neck Surg* **91**:615–19.

Strong M S, Jako G J (1972) Laser surgery in the larynx: early clinical experience with continuous CO_2 laser. *Ann Otol Rhinol Laryngol* **81**:791–8.

4

Reconstruction

Surgical defects can be filled by free grafts, by pedicled grafts, which may be axial or musculocutaneous, or by revascularized free flaps.

Free grafts

The following free grafts have been described.

1 Split-thickness skin grafts.
2 Full-thickness skin grafts.
3 Pinch grafts.
4 Dermal grafts.
5 Fascial grafts.

The first three receive their blood supply from the recipient site; the last two are avascular.

Split-skin grafts

The most common skin graft used in head and neck surgery is the split-thickness skin graft, which is used to cover donor sites and small areas of lost skin; previously it was used to line flaps.

A split-skin graft consists of epidermis and a variable thickness of dermis. Thus it can be described as thin, intermediate or thick (Fig. 4.1). Thinner grafts take more readily in difficult circumstances such as in inflammation, but thicker grafts are more stable in the long run, because of their greater quantity of dermis; also all split-skin grafts contract during healing, but thinner grafts do so more than thick ones. Obviously, therefore, each graft must be cut according to the requirements of the particular situation.

A split-skin graft has no blood supply, but, if it is firmly fixed on a vascular bed, capillaries link up between the graft and its bed within about 3 days to revascularize the graft. During this period the graft must be immobile, and to allow maximal capillary link-up there must be no collection of blood, fluid or air between the graft and its bed. Furthermore, the bed must obviously be vascular: grafts will not be taken on bare bone, cartilage or tendon. Take is also slow on fat, which is better allowed to granulate spontaneously for a few days before the graft is applied. Split skin takes readily on muscle.

Split skin can easily be taken from the thigh, the upper arm and the flat surface of the abdomen (Fig. 4.2). The site is dictated by factors such as colour

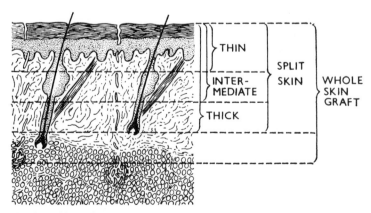

Fig. 4.1 Thicknesses of various skin grafts.

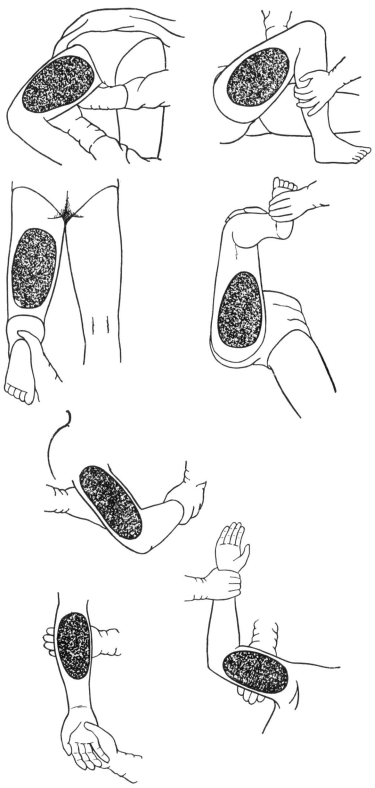

Fig. 4.2 Possible donor sites for skin grafts.

match, presence of hair, and the desirability of avoiding dressings on the leg in a patient recovering from a major operation.

Instruments

A lot of practice is needed to judge the thickness of a graft properly when using a Humby knife. The occasional plastic surgeon is better advised to use an electric dermatome which can be accurately set to a thousandth of an inch (0.025 mm), so that a graft of determined width and depth can be taken. Also a further graft can be taken from the same site if necessary. For most practical purposes the best thickness for a split-thickness skin graft is 12-1000ths of an inch (0.3 mm).

Technique of taking the graft (Fig. 4.3)

Use a non-hair-bearing area, such as the inside of the thigh, and prepare it well with a non-staining disinfectant such as hexachlorophane.

An assistant holds the limb in such a position that the muscles are relaxed, and presses the muscle mass from behind to present the maximum area of flat surface for cutting.

Set the blade of the dermatome to 12-1000ths of an inch (0.3 mm). The blade must be able to move smoothly and not drag on the skin, so lubricate it and the skin with liquid paraffin. The skin surface is held steady and flat with two boards, also lubricated with paraffin. One is put at the starting end of the donor site, and held by the surgeon; the other is moved forward just in front of the dermatome by an assistant. Press down firmly with the dermatome, cut with a continuous movement and allow the skin graft to collect on the blade. When enough skin has been raised, cut the end of the graft and place it on *tulle gras* to keep it moist. Apply swabs soaked in adrenaline or peroxide to the donor site and, when bleeding

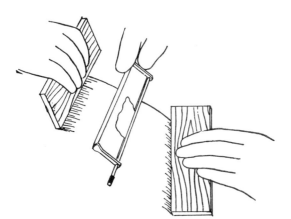

Fig. 4.3 Technique of taking a split-skin graft.

has stopped, dress it with a non-adherent dressing such as Opsite. If the site is dressed immediately, a hard cake of clotted blood forms which is painful to remove – avoid this by delaying dressing for as long as possible. Dressings are left undisturbed for 1 week and removed at the end of this time.

Application of the graft

The immediate primary method using a tie-over dressing has now given way to delayed primary skin grafting: take the skin graft at the time of operation, place it on *tulle gras* covered with a moist saline swab, roll it up and store it in a refrigerator at 4°C. Keep the recipient site moist with a sterile dressing after haemostasis has been secured; remove this dressing the next day and apply the free skin graft on *tulle gras* in the ward. Do not try to stitch it in place; provided the bed is dry, the graft sticks so well that stitching is unnecessary. Remove the *tulle gras* carefully after 48 h. This method fulfils the criteria of grafting because by the time the graft is applied the recipient area is absolutely dry; indeed take of a skin graft with this method is usually better than with the older one. Grafting may be delayed for up to 3 weeks, but take falls off gradually; furthermore the bed becomes infected after a few days. This method has the advantage of saving time at the end of a long operation, and the results are actually better than immediate grafting, because there is no danger of haematoma formation.

Secondary skin grafting

This method is used when neck skin has died and the lost skin must be replaced. The area is first allowed to granulate and, at the appropriate time, is repaired with a split-skin graft. Experience is needed to know when a granulating bed is ready for skin grafting but the following points may be helpful. The granulations ought to be flat and red and they should not bleed unduly although they should have good vascularity. The area should be totally free of slough and there ought to be evidence of marginal healing, that is a thin blue line of new skin growing in at the edge of the defect. Do not attempt to promote granulation by the use of caustics and so-called stimulating agents. All these do is kill tissue locally and cause more slough; there is no evidence to show that they improve the speed of granulation. The necrotic area is initially infected and must not be grafted until a healthy bed of granulations has formed. This usually takes at least 2–3 weeks.

Granulations that are sloughing, gelatinous or oedematous will not accept a skin graft because they are usually infected with streptococci, which kills the graft. Take swabs and if streptococci are grown give the appropriate systemic antibiotic, usually penicillin. Other organisms that may be cultured include

Pseudomonas pyocyanea, which often infects necrotic tissue, and is difficult to treat with antibiotics because there is no blood supply to the tissue in which the organism is growing. However, while the take of the graft may be reduced by perhaps 10% the best way to get rid of this infection is to graft the area: other organisms, such as the *Proteus* group and *Escherichia coli*, are opportunists and can be ignored.

The main cause of infection is slough and dead skin. *The only way to deal with infection is to remove necrotic tissue* – because the skin is dead, it is insensitive and can easily be removed with scissors and forceps while dressing the wound in the ward. Once the dead skin has been excised the area will be heavily infected at first. Systemic penicillin will deal with streptococci, but has little part in the treatment of infection with other organisms, which are best dealt with by local antiseptic dressings

Once the area is clean and granulating properly, apply the graft on *tulle gras* as before but do not attempt to stitch it in place because the stitches cut out; hold it in place with dressings and a crêpe bandage.

Full-thickness graft

A full-thickness graft requires ideal conditions, and has few uses in head and neck surgery, but it can be used for replacing small areas of skin after removal of tumours on the tip of the nose, on the auricle and in the temporal or facial areas.

A full-thickness graft must have a freshly cut, vascular bed; therefore it cannot be used on granulating surfaces. It will not take in the presence of infection or haematoma at the recipient site. Moreover, the size of the graft is limited because usually the donor site must be closed by undercutting and suture. However, the full-thickness graft does have several advantages: it usually provides a good colour match on the face and neck, and it does not contract secondarily. It is also relatively resistant to pressure, although this is not very important in the head and neck.

In head and neck work, probably the best donor site is the postauricular area. Although limited in size, this skin is hairless, and matches facial skin in colour and texture. A possible alternative is the supraclavicular skin, but here the colour match is not as good, and the donor site must usually be grafted with split skin, producing another cosmetic defect.

A full-thickness skin graft must be accurately fitted to the defect so that a pattern of the defect must first be made, using oiled silk. Make an outline of the shape using methylene blue. Moisten a sheet of jelonet on the fabric surface with spirit, and press it on the lesion outlined with the dye. Enough colour is absorbed to leave a good imprint of the outline on the fabric.

When the area is irregular, orientate the graft, before cutting it, with multiple dye tattoo punctures to fit corresponding marks in the skin surrounding the defect. This facilitates subsequent fitting of the graft (Fig. 4.4).

It is possible either to cut a full-thickness graft carefully so that no fat is left on the graft, or to cut without special regard to the fat, which is later removed with scissors. Excision of the fat after the graft has been cut is tedious but is probably easier for the occasional plastic surgeon. Cutting the graft without fat requires both skill and care; the graft can be buttonholed in the process.

To take the graft, first balloon the concavity behind the ear by injection with saline. Using the pattern already made, mark an outline on the skin with methylene blue and incise the skin. Cut the graft

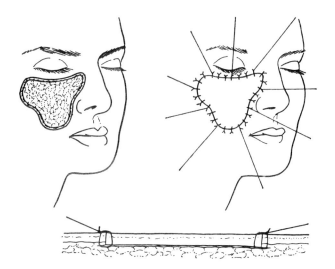

Fig. 4.4 Suturing of a full-thickness graft.

and remove carefully any fat left on it with scissors. Close the donor site by direct suture. If other sites are used close them by direct suture where possible. Where the donor site is too large to suture, use a split-skin graft to cover it.

Pinch grafts

The pinch graft leaves depressions in the donor site and elevations in the recipient site; it has no place in head and neck surgery.

Dermal grafts

Dermis was formerly popular for protecting the carotid arteries after a radical neck dissection in patients at risk of wound breakdown but is not as safe as a muscle graft. Dermis has other occasional uses, for instance to fill out a sunken defect.

Take a dermal graft by steps similar to those for split skin. First set the dermatome to 10-1000ths of an inch (approx. 0.254 mm) and shave the epidermis off, but leave it attached at one end. Then reset the dermatome to 20-1000ths (approx. 0.5 mm), and take a strip from the exposed dermis. Lastly, replace the original epidermis after bleeding has been stopped with adrenaline soaks, and apply a pressure dressing.

Fascial grafts

Temporalis fascia may also be used to cover the carotid arteries, and tensor fascia lata is used in facial slings, as described in Chapter 19.

Pedicled grafts

A skin flap is a graft which remains attached, at one or more points, by its pedicle, which provides an arterial blood supply and venous and lymphatic drainage. Pedicled skin flaps may be divided into three fundamentally different types: random, axial and musculocutaneous.

Random flaps

As its name implies a random flap may be raised anywhere, be of any size or shape and may run in any direction. Such a skin flap has a fairly poor blood supply from the subdermal vessels that pierce the underlying muscle bed and run into the skin perpendicular to it (Fig. 4.5). As a general rule the length of a random flap should not exceed that of its base, and this applies both to triangular and rectangular flaps. Irrespective of the size of the base, the flap should never exceed 5 in (approx. 12.5 cm) in length; random flaps longer than this will not survive, no matter how wide their base. Such flaps are obviously very limited in size and are now seldom used in head and neck surgery. The various types – advancement, rotation, etc. – are very well-described in MacGregor's (1982) monograph on fundamentals of plastic surgery.

Axial flaps

An axial flap is based on a named arteriovenous pedicle that runs within the skin superficial to the underlying muscle layer, parallel to the overlying skin (Fig. 4.6). Axial flaps have an extremely good blood supply, which is determined not by their

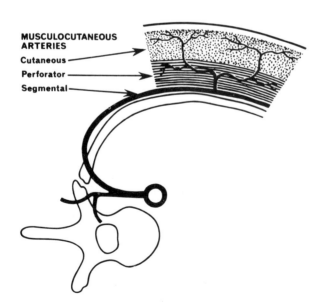

MUSCULOCUTANEOUS ARTERIES
Cutaneous
Perforator
Segmental

Fig. 4.5 Blood supply of a random flap.

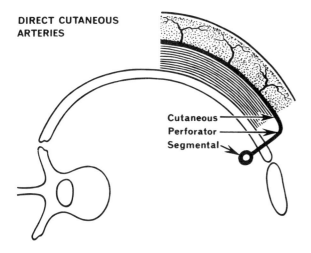

DIRECT CUTANEOUS ARTERIES

Cutaneous
Perforator
Segmental

Fig. 4.6 Blood supply of an axial flap.

length : breadth ratio but by the vascular territory of the vessels that supply them. In general they can be raised to a much greater length than random flaps and can therefore be used to move more skin over a greater distance. The use of these flaps was the first major step forward in reconstruction in head and neck surgery, but they have now largely been replaced by musculocutaneous and free flaps. However, the deltopectoral flap is still used occasionally for replacement of the skin of the lateral part of the neck.

The deltopectoral flap

This is based medially on the upper part of the chest on the upper three or four perforating branches of the internal mammary artery, which emerge through the medial end of the intercostal spaces (Fig. 4.7). Its boundaries are the clavicle superiorly, the acromion laterally and a line running through the anterior axillary fold above the nipple inferiorly. This flap will

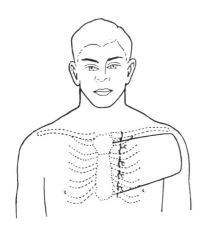

Fig. 4.7 Deltopectoral chest flap.

extend to any site in the neck and occasionally up to the level of the zygoma. In part this flexibility is explained by the fact that this flap retracts from side to side after it has been elevated but does not retract from end to end, and may indeed elongate slightly, particularly in patients over the age of 60.

Mark out the flap using the landmarks described above, then begin elevating the flap laterally. Preserve the pectoral fascia on the flap, leaving the muscle fibres absolutely bare. Also clamp the branches of the acromiothoracic axis as they are encountered, and divide and tie them 1 cm away from the flap to prevent thrombosis in the veins of the flap from a ligature applied too closely. Do not use diathermy on this flap, and have it retracted vertically upwards by an assistant using skin hooks – never double it back upon itself.

If the flap is to be left hanging, for instance when it is inset under the chin to close a pharyngeal fistula, protect it from the effects of gravity, which tend to pull its distal end away from its receptor site. Do this by non-absorbable sutures passed over a button, through the skin of the receptor site, through the fat of the flap, back through the skin and back over a button. It may be done more elegantly by the process of imbrication (Fig. 4.8), a term derived from the Latin word *imbrex*, meaning a roof tile. Excise a strip of skin about 1 cm wide from the margin of the flap and tuck this strip under the edge of the recipient site. This non-skin bearing strip is again fixed by non-absorbable sutures passing through the skin of the recipient site, through this strip of non-skin-bearing flap and out through the skin again, being tied over a button.

Axial flaps may be used as distant or local flaps: a distant flap is one in which there is an intervening area of normal skin between the donor and recipient sites; a local flap is one in which there is no intervening area, such that the flap is transposed directly from the donor to the recipient site and remains perma-

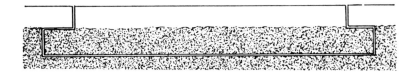

Fig. 4.8 Imbrication.

nently at that site. If there is an intervening area, the flap must usually be tubed, skin surface outwards, to protect it from infection. When the distal end has acquired a blood supply from its recipient site the tube must be divided and returned to the donor site.

There are various ways of assessing whether the flap has developed a sufficient blood supply; probably the easiest of these is to occlude the tube with a soft rubber catheter or with a special clamp that does not traumatize the pedicle. If the distal skin does not blanch after 15 min the pedicle can usually be divided with safety. In practice, if a period of 3 weeks is allowed, virtually all axial flaps can thereafter be divided with safety. The tube should be divided slowly, watching the circulation in the distal part. If the distal area becomes cold and white, division should be stopped, the divided area resutured, and the operation resumed 1 week later.

Other axial flaps

These include the temporal flap and the latissimus dorsi flap. The temporal flap was used extensively in mouth cancer but has several disadvantages: two stages are required and the cosmetic defect is very marked. Latissimus dorsi flaps have the disadvantage that it is necessary to turn the patient twice during the procedure. Both these flaps have now been almost universally abandoned in head and neck work.

Musculocutaneous flaps

The skin over most parts of the body receives its blood supply by small musculocutaneous arteries that enter it from the underlying muscle perpendicular to its surface (Fig. 4.5). It was first appreciated about 10 years ago that the obvious way to move a large area of skin is to transpose it with the underlying muscle from which it receives its nourishment. The muscles are supplied ultimately by segmental vessels that have similar perfusion pressures to the aorta. They run deeply within the muscle and give off perforators that enter the muscles and provide a communication between the segmental vessels and the musculocutaneous vessels in the skin. There may be several arterial pedicles. The artery is usually accompanied by two venae comitantes that unite after leaving the muscle to drain into a major regional vein. Five types of arterial supply to muscle have been described (Table 4.1).

The blood supply to the muscles may also be random or axial in pattern. Most of the round muscles, for example the sternomastoid, have a random supply: the perforators penetrate the belly at one end and immediately break up into small branches. The flat muscles, such as the pectoralis major, have an axial supply: the artery runs the whole length of the deep surface of the muscle giving off perforators as it goes.

A large number of musculocutaneous flaps has been described. However, the pectoralis major flap fulfils the requirements for reconstruction in 95% of cases that a head and neck surgeon will encounter.

The pectoralis major flap

The pectoralis major arises from the clavicle, from the sternum and by slips from the upper seven ribs. It is inserted into the bicipital groove of the humerus. The muscle has three major segmental subunits: clavicular, sternocostal and an external segment, the most lateral part of the muscle, which originates from the ribs.

Its main arterial supply is from the acromiothoracic artery, which springs from the first part of the axillary artery. The acromiothoracic artery gives off a superior (clavicular) branch to the clavicular segment of the muscle and a pectoral branch. The latter gives off an inferior thoracoacromial branch to the sternal segment, and a lateral thoracic trunk to the external segment (Fig. 4.9).

In 50% of cases the external segment is supplied exclusively by the lateral thoracic vessels, which spring from the second part of the axillary artery and descend along the lateral border of the pectoralis minor. In one-third of cases the muscle receives a dual supply for the lateral thoracic and thoracoacromial vessels. The sternocostal segment also gets a

Table 4.1 Patterns of vascular anatomy

Vascular pedicle		Examples used in head and neck surgery
I	One pedicle	None
II	Dominant pedicle and minor pedicles	Sternocleidomastoid Trapezius Platysma
III	Two dominant pedicles	Temporalis
IV	Segmental pedicles	None
V	One dominant pedicle plus secondary segmental pedicles	Pectoralis major Latissimus dorsi

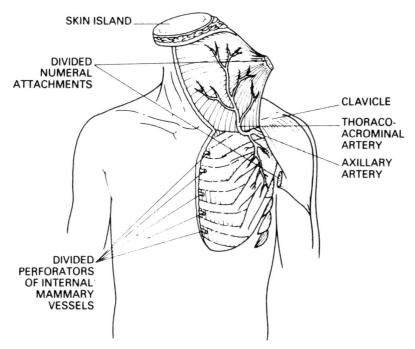

SKIN ISLAND

DIVIDED
NUMERAL
ATTACHMENTS

CLAVICLE

THORACO-
ACROMINAL
ARTERY

AXILLARY
ARTERY

DIVIDED
PERFORATORS
OF INTERNAL
MAMMARY
VESSELS

Fig. 4.9 Blood supply of the pectoralis major flap.

supply medially from a perforating branch of the internal mammary artery. The pectoralis major flap thus belongs in type V (Table 4.1).

Technique

Outline the surface markings of the pectoral branch of the acromiothoracic artery by a dotted line from the acromion to the xiphoid process. Then drop a perpendicular to this line from the centre of the clavicle. Next, mark out a skin island of appropriate size and shape over the distal end of the artery (Fig. 4.10). The borders should lie between the nipple laterally and the lateral edge of the sternum medially. Do not make the inferior edge lower than the inferior edge of the muscle, and try to make the upper edge opposite the axilla. Remember that the flap will retract by 10% in all directions when the skin is cut, and allow for this in planning.

Incise the skin on all sides down to the underlying muscle. Next divide the flat sternocostal segment about 1 cm beyond the edge of the muscle, down to the ribs. Stitch the muscle to the skin edge with several 2/0 catgut sutures to prevent shearing of the skin on the muscle. Enter the plane deep to the muscle by blunt dissection and turn the paddle laterally. Now divide the inferior muscle attachment from the ribs or rectus sheath. Again divide the muscle 1 cm distal to the skin and fix it to the skin paddle. At this point identify and divide the strips

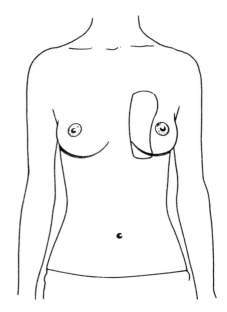

Fig. 4.10 Outline of the pectoralis major flap.

arising from the ribs, but do not confuse them with the slips of origin of the pectoralis minor muscle, which should be preserved.

You should now be able to identify the lateral border of the external segment of the muscle. Dissect

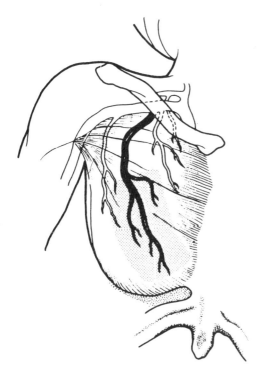

Fig. 4.11 Anatomy of upper end of pedicle of pectoralis major flap.

cleanly along this border: the only vessel crossing this space is a branch of the lateral thoracic artery – ligate and divide it. Now turn your attention to the superior edge of the flap. Prolong the incision laterally along the anterior axillary fold. The defensive incision you have now developed coincides with the lower border of a deltopectoral flap. Do not make any skin incision above this level because you may need to use the deltopectoral flap at a later date.

Using skin hooks, elevate the skin of the upper chest from the muscle layer up to the clavicle.

Now return to the flap. You should be able to lift the flap easily by blunt dissection in the fascial space between the pectoralis major and minor. Identify the pectoral vessels – the upper part of the muscle pedicle need consist solely of this arterial pedicle and a strip of the muscle about 1 cm wide on each side of it. A thin pedicle of this type is ideal if a neck dissection has not been done. But use a muscle pedicle about 10 cm wide to protect the carotid sheath if you have done a neck dissection.

Place your hand upwards behind the flap in such a position as to protect the vessels. Now divide the flat, sternal origin, medial to your hand. This part of the dissection is inelegant because the perforators are divided. Cut right up to the clavicle, dividing the clavicular segment of the muscle.

Now carry out a similar procedure through the

lateral muscle mass that forms the anterior axillary fold. Again continue right up to the clavicle but remember that the axillary vein is dangerously close.

The flap should now be fully mobile, and based solely on the vessels emerging between the clavicle and the upper border of the pectoralis minor (Fig. 4.11). The further steps of technique will depend on the intended use of the flap, and are described at the appropriate points.

Whilst the flap is being stitched into the recipient site it is usual to begin closing the donor site. It is often possible to rotate the skin of the lateral part of the chest into the defect and close it primarily. If not, rotate the lateral skin medially to close the defect as far as possible and suture it, leaving a large suction drain passing up into the cervical compartment of the dissection. Close the remaining defect with split skin, preferably using the delayed technique.

Modifications of this flap include incorporation of a segment of rib for mandibular reconstruction, or the use of two or three split flaps based over the individual segments.

Other musculocutaneous flaps

These include the sternomastoid and the trapezius. The sternomastoid flap has two main disadvantages: its upper end is dangerously close to lymph nodes that are very likely to be invaded by cancer, and secondly the blood supply to a skin paddle on its distal end is precarious. The latissimus dorsi and trapezius flaps have the disadvantage that the patient must be turned twice during the procedure. These flaps are rarely required and therefore will not be discussed here.

Free flaps

The most recent advance in reconstructive technique is major tissue transfer with reanastomosis of the artery and vein at the recipient site. A variety of tissues can be transplanted as required – skin alone, skin plus muscle, or skin plus muscle plus bone. Furthermore, a transplanted jejunal graft forms the ideal solution for pharyngeal reconstruction in many cases of hypopharyngeal cancer.

No form of surgery can be learnt from books, and microvascular surgery is the least amenable form of surgery for the armchair surgeon. Before performing anastomoses on a patient the apprentice must learn the technique by practice, firstly on artificial models and then on animals, at one of the various practical courses now available. However, the conditions in experimental animals are entirely different to humans: in the animal the vessels are always in good condition, and long-term patency is not relevant. Many a beginner, full of enthusiasm after successful anastomoses in the rat, has rediscovered the aphorism that 'man is not a rat'. In humans there are special problems of exposure, vascular disease and monitoring of vessel patency. These can to some extent be learnt by assisting.

Principles of microvascular surgery

Position

The most comfortable and stable position for prolonged sitting is to have the major joints at right angles. In other words the feet should be flat on the floor (or on a platform, in the case of the shorter surgeon), the hips and knees should also be at approximately right angles, as are the elbows. The forearm and hands or wrists at least should be supported. This is readily achieved in the laboratory but can be more awkward in the operating theatre. A roll of towels may be placed under the wrist joint, for example. Fogging of the eye pieces is reduced by placing adhesive tape at the top of the mask and by tying the lower strings of the face mask loosely. If the operating chair has arms or forearm and wrist support then this can be rendered sterile by draping it with a sterile operating gown. The instruments should be held like writing implements, with the middle finger supporting the tip. This facilitates rotation of the needle holder.

Equipment

Use of the operating microscope was introduced in 1921 by the otologist Nylen, for the treatment of otosclerosis, but the limited depth and field of vision using the operating microscope remain unsolved problems. Recent developments such as foot pedal zoom magnification and X–Y movement control make the instrument more flexible – the focal length of the objective should be around 200 mm for free flap surgery. Coaxial illumination also prevents excess of shadowing by the hand. Microvascular surgery is like any other surgery – it is more easily performed with the help of an assistant. This requires the use of a double-headed microscope. It also increases the training value of assistance. With the exception of the microscope, most microsurgical procedures do not require extensive sophisticated equipment. The majority of procedures can be carried out using no. 3 or no. 5 jeweller's forceps, vessel-dilating forceps and microvascular clamps. Suitable spring-handled needle holders include Barraquet and Castro-Viejo ophthalmic needle holders. Their spring action prevents the sudden jerky movement which follows the release of a locked needle holder. Spring-handled microscissors are required, both straight to cut vessel and curved to cut thread and connective tissue surrounding the vessels. The clamps are either single or double clamps. The double clamps have the advantage of supporting the two ends of the anastomosis but the disadvantage of obscuring the amount of tissue tension present. A commonly preferred suture is a 9/0 or 10/0 monofilament nylon with a 3/8 circle tapered-point atraumatic needle, less than 100 μm in diameter.

Basic principles

1 There must be meticulous atraumatic dissection of the blood vessel.
2 The vessel wall and intima at the site of the anastomosis must be normal under hypermagnification, and if necessary resected back for this condition to be fulfilled.
3 Adequate proximal flow must be demonstrated.
4 The anastomosis must be performed without tension.
5 Local overhanging adventitia is removed.
6 Suture placement is performed without grasping the intima.

All traces of blood, air and foreign body, e.g. sutures and threads, are thoroughly irrigated away with heparinized Ringer's solution before completing the anastomosis. A 10 ml syringe with a hypodermic needle whose tip has been bent by the surgeon is useful for this procedure and also to clear and hydrate the operative field throughout the procedure. Excessive suturing should be avoided as long sutures decrease efficiency and clutter the field of view. The ideal suture length is around 10 cm.

End-to-end anastomosis

A small sheet of background material such as fine plastic can be useful. The first stitch is placed by picking up the vessel using only the adventitia and spreading the lumen using the dilating forceps. A knot is tied either using the needle holder and one pair of forceps or two pairs of fine forceps. One end of the suture is left long and suspended from a cleat which may either be on the background, or on the frame if a double clamp is used. There are two options for positioning the second suture. The first is to place it at 180° from the first suture. This is then suspended from an opposite cleat and the front wall sewn up before the vessel is flipped over and the back wall repaired. The problem about this is that the stretching of the vessel between the two diametrically opposed stay sutures tends to flatten out the lumen and there is thus a risk of obliterating it by an inadvertent through-and-through stitch.

To obviate this the technique of eccentric biangulation was described by Cobbett in 1967. This places the second suture somewhat less than 180° from the first suture so that the back wall tends to fall away from the first pair. The first stitch is therefore applied mainly to bring both segments together and a second to dictate the final number and distribution of sutures. Where there is inequality of the vessel diameters the smaller vessel should be cut obliquely and gently spread with dilating forceps. Venous anastomosis is technically more difficult because the vein is thin-walled and therefore more easily collapsible and more easily torn. Adventitial stripping should be kept to a minimum and the vein ends permitted to flow through a small amount of heparinized saline. Fewer stitches are required than in arteries of the same diameter.

Patency test

The clip on the proximal side of the venous anastomosis is removed first, followed by that on the distal side of the venous anastomosis. The distal arterial and finally the proximal arterial clamps are then released. If the anastomosis is satisfactory the blood flow through the arterial one is readily detected and venous backflow is noted shortly thereafter. Engorgement of the tissue indicates that the venous drainage is compromised. Gently lifting the vessel distal to the anastomosis by placing the forceps underneath it demonstrates the flicker of blood flowing across this area but this is usually seen only in a thin-walled vessel. The milking test is traumatic and is therefore performed as infrequently as possible. In this test two pairs of smooth forceps occlude the vessel distal to the anastomosis. The downstream forceps is then moved gently 1 cm down the vessel, expressing fluid from the segment between the two forceps. The proximal compression is then released. The presence of a patent vessel is confirmed by rapid filling of the empty segment.

The radial forearm flap

The first free skin flap to be widely used was the forearm flap. It provides skin, or skin and bone (Fig. 4.12).

The day before the operation assess the patency of

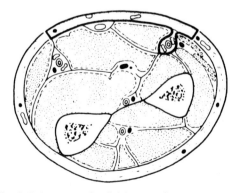

Fig. 4.12 Anatomy of radial forearm flap.

the radial artery using Allen's test. Ask the patient to open and close his or her fist rapidly 10 times, and to keep the fist closed after the tenth. Immediately after he or she closes the fist for the last time occlude the radial and ulnar arteries with your finger. The skin of the hand will be white. Then release the finger over the ulnar artery, whereupon the skin should rapidly become pink if the ulnar artery is patent. This test is not always reliable – the skin of a heavy smoker's hand is often white even before starting the test!

It is usual for the flap to be taken by a separate team working synchronously with the excisional team.

Mark out the position of the flap, usually on the distal volar surface. This might be unsuitable because of hair, and the flap might need to be sited more distally. Do not design the flap so that part of it lies on the radial or ulnar surfaces of the forearm. It is usual to use the left forearm in right-handed subjects and vice versa. Mark out the position of the radial artery and the subcutaneous forearm veins on the skin (Fig. 4.13).

Now apply a tourniquet and prepare the skin in the usual way. Incise the ulnar (medial) border of the flap, and begin elevating it from the underlying muscle. It is important to preserve the fascial layer on the flap as blood vessels run in this layer. However, the intermuscular septa that pass from the fascial layer between the muscles must be divided. Divide and ligate all large vessels in the skin, but use biopolar diathermy for small vessels, particularly the small veins running into the venae comitantes. Identify any large subcutaneous veins running across the proximal border and preserve them for anastomosis.

Continue dissection laterally until the condensation of deep fascia surrounding the radial artery and its venae comitantes is reached. Now incise the lateral, radial border and dissect in a similar manner towards the radial artery. The flap is now free apart from its fascial attachment to that artery. Follow the radial artery and any large subcutaneous veins proximally until a sufficient length of pedicle is achieved. Apply an arterial clamp to the radial artery and release the tourniquet – assess the return of colour to the hand and ensure that it can survive on the ulnar artery.

Now apply vascular clamps to any arteries and veins that are potential candidates for anastomosis, making sure that the radial artery is clamped distal to the origin of the ulnar artery from the branchial artery, just beyond the elbow joint. Only apply the clamps at the last minute when the recipient site and its vessels have been fully prepared.

Close the donor site by a split-skin graft, and immobilize the forearm for 2 weeks with a plaster of Paris cast. If a distal flap has been used the split skin will not take on tendon – this is one reason why a

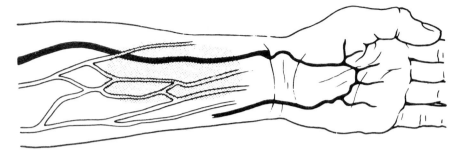

Fig. 4.13 Radial forearm flap marked out.

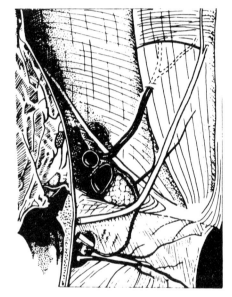

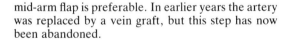

Fig. 4.14 Anatomy of rectus abdominis flap.

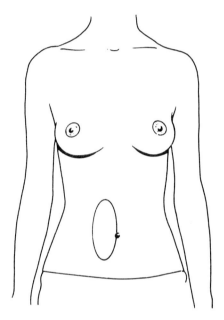

Fig. 4.15 Rectus abdominis flap marked out.

mid-arm flap is preferable. In earlier years the artery was replaced by a vein graft, but this step has now been abandoned.

Rectus abdominis flap

If you need a free flap consisting of muscle and skin there are at least two popular flaps available: the latissimus dorsi and the rectus abdominis. The former has two disadvantages: it is quite tricky to harvest properly and safely, and the patient must be turned on the side. The rectus abdominis is one of the easiest flaps to harvest, and furthermore it can be mobilized easily by a second team during the excisional phase. The rectus abdominis arises from the pubis, and is inserted into the anterior surface of the xiphoid process and the fifth, sixth and seventh ribs. It is encased in the rectus sheath, but the posterior wall of the sheath is deficient in its lower quarter,

below the arcuate line, which lies about the level of the anterior superior iliac spine. The muscle is supplied by the superior and inferior epigastric arteries: the former arises from the internal mammary and the latter from the external iliac artery. Both arteries enter the sheath and run in a vertical direction between the muscle and the posterior layer of the sheath; both pass into the muscle towards its centre where they break up into small branches to supply the muscle, and anastomose with each other (Fig. 4.14). The inferior pedicle is usually wider than the superior.

Mark out a flap of sufficient size, to one side of the umbilicus, making sure that its lower border lies above the arcuate line (Fig. 4.15). Incise the skin on all sides and expose the lateral and medial borders of the rectus sheath. Cut through the sheath to expose the lateral and medial borders of the muscle. Suture the skin to the muscle with a few 2/0 sutures to

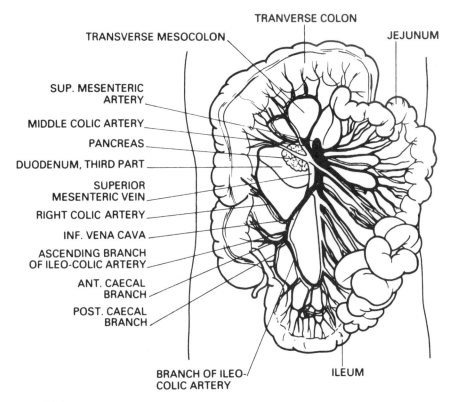

TRANVERSE COLON

TRANSVERSE MESOCOLON

JEJUNUM

SUP. MESENTERIC ARTERY

MIDDLE COLIC ARTERY

PANCREAS

DUODENUM, THIRD PART

SUPERIOR MESENTERIC VEIN

RIGHT COLIC ARTERY

INF. VENA CAVA

ASCENDING BRANCH OF ILEO-COLIC ARTERY

ANT. CAECAL BRANCH

POST. CAECAL BRANCH

BRANCH OF ILEO-COLIC ARTERY

ILEUM

Fig. 4.16 Anatomy of jejunum.

prevent shearing. Elevate the lateral border of the muscle and dissect posterior to the muscle between it and the posterior rectus sheath, searching carefully for the superior and inferior epigastric arteries and their venae comitantes. Once you have found the vessels, develop a long pedicle, preferably from the inferior epigastric artery. You can now cut transversely through the muscle, preserving the vascular pedicle carefully. When the donor site is fully prepared place vascular clamps across the pedicle, divide and ligate the other vascular pedicle and remove the flap. Usually you will be able to close the defect of the abdominal wall primarily.

Jejunal loops

The arteries to the small intestine arise from the superior mesenteric artery, by 10–16 branches. They pass between the layers of the mesentery, each dividing into two branches that anastomose with the adjacent artery to form a series of arcades, which give off secondary branches to supply the gut. The upper jejunal branches form only one or two arches, but the process of division is repeated three or four times in the ileal arteries, forming four or five tiers of arteries. This might be the reason why a jejunal loop is more reliable as a graft (Fig. 4.16).

Open the abdomen through an upper paramedian incision, and identify a suitable loop of jejunum. Choose a loop of suitable length, and identify its vessels by holding the mesentery against a light. Follow the artery and vein to their attachments to the superior mesenteric artery and vein. Divide the mesentery in a V-shape, dividing and ligating any lateral branches.

Place bowel clamps across the bowel at the proximal and distal ends and occlude the proximal and distal ends of the loop with a stapling device. Divide

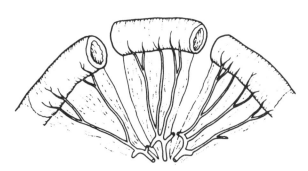

Fig. 4.17 Jejunal loop isolated.

proximally and distally, between the clamp and the stapled bowel (Fig. 4.17). Then reanastomose the bowel in the usual way in two layers. At this stage the proximal ends of the loop are occluded by staples but the vessels are still patent.

Once the recipient site is prepared, including preparation of its blood vessels, clamp the jejunal vessels and remove the loop. Close the defect in the mesentery and close the abdomen in the usual way.

References and further reading

Pectoralis major flaps

Ariyan S, Cuono C B (1980) Myocutaneous flaps for head and neck reconstruction. *Plast Reconstr Surg* **2**:321–45.

Baeck S, Biller H F, Krespi Y P *et al.* (1979) The pectoralis major myocutaneous island flap for reconstruction of the head and neck. *Head Neck Surg* **1**:293–300.

Biller H F, Krespi Y P, Lawson W *et al.* (1980) A one-stage flap reconstruction following resection for stomal recurrence. *Otolaryngol Head Neck Surg* **88**:357–60.

Krespi Y P, Wurster C F, Sisson G A (1985) Immediate reconstruction after total laryngopharyngoesophagectomy and mediastinal dissection. *Laryngoscope* **95**:156–61.

Manstein C H, Manstein G, Somers R G *et al.* (1985) Use of pectoralis minor muscle in immediate reconstruction of the breast. *Plast Reconstr Surg* **76**:566–9.

Reid C D, Taylor G I (1984) Vascular territory of the acromiothoracic axis. *Br J Plast Surg* **37**:194.

Sisson G A, Goldman M E (1981) Pectoral myocutaneous island flap for reconstruction of stomal recurrence. *Arch Otolaryngol Head Neck Surg* **107**:446–9.

Trapezius flaps

Ariyan S (1979) One-stage repair of a cervical esophagostome with two myocutaneous flaps from the neck and shoulder. *Plast Reconstr Surg* **63**:426–9.

Baek S M, Biller H F, Krespi Y P, *et al.* (1980) The lower trapezius island myocutaneous flap. *Ann Plast Surg* **5**:108–14.

Bertotti J A (1981) Trapezius-musculocutaneous island flap in the repair of major head and neck cancer. *Plast Reconstr Surg* **65**:16–21.

Daeseler E H, Anson B J (1959) Surgical anatomy of the subclavian artery and its branches. *Surg Gynecol Obstet* **108**:149–73.

Demergasso F, Piazza M V (1979) Trapezius myocutaneous flaps in reconstructive surgery for head and neck cancer: an original technique. *Am J Surg* **138**:533–6.

Goodwin W J, Rosenberg C J (1982) Venous drainage of the lateral trapezius musculocutaneous island flap. *Arch Otolaryngol Head Neck Surg* **108**:411–13.

Guillamondegui Q M, Larson D L (1981) The lateral trapezius musculocutaneous flap: its use in head and neck reconstruction. *Plast Reconstr Surg* **67**:143–50.

Krespi Y P, Baek S M, Surek C L (1983) Flap reconstruction of the upper face: free flaps vs lower trapezius myocutaneous flap. *Laryngoscope* **93**:485–8.

McCraw J B, Dibbell D G (1977) Experimental definition of independent myocutaneous vascular territories. *Plast Reconstr Surg* **60**:212–20.

McCraw J B, Magee W P, Kalwaic H (1979) Uses of the trapezius and sternomastoid myocutaneous flaps in head and neck reconstruction. *Plast Reconstr Surg* **63**:49–57.

Maruyama Y, Nakajima H, Fujino T *et al.* (1981) The definition of cutaneous vascular territories over the back using selective angiography and the intra-arterial injection of prostaglandin E1: some observations on the use of the lower trapezius myocutaneous flap. *Br J Plast Surg* **34**:157–61.

Mathes S J, Nahai F (1981) Classification of the vascular anatomy of the muscles: experimental and clinical correlation. *Plast Reconstr Surg* **67**:177–87.

Micali G, Romeo L (1982) Experience with trapezius and tensor fascia lata myocutaneous flaps. *Ann Plast Surg* **9**:94–100.

Mutter T D (1842) Cases of deformity from burns, relieved by operation. *Am J Med Sci* **4**:66–80.

Panje W R (1980) Myocutaneous trapezius flap. *Head Neck Surg* **2**:206–12.

Panje W R (1982) A new method for total nasal reconstruction. *Arch Otolaryngol Head Neck Surg* **108**:156–66.

Panje W R (1985) Mandible reconstruction with the trapezius osteomusculocutaneous flap. *Arch Otolaryngol Head Neck Surg* **111**:223–9.

Rosen H M. The extended trapezius musculocutaneous flap for cranio-orbital facial reconstruction. *Plast Reconstr Surg* **75**:318–24.

Shapiro M J (1981) Use of trapezius myocutaneous flaps in the reconstruction of head and neck defects. *Arch Otolaryngol Head Neck Surg* **107**:333–6.

Tucker H M, Sobol S M, Levine H *et al.* (1982) The transverse cervical trapezius myocutaneous island flap. *Arch Otolaryngol Head Neck Surg* **108**:194–8.

Zovickian A (1957) Pharyngeal fistulas: repair and prevention using mastoid-occiput shoulder flaps. *Plast Reconstr Surg* **19**:355–72.

Latissimus dorsi flaps

Bartlett S P, May J W, Yaremduik M J (1981) The latissimus dorsi muscle: a fresh cadaver study of the primary neurovascular pedicle. *Plast Reconst Surg* **67**:631.

Bailey B N (1979) Latissimus dorsi flaps – a practical approach. *Ann Acad Med Singapore* **8**:447.

Bostwick J, Nahai F, Wallace J G, Vasconze L O (1979) Sixty latissimus dorsi flaps. *Plast Reconstr Surg* **63**:31.

Maxwell P G (1980) Iginio Tansini and the origin of the latissimus dorsi musculocutaneous flap. *Plast Reconstr Surg* **65**:686.

Olivari N (1976) The latissimus flap. *Br J Plast Surg* **29**:126.

Principles of microvascular surgery

Acland R D (1980) *Microsurgical Practice Manual*. St Louis, Mosby.

Ballantyne D L, Razaboni R M, Harper A D (1980) *Microvascular Surgery: A Laboratory Manual*. New York, Institute of Reconstructive Plastic Surgery, New York University Medical Center.

Cobbett J R (1967) Microvascular surgery. *Surg Clin North Am* **47**:521–42.

Godina M (1979) Preferential use of end-to-side arterial

anastomoses in free flap transfer. *Plast Reconstr Surg* **64**:673.

O'Brien B M, Morrison W A (1987) *Reconstructive Microsurgery*. London, Churchill Livingstone.

Serafin D, Georgiade N G, Peters C R (1976) Microsurgical composite tissue transplantation. A method of immediate reconstruction of the head and neck. *Clin Plast Surg* **3**:447–57.

Smith J W (1966) Microsurgery: review of the literature and discussion of microtechniques. *Plast Reconstr Surg* **37**:227–45.

Free arm flaps

Lamberty B G H, Cormack G C (1982) The forearm angiotomes. *Br J Plast Surg* **35**:420.

Song R, Gao Y, Song Y, Yu Y, Song Y (1982) The forearm flap. *Clin Plast Surg* **9**:21.

Soutar D S, Scheker L R, Tanner N S B, McGregor I A (1983) The radial forearm flap: a versatile method for intra-oral reconstruction. *Br J Plast Surg* **36**:1.

Yang G *et al.* (1981) Forearm free skin flap transplantation. *Nat Med J China* **61**:139.

Rectus abdominus flaps

Boyd J B, Taylor G I, Corlett R (1984) The vascular territories of the superior epigastric and the deep inferior epigastric systems. *Plast Reconstr Surg* **73**:1.

Bunkis J, Walton R L, Mathes S J, Krized T J, Vasconez I O (1983) Experience with the transverse lower rectus abdominis operation for breast reconstruction. *Plast Reconstr Surg* **72**:819.

Scheflan M, Dinner M I (1983) The transverse abdominal island flap. Part I. Indications contraindications, results and complications. *Ann Plast Surg* **10**:24.

Scheflan M, Dinner M I (1983) The transverse abdominal island flap. Part II. Surgical technique. *Ann Plast Surg* **10**:120.

Taylor G I, Corlett R J, Boyd J B (1984) The versatile deep inferior epigastric (inferior rectus abdominus) flap. *Br J Plast Surg* **10**:24.

Jejunal flaps

Flynn M B, Acland R D (1979) Free intestinal autografts for reconstruction following pharyngolaryngo-oesophagectomy. *Surg Gyn Obstet* **149**:858.

Hester R T, McConnel F M S, Nahai F, Jurkiewicz M J, Brown R G (1980) Reconstruction of cervical oesophagus, hypopharynx and oral cavity using free jejunal transfer. *Am J Surg* **140**:487.

Katsaros J, Tan E (1982) Free bowel transfer for pharyngo-oesophageal reconstruction: an experimental and clinical study. *Br J Plast Surg* **35**:268.

Nakamura T, Inokuchi K, Sugimachi K (1975) Use of revascularised jejunum as a free graft for cervical oesophagus. *Jpn J Surg* **5**:92.

Robinson D W, MacLeod A (1982) Microvascular free jejunum transfer. *Br J Plast Surg* **35**:258.

Seidenberg B, Rosenak S S, Hurwitt E S, Som M L (1959) Immediate reconstruction of the cervical oesophagus by a revascularised isolated jejunal segment. *Ann Surg* **149**:162.

5

Complications

Complications of head and neck surgery

This section deals only with the complications peculiar to head and neck surgery; information regarding the general complications of any major operation, e.g. chest infection, deep venous thrombosis or urinary retention, can be obtained from works on general surgery. In general the incidence of these complications is inversely proportional to the care taken in the performance of the operation.

The complications after a major head and neck operation may for convenience be discussed under the three headings of immediate, intermediate and late. *Immediate* complications are those that are a direct result of technical faults during the operation, and which manifest themselves in the first 24 h after operation. *Intermediate* complications come on during the succeeding few weeks, generally as a result of failure in the healing process, and occur before the patient leaves hospital. Finally, there are *late* complications, which come on months or years after the operation when the patient has returned home. Careful follow-up and anticipation are necessary to forestall these.

Immediate complications

Bleeding

After a major head and neck operation this manifests itself either by bleeding from an anastomosis into the mouth or pharynx, or by haematoma formation under the skin flaps. In either case it is quite obvious to the trained observer and should be detected long before there are changes in the vital signs.

After resection of a carcinoma in the mouth, pharynx or larynx, bleeding may take place from the suture line. Bleeding into the mouth may also occur after a total maxillectomy if all the branches of the maxillary artery and pterygoid venous plexus have not been tied. In either of these events blood is seen trickling from the mouth, and diagnosis should be easy. This complication is one of the reasons why most patients undergoing head and neck surgery should have a temporary tracheostomy with a cuffed tube, to prevent interference with the airway by a large amount of blood, to prevent inhalation of blood into the trachea; and to allow any bleeding to be dealt with without fear of the airway being compromised.

Bleeding may also occur after a radical neck dissection, a particularly troublesome source being the posterior surface of the bridge flap used in the double horizontal incision; other potential sites of bleeding are the branches of the external carotid artery or the transverse cervical artery. Bleeding in this instance manifests itself by swelling of the neck if the suction drains are unable to cope with it; another reason why dressings should not be used after a neck operation is that this complication can then be readily recognized.

The principles of management of bleeding in these two situations are the same as those after any operation. The bleeding point should be found and ligated, and blood lost should be replaced by transfusion. Attempts to arrest the haemorrhage by applying pressure dressings to the neck, or attempting to pack a bleeding cavity, are a waste of time. The bleeding is almost always not arrested, time is lost, the patient is further exsanguinated, and infection and necrosis of skin flaps are induced. A prompt decision should be made, therefore, to return the patient to theatre, reopen the wound and secure the bleeding point. Before this is done, blood lost must be replaced, to return the patient's circulating blood volume to normal.

Airway obstruction

After extensive resection of tissue within the mouth, pharynx or larynx, there is inevitably oedema of the remaining parts, and the airway is often compromised. Furthermore, after a bilateral neck dissection, either simultaneous or staged, there is often soft tissue oedema. A tracheostomy must be done in all these cases before or during the procedure to prevent airway obstruction. Should this advice be ignored for any reason, at the first sign of airway obstruction a tracheostomy must be carried out. A very wise aphorism is that if a tracheostomy comes into your mind then that is the time to do it. Failure to do so will often later be regretted.

Pneumothorax

The cervical pleura may be damaged during any operation low in the neck, especially if the manubrium is removed; the mediastinal pleura may be damaged during oesophageal resection. If the patient has been ventilated during the anaesthetic, the presence of a pneumothorax may not be appreciated until shortly after the end of the operation. In such patients a portable chest radiograph should be taken in the operating theatre at the end of the procedure. If the patient becomes restless, cyanosed or dyspnoeic after operation he or she probably has a pneumothorax – provided the suspicion enters the surgeon's mind, the clinical diagnosis by the usual methods is usually made easily without a chest radiograph. Indeed, if a pneumothorax is extensive, it may not be to the patient's advantage to wait until a radiograph is obtained; it is preferable to introduce a catheter into the second intercostal space, and connect it to an underwater seal. If this does not restore the patient to normal it is worthwhile remembering that there may be a pneumothorax on the other side, and that if there has been extensive bleeding there may even be a haemopneumothorax.

Haemopneumothorax may be difficult to diagnose even by radiography because at the end of the operation radiographs are usually taken with the patient lying on his or her back. In these circumstances, fluid in the pleural cavity will not be shown. If there is a large quantity of fluid in the pleural cavity it can readily by aspirated, either by applying suction to the underwater seal or by inserting another catheter into the seventh or eight intercostal space in the mid axillary line and applying suction to that catheter.

Increased intracranial pressure

The intracranial pressure rises threefold when one internal jugular vein is divided, and fivefold when both are tied, but returns to near normal levels within 24 h. This rise seldom causes symptoms, but may do so after both veins have been tied or if a dominant jugular vein has been tied on one side.

The signs and symptoms of increased intracranial pressure are restlessness, headache, slowing of the pulse, a rising blood pressure, swelling of the face, and cyanosis and congestion of the skin of the face. If a patient's lips and ears are cyanosed at the end of a head and neck operation, do not presume that he or she is suffering from peripheral cyanosis due to cardiorespiratory failure before examining the other extremities. If these are found to be pink and warm the facial cyanosis is due to ligation of the major neck veins.

Prevent this complication as far as possible by avoiding dressings around the neck, by not allowing the patient to hyperextend the neck (particularly after a bilateral neck dissection) and by sitting the patient up as soon as possible after an operation. If increased intracranial pressure occurs, sit the patient up and give 200 ml of 25% mannitol intravenously as quickly as possible. If the diagnosis is correct the results of this are usually dramatic; the condition should be reversed within 10–15 min. A diuresis will occur, and the patient can be expected to pass 500 ml of urine within the next 2 h. If he or she has not done so, pass a catheter. As the intracranial pressure falls rapidly to normal within 24 h this procedure rarely needs to be repeated.

Carotid sinus syndrome

The carotid sinus is a baroreceptor; an increase in carotid arterial pressure normally causes bradycardia and decreased systemic blood pressure. This stimulus is slight compared to the manipulation at operation, which may result in a marked drop in blood pressure and slowing of the pulse. This is anticipated and dealt with by an experienced anaesthetist, but it may be alarming to one less experienced. The surgeon can help by injecting 2% lignocaine around the sinus, thereby blocking glossopharyngeal afferent fibres.

Postoperative scarring may leave the sinus in a highly sensitive state so that palpation of the neck, dressings, or even turning the head from side to side may result in faintness or even loss of consciousness due to hypotension and bradycardia. This hypersensitivity persists indefinitely. This symptom coming on some months after operation usually indicates recurrent tumour invading the glossopharyngeal nerve.

Intermediate complications

Anastomotic leak

This topic is dealt with on page 29.

Chylous fistula

There is no disgrace in damaging or cutting the thoracic duct whilst operating low on the left side of the neck; indeed it may often be necessary to do so when carrying out a thorough radical neck dissection. However, failure to recognize this complication can be disastrous.

Because the patient has fasted it may not be obvious that the duct has been cut because the fluid is clear, and small in amount.

If an injury to the thoracic duct is overlooked it will not usually manifest itself until the patient is being given tube feeds. At this time the suction drainage increases dramatically in volume and may reach 500 ml/day, the drainage consisting of thick white fluid resembling milk. If this leak is allowed to continue the flaps will not sit properly and the patient becomes emaciated within the first 24 h. Return the patient to theatre, reopen the lower part of the neck wound, find the injured duct and stitch the end with 4/0 silk. Finding the duct is usually not feasible after 24 h because of maceration of tissue. After this time the condition must be managed by stopping tube feeds, and relying on intravenous (hyper)alimentation.

Seroma

A collection of serum under the neck flap can be prevented by using suction drainage for at least 5 days. A seroma may occur in the first 48 h after the drainage tubes have been removed. Serum always collects in the supraclavicular fossa, the most dependent part of the neck.

Part of the routine daily care should be to ask the patient to hunch the shoulder, whereupon the fossa should form a pronounced dip. If the dip is absent then serum is present and must be aspirated.

Use a wide-bore needle and aspirate daily until no more serum collects – it may be necessary to do this for up to 2 weeks in order to stop serum accumulating and thus lifting the neck flaps.

After each aspiration apply a pressure dressing using fluffed-up 4 × 4 cm swabs over the lower neck held on with two overlapping strips of 7.5 cm elastic strapping (painting the front of the chest and scapular region with tincture of benzoin helps to maintain adhesion). The strapping is further fixed by placing strips of 2.5 cm adhesive tape to its margins.

If repeated aspiration and dressing are necessary, Montgomery strapping on the chest and back helps to stop the skin being abraded by repeated removal of strapping. Montgomery straps are pieces of 7.5 cm adhesive with eyelets cut in the ends through which tapes are passed. The fluffs can then be held by tying the tapes over them.

Failure of skin healing

Necrosis of the skin of the neck is a disaster that is fortunately much less common than it was a generation ago. It is caused by many factors and as a result of it the patient may die. At the very least he or she is caused discomfort because the neck flaps must be debrided, the resulting raw area must be repaired by skin grafts, the stay in hospital is prolonged, and the resulting scar is cosmetically unacceptable.

As was pointed out in the section on incisions (Chapter 3), surgery in the neck differs markedly from surgery in the abdomen or chest, because to gain access to the structures in the neck, large skin flaps must be elevated. These flaps are usually so big that their viability may be marginal, and it may be compromised by the use of unsuitable incisions, particularly in a patient who has been irradiated.

If wound infection does occur, a swab should be taken and treatment with antibiotics begun while awaiting the result. Appropriate prophylactic antibiotic measures have been discussed in Chapter 3 for patients whose pharynx has been opened.

Provided that there is no necrosis of tissue, infection is likely to be due to the Gram-positive cocci and treatment should, therefore, be with intramuscular soluble penicillin 500 000 units, 6-hourly.

There are several metabolic factors that militate against good healing including poor nutrition, metabolism of protein by the tumour, uncontrolled diabetes, renal failure and unreplaced blood loss.

With modern anaesthetic techniques, including the use of central venous pressure measurements, blood replacement should be accurate but it is worthwhile checking that the haemoglobin is normal 48 h after operation, when the blood volume has settled down to normal.

If a flap is about to necrose, it can be seen that its circulation is poor; it is congested so that finger pressure produces blanching and rapid refilling. Within the first 24 h the flap will be dark blue or black and at this stage it must be excised back to healthy bleeding skin. If this is done before infection supervenes the resulting defect can be filled with a split-thickness skin graft, but if excision of dead tissue is not carried out at this stage, infection will inevitably supervene and healing by granulation will then be required. If infection does occur, culture of the discharge will usually reveal a mixture of organisms of the Gram-negative variety such as *Pseudomonas pyocyanea*, the *Proteus* group or *Escherichia coli*. Treatment of such an infection is not by the expensive and dangerous antibiotics to which these organisms are usually sensitive. As these organisms are growing in tissues without blood supply, the antibiotic cannot be expected to reach the site of infection. If the dead tissue is not excised the organisms will continue to thrive, causing venous thrombosis in adjacent healthy tissue. This leads to further skin necrosis, a process which is accelerated by pyocyanin secreted by *P. pyocyanea*. If infection has occurred it is impossible at this stage to close the defect by grafting; it will be necessary to wait for several weeks until a healthy granulating bed has been prepared by the use of daily debridement and local dressings, as outlined in Chapter 4.

Carotid artery rupture

Rupture of one of the major blood vessels of the neck is usually the culmination of several complications – the skin wound breaks down, usually because an improper incision has been used in an irradiated patient (a vertical component and a three-point junction are often the culprits); infection supervenes, particularly if the patient is in a poor metabolic state and has an infected mouth to begin with; the carotid arteries are then exposed and gangrene of their walls occurs because infection leads to thrombosis of their vasa vasorum. Finally, the artery ruptures and the patient often dies, or at best survives with a hemiplegia.

Prevent this disaster by attention to all the points of preparation and operative technique outlined in the appropriate chapters. In particular, protect the carotid arteries in all patients at risk (i.e. those who have been irradiated) by a muscle graft (p. 102). Also do not deprive the arteries of their vasa vasorum, derived from the branches of the thyrocervical trunk, and do not strip off the adventitia of the carotid sheath during neck dissection.

Despite all precautions, some wounds break down and some patients get fistulae so that the carotid sheath is exposed from without or within. Rupture virtually never occurs unheralded; in the 48 h before rupture there is always a small prodromal bleed, and this must be respected. Protect the airway with a cuffed tracheostomy tube, put up a drip and cross-match 4 units (approx. 2 l) of blood; excise all dead tissue, and keep the artery covered by frequent moist soaks.

Warn all personnel that massive rupture may occur and instruct them what to do – control bleeding with immediate finger pressure; secure the airway by inflating the cuff on the tracheostomy tube; and give blood immediately.

Take the patient to theatre; if possible, blood volume should be restored before anaesthesia is induced. It might be necessary to remind the anaesthetist to keep the head down, the blood pressure up and the arterial P_{CO_2} normal, as carbon dioxide retention predisposes to decreased cerebral blood flow. Then isolate each end of the carotid artery under a healthy piece of skin, tie it off and stitch it. Do not try to repair it or tie it off in the middle of an infected area – it will blow again next week.

At least a third of patients on whom this tragedy falls will die; of those who survive half will have a hemiplegia.

AIDS

Acquired immune deficiency syndrome (AIDS) and human immunodeficiency virus (HIV) are of con-siderable importance to the head and neck surgeon, for several reasons. Firstly, several clinical forms of AIDS and AIDS-related complex regularly present in the head and neck. For example, in one series of 150 AIDS patients attending a San Francisco oral medicine clinic, 80% had Kaposi's sarcoma, 53 with oral involvement; 7 had oral squamous cell carcinoma; 3 had oral non-Hodgkin's lymphoma, and candidiasis was almost universal. These clinical aspects are discussed in Chapter 6. Secondly, the allied immunodeficiency may compromise the host response to surgical trauma. Finally, as in any surgical procedure, there is a risk of cross-contamination of the surgeon, and also the patient. Percutaneous injuries which could result in cross-infection occur in 2–15% of surgical procedures. Analysis of the nucleotide sequence of HIV provirus from an infected dentist in 1991 showed an unusual degree of similarity with specimens obtained from 5 of his patients – probably the first reported case of a health care worker infecting his patients. There is currently a debate in the UK between those who propose the testing of patients suspected of being at high risk – and, by inference, of the medical, dental and allied professions – and others who advocate a policy of universal anti-infective precautions for all workers and all patients. In favour of the former are the arguments of cost and dilution of alertness. Proponents of the latter quote the absence of known risk factors in 28% of almost 53 000 people who tested positive in a publicly funded USA test site in a 20-month period and the fact that heterosexual contact is the only exposure category in 10% of AIDS cases in the UK. There is, moreover, evidence that surgeons' awareness of patients' seropositivity or high-risk status does not in any case affect their exposure to blood or body fluids.

The positive measures which can be taken to reduce the risk of cross-infection include universal vaccination of medical personnel against hepatitis B, which is much more readily acquired from a carrier following percutaneous injury (6–30% incidence of seroconversion) than HIV (0.4% seroconversion). In one USA series, 60% of HIV carriers were also hepatitis B-positive. It is important to be aware of any breaches in integrity of the hand skin, and to avoid in any case cutaneous contact with blood or saliva, not only in the operating theatre, but also in the clinic, where the wearing of gloves for indirect layrngoscopy is recommended. Intraoperative precautions include the use of goggles for conjunctival protection, and a face visor during heavily contaminating procedures (e.g. the use of drills or saws.). A safe technique should be developed for the exchange of sharp instruments among operating theatre personnel and a no-touch method of inserting sutures.

Late Complications

Primary recurrence

It is axiomatic that if excision of the tumour was adequate in the first place, recurrence at the primary site should be unusual; by the same token it is usually untreatable. However, on occasion, a primary recurrence may be treatable either by radiotherapy, or by resection and extensive plastic reconstruction.

The cure rate for this sort of salvage surgery is well under 10% so consider carefully exactly what you can offer the patient in the way of palliation or cure before embarking on an enormous resection.

Lymph gland metastases

Some patients with head and neck cancer later develop a contralateral enlarged lymph node – particularly those suffering from carcinomas of the aryepiglottic fold, the epiglottis and the hypopharynx. These patients should usually be treated by radical neck dissection. However, as the first side has already been dissected, these patients are at the same risk of increased intracranial pressure and of swelling of the soft tissues causing respiratory obstruction as those undergoing bilateral neck dissection. Therefore a temporary tracheostomy should always be done to tide them over the first few days after operation.

Occasionally small infiltrated lymph nodes recur after a radical neck dissection, especially at the lower part of the posterior triangle and under the trapezius. These should be removed by local excision, but they herald a gloomy prognosis.

The place of chemotherapy in palliation is discussed in Chapter 3.

Failure of thyroid and parathyroid glands

As part of a laryngectomy the thyroid and parathyroid glands may be resected on one side of the neck. Furthermore, fibrosis often develops on the other side so that a year after operation the blood supply to both the thyroid and parathyroid glands may be compromised and, in particular, parathyroid failure may occur.

The symptoms of both thyroid and parathyroid failure come on slowly and may be indefinite, such as depression (which is to be expected in the cancer patient anyway) or lethargy. It is important in patients who have undergone extensive neck operations to check thyroid function by estimation of serum thyroxine and parathyroid function by serum calcium every few months after the first year.

Thyroid and parathyroid gland replacement are discussed in Chapter 3.

Dysphagia (see Chapter 17)

A stricture may form in the pharynx after a simple total laryngectomy, or after pharyngolaryngectomy or pharyngeal reconstruction. After a straightforward total laryngectomy, stricture is more likely if the operation was done for a piriform sinus tumour in which a large area of mucosa is sacrificed. After pharyngolaryngectomy, stricture formation often follows a skin repair but not repair by gastric transposition or jejunal loop.

In either case the stricture usually responds readily to dilatation at monthly intervals, and this should only be required on two or three occasions. If it is required more often than this, the stricture may be kept open by the patient using a Hurst mercury bougie. If these procedures are unsuccessful, and the patient is severely incapacitated, the neck should be reopened and the stricture repaired surgically.

Hypertrophy of the tail of the parotid gland

In a small proportion of patients after radical neck dissection there may appear, after a few weeks, a swelling at the amputated tail of the parotid gland. This resembles a recurrent cancer and, naturally, causes a lot of worry both to the patient and the surgeon. It should be recognized as a reasonably common complication and the patient should be reassured. Unless there is an obvious localized hard swelling indicating a recurrence, surgery should not be performed on the tail of the gland because further hypertrophy will merely occur higher up. Its importance lies just in the fact of recognizing it and doing nothing about it apart from reassuring the patient.

Lymphoedema

When both internal jugular veins are tied lymphoedema often follows, due to interruption of the lymphatic drainage channels from the head, especially those of the lateral aspect of the neck. Lymphoedema is particularly marked when neck dissection is combined with excision of a midline structure such as the larynx or pharynx. If all steps are taken to minimize oedema, such as foregoing dressings, sitting the patient upright, and using mannitol, it often subsides within a month. If it becomes established the patient can have a grotesquely oedematous head for a long time after surgery. The condition is untreatable. Lymphoedema may also follow splitting of the lip to gain access to the mouth, or an incision in the eyelid during maxillectomy.

Fistula

A fistula from the pharynx or the oral cavity to the skin can occur after an operation on the larynx or pharynx or after the removal of an oral tumour. It can also occur after a commando operation. Three aspects of such fistulae need to be considered – prevention, management in the immediate postoperative period and management of the established fistula.

A fistula, be it orocutaneous or pharyngocutaneous, is the end-product of a number of factors in the pre-operative, operative and postoperative periods. The most important of these are previous radiotherapy and inadequate control of diabetes and anaemia in the preoperative period, poor operative technique, including a poorly made suture line, and allowing a seroma, haematoma or abscess to proceed untreated or anaemia to go uncorrected in the postoperative phase.

A fistula may form because a suture line gives way or because tissue becomes necrotic. With suture failure there is no loss of tissue as there is with necrosis. A fistula on a suture line virtually always closes spontaneously, particularly if the patient has not previously been irradiated. All that is required therefore is to prevent epithelium forming along the edges of the tract and to keep the fistula covered with a dressing until it heals.

Loss of tissue occurs in the patient who has been irradiated; if not too much tissue has been lost the fistula often closes spontaneously but before it can begin to do so all dead tissue must be cut away to allow healing to begin. A long time is often needed to control local infection – at least 8 weeks should be allowed for a fistula to close spontaneously. If the fistula at that time is stable and established it may be necessary to close it electively.

Established fistulae must be closed in such a way as to provide a lining on the inside of the mouth or the pharynx and on the outside.

Technique of closure of an established fistula

We will now describe the closure of a pharyngocutaneous fistula after total laryngectomy with loss of most of the anterior wall of the pharynx and overlying skin; the same method could be used for a large hole into the oral cavity or oropharynx.

The use of the pectoralis major musculocutaneous flap is the most reliable method available now and suits 9 out of 10 such fistulae.

Mark and elevate a pectoralis musculocutaneous flap as described on page 49. Make a horizontal incision over the clavicle to allow the flap to be brought up into the neck and develop a tunnel from this horizontal incision in a superomedial direction to allow the flap to be brought to the centre of the neck (Fig. 5.1A). Incise all around the edges of the fistula and bring up the flap which is turned upon itself, bringing the skin surface inwards so that it will form the anterior surface of the pharynx. Suture the edges of the skin island all around to the cut edges of the fistula (Fig. 5.1B). Now develop a pocket all around the fistula about 2 cm wide while undermining the skin all around it. Push the muscle edges into this pocket and fix them by non-absorbable sutures passing through the skin of the neck into the pocket,

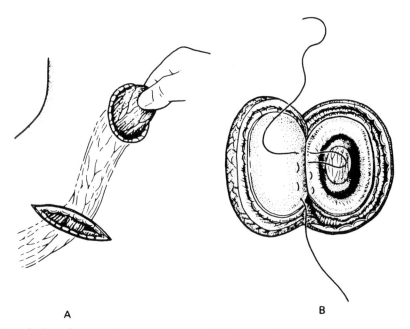

A   B

Fig. 5.1 (a) Flap brought through tunnel, skin surface inwards. (b) Suturing of skin paddle to edge of fistula.

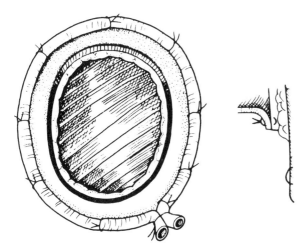

Fig. 5.2 Fixation of muscle of flap into subcutaneous tunnel.

through the muscle and out through the skin of the neck again; fasten them over rubber tubing to anchor them (Fig. 5.2). Finally, cover the outer muscle surface with a split-thickness skin graft.

Complications of radiotherapy

Acute effects

In general terms, the reactions following a course of radiotherapy can be divided into two categories – *acute* effects and *late* effects.

Acute effects occur during or shortly after the course of treatment. They are due to the killing of cells in tissues with a rapid turnover, such as mucous membranes, skin, bone marrow and gut epithelium. Enough stem cells should, however, remain alive to repopulate the tissue, and so acute effects are usually transient, leaving no permanent damage. Nevertheless, acute effects can cause considerable distress to the patient and must be taken seriously. In the treatment of head and neck malignancy, the principal acute reaction is mucositis, while the cutaneous reaction is of lesser importance. Haemopoietic disturbance and diarrhoea, which may result from irradiation of bone marrow and intestinal epithelium respectively, are not encountered in this setting.

Mucositis

As mucositis develops, it progresses through various stages. Initially there is erythema with oedema, then an adherent fibrinous exudate appears in patches which coalesce to form a confluent membrane. In severe cases this may be followed by ulceration. The reaction usually commences halfway through a 4-

week course of treatment, and gradually settles over the fortnight after completion of therapy.

The major determinant of the severity of mucositis from the patient's point of view is the amount of mucous membrane irradiated, and this in turn is dependent on the site and extent of the tumour being treated. For example, the radiation fields used on a patient with early glottic carcinoma will be approximately 5 × 5 cm and the reaction will be limited to a small section of the larynx and hypopharynx, resulting only in a mild dysphagia which is unlikely to cause any difficulty in eating or drinking. In contrast, the patient with nasopharyngeal carcinoma requires irradiation not just of the primary tumour, but also the neck nodes on both sides. The mucosa lining the nasopharynx, oropharynx, hypopharynx, larynx, posterior oral cavity and posterior nasal fossa is inevitably included in the treatment volume, and the resulting discomfort will be severe. The patient's condition must be monitored regularly during and immediately after the treatment, a soft diet is often preferred and nutritional supplements may be required. If the patient is unable to maintain an adequate oral intake of food and fluid, consideration should be given to feeding via a fine-bore nasogastric tube. This is better undertaken at the first signs of nutritional compromise, rather than left until the patient's condition deteriorates.

The duration of a course of treatment is another important factor affecting the severity of mucositis. With short overall treatment times of 3–4 weeks, reactions tend to be more severe, and a confluent fibrinous membrane usually forms over the treated area. With protracted fractionation over 6–7 weeks membranous reactions are less commonly seen, and because of this such schedules are often considered preferable when large areas of mucosa are to be irradiated. At one time it was the vogue to have a pause in treatment for perhaps 2 weeks halfway through the course to allow the mucosal reaction to subside. Unfortunately such 'split courses' allow the tumour, as well as the mucosa, to recover and this practice is therefore deplored.

The cessation of smoking and avoidance of alcohol and highly spiced food help to minimize the acute mucosal reaction. In addition, meticulous oral hygiene is essential, and Difflam mouthwashes may help. If the larynx is being treated, it is best for the patient to rest the voice. Painful dysphagia may be eased by the use of an antacid/topical anaesthetic mixture, e.g. Mucaine.

Skin reaction

The skin goes through a similar sequence of reactions to mucous membrane following irradiation. Initially there is erythema, then dry desquamation which may be followed by moist desquamation and finally ulceration. In times past, when orthovoltage was the only type of external beam irradiation available and the skin received a high radiation dose, the cutaneous reaction was severe, and could be dose-limiting. With the advent of megavoltage irradiation, however, the skin no longer need receive the full dose, and cutaneous reactions rarely proceed beyond dry desquamation, unless bolus or tissue-equivalent build-up material is used to increase the dose to the skin, as may be necessary if the tumour is infiltrating it. Under these circumstances, moist desquamation is usual. Patients should be advised not to use cosmetics, and to wear soft loose clothing around the neck which will not abrade the skin. Dry shaving with an electric razor is advised in preference to wet shaving. Traditionally patients have been advised not to wash the affected area for the duration of treatment, but the need for this restriction has lately been questioned. Oilatum cream, or alternatively 1% hydrocortisone cream, can be used to soothe the irritation of dry desquamation.

Hair loss

Epilation will occur if hair-bearing skin is treated. As the face and neck are the most commonly treated areas in most forms of head and neck cancer, this is not often a problem, unless the patient has a beard. Although the scalp is rarely treated directly, patients must be warned that hairlessness may ensue if any of the beams enter or exit through the scalp. For example, the anterior field used to treat carcinoma of the maxillary antrum exits through the back of the head, and hair will be lost at this site. Depending on the dose received by the hair follicles, regrowth usually occurs in time.

Salivary function

The flow rapidly dwindles when salivary gland tissue is irradiated, and the saliva itself becomes sticky and tenacious. Some functional recovery may occur, but this takes months or years, and is rarely complete. Loss of saliva is very uncomfortable for the patient, especially during the acute mucosal reaction, it disturbs the sense of taste and makes dental caries more likely following treatment. For these reasons, care should be taken to minimize the volume of salivary gland which is irradiated. It is usually possible to spare completely a large part of at least one gland. However, when both parotid glands and many minor glands have to be included, as is necessary when treating nasopharyngeal cancer for example, xerostomia has to be accepted as inevitable.

The eye

Because of the risk of late effects on the lens and retina, the eye is avoided if at all possible. If it is necessary to treat the eye and orbit, then acute side-effects have to be considered and minimized. The lacrimal gland should be shielded if possible, and the eye should be treated taped open, to diminish the dose to the conjunctiva. A small block can sometimes be used to protect the cornea.

Late effects
Bone

With orthovoltage irradiation, the absorption of ionizing radiation is greater in bone than soft tissue. So when an adequate tumour dose is given with orthovoltage, the dose absorbed by adjacent bone is often excessive, leading to the possibility of osteoradionecrosis. Following irradiation, although the bone might seem healthy, its situation is in fact precarious, and any insult may precipitate necrosis. The most vulnerable bone in this regard is the mandible, and extraction of a tooth is often enough to provoke necrosis. Because, moreover, many patients with head and neck cancer have bad dentition at presentation which might be made worse by radiation-induced xerostomia, dental clearance prior to radiotherapy of the oral cavity used to be recommended. With modern megavoltage irradiation, the dose absorbed by bone is not excessive, and osteoradionecrosis is now seen only rarely. If necrosis is encountered now, it is usually associated with invasion of bone by tumour. Since megavoltage irradiation is now used exclusively, clearance of healthy teeth is not required, although any diseased teeth should receive appropriate treatment before radiotherapy.

Soft tissue

Depending on the dose received, there may be some depigmentation, atrophy and telangiectasia of the skin and mucous membranes. Fibrosis may develop in muscle and connective tissue, particularly if a high dose was received. Fibrosis in the neck can be difficult to distinguish from recurrent nodal disease.

Neural tissue

The brain, brainstem and spinal cord can tolerate reasonably large doses of irradiation without ill effect, but if the limit is exceeded, the effects can be devastating. For this reason the dose to adjacent neural tissue is always considered in the planning of radiotherapy for head and neck cancer. In many of the treatment plans illustrating this book the brainstem and spinal cord have been marked on as critical structures which must not be allowed to receive more than a certain dose. The precise tolerance dose varies, depending on the size and site of the irradiated neural tissue, and on the fractionation schedule and radiation quality. As a general rule, for a given total dose, large fraction sizes are more likely to cause late effects in neural tissue, and so more protracted fractionation regimens tend to be preferred where part of the central nervous system is to be irradiated.

The eye

The lens of the eye is among the most radiosensitive structures in the body – very low total doses are required to cause a cataract. For this reason the eye is completely excluded from irradiation if possible. If it is deemed impossible to spare the eye completely, the subsequent development of a cataract may be accepted in the knowledge that this is a treatable complication. It is still, however, necessary to keep the dose to the eye as low as possible to prevent damage to the retina, which is a moderately radiosensitive structure.

Complications of chemotherapy

The complications of chemotherapy depend on the drug or combination used. Some side-effects such as nausea, vomiting, alopecia and myelosuppression occur with most, although not all cytotoxic drugs. Other side-effects are associated with particular drugs. The occurrence of complications depends not only on the drugs used, but their dose and scheduling, and on the concomitant use of radiotherapy.

General side-effects of cytotoxic drugs

Nausea and vomiting commonly accompany the use of many cytotoxics, and patients often find this the most distressing aspect of chemotherapy. The platinum drugs are the most highly emetogenic, with cisplatin worse than carboplatin. In addition to the acute vomiting at the time of treatment, patients are often nauseated and anorexic for 4 or 5 days afterwards. A high-dose metaclopramide infusion, perhaps in association with dexamethasone or lorazepam, has some effect in preventing platinum emesis, but carries the risk of dystonic reactions and should be supervised in hospital by experienced staff. Recently, new antiemetics such as ondansetron, which act by blocking the 5-hydroxytryptamine-3 receptor, have been found to be effective but cost considerations have limited their use in some hospitals. Other drugs such as cyclophosphamide, especially at lower doses, are likely to cause less severe sickness than platinum compounds, and conventional doses of metoclopramide or prochloperazine are often adequate. Some drugs used against head and neck cancer, such as vincristine and bleomycin, do not as a rule lead to sickness.

Alopecia

Unlike most cytotoxic agents, many of the drugs used against squamous cancer, such as cisplatin, bleomycin and 5-fluorouracil, do not cause hair loss. As the majority of head and neck cancer patients are elderly men, hair loss is less of a problem than it is for women with breast or ovarian cancer receiving chemotherapy. If troublesome hair loss does occur, then a wig may be prescribed.

Myelosuppression

For the clinician, bone marrow toxicity can be the most worrying problem when administering cytotoxic chemotherapy, as both neutropenia and thrombocytopenia may be rapidly fatal. Fortunately, while all cytotoxics except vincristine and bleomycin affect the bone marrow, most of the regimens used against head and neck cancer do not produce profound myelosuppression. Nevertheless a full blood count must be checked on each occasion before cytotoxics are administered. In addition, a patient who develops pyrexia or other signs of infection following chemotherapy must have a blood count performed without delay to ensure that there is not an underlying leukopenia. This is most likely to occur 7–10 days after treatment and hospitalization for bacteriological tests and broad-spectrum parenteral antibiotics are required.

Extravasation of cytotoxic drugs

Several cytotoxic drugs may cause severe tissue necrosis if they leak into the tissues during intravenous injection. As this can lead to the need for repair with skin grafting, the greatest care should be taken to ensure that extravasation does not occur in the first place. Intravenous cytotoxic drugs are best given into a newly sited freely running infusion in the forearm. The antecubital fossa should be avoided, as significant extravasation can occur here without it being immediately apparent. If pain occurs on injection, or if there is any doubt about leakage into the tissues, the infusion should be stopped immediately, and resited.

Specific drug toxicities
Methotrexate

Methotrexate, which is an antimetabolite inhibiting the enzyme dihydrofolate reductase, is widely used in head and neck cancer. In this situation, conventional doses, measured in milligrams, are used. High-dose treatment, using grams of methotrexate, is undergoing experimental evaluation in, for example, osteosarcoma treatment. In addition to myelosuppression, the principal side-effect is mucositis which is worse if the drug is given concomitantly with irradiation. Methotrexate is excreted through the kidney and may be toxic to the liver. Renal and hepatic function should therefore be checked before methotrexate is used, and if significant impairment is found this drug should be avoided. Its use is also contraindicated in the presence of pleural effusions or ascites, which may act as a 'third space', delaying excretion and enhancing myelotoxicity. Serum methotrexate levels should be checked 24 h after administration of the drug if there is any renal insufficiency or high-dose regimens have been used. If the blood level is elevated above normal limits, folinic acid must be given to terminate the action of methotrexate, and should be continued until acceptable blood methotrexate levels are reached. Alternatively, if facilities for monitoring drug levels are not available, folinic acid 'rescue' can be given routinely.

5-Fluorouracil

The drug 5-fluorouracil may be given either as an intravenous bolus injection, as an infusion over several days, or occasionally orally and is relatively non-toxic. In addition to myelosuppression, its principal side-effects are mucositis and diarrhoea, which are more common if a prolonged infusion is used.

Vinca alkaloids

Vincristine is the most commonly used vinca alkaloid. Drugs of this group interfere with mitosis causing metaphase arrest, yet their side-effects are markedly different. With vincristine, neurotoxicity, manifested as a peripheral or autonomic neuropathy, is relatively common. This usually takes the form of paraesthesiae or numbness in the fingers and toes, or abdominal bloating and constipation. If these symptoms are more than mild, the drug should be withdrawn and gradual improvement should take place. Neuropathy is rare with vinblastine – the principal adverse effect of which is myelosuppression – unlike vincristine which is only rarely associated with bone marrow suppression. The third drug of this group, vindesine, has adverse effects intermediate between those of vincristine and vinblastine.

Platinum compounds

Cisplatin, cis-diamino, dichloroplatinum or CDDP, was the first platinum drug to be introduced. It is among the most toxic of anticancer drugs available, producing profound and often prolonged emesis, nephrotoxicity, ototoxicity and neurotoxicity. Renal function should be checked prior to each course of treatment by a creatinine clearance rather than just estimation of urea and electrolytes. Intravenous hydration before, during and after cisplatin adminis-

tration is mandatory, and mannitol is often given concomitantly, in order to diminish renal toxicity. Hypomagnesaemia may occur, and so magnesium supplements are often given with the infusion. The neurotoxicity usually takes the form of a peripheral neuropathy. Pretreatment audiograms are usually recommended to provide a baseline against which ototoxicity can be assessed. Any of these adverse effects may necessitate dose reduction or withdrawal, especially if the drug is being used for palliation rather than as a treatment with curative intent. Cisplatin is relatively non-myelotoxic, and its principal effect on bone marrow is often to produce anaemia rather than thrombocytopenia or neutropenia. The newer analogue, carboplatin, is considerably more myelotoxic, yet emesis, ototoxicity, nephrotoxicity and neurotoxicity are less common than with cisplatin.

Bleomycin

Bleomycin is the most commonly used cytotoxic antibiotic in the treatment of head and neck cancer. It is unusual in that it is not myelosuppressive. The principal acute side-effect is a flu-like hypersensitivity reaction with chills, fever and rigors occurring a few hours after administration. This can be prevented by giving the drug under cover of hydrocortisone. Skin changes are relatively common with bleomycin, and may take the form of increased flexural pigmentation or sclerotic subcutaneous plaques. The most serious adverse effect with bleomycin is the development of pulmonary fibrosis. This is dose-related, more common in the elderly, and can be progressive. Suspicious changes on the chest radiograph or isolated basal crepitations are indications to stop treatment with the drug. Anaesthetists should be warned if patients have received high total doses of bleomycin, as respiratory failure may be precipitated if a general anaesthetic is given with high concentrations of inspired oxygen.

General recommendations for the use of cytotoxic chemotherapy

It can be seen from the possible adverse reactions cited above that anticancer chemotherapy is hazardous and may even be fatal. For this reason it is strongly recommended that these drugs should only be prescribed by those with appropriate training and experience in their use, and should only be administered in units where there are the necessary expertise and facilities to prevent avoidable toxicity and to provide optimal care of the patient with inescapable treatment-related morbidity.

References and further reading

Surgery

Bird A G, Gore S M, Leigh-Brown A J, Carter D C (1991) Escape from collective denial: HIV transmission during surgery. *Br Med J* **303**:351–2.

Brook I, Hirokawa R (1989) Microbiology of wound infection after head and neck cancer surgery. *Ann Otol Rhinol Laryngol* **98**:323–5.

Gerberding J L, Littell C, Tarkington A, Brown A, Schechter W P (1990) Risk of exposure of surgical personnel to patients' blood during surgery in San Francisco General Hospital. *N Engl J Med* **332**:1788–93.

Glaister D H, Hearnshaw J R, Heffron P F, Peck A W (1958) The mechanism of postparotidectomy gustatory sweating (the auriculo-temporal syndrome). *Br Med J* **2**:942–6.

Gluckman J L, McDonough J J, McCafferty G J et al. (1985) Complications associated with free jejunal graft reconstruction of the pharyngoesophagus – a multi-institutional experience with 52 cases. *Head Neck Surg* **7**:200–5.

Griebie M S, Adams G L (1987) 'Emergency' laryngectomy and stomal recurrence. *Laryngoscope* **97**:1020–4.

Hamblen D, Newton G (1990) HIV and surgeons. *Br Med J* **301**:1216–17.

Harness J K, Fung L, Thompson N W, Burney R E, Mcleod M K (1986) Total thyroidectomy: complications and technique. *World J Surg* **10**:781–6.

Hinton A E, Herdman R C, Timms M S (1991) Incidence and prevention of conjunctival contamination with blood during hazardous surgical procedures. *Ann R Coll Surg Engl* **73**:239–42.

Johansen L V, Overgaard J, Elbrond O (1988) Pharyngocutaneous fistulae after laryngectomy. *Cancer* **61**:673–8.

Kennedy P J, Poole A G (1989) Excision of the submandibular gland: minimising the risk of nerve damage. *Aust NZ J Surg* **59**:411–14.

McGuirt W F, McCabe B F, Krause C J (1979) Complications of radical neck dissection: a survey of 788 patients. *Head Neck Surg* **1**:481–7.

Milton C M, Thomas B M, Bickerton R C (1986) Morbidity study of submandibular gland excision. *Ann R Coll Surg Engl* **68**:148–51.

Ujiki G T, Pearl G J, Poticha S, Sisson G A, Shields T W (1987) Mortality and morbidity of gastric 'pull-up' for replacement of the pharyngoesophagus. *Arch Surg* **122**:644–7.

Wei W I, Lam K H, Choi S, Wong J (1984) Late problems after pharyngolaryngoesophagectomy and pharyngogastric anastomosis for cancer of the larynx and hypopharynx. *Am J Surg* **148**:809–13.

Weingrad D N, Spiro R H (1983) Complications after laryngectomy. *Am J Surg* **146**:517–20.

Wingert D J, Friesen S R, Iliopoulos J I, Pierce G E, Thomas J H, Hermreck A S (1986) Post-thyroidectomy hypocalcaemia: incidence and risk factors. *Am J Surg* **152**:606–10.

Radiotherapy

Campbell B H, Janjan N A, Byhardt R W, Toohill R J (1990) Treatment-related toxicities with Fluosol-DA 20% infusion during radiation in advanced head and neck malignancies. *Laryngoscope* **100**:237–9.

Dreizen S, Brown L R, Handler S, Levy B M (1976) Radiation–induced xerostomia in cancer patients. Effect on salivary and serum electrolytes. *Cancer* **38**:273–8.

Friedman M, Toriumi D M, Strorigl T, Grybauskas V T, Skolnik E (1988) Effects of therapeutic radiation on the development of multiple primary tumors of the head and neck. *Head Neck Surg* **Suppl I**:S48–51.

Lam K S L, Ho J H C, Lee A W M et al. (1987) Symptomatic hypothalmic–pituitary dysfunction in nasopharyngeal carcinoma patients following radiation therapy: a retrospective study. *Int J Radiat Oncol Biol Phys* **13**:1343–50.

Lindelov B, Lauritzen A F, Hausen H S (1990) Stage I glottic carcinoma: an analysis of tumour recurrence after primary radiotherapy. *Clin Oncol* **2**:94–6.

MacDougall R H, Orr J A, Kerr G R, Duncan W (1990) Fast neutron treatment for squamous cell carcinoma of the head and neck: final report of Edinburgh randomised trial. *Br Med J* **301**:1241–2.

Mintz D R, Gullane P J, Thomson D H, Ruby R R F (1981) Perichrondritis of the larynx following radiation. *Otolaryngol Head Neck Surg* **89**:550–4.

Modan B, Mart H, Baidatz D, Mast H, Steinitz R, Levin S G (1974) Radiation induced head and neck tumours. *Lancet* **1**:277–9.

O'Neill J V, Katz A H, Skolnik E M (1979) Otologic complications of radiation therapy. *Otolaryngol Head Neck Surg* **87**:359–63.

Parsons J T, Mendenhall W M, Cassissi N J, Stringer S P, Million R R (1989) Neck dissection after twice-a-day radiotherapy: morbidity and recurrence rates. *Head Neck Surg* **11**:400–4.

Thompson W B, Cassissi N J, Million R R (1987) Postoperative radiation of open head and neck wounds. *Laryngoscope* **97**:267–70.

Chemotherapy

Anonymous (1987) 5-HT3 receptor antagonists: a new class of antiemetics (editorial). *Lancet* **1**:1470–1.

Coates A, Abraham S, Kaye S B et al. (1983) On the receiving end – patients' perception of the side-effects of cancer chemotherapy. *Eur J Cancer Clin Oncol* **19**:203–8.

Jones A L, Hill A S, Soukop M et al. (1991) Comparison of dexamethasone and ondansetron in the prophylaxis of emesis induced by moderately emetogenic chemotherapy. *Lancet* **338**:483–7.

Kris M G, Gralla R J, Clark R A et al. (1985) Incidence, course and severity of delayed nausea and vomiting following the administration of high dose cisplatin. *J Clin Oncol* **3**:1379–84.

Morran C, Smith D C, Anderson D A, McArdle C S (1979) Incidence of nausea and vomiting with cytotoxic chemotherapy in a prospective randomised trial of antiemetics. *Br Med J* **1**:1323–5.

Plowman P N, McElwain T, Meadows A (eds) (1991) *Complications of Cancer Management.* Guildford, Butterworth-Heinemann.

6

Benign disease of the neck

This chapter is devoted to benign conditions in the neck, most of which cause a mass in the neck. Half of all neck masses seen in a general hospital are of thyroid origin, usually a toxic or non-toxic goitre. These will not be discussed in this chapter. A brief outline will be given of the other main causes of a lump in the neck. They can be classified as follows:

1 Congenital – lymphangiomas, dermoids, thyroglossal duct cysts, branchial cysts and branchial sinuses.
2 Developmental – laryngoceles, pharyngeal pouches.
3 Infective – bacterial, viral, tuberculous.
4 Neurogenous tumours – paragangliomas, peripheral nerve tumours.
5 Tumours of the parapharyngeal space.

Congenital neck masses

Lymphangiomas

Embryology

The lymph system arises from two jugular sacs, two posterior sciatic sacs and a single retroperitoneal sac. Endothelial outbuddings from these extend centrifugally to form the peripheral lymphatic system.

The probable cause of cystic hygroma (see below) is that endothelial fibrillar membranes sprout from the walls of the cyst, penetrate the surrounding tissue, canalize and produce more cysts. The pressure of the cysts forces the tumour along the lines of least resistance into planes or spaces between large muscles or vessels.

Pathology

Lymphangiomas are of three types:

1 Simple lymphangioma, consisting of thin-walled, capillary-sized lymphatic channels – 40%.

2 Cavernous lymphangioma, consisting of dilated lymphatic spaces – 35%.
3 Cystic hygroma, composed of cysts of various sizes – 25%.

It may be that there is no essential difference between these three, and that their apparent difference is due to their site.

Simple lymphangiomas and cavernous lymphangiomas occur in the lips, tongue, cheek and floor of the mouth, where the tissue planes are relatively tight. A cystic hygroma arises mainly in the neck where it has more space to expand into, and where the tissue planes are looser. It can spread from the neck into the cheek, floor of mouth, tongue, parotid and ear canal.

Thirty five per cent of all lymphangiomas occur in the cheek, tongue and floor of mouth, 25% in the neck and 15% in the axilla. There is no sex or side predominance. Two out of three cystic hygromas are noted at birth, three out of four before the end of the first year, and nine out of 10 before the end of the second year.

Clinical features

Most of these tumours are noted at or shortly after birth. They can present for the first time in adult life in the mouth, as can recurrences of cystic hygromas operated on originally in infancy.

If size alone is the prominent first symptom, the cyst can interfere with breathing causing stridor; in this case the trachea is seen to be displaced on radiographs and there may be widening of the mediastinum. Brachial plexus compression with pain and hyperaesthesia may also occur. Sudden increase in size due to haemorrhage may be fatal.

Treatment

The treatment of cystic hygroma and the other lymphangiomas is excision. Sclerosant injection, and incision and drainage, are worthless because only one of numerous cysts can be dealt with, and incision can provoke life-threatening infection.

No operation should be done without a preoperative chest radiograph to rule out mediastinal involvement. Damage to the facial, hypoglossal and accessory nerves may be difficult to avoid and so a nerve stimulator should be used. Because of the enormous skin stretching, and interference with the mandibular branch of the facial nerve, a good cosmetic result is difficult to achieve. Excision of excess skin will usually be needed. Multiple excisions may be needed over several years.

Intraoral lymphangiomas should be removed from an external approach because they will almost certainly be more extensive than expected.

The recurrence rate after excision of a cystic hygroma is 10–15% and usually becomes obvious within 9 months. Recurrence of cavernous lymphangiomas is more common than that of cystic hygromas.

Problems

Intraoral lymphangiomas can be confused with ranulas, of which there are two types. The simple ranula is a retention cyst arising from a minor salivary gland in the floor of the mouth. It is unilocular and relatively thick-walled; it is therefore easy to excise. The plunging ranula is probably part of a cystic hygroma. It is very thin-walled and invades the upper part of the neck, penetrating between the muscles. It is very difficult to excise completely.

Midline dermoids
Pathology

In the head and neck there are three varieties:

1 The epidermoid cyst, which has no adnexal structures. It is lined by squamous epithelium and contains cheesy keratinous material. This is the commonest variety.
2 The true dermoid cyst, which is lined by squamous epithelium and contains skin appendages such as hair, hair follicles, sebaceous glands and sweat glands. These can be congenital or acquired: the former type occurs along lines of fusion and the latter is due to implantation of epidermis at the time of a puncture wound.
3 The teratoid cyst is lined either by squamous or respiratory epithelium, and contains elements from ectoderm, endoderm and mesoderm – nails, teeth, brain, glands, etc. This is the rarest variety.

Only 2% of dermoid tumours rise in the neck, always in the midline. They form 20% of all midline neck cysts. There is no sex predominance.

Clinical features

These cysts present as solid or cystic masses in the midline of the neck between the suprasternal notch and the submental region. Painless swelling is the only symptom and obstructive symptoms are rare.

Treatment

The only treatment is complete local excision.

Thyroglossal duct cysts
Embryology

The thyroid anlage arises from the floor of the primitive pharynx between the first and second pharyngeal pouches. Originally hollow, it becomes solid as it migrates to the lower neck, the lower end dividing into two portions that become the thyroid lobes. The stalk should atrophy at the sixth week but if it persists it becomes the thyroglossal duct in which cysts can develop. It runs from the thyroid gland behind, through or in front of the hyoid bone and ends deeply at the foramen caecum of the tongue.

Pathology

There is no sex predominance and the mean age at presentation is 5 years (range 4 months – 70 years). Ninety per cent are midline and 10% lie laterally; of the latter 95% are on the left side and 5% on the right.

Three out of four cysts are prehyoid and the rest lie at the level of the thyroid cartilage, the cricoid cartilage or above the hyoid.

Spontaneous fistula formation is rare, a fistula usually being due to an attempted drainage of a misdiagnosed abscess or to an inadequate excision leaving the hyoid bone intact. A fistula is present in 15% of patients when first seen.

Clinical features

This is the commonest midline neck cyst: 95% present with a painless cystic lump that moves on swallowing or protruding the tongue. It is mobile in all directions and can usually be transilluminated. Five per cent present with tenderness and rapid enlargement due to infection.

Treatment

Treatment is by excision, including the body of the hyoid bone between the lesser horns, after the duct has been dissected to this area.

In a fistula or revision operation, the mouth of the fistula is excised in an ellipse: a double Z-plasty often gives a better cosmetic result than simple closure.

Problems

The main cause of difficulty is failure to remove the body of the hyoid bone. Incredibly, patients are still seen with recurrent thyroglossal cysts in which this essential step has been omitted.

Another unusual problem is a carcinoma in a thyroglossal cyst. This is dealt with in Chapter 7.

Branchial cysts

Embryology

There are at least four theories of origin of branchial cyst but because of the complicated development of the region none has been proven.

The *branchial apparatus theory* suggests that branchial cysts represent remains of pharyngeal pouches or branchial clefts, or a fusion of these two elements. According to this theory, cysts arise from the first pouch and have an internal opening between the bony and cartilaginous parts of the external meatus, or from the second pouch, opening at the posterior pillar at the base of the tonsil. Origin from the third and fourth pouch is unlikely because internal openings would have to be at the level of the pyriform sinus or below. Furthermore, branchial cysts are not associated with tracks or openings into the pharynx. If this theory were correct, more cysts would be present at birth. Not only has this only been described once but the peak age incidence is the third decade, which is late for a congenital lesion (cf. thyroglossal duct cyst).

The *cervical sinus theory* is an extension of the previous one and considers that branchial cysts represent remains of the cervical sinus of His, which is formed by the second arch growing down to meet the fifth.

The *thymopharyngeal duct theory* suggests that cysts are remnants of the original connection between the thymus and the third branchial pouch from which it takes origin. As a persistent thymic duct has never been described and no branchial cyst has ever been reported deep to the thyroid gland, this theory is very unlikely.

The *inclusion theory* suggests that there is not enough evidence to show that cysts arise from the branchial apparatus and goes on to suggest that the cysts are the result of epithelial inclusions in lymph nodes.

Supporting this theory is the fact that most branchial cysts have lymphoid tissue in the wall and that they have been described in the parotid gland and pharynx. This theory also explains why branchial cysts have no internal opening.

Pathology

Branchial cysts are usually lined by stratified squamous epithelium, and 80% have lymphoid tissue in the wall. They contain straw-coloured fluid in which cholesterol crystals are found.

Clinical features

The male:female ratio is 3:2 and the peak age incidence is the third decade (range 1–70 years). Two out of three are on the left side and one in three on the right; 2% are bilateral. Two out of three lie anterior to the sternomastoid in the upper third of the neck and the remainder are found in the middle and lower neck, the parotid, the pharynx and the posterior triangle. In 80% the swelling is persistent; in the remainder it may be intermittent. Pain is a feature in 30% and infection in 15%. Seventy per cent are cystic; 30% feel solid.

Treatment

Treatment is by excision (Fig. 6.1). Make a transverse incision through platysma and elevate flaps superiorly and inferiorly keeping platysma in the skin flap. The incision should be generous – about 3 in (about 7 cm) long. Divide the fascia on the anterior border of the sternomastoid and retract it laterally. Identify the cyst – it is very important to avoid rupturing it as removal after this accident is rather difficult. Free it anteriorly, inferiorly, superiorly and medially with a knife and elevate the tail of the parotid gland if necessary. If the lower pole of the gland has to be elevated then it is best to find the mandibular branch of the facial nerve and follow it backwards through the gland substance to preserve it. Then remove the cyst *in toto* – there is no need to look for an associated track.

Controversial points

The only point of controversy about branchial cysts is that they are often confused with branchial sinuses; in particular they are often described as having a track. However, careful questioning has failed to reveal a single surgeon who has ever seen this mythical track.

Branchial sinus

This is an entirely different entity from a branchial cyst. It is of congenital origin and consists of a skin-lined track, opening internally in the tonsillar fossa, and externally at the anterior border of the sterno-mastoid muscle, at the junction of its middle and lower third. It virtually always presents in young infants as a discharging sinus.

A branchial sinus should be excised in a step-ladder fashion, removing the mouth of the pit in an ellipse. Follow the track upwards – it takes a rather sharp bend upwards in most cases. It travels above the hypoglossal nerve and between the internal and

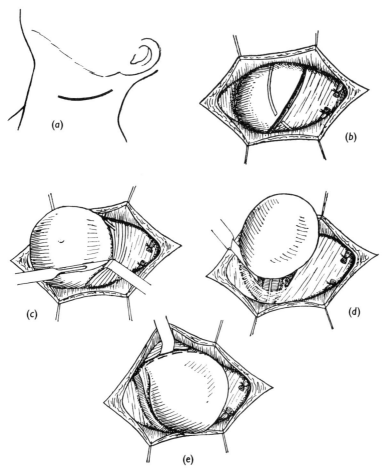

Fig. 6.1 (a) Incision for removal of branchial cyst; (b) beginning of dissection medial to sternomastoid; (c) cyst freed laterally; (d) cyst freed medially; (e) cyst freed superiorly.

external carotid arteries, usually below the postauricular and occipital branches of the external carotid. Thus no arterial branches need to be tied, but the nerve must be identified. In other instances the track goes up towards the ear, and in this condition it is necessary to remove the superficial lobe of the parotid gland. Once this lobe is removed, finding the rest of the track is easy. It may be found to enter the junction of the cartilaginous and bony external auditory meatus. Some indication of this may be gained before operation if the patient also complains occasionally of a discharging ear, for which no middle-ear cause can be found.

The most important complication of this procedure is division of, or damage to, the hypoglossal nerve. This is most likely to happen if one of the pharyngeal veins is cut and blind attempts are made to secure haemostasis. The nerve is likely to be caught in the end of artery forceps that have not been applied properly, as these pharyngeal veins disappear medially behind the hypoglossal nerve. It is unlikely that any damage will be caused to the carotid artery if care is taken; provided the operator realizes where the track goes, damage should be avoided. The facial nerve can also be damaged, especially the mandibular branch, but this will be avoided if the previous steps described have been taken.

Developmental neck masses

Laryngocele

Pathology

The incidence is only 1 per 2.5 million population per year. The sex incidence is 5 : 1 in favour of men, and the peak age incidence is in the sixth decade. Four out of five are unilateral. They can be external (30%) and expand through the thyrohyoid membrane, internal (20%) and present in the vallecula, or combined (50%).

There is no evidence to show that 'blowing' hobbies, or jobs such as trumpet-playing or glass-blowing, cause laryngoceles. Lower animals have air sacs and it is considered that laryngoceles in humans represent atavistic remnants of these. Blowing hobbies increase the intralaryngeal air pressure and bring otherwise symptomless laryngoceles to light.

Of more importance is the coexistence of a carcinoma of the larynx, which acts as a valve allowing air under pressure into the ventricle. External laryngoceles are said to be found in 1 in 6 laryngectomy specimens removed for laryngeal carcinoma, as opposed to 1 in 50 specimens removed for pyriform sinus cancer. The difficulty in interpreting this statement is the absence of a definition of the level at which an enlarged saccule becomes a laryngocele.

Clinical features

Hoarseness and neck swelling are the commonest presenting features. Others are stridor, sore throat, snoring, pain or cough. One in 10 present with infected sacs – pyoceles.

On palpation the swelling over the thyrohyoid membrane can be easily emptied. Plain radiographs show the air-filled sac in all cases.

Treatment

Laryngoceles ought to be removed, for they enlarge and eventually obstruct the larynx. Through a collar incision over the thyroid cartilage, find the sac and follow it downwards. To expose the neck of the sac, elevate the perichondrium from the upper half of the thyroid cartilage on the same side. Remove the upper half of the thyroid cartilage, which allows the sac to be removed at its origin from the saccule (Fig. 6.2). Divide the sac at its neck and stitch it as in a hernia repair. Replace the periochondrium over the defect and close the wound.

A pyocele should be treated with antibiotics before surgery.

Problems

The difference between an enlarged saccule and a laryngocele has not been defined. Therefore, we propose that the upper border of the thyroid cartilage should be taken as the dividing line. This point is of practical importance, for enlarged saccules can be found on a plain radiograph of the neck during the Valsalva manoeuvre in quite a large proportion of patients with hoarseness. If these are small (i.e. below the upper border of the thyroid cartilage), exploration is usually futile. Whether these large saccules ever develop into true laryngoceles, how many of them do so, and whether these patients should be followed up, is unknown.

Pharyngeal pouch
Pathology

There are many types of pharyngeal diverticula but the commonest type is the pulsion diverticulum of the posterior wall passing through Killian's dehiscence.

The cause is unknown but it is thought that it is related to a disorder of swallowing. The cricopharyn-

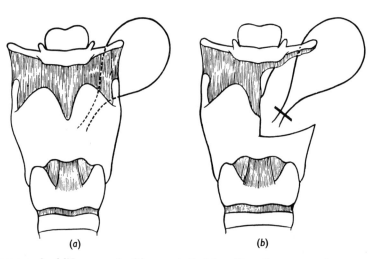

Fig. 6.2 Removal of laryngocele. (a) Laryngocele; (b) upper half of thyroid cartilage removed to expose neck of laryngocele.

geus is normally closed but opens naturally during swallowing. Manometric studies in patients with pharyngeal pouches have failed to show cricopharyngeal spasm. Manofluorometric analysis has, however, shown a restriction of upper sphincter opening. This may result in an area of increased pressure in the hypopharynx and a herniation of mucosa above the cricopharyngeus through the dehiscence of Killian.

Clinical features

Pouches are more commonly seen in the elderly. Presenting symptoms are dysphagia, halitosis, regurgitation of undigested food, weight loss, cough, occasional hoarseness and recurrent chest infection due to aspiration. A neck mass is rare.

A barium swallow demonstrates the pouch in all cases. Oesophagoscopy is necessary in every patient: firstly, to exclude a carcinoma; secondly, to look for a hiatus hernia, which often coexists; thirdly, to pass a feeding tube; and fourthly, to pack the pouch immediately before the operation. The oesophagoscope usually enters the pouch and it may be difficult to pass it over the bar that separates the pouch from the mouth of the oesophagus.

Treatment

Unless the pouch is a tiny incidental radiological finding it will require treatment.

Endoscopic diathermy has given good results in some hands but the best results are obtained by inversion and myotomy for all but the biggest pouches which require excision. If the patient is unfit for external surgery he or she is also unfit for endoscopic surgery, which must often be repeated.

To facilitate dissection and identification pack the pouch with acriflavine gauze before exploration.

Approach the pouch through a collar incision, preferably on the left side of the neck, at the level of the cricoid cartilage, that is, the level of origin of the neck of the sac (Fig. 6.3). Divide the skin and platysma, elevate superior and inferior flaps, and retract them with Joll's clamp, and use side towels. Divide the fascia along the anterior border of the sternomastoid muscle and dissect down to the prevertebral fascia between the carotid sheath and the central structures of the neck, dividing the omohyoid muscle. The pouch should be found easily, lying posterior to the oesophagus. Dissect the pouch free of the surrounding tissues (Fig. 6.3d) until its neck can be seen. Define the fibres of the cricopharyngeus muscle immediately inferior to the neck of the sac, and divide them posteriorly with scissors at this

stage. The neck of the sac will be found to be about 3 cm long.

If the pouch can be inverted into the pharyngeal lumen without opening it, this is the best treatment. Invert the pouch and oversew the site from which it arose using a polyglycol or non-absorbable suture. If the pouch is too big to invert, it must be excised. Before removing the sac, place a stay suture at its inferior and superior ends. Then excise the sac, with scissors, about 5 mm from the oesophagus. Close the inner layer of the defect with Connell's sutures, one beginning at the superior stay suture and proceeding about halfway down the defect, and the other beginning at the inferior end and proceeding superiorly to meet the point where the superior suture ended. Superior and inferior sutures are then tied to each other, cut and the end allowed to fall into the oesophageal lumen. Insert a second layer of 3/0 catgut or 3/0 black silk in a continuous running suture to reinforce this first suture line. Wash out the wound and close it with a continuous suction drain.

An alternative method to formal excision and closure of the defect is to staple the neck of the pouch with one of the 'guns' now available, and then to cut the pouch off distal to this.

Problems

The main problem in this operation is the avoidance of complications. All large series show that primary healing after routine excision is far from usual. At least one-third of these patients still suffer major complications such as infection, fistula, stenosis and vocal cord paralysis. The incidence of these can be dramatically reduced by inversion rather than excision of the pouch.

For some reason many surgeons are resistant to doing a myotomy. Why, is not clear: it is easy to do, it has no deleterious effects, and failure to do so commonly leads to recurrence.

A carcinoma in a pharyngeal pouch is dealt with in Chapter 7.

Infective neck masses

Parapharyngeal abscess

Surgical anatomy

The parapharyngeal space extends from the base of the skull to the level of the hyoid bone, where it is bounded by the sheath of the submandibular gland. Laterally lie the lateral pterygoid muscle and the sheath of the parotid gland, medially the pharynx, and posteriorly the carotid sheath.

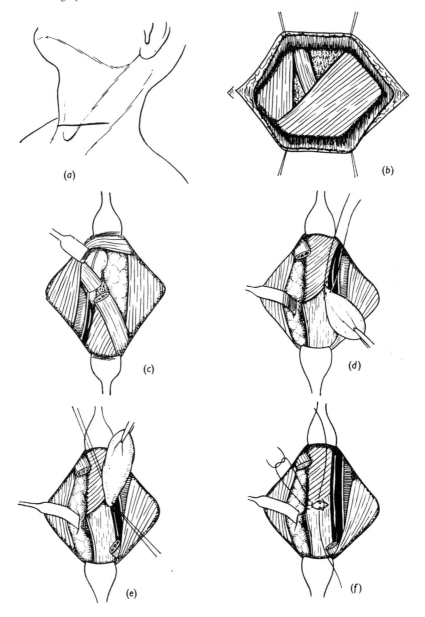

Fig. 6.3 Removal of pharyngeal pouch. (a) Incision line; (b) beginning of dissection medial to sternomastoid; (c) retraction of carotid sheath and sternomastoid muscle – omohyoid divided; (d) recurrent laryngeal nerve exposed – thyroid retracted medially, pouch exposed; (e) neck of pouch dissected out; (f) repair of pharyngeal defect.

Surgical pathology

The commonest neck swelling in children is an enlarged jugulodigastric lymph node secondary to tonsillitis. Although this can proceed to abscess formation the infection seldom extends to the parapharyngeal space. Parapharyngeal abscess is commoner in adults and is a complication of tonsillectomy or tonsillitis in 60% and of extraction of the lower third molar in a further 30%. The remaining 10% are due to extension of infection from the petrous apex or mastoid tip.

Clinical features

The temperature is elevated and the patient has marked trismus and pain. The tonsil is pushed medially but looks normal. The neck swelling is most marked at the posterior part of the middle third of the sternomastoid.

Treatment

Give the patient antibiotics for at least 48 h. If there is not a good response, incision and drainage will be required, the space being opened from a point medial to the mandible down to the clavicle. Leave the drain in for at least 72 h and continue antibiotics for 10 days.

Ludwig's angina

Surgical anatomy

The submandibular space lies below the floor of the mouth and tongue, and extends from the hyoid to the mandible. The space is divided into two by the mylohyoid muscle. The space above the muscle is called the sublingual space and contains the sublingual gland, the lingual and hypoglossal nerves and the submandibular duct. The space below the muscle is the submaxillary space, and it contains the gland.

Surgical pathology

The source of the infection is dental in 80% of cases, especially from the low molar and premolar teeth whose roots lie close to the lingual plate of the mandible; the roots of the second and third permanent molars lie below the mylohyoid line. If a dental root abscess drains into the space there will be little in the way of dental pain. The remaining 20% are due to soft tissue and tonsillar infection. The most usual microorganism in simple dental infection is *Streptococcus viridans*.

Clinical features

A brawny swelling affects the submental and submandibular regions. The floor of the mouth will become swollen and oedematous if the infection is in the sublingual space. The tongue may be pushed backwards causing respiratory obstruction. The temperature is elevated and the patient has pain, trismus and excessive salivation.

Treatment

Incision and drainage should be postponed as long as possible because pus is seldom found. Treat the patient with an antibiotic and analgesics. Tracheostomy is seldom necessary.

Tuberculous cervical adenitis

Pathology

In the western world most of the morbidity and mortality from tuberculosis are caused by postprimary pulmonary tuberculosis. The majority of cases occur in middle-aged and elderly subjects. Lymph node tuberculosis remains a very common manifestation elsewhere in the world, especially in Asians. The enlargement of the node is usually painless. When the node caseates and liquefies the swelling becomes fluctuant and sinus formation is common. The majority of infections are caused by *Mycobacterium tuberculosis* but *M. bovis*, endemic in cattle, can be spread to humans by milk. The primary infection of cervical tuberculosis is usually in the tonsil and in most people this and the associated lymph node lesions heal and calcify. Where healing is incomplete, haematogenous lesions may develop in the lungs, bones or kidneys, sometimes after many months.

Clinical features

The patient has usually had enlarged neck nodes for a long time and it is pain that brings him or her to see a doctor. However, in Asia about half the patients have sinus formation, skin involvement or cold abscesses when first seen.

Nine out of 10 cases are unilateral nodes and involve only one gland group – usually the deep jugular chain, although the posterior triangle nodes are often affected.

Diagnosis is by a positive skin test, demonstration of acid-fast bacilli in the lymph node biopsy and growth of *Mycobacterium tuberculosis* from the biopsy.

Treatment

Two clinical situations must be distinguished. The first is a patient with a single lump in the neck of unknown cause. If clinical investigations do not show a cause the mass is excised, half is sent for histology and half for culture for tuberculosis. If tuberculosis is confirmed the patient is treated with antituberculous chemotherapy. The second concerns the patient with multiple infected nodes with sinus formation, in whom the diagnosis is already known. Such a patient should be treated by antituberculous chemotherapy followed by excision of any residual disease. Short-course regimens lasting 6 or 9 months are now the usual choice in the west. For example, a 6-month course of ethambutol or streptomycin plus isoniazid plus rifampicin plus pyrazinamide for 2 months, followed by a 4-month course of isoniazid plus rifampicin. Less expensive regimes are more appropriate in developing countries but require to be continued for 12 months: for example, a combination of isoniazid and thiacetazone which can be given by daily oral doses. Other important considerations in management are isolation of patients who are excreting tubercle bacilli. Ziehl–Neelsen stain examination of sputum smears and tuberculin testing of family contacts.

AIDS

Head and neck manifestations of acquired immune deficiency syndrome (AIDS) include multicentric simple parotid cysts, benign lymphoid hyperplasia, cutaneous, oral or pharyngeal lesions of Kaposi's sarcoma, hairy leukoplakia and aerodigestive lesions of *Candida*. Pathologically, Kaposi's sarcoma lesions show an overgrowth of spindle cells in the dermis. There are intervening vascular clefts and thin vessels, with peripheral inflammatory and plasma cells – thus, peripheral biopsy may be non-diagnostic. Three histological patterns have been described: firstly, a monocellular pattern in which spindle cells predominate; secondly, a mixed pattern where spindle cells are admixed with endothelial cells, and finally an anaplastic form which is characterized by considerable pleomorphism, mitosis and areas of necrosis. Sometimes parotid enlargement is due to intraparotid lymph nodes which are usually enlarged by the same follicular hyperplasia that has been reported in other cervical nodes.

Kaposi's sarcoma was described in 1872 and was traditionally found in East Europeans, Africans or in immunosuppressed patients. African Kaposi's is not however human immunodeficiency virus (HIV)-related. Since 1981 the syndrome has increasingly been associated with homosexual males and is now recognized as one of the diagnostic criteria of AIDS. It may be a multifocal response to infection (? cytomegalovirus) rather than a true neoplasm. Almost half of the head and neck lesions are on the palate but the disease can occur on any site from the turbinates to the trachea. Clinically there are reddish-purple lesions which may be either single or multiple and occurring either on the skin or the mucosa. These may have the appearance of a macule, a papule, a nodule or an ulcer. The distribution of lesions in the upper body is of interest, as in the classical Kaposi's sarcoma, lesions affected the lower limbs in 75% of patients.

Gastrointestinal involvement also characterizes AIDS-related Kaposi's, although these lesions are usually asymptomatic. Pulmonary involvement by Kaposi's sarcoma is unusual but chronic cough and shortness of breath can be related to *Pneumocystis carinii* pneumonia or infection with *Mycobacterium avium*.

Treatment of Kaposi's sarcoma probably does not result in an increased life expectancy. Therapeutic indications therefore include obstruction of the airway or foodway, pain, bleeding or disfigurement. Radiotherapy to a dose of 16 Gy in four fractions over 4 days provides very good local control of skin lesions but this dosage results in a severe oral mucositis. The oral mucosa should not therefore be exposed to a fraction greater than 1 Gy and is probably best treated by chemotherapy, for example, vincristine, etoposide, cyclophosphamide,

adriamycin or bleomycin. A combination of vincristine in a 2 mg intravenous bolus with 30 mg bleomycin infused over 24 h every 3 weeks is reported to be well-tolerated and with a good response. The use of vinblastine as a single agent is associated with a 37% partial or complete remission. With the exception of vincristine and bleomycin all the drugs suggested cause myelosuppression. The use of vinblastine, for example, has been associated with a 22% incidence of opportunistic infection. Once a cumulative total dose of bleomycin of 210 mg has been reached the drug should be omitted and vincristine used alone, to prevent bleomycin-induced pulmonary toxicity.

Treatment of AIDS – related infection is problematic. In one series of patients with *P. carinii* pneumonia, only 15% were able to complete therapy with trimethoprim–sulphamethoxazole. This is because of the incidence of toxic reactions, including rashes, liver dysfunction and leukopenia. Treatment of disseminated *M. avium intracellulare* often requires up to six antituberculous drugs which most patients tolerate poorly. Patients with *Candida* oesophagitis and laryngitis often require ketoconazole and often amphotericin B. Progression to *Candida* septicaemia is associated with a mortality of nearly 50%.

Miscellaneous causes of lymphadenopathy

Toxoplasmosis

Toxoplasmosis is a worldwide infection caused by *Toxoplasma gondii*, a protozoon transmitted by the ingestion of cysts excreted in the faeces of infected cats, or from eating undercooked beef or lamb. The manifestations of congenital infection are principally cerebral, including hydrocephalus or microcephaly. Many patients with acquired toxoplasmosis are asymptomatic. Acute symptoms include generalized aches and pains, fever, cough, malaise and a maculopapular rash. In the more chronic form there may simply be lymphadenopathy. The peripheral blood picture shows lymphocytosis with some atypical mononuclear cells similar to those seen with Epstein–Barr infection. Reactivation of latent toxoplasmosis may cause encephalitis in immunocompromised patients. Diagnosis is confirmed by the presence of serum antibodies, by lymph node biopsy or by examination of the cerebrospinal fluid. Where treatment is indicated – in infants, immunosuppression or ocular involvement – a combination of sulphadimidine, pyrimethamine and folic acid is used and the blood count is monitored weekly.

Toxoplasmic encephalitis is now the most common cause of intracerebral mass lesions in patients with AIDS. The complication is estimated to develop in 25% of AIDS patients in much of western Europe and is thought to be due to reactivation of the chronic latent infection. Computed tomography typically shows multiple intraparenchymal lesions. Serological tests are usually negative.

Actinomycosis

This disease is now regarded as a bacterial infection and is caused by *Actinomycosis israelii*, an anaerobic organism which is a commensal in the healthy oral cavity. The organism may become pathogenic when the mucous membrane is injured. Infection usually affects the cervicofacial region and is nearly always associated with severe dental caries and periodontitis. Occasionally suppurative pneumonia and empyema may develop. A firm indurated mass with indefinite edges is found, usually lateral to the mandible. If untreated the mass spreads by direct invasion to adjacent tissue and becomes bony hard. Characteristically multiple sinuses develop which discharge pus and watery fluid containing sulphur grains. Treatment is by intravenous benzylpenicillin and may require to be continued for several weeks.

Cat-scratch disease

This is a slowly progressive chronic form of regional lymphadenopathy, associated with small pleomorphic Gram-negative bacilli within the walls of capillaries, and in lymph node macrophages, but the bacillus and its associated antibody are hard to identify. The involved lymph nodes are acutely tender. Only one-third of patients are pyrexial but about 90% give a history of contact with cats, most commonly kittens. A primary papule or vesicle develops at the site of a scratch 1–2 weeks after contact with the cat. This subsides after a few weeks and may be helpful in diagnosis. Lymphadenopathy ensues 1–2 weeks later. The former practice of cat-scratch antigen skin testing is now inadvisable because of the risk of transmission of AIDS or hepatitis B.

Brucellosis

This is primarily a disease of domesticated animals and causes contagious abortion or other reproductive problems in cattle (*Brucella abortus*), pigs (*B. suis*), goats (*B. melitensis*), dogs (*B. canis*), and sheep (*B. ovis*). Human spread occurs by direct contact of infected tissue with conjunctiva or broken skin, by ingestion of contaminated meat or dairy products and by inhalation of infectious aerosols. Pasteurization of milk and other measures have greatly reduced the incidence in the western countries, but stock producers, abattoir employees and veterinary surgeons remain at risk. The symptoms in humans are so variable that there is no characteristic clinical picture. The average incubation is 2–3 weeks and some infections are subclinical. In clinical cases most patients have drenching

sweats, chills, fever and malaise. Although classically associated with undulating fever, the commonest pyrexia pattern is a slight elevation in the morning with an increase in the afternoon. About 20% of patients have cervical and inguinal lymphadenopathy and a similar percentage have splenomegaly. Relapses occur in 5% of patients but are uncommon in appropriately treated individuals. Complications include arthritis, meningitis, depression, genitourinary symptoms, abnormal liver function tests, pulmonary symptoms and blood dyscrasias. A definitive diagnosis is made by recovering the organism from blood, fluid or tissue specimens. Blood cultures should be processed using the Castaneda biphasic medium bottle. The diagnosis can also be made serologically.

Treatment is probably best effected by combination therapy as most single agents are associated with a 30% chance of relapse. The presently favoured World Health Organization recommendation is a combination of doxycycline 200 mg and rifampacin up to 900 mg daily for 6 weeks. Prevention is by reducing the incidence of brucellosis in animal populations, e.g. the vaccination of cattle with *B. abortus* strain 19 vaccine.

Infectious mononucleosis

Epstein–Barr virus (EBV) is a member of the human herpesvirus group which is found worldwide, and frequently causes subclinical infection in early childhood. In addition to causing infectious mononucleosis, EBV has been associated with nasopharyngeal carcinoma, and African Burkitt's lymphoma, in which Epstein's group originally described the viral particles. The C3d receptor for EBV is found on B lymphocytes and nasopharyngeal epithelial cells of humans and certain primates. After attachment to the receptor (which is the receptor for the D region of the third component of complement), the virus gains entry to susceptible B lymphocytes. In the USA and the UK, EBV seroconversion occurs before the age of 5 in about 50% of the population. A second wave of seroconversion occurs midway through the second decade of life and is associated with clinical infectious mononucleosis. The virus persists in the oropharynx of patients for up to 18 months after clinical recovery and can be cultured from throat-washings of 15% of normal healthy adults and 50% of renal transplant recipients. The virus may be spread by transfer of saliva with kissing. The virus infects susceptible B lymphocytes within the pharynx and disseminates during the 1–2-month incubation period. The virus causes synthesis of antibodies directed against viral antigens and also antigens found on sheep, horse and bovine red cells (heterophile antibodies). During the first few weeks of clinical illness a mononuclear lymphocytosis is present. The white cell count comprises more than

50% mononuclear cells and more than 10% of atypical lymphocytes.

The leading clinical triad is fever, sore throat and lymphadenopathy. About 5% of patients have a rash which is almost universal if ampicillin is inadvertently administered. Up to 50% have palatal petechiae or splenomegaly. More serious complications include autoimmune haemolytic anaemia, thrombocytopenia, splenic rupture, encephalitis and cranial nerve palsies. On rare occasions the degree of pharyngeal obstruction from swelling of the lymphoid tissue is such that tracheostomy is required to prevent acute upper airway obstruction.

The vast majority of cases subside over 2–3 weeks. Elevation of hepatocellular enzymes is usually also self-limiting but alcohol is probably best avoided for a few months after the illness. Treatment is largely supportive. Contact sports or heavy lifting should be avoided during the first 2–3 weeks of illness. Corticosteroids have a part to play in impending airway obstruction, in severe thrombocytopenia or haemolytic anaemia, and sometimes in the presence of other complications. The role of antiviral chemotherapy in the management of EBV infections is likely to broaden as new agents are developed. Given the potential oncogenicity of EBV, the risk of administration of inactivated EBV as a vaccination has not yet been fully evaluated and immunization against EBV has not been established.

Neurogenous tumours

Chemodectomas

Pathology

There is a high incidence of carotid body tumour in Peru, Colorado and Mexico City, which are all high-altitude places where chronic hypoxia leads to carotid body hyperplasia. In the rest of the world it is a rare tumour.

The average age of presentation is in the fifth decade and there is no sex predominance. One in 10 patients have a positive family history and some of this group have bilateral tumours or phaeochromocytoma.

The tumour arises from the chemoreceptor cells on the medial side of the carotid bulb and is firmly adherent to this area. Histology shows cells similar to normal carotid body cells – large uniform epithelioid cells surrounded by a vascular stroma. The cells are not hormonally active. Proven metastases are rare; reported cases often proved to be metastases from papillary carcinoma of the thyroid.

Clinical features

Patients present with a long history (5–7 years) of a slowly enlarging painless lump in the region of the carotid bulb. About 30% present with a pharyngeal mass pushing the tonsil medially and anteriorly. Thus biopsy of a pharyngeal swelling must *never* be taken from within the mouth!

On palpation the mass is firm, rubbery and pulsatile and refills in steps synchronous with the pulse after compression. A bruit may be present and the mass may decrease in size with carotid compression. It is said that it can be moved from side to side but not up and down: this is also true of most other lumps in the neck.

Nerve involvement is rare.

Investigation

The length of history differentiates this tumour from a metastatic gland. Such a history is, however, compatible with a branchial cyst or a tuberculous gland.

Whenever a carotid body tumour is suspected a carotid angiogram should be done to demonstrate a tumour circulation, to determine the extent of the tumour and to see if there is a cross-circulation.

This tumour must *never* be biopsied.

Treatment

It is rare for a patient to die of an untreated carotid body tumour and metastases are exceptionally rare. Thus the mere presence of a carotid body tumour does not justify an attempt at removal. Indications for removal are patients in good health under the age of 50 years who have a small or medium-sized tumour; patients with tumours extending into the palate or pharynx interfering with swallowing, speaking or breathing; or tumours with an aggressive growth pattern.

Although these tumours were originally thought to be radioresistant, cures have been reported in recent publications. Radiotherapy should be used in patients who refuse surgery, in poor-risk cases or in metastatic disease.

Removal of a carotid body tumour

Make a long incision from the mastoid process to the clavicle down to the anterior border of the sternomastoid muscle: this is one of the few occasions when the incision is justified.

Dissect down to the carotid sheath and find the common carotid artery, the internal jugular vein and the vagus nerve. Free the common carotid artery on all sides, preserving the vagus nerve carefully. Now place a tape loosely around the common carotid artery and tag it with an artery forceps. The tape is placed at this stage to allow easy and rapid occlusion of the carotid artery if you later damage the internal carotid artery.

Now follow the common carotid artery upwards,

dissecting along the adventitia, and mobilizing the vagus nerve. When you start to approach the tumour you will encounter large numbers of thin-walled veins more brown than red in colour. These veins bleed very easily and are a source of difficulty in this procedure. This difficulty can be overcome by dissection with two dissecting forceps with fine points and no teeth. Grasp the tissue close to the adventitia of the artery with these forceps and pull it apart. Surprisingly this produces much less bleeding than attempts at sharp dissection, which are slow, tedious and attended by steady bleeding.

Continue in this fashion, freeing the tumour from the internal carotid artery in particular with great care. It should always be possible to preserve the vagus nerve but the hypoglossal nerve is often stretched and may need to be divided.

Vagal body tumours

Vagal paragangliomas arise from nests of paraganglionic tissue within the perineurium of the vagus nerve just below or at its ganglion nodosum. Characteristically the tumours lie just below the base of the skull near the jugular foramen, are contiguous with the vagus nerve and replace the ganglion nodosum. Intravagal tumours, however, are not restricted to this site and may be found at various sites along the nerve and down to the level of the carotid artery bifurcation.

Vagal paragangliomas most commonly present as slowly growing and painless masses high in the anterolateral aspect of the neck. On examination the mass is often noted near the origin of the sternocleidomastoid muscle with a concomitant medial displacement of peritonsillar structures. Approximately one-half of the patients have had symptoms or signs for more than 3 years before diagnosis. Pharyngeal pain is usually a late sign and indicates irritation of the pharyngeal plexus, often preceding the onset of cranial nerve palsies. Pulsating tinnitus, deafness, syncope and vertigo may also be noted.

The diagnosis is confirmed by arteriography. Vagal paragangliomas are surrounded by a pharyngeal plexus of veins and consequently tend to appear larger upon arteriography than they really are.

Vagal paragangliomas are more malignant than carotid body lesions, mainly because of the tendency to spread into the cranial cavity. Surgery is needed. The approach used is that described below for parapharyngeal tumours. The numerous thin-walled veins should be dealt with in the same way as for carotid body tumours. The most dangerous part of the dissection is superiorly where the internal carotid artery loops over the tumour and then immediately enters the skull. Injury is frequent at this site, so that the help of a vascular surgeon is advisable.

Peripheral nerve tumours

Pathology

Neural tumours are derived from cells taking origin from the neural crest cell. They can be divided into two main groups: the nerve sheath tumours and the tumours derived from the sympathoblast.

The normal nerve fibre is ensheathed by Schwann cells and by loosely distributed endoneural fibroblasts. The Schwann cell is the parent cell of the common clinical tumours, the schwannoma and the neurofibroma. A classification of peripheral nerve tumours is shown in Table 6.1.

Schwannomas were previously called neuromas or neurilemmomas; both terms are incorrect. Neuroma wrongly suggests an origin from nerve fibres. A nerve sheath consists of two layers; an outer layer (the neurilemma) and an inner layer (the neurolemma or sheath of Schwann), so neurilemmoma is inaccurate. Neurolemmoma would be correct but misleading; the term schwannoma should therefore be used. This tumour is solitary and encapsulated, being attached to or surrounded by the nerve. A paralysis of the associated nerve is thus unusual. Malignant change is also very unusual, if it occurs at all. The vagus nerve is the commonest site of origin of this tumour.

Usually the only symptom of these tumours is a mass which grows slowly, if at all.

Neurofibromas may form part of von Recklinghausen's syndrome of multiple neurofibromatosis or rarely may be single. Multiple neurofibromatosis is an autosomal dominant hereditary disease, often present at birth. Café-au-lait spots associated with this disease are well-known, but more important

Table 6.1 The developmental origins of peripheral nerve tumours

Neural crest cell	Schwann cell	Neurofibroma
		Neurilemmoma (schwannoma)
	Sympathicoblast	Ganglioma (ganglioneuroma)
		Chemodectoma (carotid, vagus, glomus jugulare)

are other neurological lesions such as gliomas, meningiomas, acoustic neuromas, and the neuropolyendocrine syndrome of mucosal neuromas, phaeochromocytomas and medullary thyroid carcinomas. Malignant change occurs in about 10% of these tumours, so that some patients die of this disease. These tumours incorporate nerve fibres and generally cause paralysis of their nerve of origin.

Clinical features

These tumours usually enlarge slowly over a period of years; a painless neck mass is the only sign. Diagnosis requires angiography to differentiate these tumours from paragangliomas, but the final diagnosis must usually wait until excision.

Treatment

The nerve from which the tumour arises is only evident in one in three operations. It may be stretched over the capsule of the tumour, or the tumour can be in the central core of the nerve with the fibres spread around it. All simple tumours should be excised and an attempt made to rejoin or graft the nerve.

Entry into the parapharyngeal space can be posterior to the submandibular gland, beneath the parotid – a cervical rather than a transparotid approach. Although some neurogenous tumours can be removed from the surface of the nerve it is inevitable that others are so closely integrated to the vagal trunk that a section of the cranial nerve has to be resected with secondary rehabilitation of the larynx.

References and further reading

Congenital neck masses

Cohen S R, Thompson J W (1986) Lymphangiomas of the larynx in infants and children: a survey of pediatric lymphangioma. *Ann Otol Rhinol Laryngol* **127** (suppl):1–20.

Emery P J, Bailey C M, Evans J N G (1984) Cystic hygroma of the head and neck: a review of 37 cases. *J Laryngol Otol* **98**:613–19.

Fleming W B (1988) Infections in branchial cysts. *Aust NZ J Surg* **58**:481–3.

Friedberg J (1989) Pharyngeal cleft sinuses and cysts, and other benign neck lesions. *Pediatr Clin North Am* **36**:1451–69.

Godin M S, Kearns D B, Pranksy S M et al. Fourth branchial pouch sinus: principles of diagnosis and management. *Laryngoscope* **100**:174–8.

Kennedy T L (1989) Cystic hygroma–lymphangioma: a rare and still unclear entity. *Laryngoscope* **99** (suppl):1–10.

Komisar A (1983) Pharyngoceles (lateral pharyngeal diverticula) of the hypopharynx. *Otolaryngol Head Neck Surg* **91**:450–2.

Leveque H, Saraceno O A, Tang C-K, Blanchard O L (1979) Dermoid cysts of the floor of the mouth and lateral neck. *Laryngoscope* **89**:296–305.

Mitchell O B, Irwin C, Bailey O M, Evans J N G (1987) Cysts of the infant larynx. *J Laryngol Otol* **101**:833–7.

Radkowski D, Arnold J, Healy G B et al. (1991) Thyroglossal duct remnants: preoperative evaluation and management. *Arch Otolaryngol Head and Neck Surg* **117**:1378–81.

Ricciardelli E J, Richardson M A (1991) Cervicofacial cystic hygroma: patterns of recurrence and management of the difficult case. *Arch Otolaryngol Head Neck Surg* **117**:546–53.

Shinkwin C, Whitfield B C S, Robson A K (1991) Branchial cysts: congenital or acquired? *Ann R Coll Surg Engl* **73**:379–80.

Solomon J R, Rangecroft L (1984) Thyroglossal–duct lesions in childhood. *J Pediatr Surg* **19**:555–61.

Tuffin J R, Theaker E (1991) True lateral dermoid cyst of the neck. *Int J Oral Maxillofac Surg* **20**:275–6.

Developmental neck masses

Amin M, Maran A G D (1988) The aetiology of laryngocoele. *Clin Otolaryngol* **13**:267–72.

Civantos F J, Holinger L D (1992) Laryngoceles and saccular cysts in infants and children. *Arch Otolaryngol Head Neck Surg* **118**:296–300.

Freeland A P, Bates G J (1987) The surgical treatment of pharyngeal pouch: inversion or excision? *Ann R Coll Surg Engl* **69**:57–8.

Huang B, Payne W S, Cameron A J (1984) Surgical management for recurrent pharyngoesophageal (Zenker's) diverticulum. *Ann Thorac Surg* **37**:189–91.

Knuff T E, Benjamin S B, Castell D O (1982) Pharyngoesophageal (Zenker's) diverticulum – a reappraisal *Gastroenterology* **82**:734–6.

Maran A G D, Wilson J A, Al Muhanna A H (1986) Pharyngeal diverticula. *Clin Otolargyngol* **11**:219–25.

Payne W S, King R M (1983) Pharyngoesophageal (Zenker's) diverticulum. *Surg Clin North Am* **63**:815–26.

Stell P M, Maran A G D (1975) Laryngocoele. *J Laryngol Otol* **89**:915–24.

Infective neck masses

Alessi D P, Dudley J P (1988) Atypical mycobacteria-induced cervical adenitis: treatment by needle aspiration. *Arch Otolaryngol Head Neck Surg* **114**:664–6.

Bennhoff D F (1985) Actinomycosis: diagnostic and therapeutic considerations and a review of 32 cases. *Laryngoscope* **94**:1198–217.

Chang R S, Lewis J P, Abilgaard C F (1973) Prevalence of oropharyngeal excreters of leukocyte transforming agents among a human population. *N Engl J Med* **289**:1325–7.

Deitel M, Bendago M, Krajden S et al. (1989) Modern management of cervical scrofula. *Head Neck* **11**:60–6.

Mikaelian A J, Varkey B, Grossman T W, Blatnik D S (1989) Blastomycosis of the head and neck. *Otolaryngol Head Neck Surg* **101**:489–95.

Wolf H, Haus M, Wilmer E (1984) Persistence of Epstein–Barr virus in the parotid gland. *J Virol* **51**:795–8.

Young E J (1983) Human brucellosis. *Rev Infect Dis* **5**:821–44.

Young L S, Sixbey J W, Clark D et al. (1986) Epstein–Barr virus receptor on human pharyngeal epithelia. *Lancet* 1:240–2.

AIDS

Barzan L, Carbone A, Tirelli U et al. (1990) Nasopharyngeal lymphatic tissue in patients infected with human immunodeficiency virus. *Arch Otolaryngol Head Neck Surg* 116:928–31.

Kraus D H, Rehm S J, Orlowski J P, Tubbs R R, Levine H L (1990) Upper airway obstruction due to tonsillar lymphadenopathy in human immunodeficiency virus infection. *Arch Otolaryngol Head Neck Surg* 116:738–40.

Marcusen D C, Sooy C D (1985) Otolaryngologic and head and neck manifestations of acquired immunodeficiency syndrome (AIDS). *Laryngoscope* 95:401–5.

Rothstein S G, Persky M S, Edelman B A, Gittleman P E, Stroschein M (1989) Epiglottitis in AIDS patients. *Laryngoscope* 99:389–92.

Shugar J M A, Som P M, Jacobson A L, Ryan J R, Bernard P J, Dickman S H (1988) Multicentric parotid cysts and cervical adenopathy in AIDS patients. A newly recognised entity: CT and MR manifestations. *Laryngoscope* 98:772–5.

Silverman S, Migliorati C A, Lozada-Nur F, Greenspan D, Conant M A (1986) Oral findings in people with or at high risk for AIDS: a study of 375 homosexual males. *J Am Dent Assoc* 112:187–92.

Stafford N D, Herdman R C D, Forster S, Munro A J (1989) Kaposi's sarcoma of the head and neck in patients with AIDS. *J Laryngol Otol* 103:379–82.

Stern J C, Lin P-T, Lucente F E (1990) Benign nasopharyngeal masses and human immunodeficiency virus infection. *Arch Otolaryngol Head Neck Surg* 116:206–8.

Neurogenous tumours

Diran O, Holmes W F (1981) Parapharyngeal schwannomas. *Otolaryngol Head Neck Surg* 89:77–81.

Ferlito A, Pesavento G, Recher G et al. (1984) Assessment and treatment of neurogenic and non-neurogenic tumors of the parapharyngeal space. *Head Neck Surg* 7:32–43.

Franklin D J, Moore G F, Fisch U (1989) Jugular foramen peripheral nerve sheath tumors. *Laryngoscope* 99:1081–7.

Horak E, Szentirmay Z, Sugar J (1983) Pathological features of nerve sheath tumors with respect to prognostic signs. *Cancer* 151:1159–67.

Jackson C G, Harris P F, Glasscock M E et al. (1990) Diagnostic and management of paragangliomas of the skull base. *Am J Surg* 159:389–93.

Katz A D, Passy V, Kaplan N (1971) Neurogenous neoplasms of major nerves of the head and neck. *Arch Surg* 103:51–6.

Sharp J F, Kerr A I G, Carder P, Sellar R J (1989) Facial schwannoma without facial paralysis. *J Laryngol Otol* 103:973–5.

Wilson J A, McLaren K, MacIntyre M A et al. (1988) Nerve-sheath tumours of the head and neck. *Ear Nose Throat J* 67:103–10.

7

Malignant neck masses

Squamous carcinoma

Many carcinomas of the head and neck sooner or later metastasize to the lymph nodes of the neck, which form a barrier that prevents further spread of the disease for many months. A sarcoma of the head and neck is assigned a stage that depends not only on the extent of the primary tumour (and the presence of distant metastases) but also on enlargement of the cervical lymph nodes. The International Union against cancer (UICC) classification is shown in Table 7.1. This is the best current classification but is subject to some criticism. For example, there is a great deal of observer error so that different observers only agree on the presence of the palpable nodes in about 70% of patients. Furthermore, some palpable nodes contain tumour, whereas some nodes that contain tumour are not palpable.

Sadly the new UICC classification is as complex as the American Joint Committee (AJC) scheme (Table 7.2) but differs from it. It would have been better to have a uniform system.

Careful pathological studies cast grave doubt on the significance of clinical staging. Much the most important prognostic factor is the number of nodes invaded, and in particular the presence of extranodal tumour, often called capsular rupture. Neither of these can be measured clinically. Furthermore, the clinical staging gives great weight to laterality, whereas pathological studies have shown that bilateral nodes, if they are both N_1 in the UICC/AJC category, do not carry a worse prognosis than unilateral N_1 nodes. Finally, neither scheme allows classification of massive (i.e. greater than 6 cm) nodes on both sides of the neck, which are almost universally fatal.

Table 7.1 International Union against Cancer (UICC) classification for tumour staging

Stage	Description
N_x	Regional lymph nodes cannot be assessed
N_0	No regional lymph node metastasis
N_1	Metastasis in a single ipsilateral lymph node, 3 cm or less in greatest dimension
N_2	Metastasis in a single ipsilteral lymph node, more than 3 cm but less than 6 cm in greatest dimension, or in multiple ipsilateral lymph nodes, none more than 6 cm in greatest dimension, or in bilateral or contralateral lymph nodes, none more than 6 cm in greatest dimension
N_{2a}	Metastasis in a single ipsilateral lymph node, more than 3 cm but not more than 6 cm in greatest dimension
N_{2b}	Metastasis in multiple ipsilateral lymph nodes, none more than 6 cm in greatest dimension
N_{2c}	Metastasis in bilateral or contralateral lymph nodes, none more than 6 cm in greatest dimension
N_3	Metastasis in a lymph node more than 6 cm in greatest dimension

Table 7.2 American Joint Committee (AJC) classification for tumour staging

Stage	Description
N_x	Minimum requirements to assess the regional nodes cannot be met
N_0	No clinically positive node
N_1	Single clinically positive homolateral node 3 cm or less in diameter
N_2	Single clinically positive homolateral node more than 3 cm but not more than 6 cm in diameter, or multiple clinically positive homolateral nodes, none more than 6 cm in diameter
N_{2a}	Single clinically positive homolateral node more than 3 cm but not more than 6 cm in diameter
N_{2b}	Multiple clinically positive homolateral nodes, none more than 6 cm in diameter
N_3	Massive homolateral node(s), bilateral nodes, or contralateral node(s)
N_{3a}	Clinically positive homolateral node(s), one more than 6 cm in diameter
N_{3b}	Bilateral clinically positive nodes (in this situation, each side of the neck should be staged separately, i.e. N_{3b}: right, N_{2a}: left, N_1)
N_{3c}	Contralateral clinically positive node(s) only

Table 7.3 Incidence of lymph node metastases in the International Union against Cancer (UICC) and American Joint Comittee (AJC) staging schemes

Stage	UICC	AJC
N_0	65%	65%
N_1	12%	12%
N_{2a}	7%	7%
N_{2b}	1%	1.5%
N_{2c}	5%	NA
N_3	10%	NA
N_{3a}	NA	7.5%
N_{3b}	NA	5%
N_{3c}	NA	0.2%
Not classifiable	0%	2%

NA = Not applicable

The appropriate distribution of patients between the categories using both schemes is shown in Table 7.3. These figures are only approximate and will obviously vary between centres. The various categories of the UICC classification will be used as convenient headings to discuss the management of metastatic nodes in the neck.

General treatment policy

Patients with no palpable nodes (N_0)

The treatment of patients with no clinically detectable nodal spread has long been controversial. At different times, different policies have been in fashion. In recent years a growing realization that head and neck cancer comprises a varied group of diseases with differing natural histories which require individualized treatment has replaced the belief that there must be one right treatment for all. This, coupled with the advent of investigative techniques such as computed tomography (CT) scanning and aspiration cytology, has led to the development of a more rational approach.

There are two principal ways to manage a clinically negative neck. It may either be left alone, reserving treatment for relapse, or one may choose to treat it, just in case there is occult nodal involvement. If it is decided to treat a negative neck, the modality chosen is most often that used to treat the primary tumour.

The likelihood of there being involved nodes depends on several factors. The nature of the primary tumour is clearly of importance, and the incidence of occult nodal involvement in patients with tumours at different sites is shown in Table 7.4. In addition to the site, the size and local extent of the primary are also significant, with occult nodal disease being more common with advanced primary tumours. Lastly, although this section is principally concerned with squamous carcinoma, it should be remembered that the pathology of the tumour – both its histological variety and degree of differentiation – is relevant. For example, papillary thyroid carcinoma is more likely to have occult nodal involvement than follicular, and high-grade tumours more likely than low.

Elective or prophylactic neck dissection is a neck dissection performed when there are no palpable nodes in the neck. The classical technique of radical neck dissection is considered excessive in these circumstances, and a modified dissection which preserves the sternomastoid muscle, the jugular vein and the accessory nerve is preferred. Elective neck dissection may be considered a reasonable adjuvant to radical surgery for a primary tumour when a high likelihood of occult nodal disease is indicated by the site, size or histology of the primary tumour. Other factors which may encourage an elective dissection include a patient who is likely to default from follow-up and occasions when the performance of a preliminary neck dissection will create better surgical access for the removal of the primary tumour. Many patients with locally advanced cancer now have a routine CT scan performed prior to surgery to determine the extent of the primary tumour. In some, enlarged but impalpable neck nodes will be demonstrated. In these cases, neck dissection should be undertaken, but this should be regarded as therapeutic rather than prophylactic. If the CT scan is negative it is reasonable to follow a policy of observation. Because of this, an argument can be advanced for CT examination of the neck in all patients who have a significant chance of occult nodal involvement.

It has been shown that only 5% of patients with carcinomas of the larynx, hypopharynx and mouth die of uncontrolled disease in the neck; the remainder are cured, or die of intercurrent disease, of recurrence at the primary site or of distant metastases. The only patient who can benefit by prophylactic neck dissection is the one who later dies solely of recurrent disease in the neck, and it seems therefore that the maximum possible benefit in terms of increased survival rate is about 5%. Against this it must be remembered that the mortality rate of radical neck dissection is between 1 and 2% so that the overall net improvement in 5-year survival figures that could theoretically be achieved by prophylactic neck dissection is reduced to around 2%.

For patients treated by radical radiotherapy,

Table 7.4 Incidence of occult nodes

Site	Incidence
Supraglottic larynx	15%
Pyriform fossa	35%
Base of tongue	20%
Transglottic carcinoma	10%

somewhat different considerations apply. In many cases the volume irradiated will of necessity encompass the first echelon of nodes. For example, the jugulodigastric and jugulo-omohyoid nodes are included when the supraglottis is treated, the lateral pharyngeal node is covered by the fields used for antral carcinomas, and the upper deep cervical chain and parapharyngeal nodes are treated *en bloc* with lateral oropharyngeal tumours. As the spread of carcinoma through the lymphatics is usually an orderly process, it is unlikely for more remote nodes to contain occult deposits if the proximal group is not palpably enlarged. Treatment of the primary tumour and first echelon of nodes is, therefore, often considered adequate in patients with clinically negative necks. In some cases such as nasopharyngeal carcinoma, however, the likelihood of lymphatic involvement is such that prophylactic irradiation of the whole neck should be undertaken.

The available data suggest that the principal value of prophylactic neck treatment, whether by surgery or irradiation, is to reduce significantly the chance of subsequent relapse in the neck. There is little evidence to indicate that this translates into greatly improved survival. The place of prophylactic treatment is destined to remain controversial, as a randomized trial to settle the question of survival benefit is probably impossible.

Single palpable metastases in one side of the neck less than 3 cm in diameter (N_1)

A high proportion of nodes in this category do not contain tumour, and so a fine-needle aspirate for cytology can be valuable. If malignant cells are shown, the neck can be treated appropriately. As extranodal tumour is uncommon in this group of patients, a functional neck dissection may well be justified. However, the surgeon must be experienced and have carried out many classical radical neck dissections, and should have a thorough knowledge of the pathology of cancer in the neck, and in particular the nodes most likely to be involved by any one tumour.

If a good aspirate has shown only lymphoid cells typical of a reactive node, it is probably safe to leave the neck alone, treating only the primary. The patient should, of course, be kept under very close observation, and treated appropriately if there is any sign of progression of disease in the neck.

In most patients with a solitary, small (less than 2 cm) node, radical radiotherapy remains an acceptable alternative to surgery where the preferred treatment for the primary tumour in the absence of nodal involvement would be irradiation. In these circumstances, the entire ipsilateral neck should be treated.

Large (>3 cm <6 cm) nodes (N_{2a}) or multiple unilateral nodes (N_{2b})

Nodes in this category require a classical radical neck dissection because of the high incidence of extracapsular spread of the tumour. The incidence of further recurrence in the neck is *probably* reduced by adding radiotherapy to the treatment regimen, although overall survival is not affected. However, if the patient is saved the discomfort of a further recurrence in the neck this is probably worthwhile.

Bilateral and contralateral nodes (N_{2c})

Bilateral neck nodes are not common, occurring in about 5% of head and neck cancers overall, more commonly from tumours of the base of the tongue, the supraglottic larynx and the hypopharynx. It used to be thought that the presence of bilateral neck glands was a very bad prognostic sign, but careful pathological studies have shown that this is not so – the prognosis is determined more by the size and number of nodes and by extracapsular rupture than by laterality. Small (N_1 or N_{2a}) bilateral nodes are therefore well worth treating.

Later contralateral nodes

The prognosis for a patient in whom a node appears on the second side of the neck some time after a dissection on one side is quite good. In this circumstance a radical neck dissection produces a 5-year survival of approximately 30%.

Massive nodes (>6 cm; N_3)

The presence of massive nodes is an uncommon event occurring in about 5% of all patients with head and neck cancer. These nodes used to be referred to as 'fixed', but size is now the main criterion for staging. The word 'fixed' itself is one which is subject to individual interpretation and indeed very few nodes are truly fixed. A node is unlikely to be fixed until it becomes very large, i.e., 6 cm or more in diameter, and is rarely fixed when it is smaller than this. It has generally been thought that the presence of massive glands contraindicates surgery, but this is probably not an absolute.

If the tumour is fixed to or invades the jugular vein the patient is almost certainly incurable. Likewise, fixation to the base of the skull in the region of the mastoid process and to the brachial plexus is also almost certainly a contraindication to treatment. Fixation to the skin is not necessarily a contraindication and it is possible to resect the tumour with the overlying skin, which is replaced. On occasion, this has produced long-term survival and certainly may give very helpful palliation.

When a tumour invades the arterial tree, resection of the vascular system has been practised. Replacement of the common or the internal carotid arteries by a vein graft has a high operative mortality but a few patients may survive to live a useful life for periods of up to 2 years. Anastomosis of the stumps of the internal and external carotid arteries has a lower operative mortality and some patients may survive for long periods.

In patients with inoperable disease in the neck, radical radiotherapy is very seldom curative, but may provide good palliation. Low-dose irradiation is of little value. Great care should be taken in the assessment of patients with very advanced disease when selecting their treatment. For some, no treatment other than adequate analgesia and appropriate nursing care is the best policy.

Surgery

The classic technique of radical neck dissection was described by Crile in 1906 and later popularized by Martin. It remained essentially unchanged for several decades but with the introduction of new conservative techniques modifications began to be introduced to the classic technique. Unfortunately a multitude of terms have been used to describe these techniques; the majority have been proposed by individuals and there has been no standard classification until recently.

The Committee for Head and Neck Surgery and Oncology of the American Academy of Otolaryngology, Head and Neck Surgery published a standardized terminology for neck dissection in 1991.

The following definitions are recommended for the boundaries of the lymph node groups removed in radical neck dissection (Fig. 7.1).

Level I

This consists of the submental group of lymph nodes within the triangle bounded by the anterior belly of digastic and the hyoid bone and the submandibular group of nodes bounded by the posterior belly of digastric and the body of the mandible.

Level II – upper jugular group

This consists of the lymph nodes located around the upper third of the internal jugular vein and adjacent spinal accessory nerve extending from the level of the carotid bifurcation to the skull base.

Level III – middle jugular group

This consists of lymph nodes located around the middle third of the internal jugular vein extending from the carotid bifurcation superiorly to the cricothyroid notch inferiorly.

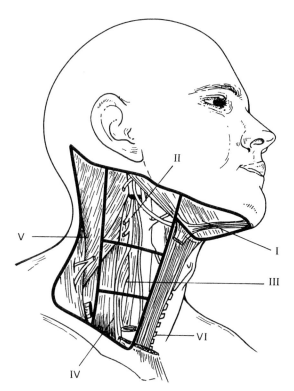

Fig. 7.1 The level system for describing the location of lymph nodes in the neck. I = Submental and submandibular group; II = upper jugular group; III = middle jugular group; IV = lower jugular group; V = posterior triangle group; VI = anterior compartment group.

Level IV – lower jugular group

This consists of the lymph nodes located around the lower third of the internal jugular vein extending from the cricothyroid notch to the clavicle inferiorly.

Level V – posterior triangular group

These nodes are located along the lower half of the spinal accessory nerve and the transverse cervical artery. The supraclavicular nodes are also included in this group. The posterior border is the anterior border of the trapezius and the anterior boundary is the posterior border of the sternomastoid muscle.

Level VI – anterior compartment group

This consists of lymph nodes surrounding the midline visceral structures of the neck extending from the hyoid bone superiorly to the suprasternal notch inferiorly. The lateral boundary in each side is the medial border of the sternomastoid. It contains the perithyroid, the paratracheal, the perilaryngeal and precricoid lymph nodes.

Neck dissection classification

The following classification is now recommended for neck dissection.

Radical neck dissection

This is the classical operation which includes removal of all the cervical lymph node groups extending from the inferior border of the mandible superiorly to the clavicle inferiorly and from the midline anteriorly to the anterior border of the trapezius muscle posteriorly. All the lymph node groups from levels I through to VI are included, as are the spinal accessory nerve, internal jugular vein and the sternomastoid muscle.

Modified radical neck dissection

This refers to the excision of all lymph node groups removed by the radical neck dissection with preservation of one or more of the following structures – spinal accessory nerve, internal jugular vein and sternomastoid muscle.

Selective neck dissection

This refers to any type of lymph node removal where there is preservation of one or more lymph node groups removed by the radical neck dissection. Five subtypes are allowable:

1 Supraomohyoid neck dissection refers to the removal of lymph nodes from levels I, II and III. The posterior limits of the dissection are the cutaneous branches of the cervical plexus and the posterior border of the sternomastoid muscle. The inferior limit is the superior belly of the omohyoid muscle where it crosses the internal jugular vein.
2 Posterolateral neck dissection refers to removal of lymph nodes in levels II, III, IV and V. The procedure is mostly used to remove nodal disease from cutaneous melanoma of the posterior scalp and neck.
3 Lateral neck dissection refers to removal of nodes in levels II, III and IV.
4 The anterior compartment neck dissection refers to removal of lymph nodes from the anterior triangle of the neck, i.e. level VI.
5 Extended radical neck dissection refers to the removal of one or more additional lymph node groups and/or non-lymphatic structures not encompassed by the radical neck dissection. This may include the parapharyngeal, superior mediastinal and paratracheal lymph nodes. Non-lymphatic structures might include the carotid artery, the hypoglossal nerve, the vagus nerve and the paraspinal muscles.

Radiotherapy

The technique employed for treatment of metastatic carcinoma in neck nodes depends on whether or not the primary tumour is receiving concurrent radiotherapy. The appropriate method of neck irradiation to be used in conjunction with the treatment of various primary tumours is described in the relevant chapters. The technique described here may be used postoperatively after neck dissection, prophylactically when the primary has been treated surgically, or for inoperable or recurrent disease.

The patient should be treated lying supine with the neck extended, immobilized in a beam-directing shell. The upper limit of the field will be along the mentomastoid line and the field extends down to the clavicles. Laterally the beam will extend to include the skin. Great care is needed to ensure that the cervical cord is not included in the high dose volume. If both sides of the neck are being treated, a midline lead block is used to shield this critical structure, and there is the added advantage of sparing of the laryngeal and oesophageal mucosa. If one side only requires treatment, the medial edge of the field should be 1 cm away from the midline, and the beam may be angled 5° to take account of beam divergence. The accurancy of the set-up should be checked with portal verification films. If there is skin involvement by tumour, 0.5 cm of wax bolus should be applied to the shell over the affected area to circumvent the skin-sparing effect of megavoltage irradiation.

Treatment is given with 4–6 MV photons from a linear accelerator. A dose of 50 Gy in 20 fractions over 4 weeks is adequate for the sterilization of microscopic disase, such as after a radical neck dissection or when electively irradiating the clinically negative neck. If there is macroscopic disease, a smaller field should be used to boost the site of initial bulk disease. A further 15 Gy in 10 fractions may be given over 2 weeks. Electrons may be useful here, because of their limited penetration. The effective treatment depth of 10 MeV electrons is 3 cm. If greater penetration is required it is better to use photons for this purpose.

Lymphoma

The lymphomas are tumours arising primarily from lymphatic tissue, usually lymph nodes but also other sites including the alimentary tract. The two principal groups are Hodgkin's and non-Hodgkin's lymphoma. The relatively common occurrence of lymphoma in head and neck nodes exemplifies the potential benefits of fine-needle aspiration cytology. The early detection of lymphoma redirects subsequent investigations down a very different path from that which would be followed if, for example, squamous carcinoma had been detected. Preoperative diagnosis in this way also indicates that any biopsy material should be sent fresh to the pathologist for cytogenetic studies and subtyping; these give prognostic and therapeutic information. Only a limited amount of typing is possible on an aspirate which gives no information on nodal architecture. Furthermore, the morphological appearance of the cells of the non-Hodgkin's lymphomas bear sufficient resemblance to their normal counterpart cells to make a diagnosis of malignant lymphoma on cytological grounds problematic.

Hodgkin's disease

This lymphoma is more frequently localized than the non-Hodgkin's variant. The 10-year survival in localized disease is 40%. The probable cell origin is the T lymphocyte and involved lymph nodes characteristically show multinucleate Reed–Sternberg cells. In contrast to the confusion surrounding the classification of non-Hodgkin's lymphoma. Hodgkin's disease is classified into four morphological groups. One of these, lymphocyte depletion, which is associated with a large number of Reed–Sternberg cells and diffuse fibrosis, is associated with a poor prognosis. The remaining variants – lymphocyte predominance, nodular sclerosis and mixed cellularity – do not differ significantly in prognosis. Much the commonest variant in Europe and North America is nodular sclerosis, which accounts for up to 75% of cases. The disease relapses and remits in at least 25% of patients. The commonest site for presentation is the neck, although deposits may also be present in the mediastinum, liver and bone marrow. Two symptoms which remain unexplained are pruritus and alcohol pain, the latter being associated with nodular sclerotic Hodgkin's disease. The three symptoms which are generally regarded to be associated with a poor prognosis are pyrexia, night sweats and weight loss.

The practice of diagnostic laparotomy and splenectomy, introduced in 1968, has now fallen out of favour, as the staging benefits were offset by an 8% incidence of overall serious complications, of which half were fatal. Although the majority of centres now favour CT scanning to assess subdiaphragmatic disease, lymphography is still occasionally used to show the shape, size and filling pattern of potentially involved nodes.

Localized Hodgkin's responds very well to radiotherapy and surgery has little part to play except in the establishment of the diagnosis. Combination chemotherapy is the initial treatment of choice in patients with stage IV disease, i.e. diffuse or disseminated involvement of one or more extralymphatic sites, and in patients with nodal disease on both sides of the diaphragm and involvement of the spleen. One current regime, for example, is the use of chlorambucil, vincristine, procarbazine and prednisolone (LOPP). Fortunately Hodgkin's disease rarely presents in Waldeyer's ring as, if this area requires to be irradiated, the whole pharynx up to the skull base is involved in the field. The patient may suffer for many months from anorexia, dysphagia and mucositis.

Non-Hodgkin's lymphoma

Non-Hodgkin's lymphomas account for 3–5% of malignant deaths in the developed countries. High-grade tumours are more common in younger age groups and the relative 5-year survival rate in the USA has improved from 28% in the early 1950s to almost 50% in the early 1980s. The Rappaport classification, developed in the 1950s, retained its prognostic relevance in the era of combination chemotherapy and is therefore still used in some centres. Non-Hodgkin's lymphomas appear to arise from all lymphoid cell subpopulations, including B and T cells and their precursors. In other words there are at least four major subgroups. Neoplasms caused by genetic changes in precursor cells are more likely to occur during childhood while those in mature cells undergoing antigen-dependent differentiation are more likely to arise in adulthood. Neoplasms arising in B cell precursors are frequently categorized as acute leukaemia while those of T cell precursors often present as enlargement of the thymus. B cell neoplasms include small cell lymphomas and small non-cleaved cell lymphomas, which are prefollicle centre cell neoplasms, but the majority of lymphomas in the more developed countries arise from follicle centre cells. The various neoplasms of peripheral T cell origin usually express helper or suppressor antigens (CD4 or CD8).

Malignant lymphomas are derived from a single clone whose lineage is identified by the use of monoclonal antibodies. Since the processing of tissue for paraffin embedding often alters antigenic determinants, most antibodies are used on viable cell suspensions or on frozen sections. The Rappaport classification was developed before there was knowledge of the division of lymphocytes into B and T cells, and while later systems such as the Lukes and Collins classification attempted to find morphological features which correlated with immunological subtypes, the associations were inconstant. None the less, the histological appearance of a lesion is the single most important predictor of clinical behaviour. Most lymph nodes involved by malignant lymphoma show replacement of normal nodal architecture by neoplastic elements in either a nodular or a diffuse pattern. Follicular lymphomas are always of B cell origin, the commonest variant being of a predominantly small cleaved cell type.

Individuals with Sjögren's syndrome are at increased risk of developing high-grade B cell lymphomas whose development is usually accompanied by the disappearance of polyclonal hypergammaglobulinaemia and rheumatoid factor from the serum; the reactive lymphoid cell population seems to disappear and be replaced by a neoplastic lymphoid proliferation. Small monoclonal proliferations of lymphocytes can be detected in the minor salivary gland lesions which probably represent a preneoplastic event. The majority of affected salivary glands contain detectable B cell clones which probably represent the first stage in neoplasia.

Hashimoto's thyroiditis patients are also at increased risk of developing malignant lymphoma as are patients with immunosuppression.

Unlike Hodgkin's disease, the non-Hodgkin's lymphomas include a wide range of tumours with histological, immunological and cytogenetic heterogeneity. Cytogenic studies have correlated chromosomal abnormalities with specific immunophenotypes and histology. Structural rearrangements of chromosome 14 at bands q11–13, q22;q24 and q32 are the most common abnormalities found in the lymphomas. The high frequency of involvement of 14q32 has led to the suggestion that rearrangements in this region may be important in the initiation of lymphoid malignancies. Furthermore, the 14q11–13 region may contain genes responsible for the promotion of the malignant processes. Deletion of 6q is another common chromosome abnormality. Clonal chromosomal abnormalities have been reported in up to 100% of patients with non-Hodgkin's lymphoma. The cytogenic findings do appear to be of prognostic significance. For example, survival is significantly longer in patients with more than 20% normal cells.

More than 80% of Burkitt's lymphomas carry a translocation from the chromosome 8 to chromosome 14. Another specific subtype of non-Hodgkin's lymphoma – adult T cell leukaemia/lymphoma – appears to have a relationship with the human T cell lymphotrophic virus (HTLV-1). The lymphomas in human immunodeficiency virus (HIV)-infected patients are usually extranodal with involvement of the gastrointestinal tract, including intraoral and anorectal lymphomas as the second most frequent site after the central nervous system. The recently isolated human B cell lymphotrophic herpesvirus (HBLV) may be the oncogenic agent in patients with acquired immune deficiency syndrome (AIDS).

Non-Hodgkin's lymphoma is most frequently found in the fifth to seventh decades and is associated with diffuse invasion of the bone marrow in up to 80% of patients. The commonest site of extranodal non-Hodgkin's lymphoma is Waldeyer's ring and the disease may also affect the salivary glands, paranasal sinuses, orbit or thyroid. Diagnostic staging laparotomy was never very popular in this type of lymphoma and CT scanning is the systemic examination of choice.

As with primary nodal non-Hodgkin's disease, extranodal early lymphomas respond well to a radiation dose of 3500–4000 cGy. The CHOP therapy regime remains popular for disseminated disease and comprises cyclophosphamide, hydroxydaunorubicin, Oncovin (vincristine) and prednisolone. Chemotherapy may also be preferred because of technical reasons which make radiotherapy difficult – for example, in gastrointestinal involvement.

The 'occult' primary

This section will discuss the common clinical situation of the patient over the age of 45 who presents with a single lump in the upper part of the lateral side of the neck, which may be a secondary malignancy. The diagnosis should be tackled by thinking what tissues are present at the appropriate site and what diseases may arise from each of these tissues.

Pathology

The tissues present at this site are skin, subcutaneous tissue and fat, the sternomastoid muscle, the contents of the carotid sheath – that is, the internal jugular vein, the carotid artery, the vagus nerve and the deep cervical lymphatic chain – the parotid gland, and finally the cervical spine. From the skin arise sebaceous cysts but these are unlikely to cause any diagnostic difficulty. From the subcutaneous tissue can arise lipomas, and neurofibromas in von Recklinghausen's disease. Other unusual causes of a lump in this area of the neck are a paraganglioma of the carotid body or the vagal bodies, a laryngocele, a pleomorphic adenoma of the tail of the parotid gland, and a large osteophyte of the cervical spine. These conditions are dealt with elsewhere. The sternomastoid muscle does not give rise to any specific disease, but the carotid sheath medial to it is a common source of such swellings. The vast majority arise from the lymph nodes, and may be due to inflammatory disease, neoplasia, or miscellaneous disorders, as discussed above. They may also be due to a secondary malignancy, which can arise from a tumour in virtually any part of the body, although obviously there are certain sites of predilection. Most carcinomas of the head and neck metastasize to the lymph nodes in the deep cervical chain but an enlarged lymph node in the neck may be the only presenting symptom in carcinomas, particularly of the pharynx, that is the nasopharynx, the oropharynx and the hypopharynx (Table 7.5), the larynx and the thyroid gland being other sites.

A secondary malignant node in the neck may also be due to a tumour below the clavicle – the lung, the stomach and the breast being common sites – though on occasion such a node may arise from a primary elsewhere in the body. A cancer presenting with a

Table 7.5 Neck node as a sole presenting symptom – site of primary

Site	Incidence
Nasopharynx	60%
Oropharynx	20%
Pyriform fossa	10%

node in the neck is mainly a disease of men, being four times more common in men than in women, with a maximum age incidence of 65 years in men and 55 years in women.

The histology of the tumour obviously varies depending on the interest of the surgeon, but between one-third and one-half of all such nodes are infiltrated by squamous carcinoma, a quarter by undifferentiated or anaplastic carcinoma, and a similar number by adenocarcinoma if the supraclavicular nodes are involved.

A small number of nodes is involved by miscellaneous tumours, including malignant melanomas, thyroid tumours, etc. In about one-third of patients a primary tumour can be found by careful investigation at the time of presentation, the primary sites in order of frequency being the nasopharynx and the tonsil, the base of the tongue and other miscellaneous sites in the head and neck, followed by the bronchus, the breast, the stomach and other sites. Careful follow-up will later show the primary site in one-third of these patients. The primary site is more commonly found in the head and neck than anywhere else and the sites are the same as described above. It is worth noting that a carcinoma of the tonsil may not declare itself for several years after the gland appears in the neck.

Finally a branchogenic carcinoma should be remembered – this usually occurs at a younger age, but can occur at any age, and may feel clinically exactly like a malignant lymph node.

Investigation

Investigation of such a patient should follow the five well-known steps of history, examination, radiology, laboratory tests and endoscopy.

History

The history does not usually help very much in arriving at a diagnosis. It is usually that of a mass for several weeks, which has increased quickly in size but which is otherwise painless. It is important to ask about other symptoms of disease in the head and neck, particularly dysphagia, hoarseness and sore throat, and for pulmonary and gastric symptoms such as cough, haemoptysis, indigestion and a loss of weight. The rare laryngocele fluctuates in size and a

tumour arising from the vagus nerve may cause hoarseness due to paralysis of the vagus nerve, but otherwise the history is of little help in making the diagnosis.

Examination

The lump itself should be examined for size, mobility and fixation to deep tissues. It is said that a carotid body tumour is mobile from side to side and not up and down, but this is also true of virtually every other lump in this area. A lump in the neck in a patient with a tumour of the pyriform fossa may not be a secondary in a lymph gland but may be a direct extension of the tumour through the thyrohyoid membrane; this should be assessed by asking the patient to swallow, when a lump due to direct extension will move up and down. A carotid body tumour can be compressed and can be made smaller by pressure on the carotid artery; it refills in bounds with each pulsation of the artery.

Examine the other lymphatic sites, notably the axillae, the groins, the liver and the spleen. Palpate the abdomen for enlargement of the stomach, liver and spleen. Finally, it is vitally important that the head and neck be examined thoroughly – particularly the nasopharynx, the oropharynx and the hypopharynx – before the investigation proceeds further, and particularly before a biopsy is carried out. Tumours at these sites may have one presenting symptom only, that is, a gland in the neck. Many of these tumours are eminently treatable but if the first investigation to be carried out is an incisional biopsy the result may be disastrous.

Radiology

Radiographs of the neck may show calcification in a tuberculous lymph node, an osteophyte or a laryngocele. A thyroid scan also is very seldom of benefit: if a lump cannot be felt it is rarely demonstrated by a scan. A chest radiograph should always be taken to show the mediastinal lymph nodes, to demonstrate another secondary deposit, to assess the general health, and to show if there is a primary bronchial tumour. It is worth remembering that a tumour on the left side of the lung may present with a gland in the right side of the neck because of the paucity of the lymphatics on the left side of the superior mediastinum. It may also be thought that other radiological investigations, such as a barium swallow, barium meal, barium enema and follow-through, or intravenous pyelogram, would be helpful, but if the primary tumour is below the clavicle then this information is of academic interest only since the patient is untreatable.

If there is any clinical suspicion that the mass may arise from, invade or displace the carotid artery, an angiogram, probably by the femoral route, should be carried out.

A CT scan seldom reveals an 'occult' primary tumour.

Haematology

The usual full blood count and erythrocyte sedimentation rate should be carried out to ensure that the diagnosis is not chronic lymphatic leukaemia, but this seldom turns out to be the case. In certain specific infections there are specific laboratory tests such as the Kveim test for sarcoid, and the Paul-Bunnell test for infectious mononucleosis.

Needle biopsy

Take a fine-needle aspirate as part of the patient's first work-up. This will provide the diagnosis in a high proportion of patients, particularly if the tumour is a squamous carcinoma. The result is unreliable, however, in the lymphomas.

Endoscopy

Finally the patient should be examined under anaesthetic, which allows the entire upper respiratory tract to be palpated; some small tumours, particularly in the base of the tongue and the tonsil, can often be better felt than seen. The nasopharynx can also be more closely examined than in the outpatient department. If a tumour is found, biopsy is taken, and a bronchoscopy and oesophagoscopy performed.

Finally if no tumour has been found, take a blind biopsy of the posterolateral wall of the nasopharynx, and of the base of the tongue on the same side, and remove the tonsil on the same side for multiple sections.

Treatment

The above scheme will produce a diagnosis in a large proportion of patients, but there will still be a proportion in whom the diagnosis has not been made. As a practical guide it is suggested that the following should be done. The patient's permission should be obtained for carrying out a radical neck dissection. He or she is then anaesthetized, and an incision is made over the lump, through which a radical neck dissection can be carried out, if necessary, and the lump is removed by excisional biopsy; the lump must be excised entirely and an incisional biopsy must not be done. If a frozen section of the node shows squamous carcinoma and the node is single and discrete, a radical neck dissection should be carried out. Such a node must have arisen from the head and neck, from the lung, or from the cervix in a woman, and if no tumour has been found in lung or cervix there is a fairly high chance that the primary tumour is in the head and neck. Although it cannot be found at the time of examination, there is a reasonable chance of curing it. The patient should thereafter be followed up at regular intervals for 5 years, looking for the primary site, which should be treated appropriately if and when it appears. Such a policy cures about 25% of patients.

If, on the other hand, there are several nodes, if the tumour has ruptured the capsule, or if the histologist is uncertain of the nature of the tumour, close the neck and ask a radiotherapist to see the patient. If the tumour is multiple or has ruptured the capsule it is not curable by surgery, and if the histologist is uncertain of its nature on frozen section it is extremely unlikely to be a squamous carcinoma and therefore it probably arose beyond the head and neck. Finally, an adenocarcinoma, an anaplastic carcinoma, or a squamous carcinoma in the supraclavicular nodes should not be treated radically because the primary site is presumably below the clavicle; palliative radiotherapy might help if the tumour is fungating.

Branchogenic carcinoma

This is a rare condition but a definite entity presenting as a single mass in the upper neck. It was at one time thought to be fairly common but it is now known that most are secondary malignancies. Four criteria are laid down for a diagnosis to be accepted but only a handful of cases have fulfilled these. They are:

1 The carcinoma should be demonstrated as arising in the wall of a branchial cyst.
2 The tumour should occur in a line running from a point just anterior to the tragus along the anterior border of sternomastoid to the clavicle.
3 The histology should be compatible with an origin from the tissue found in branchial vestiges.
4 No other primary should become evident in a 5-year follow-up.

Thyroglossal duct carcinoma

This is rare but nearly 100 cases have been described. The tumour is nearly always a papillary thyroid carcinoma. Most cases have presented as benign cysts and the diagnosis was made histologically. There is no sex predominance and the peak age incidence for women is the fourth decade and for men the sixth decade. Only 10% had evidence of metastatic disease as compared to 50% for carcinoma arising in an ectopic thyroid.

Treatment is by local excision followed by suppressive doses of thyroxine.

Carcinoma in a pharyngeal pouch

This is a rare disease of which only about 30 cases have been reported in the English literature. The incidence of malignancy is probably between 0.5 and 1%. It affects men predominantly in a ratio of about 5:1 and usually occurs in a long-standing diverticulum, the average duration of symptoms being greater than 7 years. The age of diagnosis is usually over 50 years. The main predisposing factor is thought to be chronic irritation and inflammation of the diverticulum lining from food retention. Symptoms indicating carcinomatous change are increased dysphagia, weight loss and occasionally blood in the regurgitated food. A mass may be found in the neck.

The usual lesion is an invasive squamous cell carcinoma, but a few cases of carcinoma-*in-situ* have been reported in the literature.

Barium studies show a constant filling defect, unlike food debris which changes between films or repeat swallows. It is usually seen in the distal two-thirds of the pouch but can easily be missed. The diagnosis may be first made at operation.

The unusual case with a tumour confined to the pouch should be treated by diverticulectomy. Most cases require total pharyngolaryngectomy as for a postcricoid carcinoma. The outlook is dismal.

Malignant neurogenic tumours

Most malignant tumours of peripheral nerve origin arise from the Schwann cell. These malignant schwannomas are malignant *ab initio* and do not represent malignant change in a benign schwannoma.

The neoplasms derived from the primitive sympathetic cells of the neural crest are shown in Table 7.6. Neuroblastomas are tumours of childhood, and in the head and neck may be secondary from an abdominal tumour or may arise primarily from the cervical sympathetic chain.

These tumours form only 1% of head and neck tumours, but nerve tumours are commoner in the head and neck than in the rest of the body. They can arise from any of the cranial nerves or plexuses but the vast majority arise from the vagus within the carotid sheath.

References and further reading

Squamous carcinoma

Alexander P (1976) Metastatic spread and 'escape' from the immune defenses of the host. *Natl Cancer Inst Monogr* **44**:125.

Ballantyne A J, Jackson G L (1982) Synchronous bilateral neck dissection. *Am J Surg* **144**:452.

Barker J L, Fletcher G H (1977) Time, dose, and tumor volume relationships in megavoltage irradiation of squamous cell carcinomas of the retromolar trigone and anterior tonsillar pillar. *Int J Radiat Oncol Biol Phys* **2**:407.

Beahrs O H, Devine K D, Henson S W Jr (1959) Treatment of carcinoma of the tongue: end results in 168 cases. *Arch Surg* **79**:399.

Bekheit F, Isrander F (1964) Bilateral radical neck dissection. *J Egypt Med Assoc* **47**:573.

Berger D S et al. (1971) Elective irradiation of the neck lymphatics for squamous cell carcinomas of the nasopharynx and oropharynx. *Am J Radiol* **111**:66.

Berlinger N T et al. (1976) Prognostic significance of lymph node histology in patients with squamous cell carcinoma of larynx, pharynx, or oral cavity. *Laryngoscope* **86**:792.

Biller H, Davis W, Ogura J H (1971) Delayed contralateral metastasis with laryngeal and laryngopharyngeal cancers. *Laryngoscope* **81**:1499.

Campos J L, Lampe I, Fayos J V (1971) Radiotherapy of carcinoma of the floor of the mouth. *Radiology* **99**:677.

Cassisi N, Dickerson D, Million R (1978) Squamous cell carcinoma of the skin metastatic to parotid nodes. *Arch Otolaryngol* **104**:336.

Conley J (1970) *Concepts in Head and Neck Surgery*. New York, Grune Stratton.

del Regato J A (1977) Pathways of metastatic spread of malignant tumors. *Semin Oncol* **4**:33.

DeSanto I et al. Neck dissection: is it worthwhile? *Laryngoscope* **92**:502.

Djannan M et al. (1973) Significance of jugular vein invasion by metastatic carcinoma in radical neck dissection. *Am J Surg* **126**:666.

Fisher B, Saffer E A, Fisher E R (1972) Studies concerning the regional lymph node in cancer. IV Tumor inhibition by regional lymph node cells. *Cancer* **33**:631.

Fletcher G H (1972) Elective irradiation of subclinical disease in cancers of the head and neck. *Cancer* **29**:1450.

Fletcher G H, MacComb W S, Braun E (1960) Analysis of sites and causes of treatment failures in squamous cell carcinomas of the oral cavity. *Am J Radiol* **83**:405.

Fletcher G et al. (1973) Neck nodes. In: Fletcher G (ed) *Textbook of Radiotherapy*, 2nd edn. Philadelphia, Lea & Febiger.

Frazell E L, Lucas J C Jr (1962) Cancer of the tongue: report of the management of 1554 patients, *Cancer* **15**:1085.

Futrell J W et al. (1971) Predicting survival in cancer of the larynx or hypopharynx. *Am J Surg* **122**:451.

Table 7.6 Neoplasms derived from primitive sympathetic cells

Benign tumours	Malignant tumours
Ganglioneuroma	Neuroblastoma
Phaeochromocytoma	Ganglioneuroblastoma
	Phaeochromocytoma

Gius J A, Grier D H (1950) Venous adaption following bilateral radical neck dissection with excision of the jugular vein. *Surgery* **28**:305.

Henschke U R *et al.* (1964) Local recurrences after radical neck dissection with and without preoperative x-ray therapy. *Radiology* **82**:331.

Jesse R H *et al.* (1970) Cancer of the oral cavity: is elective neck dissection beneficial? *Am J Surg* **120**:505.

Jesse R H, Fletcher G H (1963) Metastases in cervical lymph nodes from oropharyngeal carcinoma: treatment and results. *Am J Surg* **90**:990.

Johnson J T (1990) A surgeon looks at cervical lymph nodes. *Radiology* **175**:607–10.

Leipzig B, Hokanson J (1982) Treatment of cervical lymphoma in carcinoma of the tongue. *Head Neck Surg* **5**:3.

Lindberg R D (1972) Distribution of cervical lymph node, metastases from squamous cell carcinoma of the upper respiratory and digestive tracts. *Cancer* **29**:1446.

Lindberg R D, Jesse R H (1968) Treatment of cervical lymph node metastases from primary lesions of the oropharynx, supraglottic larynx, and hypopharynx. *Am J Radiol* **102**:132.

McGavran M, Bauer W, Ogura T (1961) The incidence of cervical lymph node metastases from epidermoid carcinoma of the larynx and their relationship to certain characteristics of the primary tumor. *Cancer* **14**:55.

McGuire F, McCabe B (1980) Bilateral neck dissections. *Arch Otolaryngol* **106**:427.

Marshall K, Edgerton M (1977) Indications for neck dissection in carcinoma of the lip. *Am J Surg* **133**:216.

Mooney C S *et al.* (1969) Simultaneous bilateral radical neck dissection following high level radiation therapy. *J Surg Oncol* **1**:335.

Moore O, Frazell E (1964) Simultaneous bilateral neck dissections: experience with 151 patients. *Am J Surg* **107**:565.

Ogura J H, Biller H F, Wette R (1971) Elective neck dissection for pharyngeal and laryngeal cancers: an evaluation. *Ann Otol Rhinol Laryngol* **80**:646.

Putney F J (1961) Elective versus delayed neck dissection in cancer of the larynx. *Surg Gynecol Obstet* **112**:736.

Reed G F, Mueller W, Snow J P (1959) Radical neck dissection. *Laryngoscope* **69**:702.

Sako K (1964) Fallability of palpatation in diagnosis of metastasis to nodes. *Surg Gynecol Obstet* **118**:989.

Shah J P, Candela F C, Poddar A K (1990) The patterns of cervical lymph nodes metastases from squamous carcinoma of the oral cavity. *Cancer* **66**:109–13.

Snow G B, Annyas A A, Van Scooten E A, Bartelink H, Hart A A M (1982) Prognostic factors of neck node metastasis. *Clin Otolaryngol* **7**:185–93.

Southwick H W (1971) Elective neck dissection for intraoral cancer. *JAMA* **217**:454.

Spiro R H *et al.* (1974) Cervical node metastasis from epidermoid carcinoma of the oral cavity and oropharynx. *Am J Surg* **128**:562.

Spiro R H, Strong E W (1973) Discontinuous partial glossectomy and radical neck dissection in selected patients with epidermoid carcinoma of the mobile tongue. *Am J Surg* **126**:544.

Stell P M, McCormick M S (1987) Prognosis in cancer of the head and neck. In: Taylor I (ed) *Progress in Surgery*, vol 2. Edinburgh, Churchill Livingstone, pp. 1–17.

Strong E W (1969) Preoperative radiation and radical neck dissection. *Surg Clin North Am* **49**:271.

Sugarbaker E V, Wiley H (1951) Intracranial pressure studies incident to resection of the internal jugular veins. *Cancer* **4**:242.

Teichgracher J, Clairmont A (1984) The incidence of occult metastasis for cancer of the oral tongue and floor of mouth: treatment rationale. *Head Neck Surg* **7**:15.

Vikram B (1984) Changing patterns of failure in advanced head and neck cancer. *Arch Otolaryngol* **110**:564.

Vikram B *et al.* (1980) Elective postoperative radiation therapy in stage III & IV epidermoid carcinoma of the head and neck. *Am J Surg* **140**:580.

Wang C, Meyer J (1971) Radiotherapeutic management of carcinoma of the nasopharynx: an analysis of 170 patients. *Cancer* **28**:566.

Welsh I W, Welsh J I (1966) Cervical lymphatics: pathological conditions. *Ann Otol Rhinol Laryngol* **75**:176.

Weymuller E A Jr, Kiviat N B, Duckett L G (1983) Aspiration cytology and cost effective modality. *Laryngoscope* **93**:561.

The 'occult' primary, branchogenic and pharyngeal pouch carcinomas

Baraka M E, Sadek S A A (1985) Carcinomatous changes in pharyngeal diverticula. *J Laryngol Otol* **9**:297–9.

Glynne-Jones R G, Annand A K, Young T E, Berry R J (1990) Metastatic carcinoma in the cervical lymph nodes from an occult primary: a conservative approach to the role of radiotherapy. *Int J Radiat Oncol Biol Phys* **18**:289–94.

Kristensen S, Juul A, Moesner J (1984) Thyroglossal cyst carcinoma. *J Laryngol Otol* **98**:1277–80.

McCarthy S A, Turnbull F M (1981) The controversy of branchogenic carcinoma. *Arch Otolaryngol* **107**:570–2.

Micheau C, Klijanienko J, Luboinski B, Richard J (1990) So-called branchiogenic carcinoma is actually cystic metastases in the neck from a tonsillar primary. *Laryngoscope* **100**:878–83.

Strasnick B, Moore D M, Abemayor E, Julliard G, Fu Y S (1990) Occult primary tumours. The management of isolated submandibular lymph node metastases. *Arch Otolaryngol Head Neck Surg* **116**:173–6.

Lymphoma

Burres S A, Crissman J D, McKenna J, Al-Sarraf M (1984) Lymphoma of the frontal sinus: case report and review of the literature. *Arch Otolaryngol* **110**:270–3.

Hamburger J I, Miller M, Kini S R (1983) Lymphoma of the thyroid. *Ann Intern Med* **99**:685–93.

Jelliffe A M (1986) Hodgkin's disease and non-Hodgkin's lymphomas. In: Hope-Stone H F (ed) *Radiotherapy in Clinical Practice*. London, Butterworths, pp. 177–202.

Kang J S, Robbins K T, Fuller L M *et al.* (1984) Stages I and II non-Hodgkin's lymphomas of Waldeyer's ring and the neck. *Am J Clin Oncol* **7**:629–39.

Lukes R J, Collins R D (1975) New approaches to the classification of the lymphomata. *Br J Cancer* **3** (Suppl):1.

Lukes R J, Butler J J, Hicks E B (1966) Natural history of Hodgkin's disease as related to its pathology picture. *Cancer* **19**:317.

Magrath I T (ed) (1990) *The Non-Hodgkin's Lymphomas*. London, Edward Arnold.

Ogden G R (1986) Lymphoma of the oral soft tissues. *Br Dent J* **161**:9–12.

Rappaport H, Winter W J, Hicks E B (1956) Follicular lymphoma: a revaluation of its position in the scheme of malignant lymphomas. *Cancer* **9**:792.

Steward W P, Todd I D H, Harris M *et al*. (1984) A multivariate analysis of factors affecting survival in patients with high-grade histology non-Hodgkin's lymphoma. *Eur J Cancer Clin Oncol* **20**:881–9.

Swerdlow J B, Merl S A, Davey F R, Gacek R R, Gottlieb A J (1984) Non-Hodgkin's lymphoma limited to the larynx. *Cancer* **53**:2546–9.

8

Neck dissection

Radical neck dissection

Preoperative preparation

A patient undergoing a unilateral neck dissection does not require a tracheostomy unless the operation is combined with removal of a primary tumour in continuity; it is advisable to do an elective tracheostomy for a patient undergoing a bilateral or second neck dissection.

Position

The patient is intubated and laid supine on the table, with the head extended and turned to the opposite side, and a flat pillow is placed under the ipsilateral shoulder to make dissection of the posterior triangle easier.

Incision

The incision will depend on whether the patient has been irradiated or not. If the patient has not been irradiated use the Y-incision with a lazy S on the vertical limb to reduce scar tissue contracture (Fig. 8.1). If the patient has been irradiated, two incisions are suitable: the half-H (or T on its side) described by Hetter (Fig. 8.2) and the double horizontal incision described by McFee (Fig. 8.3).

The vertical limb of any of these incisions must not cross the clavicle as this compromises any future chest flaps.

The McFee incision consists of two horizontal limbs: the first begins over the mastoid process, curves down to the hyoid bone and then up again to the point of the chin. The second lies about 2 cm above the clavicle; it starts laterally at the anterior border of the trapezius and ends medially at the midline. The lateral end of this lower incision can be turned up if necessary to improve access.

The order of the steps may vary, but what is described below is considered to be the simplest and safest technique for a beginner. It is presumed here

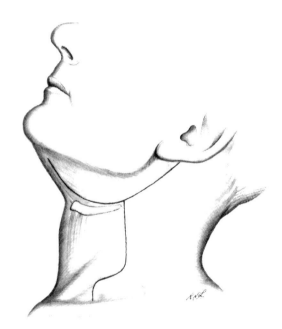

Fig. 8.1 Y-type incision.

that the operation is being carried out alone, not in continuity with resection of a primary tumour.

Raising the flaps

Mark out the incision with a skin dye using either a mapping pen or a sharpened orange stick. If mistakes are made in marking the incision the dye can usually be erased with alcohol. Do not scratch the skin with a needle to indicate suture marks; it is better to dip the tip of an intramuscular needle in dye and make dots on the skin in three or four places for critical sutures.

With traction and countertraction incise the skin in one movement with a no. 10 blade down to and through the platysma muscle, the fibres of which spring apart if strong tension is applied. In the posterior part of the neck, the fibres of the sterno-

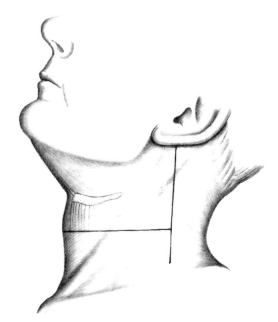

Fig. 8.2 Half-H incision.

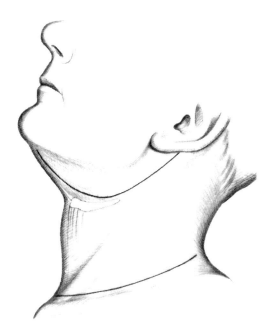

Fig. 8.3 Double horizontal incision (McFee).

mastoid are inserted directly into the skin, resulting in a little more bleeding in this area. Keep the platysma on the skin flaps as it increases the strength of the wound, and increases the blood supply to the skin flaps. It has been said that the platysma should

be removed because there are lymphatics within it. If these lymphatics are invaded by cancer, the patient is incurable by surgery.

The assistant places double skin hooks underneath the platysma and applies traction directly upwards – toothed forceps or Allis forceps must never be applied to the skin edge. Apply countertraction to the specimen to show the subplatysmal plane: dissection here causes no bleeding, provided the branches of the external and anterior jugular veins are tied; bleeding usually signifies that a wrong plane has been entered.

In a double horizontal incision raise the lower flap and the lower half of the middle flap from below, and the upper flap and the upper half of the middle flap from above. Then gain access by retracting the middle bridging flap with tapes. Stop any bleeding from the inner surface of the bridge flap at this point.

During dissection in the upper part of the neck, two branches of the facial nerve must be preserved – the cervical and the marginal mandibular (Fig. 8.4).

The first supplies the part of the platysma that crosses the mandible and is inserted into the corner of the mouth, and the second supplies the muscles around the mouth. Division of either nerve therefore leads to a weakness of the lower lip. Both nerves curve downwards below and in front of the angle of the mandible across the facial vessels about one finger's breadth below the mandible. The marginal mandibular branch then runs immediately superior to the submandibular gland while the cervical branch runs lateral to this gland. Both the nerves then curve upwards again to reach their destination.

The usual method of protecting these nerves by ligating and dividing the facial vessels on the submandibular gland and lifting them over the mandible does not work when the nerves' course is lower than usual; this manoeuvre also compromises removal of the pre- and postfacial nodes, which are often affected in oral tumours. It is also dificult to preserve these branches if the platysma is left on the specimen.

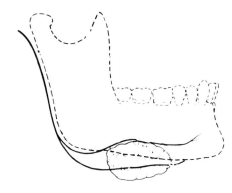

Fig. 8.4 Cervical and marginal mandibular branches of facial nerve.

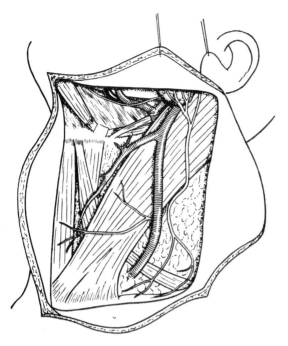

Fig. 8.5 Flaps raised.

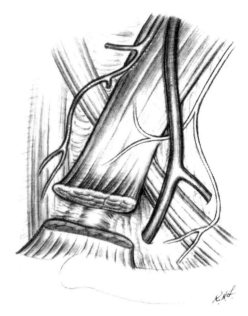

Fig. 8.6 Division of lower end of sternomastoid.

The easiest way to preserve the branches of the facial nerve is to cut right through the fascia at the level of the hyoid bone down to the capsule of the submandibular gland, elevate the resulting flap over the mandible and stitch it to the skin flap, taking care not to transfix the nerve.

If there are metastatic glands in close relationship to the nerve do not compromise the cancer operation and do not attempt to preserve the nerves, as the resulting weakness to the corner of the mouth is acceptable if cure is obtained.

Stitch the upper and lower skin flaps back to the towels taking care not to pass the needle through the epidermis (Fig. 8.5).

Lower end of the internal jugular vein

It is a basic principle of cancer surgery that the main vein draining the area being operated upon must be divided first. This step reduces the number of systemic metastases because small tumour emboli released by manipulating the tumour are unable to find their way into the general circulation. Whether this is very important in head and neck cancer is uncertain.

The lower end of the internal jugular vein must therefore be divided first after exposing it by dividing the sternomastoid muscle (Fig. 8.6). The assistant applies traction to the lower end of the muscle, at the same time flattening it, while the surgeon does the same to the upper end. With a no. 10 blade cutting on

this flat surface the muscle fibres separate very easily as long as firm traction is applied until the blueness of the vein is seen. Usually one vessel needs to be tied in the deep part of the sternomastoid. Do not transfix the lower, divided end of the sternomastoid muscle. This produces a large mass of necrotic muscle that will almost certainly form an abscess leading to breakdown of the wound.

With a no. 15 blade, open the carotid sheath right down to the vein wall. When the vein is free, retract it laterally with a small retractor and identify the vagus nerve on the wall of the common carotid artery. Then pass ligatures of 2/0 silk round the vein (Fig. 8.7). Use three ligatures, two at the lower end and one at the upper end, and transfix each end with 3/0 silk. Then hold up the vein by the long ends of the sutures and divide it with a knife between the transfixion stitches. If there is a tributary at the point of section divide it and tie it with 3/0 silk before working on the main vein.

The internal jugular vein can be torn either by passing artery forceps beneath the sternomastoid muscle to mobilize it before division or by opening the forceps longitudinally next to the vein; this manoeuvre tears off small tributaries which bleed alarmingly.

On no account allow an assistant to snatch a large bleeding vessel in this area with artery forceps; this converts a small hole into a large one. Define the injured vessel, occlude it temporarily with arterial clamps and repair the defect.

The danger of tearing the lower end of the vein is not blood loss but air embolism. If the vein is torn before it is divided put a finger on the hole and ask

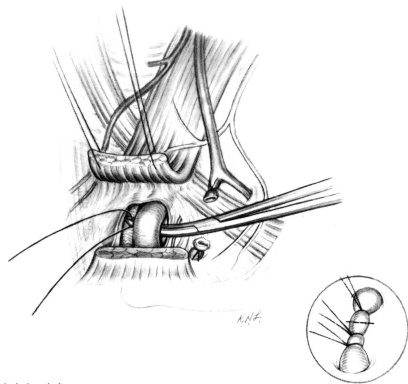

Fig. 8.7 Internal jugular vein being tied.

the anaesthetist to tilt the patients head downwards. Tie the area of the vein above and below the hole and pass ligatures above and below the tear. When these are tied the finger may be lifted off the vein.

If sutures slip off the lower end of the vein after it has been divided, again put a finger on the hole, tilt the patient feet down and when the sucker is turned up to full power gradually slide your finger off the hole, apply arterial clamps and stitch the hole with 5/0 arterial silk.

On the left side the thoracic duct passes medial to the jugular vein, then posterior to it, and finally curves round to enter the junction of the internal jugular vein and subclavian vein (Fig. 8.8). If it is seen tie it off, and if there is chylous leak (recognized as milky fluid), stop the operation, find the torn duct and oversew it with 5/0 silk.

Supraclavicular dissection (Fig. 8.9)

Divide the omohyoid muscle without clamping – it will not bleed if cut through its tendon. Incise the fascia over the fat pad lateral to the internal jugular vein and, with a finger wrapped inside a swab, push up this fat pad and identify the phrenic nerve passing over the scalenus anterior muscle from lateral to

medial. It lies behind the prevertebral fascia – do not incise this as it protects the phrenic nerve and also the brachial plexus, which is encountered next. Do not use diathermy over the fascia as this can also damage these nerves.

Pass a finger laterally, anterior to the prevertebral fascia as far as the anterior border of trapezius and during this manoeuvre divide and ligate the transverse cervical artery and vein. Also divide and tie the external jugular vein in this area. The fat in the supraclavicular fossa can be divided without bleeding by cutting down on to the finger, but take care not to cut the subclavian vein as it is pulled out of the thorax by the upward finger retraction.

Now turn to the anterior part of the specimen and elevate the internal jugular vein out of the carotid sheath (Fig. 8.10) with care so as not to tear a high thoracic duct on the left side. Establish a plane on the wall of the common carotid artery; always keep the vagus nerve in view while doing this. If the specimen is pulled up too hard at this point it is possible to tear off the thyrocervical trunk because of traction on its inferior thyroid branch; this tears a hole in the side of the subclavian artery. If this happens never try to catch the hole with artery forceps as this merely converts one fairly small hole into several large

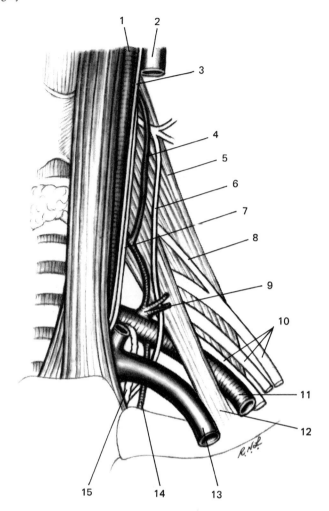

Fig. 8.8 Anatomy of the root of the neck. 1 = Common carotid artery; 2 = internal jugular vein; 3 = vagus nerve; 4 = ascending cervical artery; 5 = scalenus medius muscle; 6 = phrenic nerve; 7 = inferior thyroid artery; 8 = C5 nerve; 9 = thyrocervical trunk; 10 = brachial plexus; 11 = subclavian artery; 12 = scalenus anterior muscle; 13 = subclavian vein; 14 = internal thoracic artery; 15 = thoracic duct.

holes; control the bleeding with finger pressure, dissect out the surrounding area of the subclavian artery and its branches, occlude these branches and the subclavian artery on each side of the tear with tapes or soft rubber catheters, and then repair the defect in the subclavian artery with arterial sutures.

Dissection of the posterior triangle (Fig. 8.11)

Ascending branches of the transverse cervical artery and vein run up the anterior border of the trapezius muscle and make a bloodless dissection along this part of the muscle difficult. Bleeding can be avoided by running a finger up underneath the fat in front of the prevertebral fascia, applying large artery forceps along the junction of the muscle and fat, and dividing

between the forceps. This manoeuvre inevitably cuts the accessory nerve, which is an essential part of a routine classical neck dissection. However, if you wish to preserve the function of the shoulder it is wise to preserve the branches to the trapezius muscle from the third and fourth cervical nerve. These lateral branches arise from the cervical plexus, being ultimately derived from C3 and C4. They arise deep in the sternomastoid muscle and pass laterally beneath the fascia covering the floor of the posterior triangle to supply the trapezius muscle and also to give off a communicating branch to the accessory nerve. If you wish to preserve these nerves it is essential therefore to preserve the fascia on the floor of the posterior triangle. Furthermore, the technique just described of placing artery forceps across the

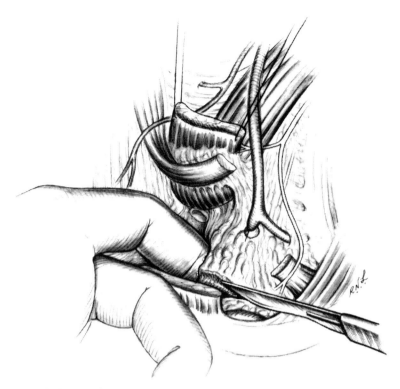

Fig. 8.9 Creating a supraclavicular tunnel.

anterior border of the trapezius inevitably divides these nerves.

The specimen is now freed inferiorly and posteriorly. Pull it medially and elevate the fat pad off the prevertebral fascia covering the floor of the posterior triangle. This is best accomplished by an assistant taking the specimen in a swab and pulling it upwards very hard. Free the specimen by sharp dissection with a knife together with countertraction. It is tacked down in three places by three neurovascular bundles consisting of a vein, an artery and a cutaneous branch of the cervical plexus (Fig. 8.12). These are best clamped, divided and tied high on the specimen to avoid damage to the phrenic nerve, which can happen if the cutaneous branches of the cervical plexus are not identified, or are tied low on the specimen, or if the coagulation diathermy is used in this area.

Continue the dissection along the common carotid artery on the adventitial plane up to the bifurcation, taking care to preserve the vagus nerve.

Damage is unlikely if the nerve is kept under vision. Also remember the posterior inclination of the internal carotid artery and vagus nerve above the bifurcation.

Do not preserve the accessory nerve during this part of the dissection; attempts to dissect out this

nerve to preserve it infringe the integrity of the *en bloc* removal.

Division of the upper end of the internal jugular vein

Divide the sternomastoid muscle from the mastoid process (Fig. 8.13). This causes some bleeding and the beginner may tend to lose the way at this point – put the index finger of the left hand on the transverse process of the first cervical vertebra and cut through the sternomastoid muscle towards this finger. The internal jugular vein is directly anterior to the transverse process of the first cervical vertebra and the finger protects it. Carry the dissection a little further forward, again under finger control, until the internal jugular vein is seen. Next follow the internal jugular vein upwards to the transverse process of the first cervical vertebra from below, dividing the fascia of the carotid sheath with scissors. This frees the jugular vein on three sides, and by keeping close to the wall it is an easy matter to pass right-angled forceps round it anteriorly and put on the three 2/0 silk ties – two above and one below the point of division.

An alternative way of identifying the internal jugular vein is to cut down on to the posterior belly of the digastric muscle – there are no vital structures

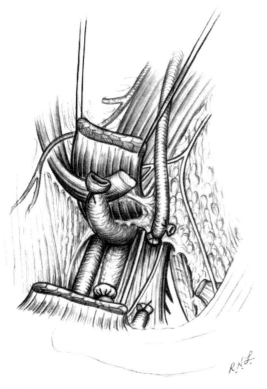

Fig. 8.10 Lower end of internal jugular vein freed from carotid sheath.

superficial to it at this point except the common facial vein. Retract the muscle upwards (Fig. 8.14), and the vein will be seen emerging from beneath it with the accessory nerve overlying it.

It is often not necessary to remove the posterior belly of the digastric muscle as it is so helpful in reinforcing closure lines and for carotid artery protection. However, in order to remove as much jugular vein as possible, retract the posterior belly of the digastric upwards to allow the ligatures to be slid up as high as possible. Before tying the ligatures identify the vagus and hypoglossal nerves. If any tributaries are seen, divide and tie them (Fig. 8.15) before tying the main vein. The occipital artery crosses the posterior part of the vein; ligate and divide it to prevent troublesome bleeding. After transfixing with 3/0 silk divide the upper end of the internal jugular vein. The upper end may be torn if the vein is not clearly seen, if small tributaries are torn off, and if poor technique is used in attempting to stop bleeding from a torn occipital artery. However, the pressure inside the upper end of the vein is only about 4 cm of water, so bleeding can be controlled by firm packing of the jugular foramen with gelfoam; if the tear can be found, repair it with arterial sutures.

Dissect forwards and find the posterior branch of

the posterior facial vein half an inch (1.2 cm) anterior to the internal jugular vein; ligate and divide it. Then divide the tail of the parotid gland in a line between the mastoid tip and the angle of the jaw. If at this point the knife is angled upwards the facial nerve may be cut. Angle the knife slightly downwards to the transverse process of the first cervical vertebra, thus cutting the parotid gland obliquely. Then find the hypoglossal nerve anteriorly and trace it to the bifurcation of the common carotid artery. Bleeding may occur at this point from veins accompanying the hypoglossal nerve. These veins generally run medial to the nerve but send three or four anastomotic branches lateral to it. Dissect along the hypoglossal nerve on the perineural sheath, clamp, divide and tie these anastomotic vessels with 3/0 silk; never use diathermy in this area. If bleeding occurs from these veins it is important to realize that the bleeding point will retract medial to the hypoglossal nerve. The way to stop this bleeding without damaging the hypoglossal nerve is to lift the nerve, either up or down, with a blunt hook, find the bleeding point, put on a small artery forceps and tie it.

Finally trace the hypoglossal nerve forwards into the submandibular triangle.

Dissection of the submandibular triangle (Fig. 8.16)

Divide the fat in the submental area and display the anterior belly of the digastric muscle. Then identify the anterior part of the submandibular gland and dissect it to the posterior border of the mylohyoid muscle. Free the upper border of the submandibular gland by dividing and tying the vessels, including the facial artery, that cross the lower border of the mandible.

Retract the mylohyoid muscle forward to show the submandibular duct, pulling the lingual nerve down in a curve. Free the latter by dividing the fascia around the submandibular ganglion with a knife. The lingual nerve gives off a small but constant branch to the submandibular ganglion, and this branch is accompanied by a vessel that can cause troublesome bleeding. Identify this nerve, place two artery forceps across it and divide between them. This allows the lingual nerve to spring upwards behind the body of the mandible. If bleeding is encountered here do not use artery forceps to stop it as they will almost certainly paralyse the lingual nerve. Pressure with adrenaline swabs will always control the bleeding. Tie the submandibular duct with 3/0 silk and divide it. During each procedure keep the hypoglossal nerve running parallel and inferior to the duct in view. Then remove the specimen by transfixion and division of the facial artery at the posteroinferior border of the submandibular gland.

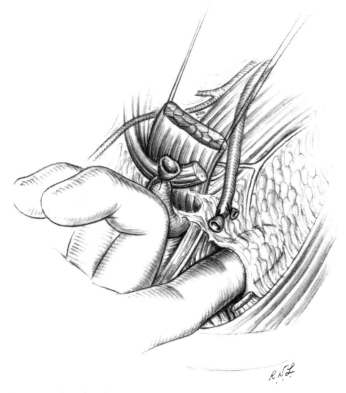

Fig. 8.11 Dissection of the posterior triangle.

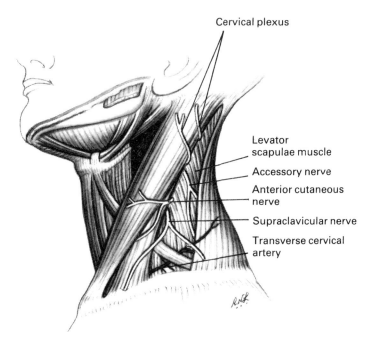

Fig. 8.12 Anatomy of cervical plexus and its cutaneous branches.

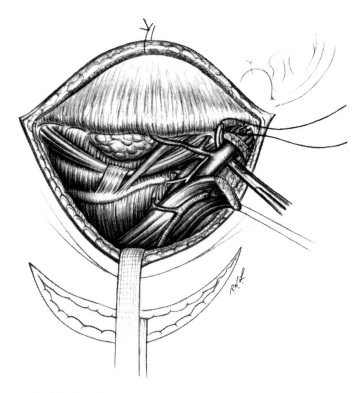

Fig. 8.13 Ligation of upper end of jugular vein.

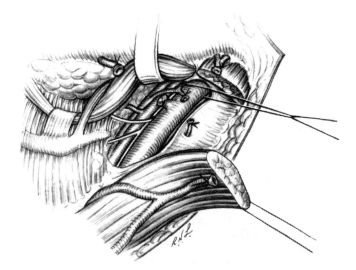

Fig. 8.14 Retraction of posterior belly of digastric to show jugular vein.

Carotid artery protection

The carotid artery must be protected in any patient whose skin wound is likely to break down or who is likely to develop a fistula; this includes patients who have been irradiated, poorly nourished patients and diabetics. Several methods of protection of the carotid sheath have been described but the only completely reliable one is that using the levator scapulae muscle (Fig. 8.17).

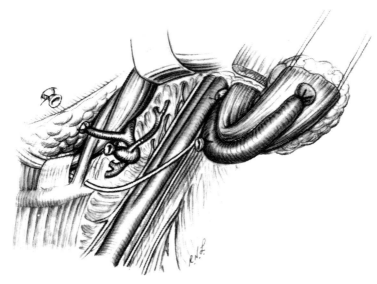

Fig. 8.15 Division of veins related to the hypoglossal nerve.

Once bleeding has stopped, identify the levator scapulae and free its posterior border. Free the lower border as near to the scapula as possible and divide it. It is then easy to swing the muscle forwards pedicled on its anterior border like a page of a book; this preserves its blood supply entering from its anterior border. Take care not to injure the brachial plexus during division of the lower end. Stitch the muscle over the carotid arteries using interrupted 3/0 chromic catgut sutures, usually to the sternohyoid muscle (Fig. 8.18). When stitching the lower end do not include the phrenic nerve in the stitch. This technique is unsuitable if the cervical nerves arising from C3 and C4 have been preserved, as they are inevitably cut in the process of lifting the muscle.

Closure

Wash the wound, discard dirty instruments and instruct the entire operating team to change their gowns and gloves. Haemostasis is completed with coagulation diathermy. Blood always pools at the

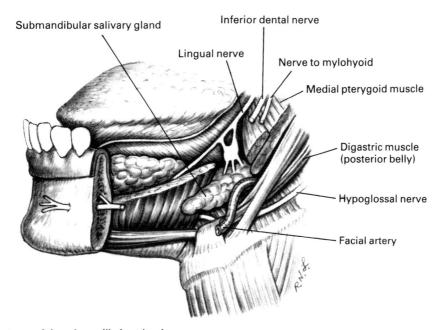

Fig. 8.16 Anatomy of the submandibular triangle.

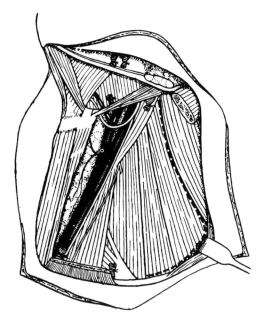

Fig. 8.17 Levator scapulae flap marked out.

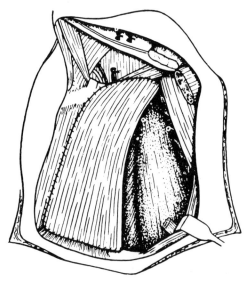

Fig. 8.18 Levator scapulae flap stitched into place.

insertion of the trapezius muscle to the clavicle because any bleeding that occurs in the neck will run down to this point.

Put in two Haemovac drains with the introducer, from the undersurface of the lower flap to the outside – it is safer to put them in from within out because if they are put in the opposite direction the sharp introducer may damage the carotid artery if it slips. Two drains are held with 3/0 chromic sutures, one along the anterior border of the trapezius, and the

other in front of the carotid artery, curving upwards into the submandibular region. Drains should never cross the carotid sheath, and they should be cut to the correct length so that there are no holes outside the skin, or else an airtight closure will not be possible. Secure the drains to the skin with a Roman garter stitch of 3/0 silk. Now make a final check for:

1 a chylous leak;
2 bleeding from the veins accompanying the hypoglossal nerve;
3 bleeding on the undersurface of the middle flap, if a double horizontal incision has been used.

These are the three commonest causes of trouble in the postoperative period.

Place buried sutures of 3/0 chromic catgut at the skin marks and further similar interrupted sutures until the flap is airtight. In order to check for this apply the suction to the Haemovac drains. If any air leaks, insert further sutures.

Close the skin with a blanket stitch of 4/0 Prolene or staples and again check for air-tightness.

No dressing is needed if all bleeding has been stopped and the wound closed so that it is airtight. Do not use Nobecutaine on the wound as this sticks to the skin and the stitches, so that when the stitches are removed, removal of the film of Nobecutaine may drag the wound edges apart.

Radical neck dissection as part of a combined procedure

When a primary tumour is removed in continuity with a neck dissection it is important to keep a band of continuity between the neck dissection and the primary growth.

Laryngeal cancer

In a total laryngectomy, the neck dissection should be left attached along the whole length of the larynx to include the superior and inferior lymphatic pedicles. A neck dissection is never done with a hemilaryngectomy but when done with a supraglottic laryngectomy it is pedicled on the thyrohyoid membrane.

Pharyngeal cancer

When a laryngopharyngectomy is performed the pedicle must be as broad as possible and it is best if it is left along the whole length of the pharynx.

Oral cancer

Oral cancers drain to the submandibular, submental and upper deep cervical nodes. Therefore, leave the specimen attached along the lower border of the mandible and include the inner layer of periosteum to preserve continuity.

Oropharyngeal cancer

Tumours of the oropharynx drain by a pedicle to the upper deep cervical nodes. Leave the specimen attached therefore near the tail of the parotid gland.

Postoperative care

No specific postoperative care is needed other than that already outlined in Chapter 3.

Complications

Most of the complications of a radical neck dissection have already been discussed in Chapter 5.

The most crippling long-term complication is the 'shoulder syndrome'. The main effects of this syndrome are long-standing pain in the shoulder and the inability to perform certain manoeuvres such as putting on a jacket. Two important movements at the shoulder joint must be considered: abduction and flexion.

Denervation of the trapezius muscle allows the shoulder girdle to rotate through 30° anteriorly. Abduction in these patients then becomes the equivalent of extension in the normal subject. The normal subject is unable to extend the arm beyond 45° because of locking of the glenohumeral joint. Abduction of the shoulder beyond 45° is therefore physically impossible in the patient with a denervated trapezius muscle. Flexion at the shoulder joint in the patient with a denervated trapezius is the equivalent of abduction in the normal subject. Abduction of the arm is a compound of two movements: firstly, elevation and rotation of the scapula on the trunk achieved by the trapezius muscle, and secondly, abduction of the humerus on the scapula mainly achieved by the deltoid muscle, assisted by the supraspinatus muscle, which helps to prevent displacement of the head of the humerus during strong deltoid action. The first 90° of the movement takes place at the shoulder joint under the control of the deltoid muscle and remains possible in the patient with a denervated trapezius. However, this 90° of movement only brings the arm to about 75° from the trunk because the shoulder girdle is tilted downwards. Furthermore, the remaining 90° of movement due to movement of the shoulder girdle on the trunk by the trapezius muscle is no longer possible. In summary, therefore, a patient with a denervated trapezius muscle can only abduct the arm from the trunk to an angle of 75° and abduction beyond that point is prevented by locking of the glenohumeral joint. He or she can flex the arm from the trunk to an angle of about 45° by the action of the deltoid muscle, but further flexion is prevented by a downward tilt of the shoulder girdle and the loss of the rotation of the shoulder girdle on the trunk by the trapezius.

References and further reading

Ballantyne A J, Guinn G A (1966) Reduction of shoulder disability after neck dissection. *Am J Surg* **112**:662.

Barkley H T, Fletcher G H, Jesse R H, Lindberg R D (1972) Management of cervical lymph node metastases in squamous cell carcinoma of the tonsillar fossa, base of tongue, supraglottic larynx and hypopharynx. *Am J Surg* **124**:462–467.

Bocca E (1953) Functional problems connected with bilateral radical neck dissection. *J Laryngol Otol* **67**:567.

Bocca E, Pignataro O (1967) A conservation technique in radical neck dissection. *Ann Otol Rhinol Laryngol* **76**:975.

Brandenburg J H, Lee C Y (1981) The eleventh nerve in radical neck surgery. *Laryngoscope* **91**:1851.

Calearo C V, Gianpietro T (1983) Functional neck dissection: anatomic grounds, surgical technique, clinical observations, *Ann Otol Rhinol Laryngol* **92**:215.

Crile G (1906) Excision of cancer of the head and neck: 132 cases. *JAMA* **47**:1780–1786.

Freeland AP, Rogers BM (1975) The vascular supply of the cervical skin with references to incision planning. *Laryngoscope* **85**:714–719.

Goffinet D R, Fee W E, Goode R I (1984) Combined surgery and postoperative irradiation in the treatment of cervical lymph nodes. *Arch Otol* **110**:736.

Grodinsky M, Holyoke E A (1938) The fasciae and fascial spaces of the head, neck, and adjacent regions. *Am J Nature* **63**:367.

Jesse R H, Ballantyne A J, Larson D (1978) Radical or modified neck dissection: a therapeutic dilemma. *Am J Surg* **136**:516–519.

Lindberg R (1972) Distribution of cervical lymph node metastasis from squamous cell carcinoma of the upper respiratory and digestive tracts. *Cancer* **29**:1446.

Lingeman R E, Helmus C, Stephens R, Ulm J (1977) Neck dissection: Radical or conservative. *Ann Otol Rhinol Laryngol* **86**:737–744.

McGuirt W F, McCabe B F, Krause C J (1979) Complications of radical neck dissection: a survey of 788 patients. *Head Neck Surg* **1**:481–487.

Molinari R, Chiesa-Sausto F, Cantu G, Grandi C (1980) Retrospective comparison of conservative and radical neck dissection in laryngeal cancer. *Ann Otol Rhinol Laryngol* **89**:578–581.

Razack M S, Silapasvang S, Sako K, Skedd D P (1978) Significance of site and nodal metastases in squamous cell carcinoma of epiglottis. *Am J Surg* **136**:520–524.

Razack M, Balli R, Saro R (1981) Bilateral radical neck dissections. *Cancer*, **47**:197–206,

Schuller D E, Platz C E, Krause C (1978) Spinal accessory lymph nodes: a prospective study of metastatic involvement. *Laryngoscope* **88**:439.

Snow G B, Annyas A A, Van Scooten E A, Bartelink H, Hart A A M (1982) Prognostic factors of neck node metastasis. *Clin Otolaryngol* **7**:185–193.

Spiro R H, Alfonso A E, Farr H W, Strong E W (1974). Cervical node metastases from epidermoid carcinoma of the oral cavity and oropharynx. *Am J Surg* **128**:562–567.

Stell P M (1983) Fixed bilateral cervical nodes. *J Laryngol Otol* **97**:851–856.

Stearns M P, Shaheen O H (1981) Preservation of the accessory nerve in block dissection of the neck. *J Laryngol Otol* **95**:1141.

9

Tumours of the larynx

Surgical anatomy

The larynx is divided into three sites and each of these sites is divided into subsites. The sites and subsites laid down by both the International Union against Cancer (UICC) and the American Joint Committee (AJC) are shown in Table 9.1.

The larynx also encompasses several spaces, or rather potential spaces, which are important in the spread of disease. These include the pre-epiglottic, paraglottic and Reinke's spaces. The pre-epiglottic space is bounded superiorly by the hyoepiglottic ligament, posteriorly by the epiglottis and anteriorly by the thyrohyoid ligament. Its apex inferiorly is limited by the attachment of the inferior end of the epiglottic cartilage by a strong fibrous band, the thyroepiglottic ligament, to the posterior surface of the thyroid cartilage below the median notch at the anterior commissure. The epiglottic cartilage has numerous foramina through which carcinoma can pass from its posterior surface into the pre-epiglottic space (Fig. 9.1).

The paraglottic space, or rather potential space, lies lateral to the true and false cords. Its lateral

relation is the thyroid cartilage, medially it is bounded by the vestibular fold and the quadrate ligament and more inferiorly by the conus elasticus, which is covered by the mucosa of the subglottic space. Medially the paraglottic space is continuous with the pre-epiglottic space, and superiorly it is bounded by the vallecula and the aryepiglottic fold. Its lateral relation is the mucosa of the medial wall of the pyriform fossa posteriorly, and the thyroid cartilage anteriorly. Inferolaterally the space is bounded by the cricothyroid ligament (Fig. 9.2).

Reinke's space lies immediately beneath the laryngeal epithelium, i.e. superficial to the thyroarytenoid muscle, and is bounded superiorly and inferiorly by the junction of the columnar and squamous epithelium, that is the superior and inferior arcuate lines.

The important tendons and ligaments of the larynx are the vocal ligament, the cricovocal membrane (conus elasticus), the vestibular ligament (quandrangular membrane) and the anterior commissure tendon. The cricovocal membrane (conus elasticus) is attached below to the entire border of the arch of the cricoid cartilage running round from one arytenoid facet to the other. Its median part, called the cricothyroid ligament, is tense and strong and triangular in shape. Its apex is inserted into the prominence of the thyroid cartilage at the anterior commissure. The upper edge of the cricovocal membrane extends from this point backwards to be inserted into the inferior border of the vocal process of the arytenoid cartilage. This upper free border is thickened and forms the vocal ligament, which is the supporting ligament of the vocal cord.

The vestibular ligament (quadrate membrane) is attached anteriorly to the depression between the two laminae of the thyroid cartilage above the vocal ligament and close to the attachment of the thyro-epiglottic ligament. It extends backwards to be inserted into the tubercle on the anterolateral surface of the arytenoid cartilage. It is composed of elastic fibrous tissue continuous with the aryepiglottic fold. Medially it is covered loosely by mucosa and

Table 9.1 Anatomical classification of the larynx (International Union against Cancer; UICC)

Regions	Sites
Supraglottis including epilarynx (including marginal zone)	Suprahyoid epiglottis (including the tip) Aryepiglottic fold Arytenoid
Supraglottis excluding epilarynx	Infrahyoid epiglottis Ventricular bands (false cords) Ventricular cavities
Glottis	Vocal cords Anterior commissure Posterior commissure
Subglottis	

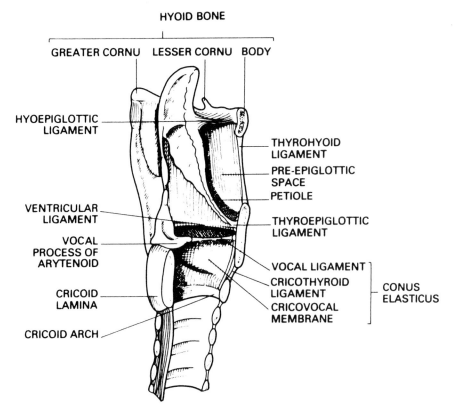

Fig. 9.1 The pre-epiglottic space (sagittally bisected larynx).

laterally it is bounded by the paraglottic space. The anterior commissure tendon is formed by the fusion of the two vocal ligaments anteriorly to form a tendon inserted into the thyroid cartilage.

The supraglottic portion of the larynx is derived from the buccopharyngeal anlage (arches III and IV), whereas the glottic and subglottic portions derive from the pulmonary anlage (arch IV). Thus each major component has an independent lymphatic circulation, separated into an upper and lower drainage system. They are collected together on the posterior wall of the cavity, but are separated laterally and anteriorly by the vocal folds. It is generally said that the vocal folds contain only a few fine capillary vessels, although some authorities disagree with this. The lymph vessels of the upper part pass alongside the superior laryngeal artery, pierce and thyrohyoid membrane and end in the upper deep cervical glands along with the lymph vessels of the pharynx. The efferent vessels from the anterior part of the lower segment of the larynx pierce the cricothyroid ligament and end in the prelaryngeal, pretracheal and deep cervical chain. The efferents from the posterolateral region pierce the cricotracheal membrane and end in the paratracheal and lower deep cervical nodes.

The free edge of the vocal cord is covered by squamous epithelium. Its superior and inferior surfaces are covered by respiratory epithelium and the junction between the respiratory and squamous epithelium above and below is marked by the superior and inferior arcuate lines respectively.

The subglottis can be divided into two parts. The anterior, fixed part is a triangle whose apex superiorly lies at the anterior commissure. Here the mucosa is tightly bound down to the cartilage, which has foramina through which tumour can pass. Laterally the subglottic mucosa covers the conus elasticus and is mobile.

The nerve supply of the larynx is more important in vocal cord paralysis and will be discussed in Chapter 10.

The staging of laryngeal carcinoma under the TNM system will be discussed in the next section. Although their wording differs, the classifications laid down by the UICC and the AJC are the same. Before we pass on to discuss pathology there are several anatomical points that are important in the TNM classification. The supraglottis requires no comment, but there is quite a lot to be said about the anatomical definition of the glottis. Firstly, a glottic tumour is describing as being T_2 when the tumour

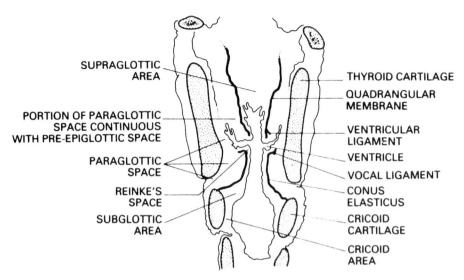

SUPRAGLOTTIC
AREA

THYROID CARTILAGE

QUADRANGULAR
MEMBRANE

PORTION OF PARAGLOTTIC
SPACE CONTINUOUS
WITH PRE-EPIGLOTTIC SPACE

VENTRICULAR
LIGAMENT

PARAGLOTTIC
SPACE

VENTRICLE

VOCAL LIGAMENT

REINKE'S
SPACE

CONUS
ELASTICUS

SUBGLOTTIC
AREA

CRICOID
CARTILAGE

CRICOID
AREA

Fig. 9.2 The paraglottic space.

extends to the supraglottis or the subglottis. Unfortunately, the classification does not define where the glottis becomes the supraglottis above and the subglottis below. It is clear from the writings of different authors that there are many different definitions of these two boundaries. Some regard the superior border of the glottis as being the superior arcuate line, whereas others include all the superior surface of the vocal cord and the floor of the vestibule in the glottis. Some place the lower border of the glottis at the inferior arcuate line, some 1 cm inferior to the free edge of the vocal cord, and some at the level of the superior border of the cricoid cartilage. The strict anatomical definition of the vocal cord is that part of the free edge of the cord, covered by squamous epithelium, which has a vertical height of about 5 mm, being bounded superiorly and inferiorly by the superior and inferior arcuate lines. If tissue above and below these lines is included in the glottis the tumour has already spread into an area of much richer lymphatic drainage than the true vocal cords, and inevitably this change in anatomical classification will dramatically affect results.

The glottis is said to consist of the vocal cords, the anterior commissure and the posterior commissure, but again these structures are not defined accurately. Strictly speaking, commissure means a point, so that the anterior commissure presumably means the point anteriorly where the vocal cords come together. It is clear, however, that many authors regard the anterior commissure as an area from which a tumour can arise. As we pass along the vocal cords to their anterior end the strip of squamous epithelium narrows, so that at the anterior end of the cord the strip of squamous epithelium is only about 1 mm

high. It may join with its fellow of the opposite side, or there can be a narrow strip 1 or 2 mm wide covered by respiratory epithelium passing between the anterior end of the two vocal cords. Indeed such an area is necessary on physiological grounds to allow mucus to pass up by ciliary action from the trachea to cross the vocal cords. At this point the vocal cords are very narrow so that a tumour that crosses the anterior commissure readily spreads off the vocal cords, in particular below the cord into the apex of the anterior central part of the subglottic space. At this point the mucosa is tightly bound to the thyroid cartilage, which has foramina for the passage of vessels providing an easy route of escape for cancer through the cartilage into the prelaryngeal tissues.

The posterior commissure is not defined, but presumably it consists of the squamous epithelium lining the anterior surface of the arytenoid cartilage and that over the vocal processes of the arytenoid cartilage. In fact, the vocal cords form only a little over a half of the glottis, the remaining part being formed by the mucosa over the vocal processes of the arytenoid cartilage and over the anterior surface of the arytenoid cartilage. Tumours seldom arise from this area.

Surgical pathology

Tumours of the larynx may be benign or malignant, but true benign tumours constitute 5% or less of all laryngeal tumours. The relative incidence is shown in Table 9.2.

Table 9.2 Benign tumours of the larynx

Tumour	Incidence
Papilloma	85%
Adenoma	5%
Chondroma	5%
Miscellaneous (granular cell myoblastomas, lipomas, haemangiomas, neurofibromas)	5%

Benign tumours

Papillomas

True papillomas are much the commonest benign laryngeal tumour. They can be divided into two types: the juvenile, which is multiple and usually regresses after puberty; and the adult, which is usually single and does not undergo spontaneous resolution.

The juvenile papilloma arises mainly on the true and false cords and the anterior commissure, but often extends into the subglottic space, the trachea, bronchi and epiglottis. It has often been thought that these lesions are not true tumours but are an abnormal tissue response to an initiating viral factor. However, electron microscopy has failed to reveal inclusion bodies. Malignant change may occur in a juvenile papilloma but *only* if the patient has been irradiated. The hallmark of the juvenile papilloma is its multiple nature and notorious propensity to recur.

Although there are no histological differences between an adult and a juvenile papilloma the former rarely recur after local removal.

The treatment of juvenile laryngeal papillomas is repeated and careful removal with a laser. Tracheostomy should be avoided if at all possible. Every effort should be made to avoid recurrence in the trachea or bronchi and if laryngeal trauma can be minimized, dysphonia and respiratory difficulty may be slight.

Haemangiomas

Capillary haemangiomas are usually tiny and present in any part of the larynx. They are usually seen in adults and can be dealt with endoscopically.

Cavernous haemangiomas are usually congenital and are rare in adults. They usually present between the third and 16th week of life with dyspnoea. Five per cent of patients will also have other congenital abnormalities. Some 80% of cavernous haemangiomas arise from the posterior wall of the larynx or trachea and involve one side of the subglottis. They are radiosensitive but the long-term effects of radiotherapy are unacceptable. Excision via a laryngofissure or excision with laser or cryotherapy has been tried but probably the best treatment option is a tracheostomy and to await resolution and growth of the trachea.

Cartilaginous tumours

This term is used deliberately to emphasize the fact that there is no clear-cut histological or clinical distinction between chondromas and chondrosarcomas. Of those reported in the literature, 20% have been considered to be malignant. This is a distinctly male disease (sex ratio 5 : 1), occurring between the ages of 40 and 60. Seventy per cent of cartilaginous tumours arise from the cricoid cartilage, 20% from the thyroid, and most of the remainder from the arytenoid. Clinically these tumours are smooth and encapsulated, and radiographs often show mottled calcification.

Irrespective of the histological appearances these tumours grow and extend locally, and require removal with a good margin. Local or distant metastases have only been recorded very rarely.

Schwannoma

Schwannomas of the larynx arise almost exclusively from the aryepiglottic fold close to the apex of the arytenoid cartilage. They usually occur in the fourth and fifth decades of life and are commoner in women. They are usually small and can be dealt with endoscopically but occasionally a lateral pharyngotomy is required for access. The necessity for a total laryngectomy is very rare. Only one case of a malignant schwannoma has been described.

Neurofibroma

Most neurofibromas are part of a generalized von Recklinghausen's syndrome. Most cases arise in children and adolescents. They mainly arise in the supraglottis but can occur as far down as the subglottis. They are not suitable for endoscopic resection because of indistinct borders and a lateral pharyngotomy or a thyrotomy is necessary for access.

Neurofibrosarcoma occurs in 10% of neurofibromas, especially in fully developed von Recklinghausen's disease.

Granular cell myoblastoma

This uncommon lesion may not be a true tumour but a degenerative disease of mature striated muscle cells. The vast majority of laryngeal granular cell tumours arise within the substance of the vocal cord and cause hoarseness. The most important point about them is that the overlying epithelium may show the appearances of pseudoepitheliomatous hyperplasia, which the pathologist may report as squamous carcinoma. If the clinician and the pathologist are unaware of this, unnecessary radical surgery may be advised.

Paraganglioma

Glomus tumours of the larynx arise from laryngeal paraganglia. These are paired structures on the internal branch of the superior laryngeal nerve and a second pair lie on the terminal branch of the posterior branch of the recurrent laryngeal nerve at the lower level of the larynx. Most patients are aged between 50 and 70 and men are affected slightly more than women. The paraganglia look like haemangiomas and cause non-specific symptoms but occasionally can cause pain. They grow slowly and destroy the laryngeal skeleton. Most are relatively radioresistant and the preferred treatment is either endoscopic excision or supraglottic laryngectomy.

Malignant tumours

Squamous carcinoma forms the vast majority of malignant laryngeal tumours. This is rather surprising in an organ lined by respiratory epithelium, and presumably indicates that squamous metaplasia is common. The relative incidence of malignant tumours is shown in Table 9.3.

Squamous carcinoma

Carcinoma-*in-situ* only occurs on the vocal cord; its treatment is discussed on p. 134. Frankly invasive squamous carcinoma is usually moderately to well-differentiated, and the incidence of lymph node metastases and survival depends on this degree of differentiation. The incidence of these metastases varies from 10% for well-differentiated tumours to 20% for moderate differentiation to 50% for poorly differentiated tumours. The survival at 5 years also falls from 80% for well-differentiated tumours to 20% for poorly differentiated tumours.

Carcinoma of the larynx may arise from the supraglottic, glottic or subglottic areas. The definition of these three areas has been given in Table 9.1.

Epidemiology

The age-adjusted mortality rate for laryngeal carcinoma in 1975 was approximately 25 cases per million per year for men and 8 per million per year for women. This represented a steady decline from the maximum mortality rate, in 1925, when it was 60 per million per year in men and 20 in women.

There is a marked social class difference, carcinoma of the larynx being twice as common in men in social class V than in men in social class I. There is also an urban variation, carcinoma of the larynx being more common in people residing in urban areas than in rural districts. Finally, there is a fairly marked international variation, the incidence being about five times as common in some parts of Spain (Zaragoza), for example, than in England and Wales.

Approximately 90% of laryngeal carcinomas occur in men, with a peak incidence between 55 and 65 years of age.

Supraglottic carcinoma

The relative proportion of laryngeal carcinomas arising in the supraglottic area varies between 15 and 60%, but 40% appears to be a reasonable figure for the UK and 30% for North America. For some unexplained reason the incidence is much higher in continental Europe.

The commonest supraglottic carcinoma is that occurring in the centre of the infrahyoid epiglottis.

These tumours nearly always (90%) invade the fenestrae in the cartilage. About 50% invade the thyroid cartilage anteriorly or along its upper lateral edge. About half of these tumours also invade the pre-epiglottic space either by spreading through the fenestrae, or more commonly by destroying the thyroepiglottic ligament and passing through the resulting breach into the pre-epiglottic space. Tumours of the base of the epiglottis invade the pre-epiglottic space frequently but the paraglottic space virtually never. It is thus safe to carry out a horizontal supraglottic laryngectomy.

A small proportion, perhaps 5% or less, of the tumours extend inferiorly to invade the floor of the ventricle or the vocal cords.

Carcinoma of the lateral part of the supraglottic space, i.e. of the ventricular bands, is much less common. These tumours tend to spread superficially on the mucosal surface to the laryngeal surface of the epiglottis and to the aryepiglottic fold. More important, however, is spread into the paraglottic space. Involvement of this space is inferred from radiography or clinical examination, which shows oedema or swelling increasing the distance between the pyriform fossa and the false cord. Radiographic reversal of the subglottic contour is due to inferior paraglottic extension of disease. Extension to this space can occur in tumours of the false cord or of the ventricle (the only mucosa embraced by this space), and in tumours of the glottis and of the medial wall of the pyriform fossa. This is the cause of vocal cord

Table 9.3 Malignant tumours of the larynx

Tumour	Incidence
Squamous cell carcinoma	85%
Carcinoma-*in-situ*	3%
Verrucous carcinoma	3%
Undifferentiated carcinoma	5%
Adenocarcinoma	0.5%
Miscellaneous carcinomas (adenoid cystic, spindle cell, etc.)	1.5%
Sarcomas (including reticulosis)	2%

Table 9.4 (UICC) classification of supraglottic tumours

T	Primary tumour
T_{is}	Carcinoma-*in-situ*
T_1	Tumour limited to one subsite of supraglottis with normal mobility
T_2	Tumour invades more than one subsite of supraglottis or glottis, with normal vocal cord mobility.
T_3	Tumour limited to larynx with vocal cord fixation and/or invades postcricoid area, medial wall of pyriform sinus or pre-epiglottic tissues
T_4	Tumour invades through thyroid cartilage and/or extends to other tissues beyond the larynx, e.g. to oropharynx, soft tissues of neck

fixation seen in the latter tumours. The UICC staging of supraglottic carcinoma is shown in Table 9.4.

Lymph node metastases are classified in the usual way. Lymphatic spread occurs via the superior lymphatic pedicle, which accompanies the superior laryngeal artery and nerve, to the immediately adjacent upper deep cervical nodes.

The incidence of lymph node metastases is shown in Table 9.5.

Glottic carcinoma

The glottis is the site of the white lesions called variously keratosis and leukoplakia. These are descriptive terms with no pathological significance. Histology shows that these lesions can be divided into three grades. Firstly, squamous cell hyperplasia with or without keratosis; this lesion requires complete removal by decortication but no other treatment. Secondly, hyperplasia with atypia; this lesion also requires decortication and careful follow-up. Finally, carcinoma-*in-situ*, which should be regarded as at least as potentially lethal as squamous carcinoma and should be treated by irradiation, or perhaps laser excision. A neighbouring frank carcinoma should, of course, be excluded carefully if a histology report of carcinoma-*in-situ* is received.

The incidence of glottic carcinoma varies in different series, but 60% would be a reasonable estimate for North America and 50–55% for the UK. Glottic carcinoma may be divided into those small tumours that arise on one vocal cord and remain localized to it for long periods, and those tumours, often called transglottic, that involve a large part of the laryngeal surface crossing the vocal cord, and which are exten-

Table 9.5 Supraglottic carcinoma: lymph node metastases (UICC classification)

N_0	80%
N_1	10%
N_2	5%
N_3	5%

sive when first seen. These tumours are *not* a later stage of a smaller tumour but probably represent a wide-field malignant degeneration.

Glottic carcinomas are classified according to the UICC, as shown in Table 9.6.

It should be noted that tumours may also arise from the posterior third of the glottis, i.e. that part of the glottis lying over the vocal process. For some reason such tumours are omitted from the classification of laryngeal tumours by the UICC and the AJC.

Glottic carcinomas arise on the vocal cord and spread along the cord in Reinke's space. These tumours may spread superficially into the neighbouring supra- or subglottic areas in 10% of patients. The tumour may also spread across the anterior commissure to the opposite cord. Invasion of the intrinsic laryngeal muscles is common, notably the thyroarytenoid muscle.

Small glottic tumours do not invade cartilage but larger ones may involve the arytenoid cartilage, or the thyroid cartilage at the anterior commissure. Once a carcinoma extends more than 1 cm inferior to the free edge of the vocal cord it may invade the cricoid cartilage.

Tumours limited to the glottis without fixation virtually never transgress the conus elasticus.

If a glottic carcinoma reaches the anterior commissure it can easily extend into the subglottis. It then lies close to the cricothyroid membrane and can escape by this route early and often. This appears to be related to the close proximity of the mucosa to the thyroid ala at the anterior commissure and to the presence of the anterior commissure tendon. Tumour may spread along this route to invade the anterior supraglottis and subglottic larynx in the midsagittal plane.

The larger transglottic tumour is one which crosses the ventricle to affect two or three regions of the larynx. It is possible that some of these tumours originate in the ventricle. This tumour invades the paraglottic space; it is an aggressive tumour that almost always invades the laryngeal framework and emerges from that cartilaginous framework between

Table 9.6 (UICC) classification of glottic tumours

T_1	Tumour limited to vocal cord(s) (may involve anterior or posterior commissures) with normal mobility
T_{1a}	Tumour limited to one vocal cord
T_{1b}	Tumour involves both vocal cords
T_2	Tumour extends to supraglottis and/or subglottis, and/or with impaired vocal cord mobility
T_3	Tumour limited to the larynx with vocal cord fixation
T_4	Tumour invades through thyroid cartilage and/or extends to other tissues beyond the larynx, e.g. to oropharynx, soft tissues of the neck

Table 9.7 Incidence of lymph node metastases in transglottic carcinoma

N_0	70%
N_1	20%
N_2	2%
N_3	5%

the thyroid and cricoid cartilages at the cricothyroid membrane. Fifty per cent invade the ipsilateral lobe of the thyroid gland and the strap muscles.

Transglottic tumours also extend posteriorly through the cricoarytenoid joint to invade the pharyngeal mucosa overlying this area – an important surgical point.

Lymph node metastases are rare in true glottic tumours; their incidence in transglottic tumours is shown in Table 9.7.

Distant metastases are rare, as in all forms of laryngeal carcinoma, being found in 1.5% of patients when first seen.

Subglottic carcinoma

Two types of subglottic tumour are to be distinguished: firstly, a tumour arising primarily in the subglottic space and secondly, a tumour arising on the vocal cords and extending into the subglottic space – some authorities claim that the former do not occur.

Subglottic carcinoma is uncommon in all published series, forming 5% or less of the total; indeed, subglottic extension of a glottic carcinoma is as common as true subglottic carcinoma.

The classification of these tumours is shown in Table 9.8.

True subglottic carcinoma is usually unilateral, virtually always ulcerofungating (i.e. not exophytic as are many epiglottic carcinomas). It quickly invades the perichondrium of the thyroid and cricoid cartilages and always extends to and frequently through the cricothyroid membrane.

These tumours virtually always spread through the conus elasticus to the glottic region, where the tumour margins tend to invade the intrinsic muscles of the true cord, producing the effect of a thickened

Table 9.8 Classification of subglottic tumours

T_1	Tumour limited to the subglottis
T_2	Tumour extends to vocal cord(s) with normal or impaired mobility
T_3	Tumour limited to the larynx with vocal cord fixation
T_4	Tumour invades through the cricoid or thyroid cartilage and/or extends to other tissues beyond the larynx, e.g. to oropharynx, soft tissues of the neck

and fixed cord, but not invading the free margin of the mucosa.

True subglottic carcinoma usually presents with stridor, as distinct from subglottic spread of a glottic tumour, which usually causes hoarseness. Vocal cord fixation occurs in about 30% of both groups; 20% of true subglottic tumours have lymph node metastases, against only 5% of the group with subglottic spread.

Unusual tumours

Verrucous carcinoma

This tumour was first described in the mouth but it may also arise from the supraglottis or glottis. It is a relatively non-aggressive tumour which seldom metastasizes in the neck. The characteristics of the tumour are as follows.

1 It comprises unusually well-differentiated keratinizing squamous epithelium arranged in compressed invaginating folds.
2 It has a warty papillary surface.
3 The clefts between adjacent papillary folds can be traced to the depths of the tumour.
4 Infiltration is on a broad basis with pushing margins against a stroma containing a prominent inflammatory reaction.
5 The usual cytological and infiltrating growth pattern of squamous carcinoma is absent.

There are two principal controversies relating to verrucous carcinoma. Firstly, otolaryngologists and pathologists cannot agree about which cases should be included in this category, and some respected authorities even deny that it is a true tumour. Secondly, there is argument about whether the apparent transition which is sometimes observed from a relatively benign to a highly malignant tumour is due to irradiation or is an independent phenomenon.

Verrucous carcinoma, which accounts for only about 1% of cases of laryngeal carcinoma, was first described in 1948. Its characteristic exophytic, fungating macroscopic appearance, likened to white fronds of seaweed, is distinct from that of typical squamous carcinoma. Many cases described as verrucous by the surgeon do not, however, fulfil the established criteria for a histopathological diagnosis of verrucous carcinoma. Because of its gross morphology, biopsies of verrucous carcinoma are often superficial, and the microscopic appearances are of mature squamous epithelium with hyper- and parakeratosis. However, 20% of cases of verrucous carcinoma have a hybrid nature with foci of poorly differentiated non-verrucous carcinoma. While it is true that some patients with verrucous disease treated by radiotherapy have subsequently succumbed to metastatic anaplastic carcinoma, it is not proven that irradiation has caused malignant transformation in a benign tumour. It is equally possible that the treatment has caused satisfactory regression of the well-differentiated component but a pre-existing focus of anaplastic carcinoma has escaped cure. Certainly this aggressive behaviour has been noted in patients treated by other modalities. It is not unreasonable to regard verrucous carcinoma as a tumour with malignant potential from the start, and to treat it as one would any squamous carcinoma. Thus a tumour sufficiently large at presentation to compromise the airway would be treated by laryngectomy, and smaller tumours would be irradiated. On the other hand only larynges, not lives, will be lost if radiotherapy is considered contraindicated, and a policy of primary radical surgery is followed.

Adenocarcinoma

True adenocarcinoma is a very uncommon lesion in the larynx. The tumour mainly affects men, is generally large on presentation, and about half the patients have lymph node metastases. Distant metastases are also fairly common and the prognosis, whatever the treatment, is poor.

The salivary adenocarcinomas, mainly adenoid cystic carcinoma, are probably equally as common; they behave in the same way as elsewhere.

Fibrosarcoma

This interesting tumour is polypoidal, with a stroma of dysplastic spindle cell material (the pseudosarcomatous element) covered by a squamous cell carcinomatous component. It is probably of epithelial origin and the sarcomatous element is probably an unusual proliferative response to the carcinoma.

Much the commonest site of origin is the vocal cord and anterior commissure. About 20% of these tumours metastasize to the cervical glands; contrary to what is often said, both histological elements may metastasize.

This tumour is treated surgically; it is becoming clear that the prognosis is not as good as was once thought.

Carcinoid tumours

Less than 30 carcinoid tumours of the larynx have been described but it is possible that this tumour is not as rare as it appears. Many are probably incorrectly classified as undifferentiated adenocarcinomas, undifferentiated carcinomas and possibly also paragangliomas and adenoid cystic carcinomas. It usually affects men between the ages of 50 and 70 and most cases are in the supraglottis. No cases of carcinoid syndrome with endocrine function have been described in the larynx. The tumours are radioresistant and produce early cervical node metastases. Surgery is the only effective form of

treatment either in the form of partial or total laryngectomy. The prognosis of carcinoids of the larynx is not good because of early metastases and most described cases have had a fatal outcome.

Mucoepidermoid tumours

Less than 40 mucoepidermoid tumours of the larynx have been described. They usually arise in the supraglottis but are not uncommon in the vocal cords or subglottis. Treatment is always by surgery since they are radioresistant.

Adenoid cystic carcinoma

Of all cases of adenoid cystic carcinoma, 1.5% occur in the larynx as compared with 6.6% in the trachea, 22.8% in the nose and paranasal sinuses and 34% in the oral cavity and pharynx. Of these tumours, 80% lie in the subglottis and most occur in males between the ages of 40 and 70. No survivor has been reported in the literature from an adenoid cystic carcinoma of the larynx. Because of the spread along perineural and perivascular planes the preferred treatment is total laryngectomy.

Rhabdomyosarcoma

This is the most frequent sarcoma of infants and adolescents but although 30% of all laryngeal rhabdomyosarcomas have been seen in children between the ages of 5 and 15 and 2 cases have been reported in neonates, the majority of patients are between the ages of 40 and 70. Rhabdomyosarcomas occur in any part of the larynx and the preferred treatment is removal of tumour bulk followed by radiation and combination chemotherapy. A survival rate of 50–70% can now be achieved with this therapeutic regime.

Plasmacytoma

About 25% of extramedullary (primary or soft tissue) plasmacytomas occur in the larynx, but even so they are a rare laryngeal tumour. They are usually single, and in appearance vary from polypoid to sessile. Lymph node metastases can occur, and ultimately a small proportion develop disseminated medullary disease. If the tumour cannot be managed endoscopically, radiation should be used.

Malignant synovioma

These usually occur on the extremities, particularly the hands and feet, but about 50 have now been described in the hypopharynx and larynx. Most of the patients were between 20 and 30 years of age and the tumours are usually supraglottic or in the pyriform fossa or posterior wall of the hypopharynx. The prognosis is better than similar tumours in the extremities and a survival rate of 20–30% is quoted. The tumours are radioresistant and the preferred treatment is radical surgery.

Kaposi's sarcoma

This disease was rare in Europe and America until recently, when it has become more and more common in association with acquired immune deficiency syndrome (AIDS). A review of 13 cases of Kaposi's sarcoma in the larynx showed that all of these patients also had skin tumours. Involvement of the larynx is thus only to be expected in the late stages when the disease has already been diagnosed from the skin lesions.

Investigations

History

Ask the patient how long he or she has been hoarse, whether he or she smokes, what his or her job is, whether he or she has any trouble with the nose or chest, and about general health. All these factors have some bearing on subsequent treatment. Dysphagia or referred otalgia indicates spread into the pharynx.

Examination

Examine the larynx with a mirror and draw your findings. Do a general head and neck examination and be particularly meticulous about feeling for lymph nodes. Take particular note of bad teeth or sepsis of the nose or postnasal space. An assessment of the respiratory function is also necessary if a partial operation is being contemplated.

If the patient has a hypersensitive throat or over-hanging epiglottis, the fibreoptic laryngoscope is a very useful adjunct.

Radiology

The most accurate preoperative assessment of the extent of a laryngeal tumour is provided by radiology. Firstly, take a plain film of the neck to demonstrate destruction of cartilage. The thyroid cartilage calcifies in an irregular manner so that it may be difficult to be certain that destruction has occurred. However, if cartilage destruction has taken place, it is almost always by extension of the tumour along the thyroepiglottic ligament to involve the part of the cartilage adjacent to the anterior commissure. In a lateral film the anterior edges of the thyroid laminae, if they are calcified, present an appearance resembling a figure-of-eight. The part of the cartilage almost always involved by a tumour is at the waist of

the eight, and expansion of this point is indicative of cartilaginous destruction.

Tomograms give more detailed information than plain films but they do not demonstrate immobility of any part of the larynx. Furthermore, the definition is not as good as it is sometimes thought to be.

Laryngograms and xerograms have now been virtually abandoned in the assessment of laryngeal carcinoma.

Conventional tomography does not demonstrate the submucosal margins of the tumour, nor does it demonstrate cartilage invasion accurately. It has therefore largely been supplanted by computed tomography (CT) scanning. This method provides helpful information about areas hidden from view by bulky tumours, such as the subglottis, the apex of the pyriform fossa and the laryngeal ventricle. However, it too does not demonstrate cartilage invasion accurately, and it has been shown that the correlation between CT scans and pathology is at best 70%. A further advantage of the CT scan is that it can demonstrate lymph node metastases before they are clinically evident.

Magnetic resonance imaging (MRI) is now becoming available in many centres but its place has not yet been fully delineated. This method is very good for demonstrating intralaryngeal structures, particularly the intrinsic muscle, and it clearly differentiates non-ossified from ossified cartilage. However, it is not able to distinguish recurrent tumour from radiation fibrosis and oedema. It has been shown that the specificity of CT and MRI with respect to the detection of cartilaginous invasion is roughly equal, at 90% (i.e. there are only 10% false-positive findings). None the less, the sensitivity of CT imaging is only half that of MRI (45% against 90%), i.e. the incidence of false-negative findings with CT scanning is much greater than with MRI scans. MRI also demonstrates invasion of the pre-epiglottic and para-glottic spaces very well. It is, of course, important to detect the extent of the tumour before treatment so that the tumour can be classified correctly. However, many surgeons regard radiology with a certain air of scepticism because it very rarely affects the decision as to how to treat the patient.

Laboratory investigations

The usual preoperative checks are made; in addition it is occasionally advisable to do a Wasserman reaction, especially in a young person.

Biopsy

Biopsy of a laryngeal tumour is obtained at laryngoscopy, under general anaesthetic.

Laryngoscopy under general anaesthetic obviously presents problems, because the anaesthetist and the surgeon both wish to monopolize the airway in a patient whose upper respiratory tract may often be compromised because of a tumour. If the patient does not have respiratory obstruction, the most satisfactory method is to examine the larynx under general anaesthetic given through a stiff, wide catheter (the insufflation technique). This ensures a good airway and allows the anaesthetist to oxygenate the patient, but because the catheter does not occupy all the lumen of the larynx it is possible to examine it satisfactorily.

A laryngoscopy should not be confined to confirming that there is a tumour present and taking a biopsy. It is vital to establish the limits of the tumour in three dimensions. Some of the important points are as follows.

In supraglottic tumours we wish to know how close the tumour comes to the true cords, in particular at the anterior commissure; in glottic tumours we wish to know particularly if the tumour has spread to the anterior commissure or over the vocal process and if there is subglottic or supraglottic spread. Therefore, retract the false cords with a beak of the laryngoscope and inspect the ventricle; no examination is complete without using the anterior commissure laryngoscope to inspect the subglottic space. Also, always examine the postcricoid region and cervical oesophagus, the valleculae and the pyriform fossae. Make drawings showing the exact extent of the tumour, with measurements.

Take a biopsy of the tumour, using as large a pair of forceps as possible, and do not crush the specimen. It is not necessary and indeed may be misleading to take a biopsy specimen including an area of apparently normal epithelium, because the epithelium of this area may only show premalignant changes and an indefinite report may be issued. Therefore, take several biopsies from the growing edge of the tumour – material at the centre of the tumour may be necrotic.

The authors believe there is no place for microlaryngoscopy in the assessment of laryngeal carcinoma.

Treatment policy

Over 95% of patients with laryngeal carcinoma are treatable. Causes of untreatability include distant metastases (less than 1%), extremely bad general health and the rare refusal by the patient. Very advanced tumours, involving all compartments of the larynx with a fixed cord and nodes that are bilateral and fixed, do very badly, having a 5-year survival of less than 5%. Radical surgery for these patients is therefore probably not justifiable.

The policy in many centres in the UK is to irradiate virtually all tumours and carry out a total laryngectomy for recurrent disease. For small glottic tumours this is excellent treatment as the cure rate is very high

and, as recurrence is very unlikely, the patient retains a normal voice. The only slight exception to this is the patient with a chronically inflamed larynx due to chronic laryngitis, heavy smoking, nasal sepsis or chronic bronchitis. Radiotherapy in such a patient often leads to a severe reaction, progressing sometimes to radiation necrosis. The patient then must lose the larynx in difficult circumstances and would have stood as good a chance of being cured with a retained voice if he or she had had a partial laryngectomy.

Although the results at other sites are not so good, primary radiotherapy with careful follow-up and salvage laryngectomy gives results which are just as good as primary surgery, with the advantage that the patient often keeps the larynx. Thus, despite the enthusiasm for surgery in many parts of the world, all the evidence is that the vast majority of patients should be treated primarily by radiotherapy with the exception of three specific instances: primary surgery should be used for patients with cartilage destruction, lymph node invasion or stridor as a presenting symptom.

A résumé of a reasonable league table of methods of treatment is shown in Table 9.9. This only considers treatment of the primary tumour. The policy for individual types of node involvement has already been discussed in Chapter 7.

Table 9.9 Résumé of treatment of squamous carcinoma of the larynx

| | N_0 | Supraglottis | | |
		N_1	N_2	N_3
T_1	RT	Supraglottic laryngectomy		
T_2	RT	Total laryngectomy		
T_3	?RT ?Total laryngectomy	Total laryngectomy		
T_4		Total laryngectomy		
		Glottis		
T_1	?RT ?Laser	NA	NA	NA
T_2	RT	NA	NA	NA
T_3	?RT ?Total laryngectomy	Total laryngectomy		
T_4		Total laryngectomy		
		Subglottis		
T_1	RT	Total laryngectomy		
T_2	RT	Total laryngectomy		
T_3		Total laryngectomy		
T_4		Total laryngectomy		

RT = Radiotherapy; NA = not applicable.

Technique of total laryngectomy

Preparation

If endotracheal anaesthesia is used the anaesthetic tube should be led out over the patient's head and this is where the anaesthetist should place him- or herself. Sterilize the skin of the whole neck, the lower half of the face, and the chest and shoulders down to the nipple line. Stitch a sterile anaesthetic connecting tube to the chest skin so that it is ready in place for quick connection to the tracheostomy tube when the trachea is divided. This prevents the anesthetist contaminating the area at the time of the tracheostomy later in the operation.

Incision

The incision depends on whether the patient has or has not been irradiated and whether a radical neck dissection is to be carried out.

If the patient has not been irradiated the best approach is a collar incision (Fig. 9.3) situated halfway between the hyoid bone and the upper edge of the sternum, extending laterally on each side to the anterior border of the sternomastoid muscles. This incision has many advantages: it gives good access; it leaves a good cosmetic scar that heals well because it is in a skin crease; the skin incision is at right angles to the line of pharyngeal repair; and there is a large inferior flap in which to make a hole for the permanent tracheostomy. If a radical neck dissection is required either at the time or later, this incision can be extended (Fig. 9.4) by lateral limbs, one running upwards to the mastoid process and one downwards to the junction of the trapezius and the clavicle.

Other incisions have been described but they are less satisfactory. The midline vertical incision is not satisfactory for a laryngectomy because it gives a poor cosmetic result, it lies immediately over the pharyngeal repair, and the final tracheostomy is included in the incision. The final tracheostomy after

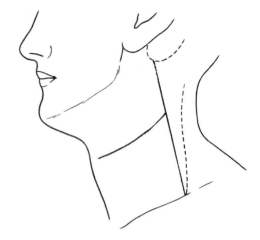

Fig. 9.4 Total laryngectomy: incision for non-irradiated patient with neck dissection.

laryngectomy should never be thus included because this leads to infection and wound breakdown – it should always be brought out through a hole in the lower skin flap.

Although the Gluck–Sorensen U-shaped flap seems attractive because it gives a large skin flap to cover the pharynx, it also suffers from disadvantages: firstly, the final stoma is usually included in the incision and secondly, the vertical limbs almost certainly cut off a large part of the blood supply to the central flap. Also if a radical neck dissection is required later it is not easy to reopen this incision in such a way as to give good access to the neck.

Mobilization of the larynx

Raise the skin flaps, including the platysma, and stitch them out of the way. If a radical neck dissection has been carried out leave it attached to the larynx with as wide a pedicle as possible.

The basic principle of total laryngectomy is that it is used for those large tumours that are known to extend into the surrounding structures, in particular the thyroid gland, the strap muscles, and the pre-epiglottic space. Remove the larynx, therefore, in a block including the strap muscles, the hyoid bone and at least one lobe of the thyroid gland.

Identify the medial border of the sternomastoid muscle and begin mobilizing the larynx by dissecting in the plane medial to the muscle (Fig. 9.5); dissect posteriorly to identify the carotid sheath and retract this laterally. Dissect down to the clavicle and up to the hyoid bone; tie the branches of the anterior jugular veins with 3/0 silk. On the side on which the thyroid lobe is to be removed, identify, divide and transfix the superior and inferior thyroid artery and vein, and the middle thyroid vein.

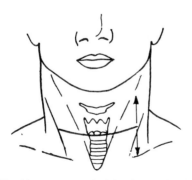

Fig. 9.3 Total laryngectomy: incision for non-irradiated patient with no neck dissection.

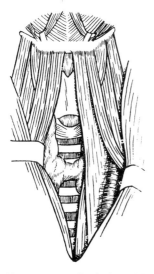

Fig. 9.5 Total laryngectomy: beginning of dissection medial to carotid sheath.

Next divide the strap muscles immediately above the sternum (Fig. 9.6) and the muscles above the hyoid bone; dissect through the fat lateral to the trachea until the tracheal wall is exposed. Dissect out the paratracheal chain of nodes at this point, if necessary following them blindly with a finger into the superior mediastinum. This is also a good opportunity to practise exposure of the recurrent laryngeal nerve lying in the tracheo-oesophageal groove. Divide this nerve, and dissect sharply in the groove separating the oesophagus from the posterior membranous wall of the trachea.

At this point be careful not to enter the pre-epiglottic space. Also do not attempt to preserve any part of the hyoid bone. Ligate and divide the inferior thyroid veins.

On the other side of the larynx on which one lobe of the thyroid gland is to be preserved dissect medial to the sternomastoid muscle, again identifying the carotid sheath and retracting it laterally. Find the superior thyroid artery and vein, divide, transfix and tie them with 3/0 silk. This mobilizes the larynx up to the level of the hyoid bone. Do not divide the inferior thyroid artery on this side, however, as it is the only blood supply to the lobe that is to be preserved. Mobilize this lobe by dividing the isthmus, and peel the thyroid lobe laterally off the trachea, dividing the numerous small vessels that run into the thyroid gland here with cutting diathermy. Dissect the strap muscles off the lobe of the thyroid gland and leave them in continuity with the specimen; this is the only point during the operation at which it is justifiable to dissect the strap muscles. If there is any doubt that the tumour may have spread into the thyroid lobe on the second side, do not hesitate to mobilize the lobe completely by dividing the inferior thyroid artery, leaving the lobe attached to the specimen. It is much easier to give a patient thyroid and calcium supplements than to treat for a recurrence.

Division of the trachea (Fig. 9.7)

The trachea can be divided at any stage in the operation from now onwards, but the easiest method is to divide it now. Make sure that all the inferior

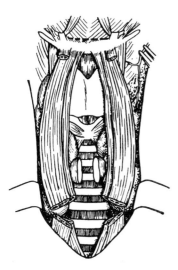

Fig. 9.6 Total laryngectomy: division of muscles and thyroid isthmus.

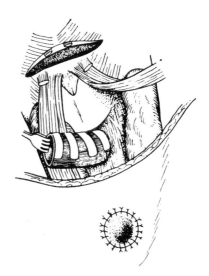

Fig. 9.7 Total laryngectomy: division of trachea and creation of stoma.

thyroid veins running next to the trachea have been divided, and mobilize the cervical trachea by dissecting in the plane between the trachea and the oesophagus. Next, estimate the position on the skin flap for the final tracheostomy and make a hole at this site about an inch in diameter, by developing upper and lower flaps.

Before proceeding further, make sure that the anaesthetist is ready to change the connections, that the connecting tube stitched on the chest at the beginning of the operation is still in a good position, that a tracheostomy tube of appropriate size (usually size 39) is available, and that its cuff has been tested and then deflated. Then divide the trachea. It is often said that the cut through the trachea should be bevelled from below upwards so that the end of the trachea will be vertical when it is swung forwards. However, this technique cuts through cartilage, which often then becomes necrotic and is expelled leading to stomal stenosis. It is much better to divide cleanly through one of the spaces between the tracheal rings.

If the anaesthetist has withdrawn the endotracheal tube, and if you have mobilized the oesophagus from the trachea, the trachea can be divided in one movement at this point; pull it forwards through the hole in the lower skin flap. Before proceeding further, place a small swab in the laryngeal remnant to prevent contaminated secretions running down into the wound. Put the cuffed tube in the trachea and connect it to the tube that was placed on the chest at the start of the operation.

Making the stoma is a very important step and it should be done as carefully as possible in two layers in order to ensure an airtight junction. Use catgut sutures to stitch the peritracheal fascia to the subcutaneous tissues in the lower skin flap. There should now be a small excess of the trachea projecting above the level of the skin and there should be an airtight closure of subcutaneous tissue to peritracheal fascia. Finally, reinforce the subcutaneous layer with a meticulous skin-to-mucosa closure using interrupted vertical mattress sutures of 3/0 nylon on a cutting needle. Put the needle in about 5 mm away from the skin edge and then into the tracheal wall but not through it. Then come vertically upwards in the tracheal wall for a distance of 3–4 mm, emerging right at the edge of the mucosa; then put the needle back through the skin edge and tie a knot loosely to allow for later swelling of the skin edge (Fig. 9.8).

Do not put sutures right through the wall of the trachea as this could lead to cartilage necrosis and contraction of the stoma. These sutures can easily be inserted with the endotracheal tube in place and it should not be necessary to disturb the anaesthetist, who continues the anaesthetic through the tracheostomy.

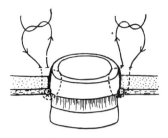

Fig. 9.8 Method of suture for tracheostome.

Removal of the larynx

The larynx can be removed from below upwards or above downwards, but the latter is safer because the inside of the larynx can be seen, and there is no danger of cutting into tumour.

Grasp the body of the hyoid bone with a large forceps and pull it forwards. With a knife cut through the base of the tongue until the pharynx is opened into; beginners are often surprised at how deep they have to go to enter the pharynx. Be careful at this point not to open into the pre-epiglottic space. As soon as the pharynx is opened the first assistant retracts the base of the tongue with a retractor placed through the hole in the pharyngeal mucosa. Then grasp the tip of the epiglottis with Allis forceps and pull it anteriorly and inferiorly. Cut the pharyngeal mucosa with scissors laterally on each side of the epiglottis, aiming towards the superior cornu of the thyroid cartilage.

Now change position and stand at the head of the table, so that you can see downwards into the larynx. Have the epiglottis held with the Allis forceps and pulled forwards by an assistant, release the larynx by dividing the constrictor muscles along the posterior edge of the thyroid cartilage with scissors. Then divide the pharyngeal mucosa on each side in the region of the superior cornu of the thyroid cartilage, aiming downwards for the posterior part of the arytenoid cartilage.

These two cuts are joined posteriorly, inferior to the cricoarytenoid joint, where there is a good plane of cleavage on the posterior cricoarytenoid muscle. Be careful to keep below the cricoarytenoid joint, and its overlying mucosa, because cancer can spread posteriorly through this joint. By following this plane downwards between the trachea and the oesophagus the larynx can be removed. Do not remove the lobe of the thyroid gland which it is intended to preserve by careless dissection during this stage. Make sure that the retained lobe of the thyroid gland is well clear of the tracheostomy or it may cause tracheal stenosis.

If a sucker is put into the lumen of the pharynx whilst removing the larynx do not allow it to be taken out, to prevent cancer cells being spilled into the tissues of the neck. Also do not contaminate the wound with instruments or suckers that have been used during removal of the tumour, but place these in a separate receiver. Discard them after removal of the tumour.

Repair of the pharynx (Fig. 9.9)

After the larynx has been removed, all personnel must change their gowns and gloves, instruments used in the dissection should be changed and resterilized, and clean towels should be placed over those already in position as they are now probably contaminated. The wound should also be washed at this stage.

Most text books describe the repair of the defect in the pharynx in the shape of a T. This inevitably produces a three-point junction, which is bad surgical technique, and is one of the factors causing a fistula. Therefore, repair the pharynx in three layers in a straight line as follows.

Before starting to close the pharynx pass a nasogastric tube and confirm that it is definitely in the oesophagus. If the mucosal edges are lacerated or have holes in them, tidy up the edges: never use damaged mucosa for a closure. Start at the lower end of the pharyngeal defect with a 3/0 catgut suture and put in a running extramucosal stitch, which picks up the edges of the pharyngeal mucosa but does not pierce the mucosa. The submucosal edges must stick together and for this an inverting suture is essential.

Continue upwards uniting the edges of the defect until the superior end is reached; tie the end of the suture and tag it with artery forceps. One layer is now completed and the defect has been closed in a straight line with no three-point junctions. Reinforce this layer with two more layers of continuous 3/0 black silk, the first being through the fascia and the second through the constrictor muscles.

Closure

Before closing the skin, if the patient has been irradiated, protect the carotid sheath with a muscle flap of the levator scapulae if a neck dissection has been done, or the sternomastoid if not.

Stitch two suction drains in place and close the skin in two layers.

Specific aftercare

In order to check that there is no fistula present give the patient a glass of milk or methylene blue in water to take before removing the nasogastric tube. If he or she can drink the whole glass without any milk appearing from the neck then the nasogastric tube can be safely removed and a soft diet begun. It is wise, however, to watch the wound for the first 12 h of feeding because a fistula is still possible. Begin feeding by mouth with a soft diet when the tube has been taken out, usually after 7–10 days.

A very important part of the rehabilitation of a patient after total laryngectomy is the restoration of the voice. This may be done by teaching the patient oesophageal speech or by various artificial devices.

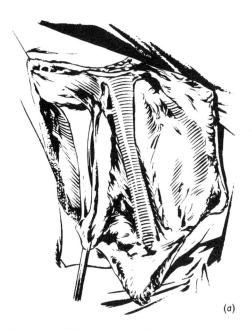
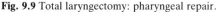
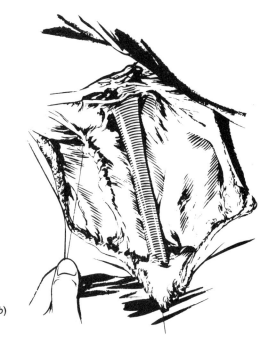

(a)   (b)

Fig. 9.9 Total laryngectomy: pharyngeal repair.

Oesophageal speech is much the best method of alaryngeal speech because the patient can use it at all times and no artificial devices which must be carried are needed. Although the voice achieved by this method can be very good it is naturally never as good as the normal voice and many women dislike it because it sounds gruff and masculine. However, many men who need their voice for work have returned to work by the use of this method. The principle of oesophageal speech is that air is passed into the oesophagus either by swallowing or by pressing with the tongue and is then regurgitated so that it causes the cricopharyngeus or other pharyngeal structures to vibrate, producing a sound that is modulated by the articulating mechanism in the usual way. It is thought that development of good oesophageal voice depends on the following factors: sex, age (elderly patients sometimes do not bother to develop this type of voice), motivation, intelligence, local factors in the pharynx (such as scarring), the formation of diverticula and the shape of the pharynx (a wide pharynx is thought to be necessary), and the condition of the oesophagus (if the patient has a hiatus hernia he or she may find it difficult to control the air stream in the oesophagus).

It is difficult to assess how many patients develop a satisfactory oesophageal voice. Although more than 60% may do so if given intensive treatment, this is not the usual figure. Certainly very good results can be obtained by keeping the patient in hospital until he or she has developed satisfactory speech and giving lessons two or three times a day. This system is used in the Netherlands with extremely good results, but in countries with limited facilities, particularly in the UK, where this is not possible, the results are not nearly so good and probably not more than a third develop really satisfactory speech. For these patients various alternatives are available. These include external machines that produce a sound which the patient can then modify by articulation. Such machines include the Cooper Rand electronic speech aid, the Servox transcervical vibrator, the Tait oral vibrator mounted on a dental plate, and the Bart's vibrator. Most of these devices consist of a machine held to the patient's throat which produces a buzzing sound. The theory is that the patient then modifies the sound by articulation to produce intelligible speech; in practice the noise produced is monotonous, metallic and often scarcely intelligible.

The alternatives are some form of tracheopharyngeal fistula and the neoglottis procedures. These will be discussed below.

Complications

1 Fistula – the principles involved in this are dealt with in Chapter 5.
2 Stenosis of the pharynx. This usually responds to dilatation but on occasion pharyngeal augmentation with a pectoralis major flap is required.
3 Stenosis of the tracheostomy.
4 Recurrence within the pharynx or at the site of the tracheostomy. Recurrence within the pharynx may respond to radiotherapy. If not, the pharynx should be resected and reconstituted by a jejunal loop as described in the chapter on the hypopharynx.
5 Stomal recurrence has four causes: implantation in the track of a preoperative tracheostomy, inadequate excision, tumour in paratracheal nodes, and a second tumour in the cervical trachea. If the recurrence invades the anterior part of the stoma it is virtually always untreatable because the lesion on the surface is the tip of the iceberg wrapped around the great vessels in the mediastinum. If the lesion affects the upper, posterior part of the stoma it can sometimes be managed successfully by a thoracotracheostomy (p. 128).

Technique of supraglottic laryngectomy

Anaesthetic

Use an endotracheal general anaesthetic as for the neck dissection, do a tracheostomy just before the laryngectomy and continue the anaesthetic through this.

Incision and radical neck dissection

Halfway through, this operation may need to be modified to a total laryngectomy, and also a contralateral neck dissection may be needed later. For these reasons use a collar incision with two lateral limbs as described previously; this meets all eventualities. As the operation must not be done for failed radiotherapy, this problem need not be considered.

Elevate the flaps and stitch them in the usual way. Carry out a radical neck dissection leaving the specimen attached by the superior lymphatic pedicle at the thyrohyoid membrane, taking great care to ensure that the specimen does not become detached because the pedicle is too narrow.

Do not include the thyroid gland in the radical neck dissection; this is unnecessary and exposes the recurrent laryngeal nerve to damage.

Be careful not to injure the vagus nerve – paralysed vocal cords after a supraglottic laryngectomy are a tragedy that may well end with the patient requiring total laryngectomy because of inhalation.

Mobilization of the supraglottic larynx

The principle of this part of the operation is to mobilize all of the supraglottic larynx in continuity with the pre-epiglottic space and the lymph nodes.

Divide the strap muscles (Fig. 9.10) on both sides at the level of the superior border of the thyroid cartilage and turn them down to the lower border of the cartilage. Identify the lower border of the thyroid cartilage and the notch on the upper border. Measure this distance, and make a mark halfway between the two points with methylene blue. This marks the position of the anterior commissure in men. In women the commissure is slightly higher, being one-third of the distance between the two above points from the notch. From this point, mark a horizontal line posteriorly along the cartilage perpendicular to the posterior edge of the thyroid cartilage, using needles soaked in dye. Cut through the perichondrium along the upper edge of the cartilage and elevate it down to the level of the marks in the cartilage (Fig. 9.11). Be careful not to tear the perichondrium – this is particularly likely to happen at the midline where it is very thin.

With a Stryker saw or dental fissure burr divide the cartilage along the line marked with dye, taking care to divide only the cartilage and not the mucosa of the larynx. Divide both sides of the thyroid cartilage.

Next divide the muscles attached to the upper border of the hyoid bone.

Divide and transfix the superior thyroid artery and vein on either one or both sides depending on the extent of the operation.

Removing the tumour (Figs 9.12 and 9.13)

This step is best carried out from the top of the table, and it is wise at this stage to wear a head lamp.

Cut down with scissors towards the vallecula, just above the hyoid bone, on the side of the radical neck

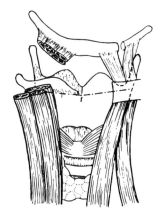

Fig. 9.11 Supraglottic laryngectomy: cartilage cuts marked and perichondrium turned down.

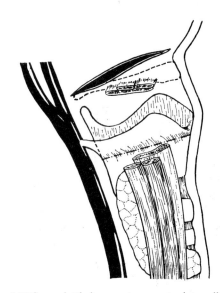

Fig. 9.12 Supraglottic laryngectomy: entry into vallecula.

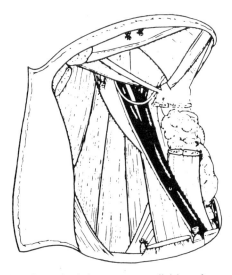

Fig. 9.10 Supraglottic laryngectomy: division of strap muscles.

dissection, and enter into the pharynx. If there is a tumour in the vallecula then enter the pharynx through the pyriform fossa on the side of the radical neck dissection.

Divide the mucosa at the base of the tongue with scissors, working from side to side through the vallecula, keeping well clear of the tumour. Retract the base of the tongue and have the epiglottis held forward with an Allis forceps. Standing at the head of the table you can now look down into the larynx and assess the extent of the tumour accurately.

For an epiglottic tumour divide each aryepiglottic fold immediately anterosuperior to the arytenoid cartilage, well clear of tumour; for a tumour on the aryepiglottic fold divide the uninvolved fold above

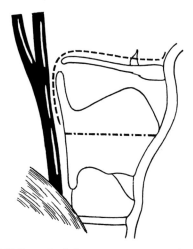

Fig. 9.13 Supraglottic laryngectomy: extent of excision.

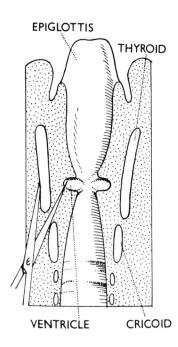

Fig. 9.15 Schematic diagram to show division through the ventricle and the thyroid cartilage.

the arytenoid cartilage but, on the side of the tumour, incise through the cricoarytenoid joint.

It is now necessary to see the ventricles, so have the assistant retract the arytenoids laterally with two skin hooks. Place one blade of the scissors inside the ventricle superior to the vocal cord, and the other blade outside the thyroid cartilage opposite the incision in the cartilage. Carry the cuts forward through the ventricles and remove the specimen with the radical neck dissection in continuity (Figs. 9.14 and 9.15).

Cricopharyngeal myotomy (Fig. 9.16)

The next step in the operation is to divide the cricopharyngeus muscle. Pass a finger into the oesophagus – the muscle will be felt in spasm, which later causes difficulty in swallowing if it is not relieved. With a finger in the oesophagus cut down through the muscle fibres as far as the mucosa. The upper part of the oesophagus should then feel loose and capacious. Do the myotomy posteriorly to avoid damage to the recurrent laryngeal nerves.

Repair of the pharynx (Figs. 9.17 and 9.18)

Make absolutely sure that all bleeding has stopped. Leave any raw surface to heal by granulation and do not attempt to close any gaps with mucosal flaps as this leads to laryngeal immobility from fibrosis.

Close the pharynx in three layers, the first one of which is under some tension. Using 2/0 silk place a stitch at the apex of the wound on the opposite side of entry into the pharynx – tie this stitch, tag it with an artery forceps and give it to the assistant, who puts the handles over the point of another artery forceps. Then place stitches about 8 mm apart, taking a big extramucosal bite in the base of the tongue above, and in the perichondrial flap below. Do not tie any of these stitches but tag each of them and store them in order on the upturned artery forceps. After placing stitches over halfway across the defect, reverse the order of the forceps by passing them on to another forceps, the last being passed first and so on.

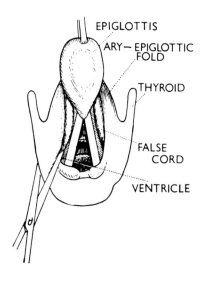

Fig. 9.14 Larynx from above to show line of division through the ventricle.

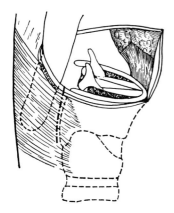

Fig. 9.16 Cricopharyngeal myotomy.

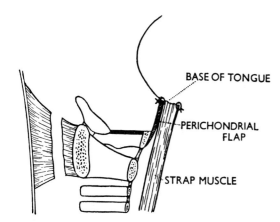

Fig. 9.17 Pharyngeal repair.

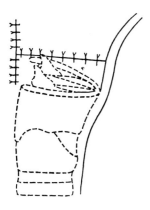

Fig. 9.18 Pharyngeal repair completed.

The first stitch has been tied already – leave this hanging on an artery forceps as a marker. Then cross the third stitch, but do not tie it – this takes the tension off the second stitch, which the assistant ties and cuts on the knot. He or she then takes the fourth stitch and crosses it to take the tension off the third stitch, which you must not release until now – tie it, and take the fifth stitch, taking the tension off the fourth held by your assistant. Proceed in this fashion until you have closed over half the defect. The remainder of the defect on the side of entry into the pharynx is now nearly vertical – place stay sutures at the top and bottom of this and close the rest of the defect with extramucosal inverting sutures. While closing the lower end of this part of the defect be careful not to catch any of the mucosa over the arytenoid cartilage in the stitch. There should be no tension on these sutures.

Now put a second row of interrupted sutures from the base of the tongue above to the sternothyroid muscle remnant below, and finally a third row of interrupted sutures from the sternohyoid muscle below to the bellies of the digastric muscle above, using 2/0 silk for each layer.

Close the skin in the usual fashion leaving a suction drain in the wound, leave the tracheostomy in place and a nasogastric tube down the nose.

Specific aftercare

1 Cork the tracheostomy tube as soon as this can be tolerated – usually between 7 and 10 days.
2 When the tracheostomy has been fully corked and the patient breathes easily, begin feeding by mouth.

The patient has lost many of the protrective mechanisms of the respiratory tract – the epiglottis, the aryepiglottic folds, the false vocal cords and the supraglottic sensory reflex. In order to be able to swallow without inhaling, he or she must, therefore, be able firstly to approximate the vocal cords, and secondly to develop a positive subglottic pressure.

Begin feeding with a semisolid diet such as rice pudding, ice cream or jelly. Tell the patient to take a deep breath before each mouthful, then bolt it in one rather than allowing it to trickle down.

During this early phase many patients have difficulty, inhale some of their food and cough. Be prepared at this stage to sit with them and encourage them to persevere. Intake and output charts must be kept meticulously and fluid shortages made good with an intravenous infusion. Weigh the patient every 2 or 3 days to make sure that he or she is getting enough to eat. When the patient is taking a reasonable amount remove the tracheostomy tube and sew up the stoma. This stage should be reached about a week after the patient starts feeding and thereafter the type and quantity of food that the patient can take is rapidly increased. Some patients take longer than this but all swallow eventually.

Specific complications

1 *Persistent oedema.* This usually occurs over the arytenoid cartilage because the lymphatic drainage of the mucosa in this area is via the aryepiglottic folds, which are divided during the operation. If this completely occludes the airway the patient can often swallow well because he or she cannot inhale. In this case allow the patient home with the tracheostomy in place and the larynx will slowly open up.
2 *Paralysis of the recurrent laryngeal nerve.* This may occur during the cricopharyngeal myotomy. If it does the patient will almost certainly need a total laryngectomy because of inhalation.

Extensions and modifications of the supraglottic laryngectomy

1 *Cord fixation in aryepiglottic fold lesions.* If this operation is done for a tumour of one aryepiglottic fold, one arytenoid is removed, paralysing the vocal cord on that side. Suture the cord remnant in the midline to ensure glottic closure. If this fails to close the gap, it can be easily closed by an injection of Teflon.
2 *Suprahemilaryngectomy.* This is an extension of the supraglottic laryngectomy in which an additional half of the larynx including the vocal cord is removed. Attempts have been made to reform this vocal cord by infracturing the upper half of the thyroid cartilage. If this is done with a high degree of skill and very accurately, the results can be very gratifying but in the average otolaryngologist's hands if a tumour is so big as to require this operation then it would be safer to do a total laryngectomy.
3 *Supraglottic laryngectomy for pyriform sinus lesions.* Unlike the USA, it is very rare in the UK to find small pyriform sinus tumours that can be safely removed by a supraglottic laryngectomy. Again it is unsafe for the average otolaryngologist to consider supraglottic laryngectomy for this tumour and these patients should have a total laryngectomy and partial pharyngectomy.

Technique of vertical hemilaryngectomy

Anaesthetic

The patient is laid in the supine position on the operating table and a general anaesthetic begun through an oral endotracheal tube. Then make a tracheostomy between the third and fourth tracheal rings, insert a size 36 cuffed Portex tracheostomy tube and continue the general anaesthetic via this. Resterilize the skin and apply new towels.

Incision

If the strict criteria of selection for this operation are applied, a neck dissection will not be needed. For this reason use a collar incision about 8 cm long across the prominence of the thyroid cartilage (mark out the incision with methylene blue first to prevent an asymmetrical scar). Incise down to the platysma and elevate flaps up to the hyoid bone superiorly and down to the second tracheal ring inferiorly, taking care not to encroach on the tracheostomy wound.

Mobilization of muscle flaps

After raising the flap, exclude the skin surface from the wound with small towels and a Joll's clamp. Then free and identify the anterior borders of both sternomastoid muscles; free the sternohyoid muscle on the involved side only down its whole length anteriorly and posteriorly but do not detach it from either its insertion or its origin. Pass a tape round this muscle to retract it laterally and free the thyrohyoid and sternothyroid muscles (again on the involved side only) in a similar manner up to their attachments to the oblique line. Cut them off the oblique line, using sharp dissection, as close to their insertion as possible and retract them laterally (Fig. 9.19).

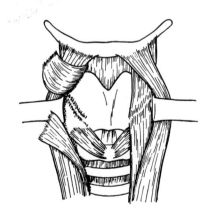

Fig. 9.19 Vertical hemilaryngectomy: detachment of strap muscles.

Formation of the perichondrial flap

Place a finger behind the posterior lamina of the thyroid cartilage and with a no. 15 blade incise along the superior border of the thyroid cartilage to the thyroid notch, then down the prominence at the midline and then along the lower margin to just in front of the posterior lamina (Fig. 9.20). Elevate the flap thus marked out, using a Freer elevator and non-toothed dissection forceps. Leave the flap attached to the posterior lamina of the thyroid cartilage.

Removal of the tumour

With a Stryker saw or dental fissure burr cut the midline of the thyroid cartilage (Fig. 9.21) but do not enter the lumen at this point. Rotate the involved side of the larynx forward and make another vertical cartilaginous cut just in front of the posterior lamina, where the perichondrial flap is attached.

The point of entry into the larynx depends on whether the tumour affects the anterior commissure or not. If it does not come up to the commissure then open into the larynx in the midline, either with

scissors or with a knife blade passed through the thyrohyoid membrane in the superior thyroid notch. If the growth comes up to the anterior commissure remove one-fifth of the opposite vocal cord by making the laryngofissure slightly to the opposite side.

When the larynx has been divided, retract the healthy side and grasp the involved side with an Allis forceps. Cut through the cricothyroid membrane along the lower border of the thyroid cartilage on the involved side; tie the cricothyroid artery. Similarly cut along the upper border of the thyroid cartilage through the thyrohyoid membrane. If the growth affects the vocal process, disarticulate the arytenoid cartilage from the cricoid and remove it. If, however, the growth does not come up to the vocal process it is better to retain the arytenoid. Do not cut across the arytenoid cartilage, especially if the patient has been irradiated, as this causes mucosal oedema after operation. The specimen is finally detached posteriorly by cutting with one blade of the scissors inside and one blade outside the posterior saw cut. Secure haemostasis with coagulation diathermy after transfixing the superior laryngeal artery.

If there is a subglottic extension of less than 5 mm remove the upper half of the ring of the cricoid cartilage to increase the margin of clearance.

Closure (Fig. 9.22)

There is no need to do a mucosal closure, but it is possible to do so by creating a flap of the mucosa of the pyriform sinus, rotating it into the laryngeal defect and stitching it into the mucosal defect.

Next, take the thyrohyoid and sternothyroid muscles and bring their cut ends together, everting them into the larynx exactly opposite the remaining vocal

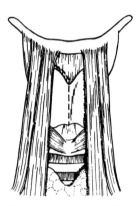

Fig. 9.20 Vertical hemilaryngectomy: cartilage incisions.

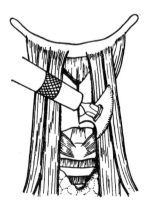

Fig. 9.21 Vertical hemilaryngectomy: division of cartilage.

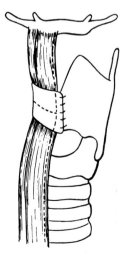

Fig. 9.22 Vertical hemilaryngectomy: laryngeal repair.

cord. Stitch them in this position with two vertical mattress sutures of 3/0 chromic catgut. The idea is to evert the ends into the form of a cord in the correct position. At this point the two sutured muscles will tend to point anteriorly but they can be rotated and sutured into the correct position by suturing them anteriorly to the remaining mucosa on the other side of the larynx and posteriorly to the mucosa that remains over the arytenoid area.

Then bring in the sternohyoid muscle to add bulk to the newly formed vocal cord. Pass the perichondrial flap outside the sternohyoid muscle and suture it to the cartilage and perichondrium on the remaining side, holding the muscles in like a belt. Close any gaps remaining above and below the closure with pursestring sutures of 3/0 chromic catgut. Close the skin in the usual fashion with drainage.

Specific aftercare

1 The tracheostomy is half corked at the end of a week, and can be fully corked and removed in about 10 days – earlier or later depending on the amount of swelling that occurs within the larynx and also depending on how much cord has been removed on the opposite side.
2 The patient is not allowed to speak for at least a week and then is helped to speak by a speech therapist. The speech ought to be quite normal from an early stage.

Specific complications

1 *Air leak.* If the closure has not been properly performed surgical emphysema occurs, even after a week, every time the patient coughs or tries to speak. This usually settles well with a pressure bandage and voice rest.
2 *Laryngeal stenosis.* If more than one-fifth of the opposite vocal cord has been removed, a Silastic keel should be put in place and left there for at least 5 weeks. An alternative is a McNaught keel made from tantalum plate, which can be cut with heavy scissors. It has a vertical plate that lies in the laryngeal lumen, to separate the raw edges, and three flanges for fixation. Its design is shown in Figure 9.22. It is often tempting to do the closure without this in order to get the patient out of hospital sooner, but this inevitably leads to a laryngeal stenosis if much of the opposite cord has been removed.

   If stenosis does occur, reopen the larynx, divide the stenosis and put a keel in place for 5 weeks. There will be no need to do another tracheostomy as the first one will still be in place.
3 *Polyp formation.* If the arytenoid cartilage has been cut, particularly in an irradiated patient, oedematous mucosa forms over the area. This looks like a large supraglottic polyp, and it can be

removed by direct laryngoscopy. Polyp formation on the newly formed vocal cord may occur but when this is stripped off at direct laryngoscopy, which is easy, a good fibrous cord is seen underneath it.

Extensions and modifications of vertical hemilaryngectomy

1 *Cordectomy.* This operation can be done if the tumour does not involve either the vocal process of the arytenoid cartilage or the anterior commissure. Split the thyroid cartilage in the midline as described previously but do not develop an external perichondrial flap and do not remove any cartilage. Once the larynx is open, retract the sound side and remove the involved cord. Transfix the superior laryngeal artery.

   Do a mucosal closure and slide the sternohyoid muscle inside the larynx on the internal perichondrium of the thyroid cartilage to replace the lost bulk.
2 *Frontal laryngectomy.* This operation is performed for tumours that only affect the anterior commissure.

   The area to be removed is the anterior commissure and anterior one-fifth to one-third of both vocal cords with the adjacent cartilage. If the laryngeal remnant is closed primarily, laryngeal stenosis will almost certainly occur, and a McNaught keel should be used to prevent this occurring (Fig. 9.23).

   Once the specimen is removed, insert the keel and close the cartilages over the limb of the keel that enters the larynx, and suture the side arms of the keel on to the perichondrium of the thyroid cartilage. Leave this in for 5 weeks, reopen the neck and remove the keel. During this time leave the tracheostomy in place.

Neoglottis procedures

Ever since the first laryngectomy was described in 1874, attempts have been made to rehabilitate the

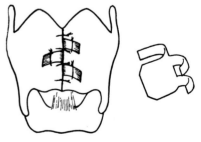

Fig. 9.23 Vertical hemilaryngectomy: McNaught keel.

speaking voice of laryngectomized patients. Most of these efforts have failed to gain popular acceptance until the development of the valves by Drs Blom, Singer and Panje.

Prior to the development of these valves, the procedures designed for producing a voice after laryngectomy could be divided into those involving the creation of tunnels by means of surgery and those involving the use of a prosthetic device to produce a sound source.

The surgical tunnels could be long ones, as described by Asai, or short ones as described by Staffieri. Although these procedures seem to work well in the hands of the originators, they did not carry the same success when used by other surgeons.

Voice prostheses could be fitted via a distant fistula, such as those described by Briani, Goode, Bryant, and Edwards, and those with a short fistula involving the Blom–Singer valve and the Panje valve.

Although the neoglottis procedures have achieved wide popularity at the present time, it is important to keep in mind that there is no need for a neoglottis procedure if the tumour has been cured by radiotherapy, if there has been a successful partial laryngectomy or if the patient has developed oesophageal voice. The usual reasons for a patient wanting a neoglottis procedure are lack of volume, lack of intelligibility, and lack of fluency in the oesophageal voice or the voice produced with a vibrator.

The tunnel for the Blom–Singer or Panje valves can be created either at the time of the primary laryngectomy or at a later date. If the procedure is done at the time of the original laryngectomy then a small fistula is made in the posterior wall of the trachea and a nasogastric tube placed in the fistula and down the oesophagus. This tube is used for feeding and, when healing is complete, the tube is removed and replaced with a speaking valve.

If it is performed as a secondary procedure then it is best done under general anaesthesia and either an oesophagoscope or a Hurst bougie passed. A fistula is made by cutting down on to this rigid instrument in the posterior wall of the trachea. A nasogastric tube is inserted for 2–3 days and then it is replaced with a valve. This, however, is only the beginning of the treatment for the patient. It is absolutely essential that the patient works with a speech therapist over the ensuing few weeks or months to get the valve fitting properly and to develop fluency in manipulation of the valve.

Although valved speech draws attention to the laryngectomized condition it compares more closely to laryngeal speech in terms of fundamental frequency and phonation time than it does to oesophageal speech.

The usual causes of failure of the speaking valve are as follows:

1 *Fixation.* If the patient has not had a radical neck dissection then prominent tendons of the sternomastoid muscle may make fixation of the Blom–Singer valve difficult. Similarly, the presence of large osteophytes can displace the valve frequently during neck turning. Generally, the Panje valve is easier to keep in place because it is shaped like a grommet, but there are too many other variables to make this as reliable as the Blom–Singer valve.
2 *Variable length.* There may be scarring at the tracheo-oesophageal area, which makes the distance between the skin and the oesophagus too great, or there may be osteophytes that narrow the pharynx. For the successful use of a valve, the tracheal stoma ought to be at least 2 cm and any degree of stomal stenosis will militate against success of a prosthesis.
3 *Patient factors.* It is very difficult for a lot of patients to learn to use these valves. They may have difficulty in removing them, replacing them and cleaning them, and their dexterity is important. Also important is the patient's interest and enthusiasm. Some patients do not like putting a finger over the trachea, especially women, and the authors have had patients reject apparently successful valves on these grounds.
4 *Pharyngo-oesophageal spasm.* Distensions of the oesophagus during airflow may produce a secondary spasm. It occurs in the majority of laryngectomized patients in varying degrees with consequent strained speech and lack of fluency. A pharyngeal nerve plexus block can temporarily eliminate the hypertonicity and should always be performed prior to a pharyngeal constrictor myotomy which will permanently reduce hypertonicity.

Near-total laryngectomy

The technique of near-total laryngectomy was introduced a decade ago. It initially did not achieve widespread acceptance because of doubts about its oncological effectiveness Results are now beginning to emerge which show that the procedure for T_3 carcinoma of the larynx is at least comparable to other modalities and it has the advantage of voice preservation.

The technique is essentially an extended hemilaryngectomy. One-half of the larynx is completely removed together with about two-thirds of the other side, leaving an arytenoid on the unaffected side. This effectively removes both paraglottic spaces. Closure is via a small mucosal tube in which the arytenoid is integrated and the patient is usually able to speak without aspirating.

In view of recent good results, although its place in the therapeutic spectrum is not yet clearly established, more attention will have to be given to it than formerly.

Stomal recurrence

The incidence of stomal recurrence ranges from 5 to 15%. The causes are:

1 inadequate resection with positive margins;
2 residual disease in the paratracheal nodes;
3 subglottic extension; and
4 tracheostomy performed prior to the resection.

Only 3% of patients with N_0 tumours have stomal disease develop as compared with 8% of N_1 tumours and 33% of N_2 tumours. The risk of stomal recurrence after emergency tracheostomy ranges from 8 to 26%. This risk drops dramatically if the subsequent laryngectomy is done within 48 h of the initial tracheostomy.

Classification

The classification is illustrated in Figure 9.24. Type 1 is localized and usually presents as a discrete nodule in the superior aspect of the stoma. The prognosis is very good if detected early. Type 2 indicates an oesophageal involvement but no inferior involvement. Prognosis for type 2 is fair to good depending on the amount of oesophageal involvement. Type 3 originates inferiorly to the stoma and usually has direct extension into the mediastinum. Type 4 indicates there is an extension laterally and often under either of the clavicles. Types 3 and 4 have had long-term controls described but no cures.

In types 1 and 2 radical therapy results in an approximate 20% 2-year cure rate. The 5-year prognosis is dismally poor but survival rates quoted are better than no survival at all. The survival of patients who are not operated on is an average 6 months with an extremely poor quality of life.

Technique of thoracotracheostomy

Incision (Fig. 9.25)

Use a T-shaped incision to create access. The first incision starts laterally in the lower neck, about 1 in (2.5 cm) above the clavicle, at the insertion of the trapezius. It extends, at this level, across the neck to a similar site on the opposite side. It includes an ellipse of skin around the stomal recurrence. The second incision is made at right angles to this in the midline and runs to the xiphisternum.

Raise the chest flaps, tying the branches of the upper internal mammary artery with other bleeding points. Strip the periosteum over the left half of the manubrium and the medial end of the clavicle, and divide the medial end of the clavicle with a Gigli saw. Then divide the first costal cartilage, usually with a knife, taking care not to injure the pleura or the internal mammary artery. Now divide the manubrium vertically in the midline with a sternal chisel and remove half of it with the medial end of the clavicle and first rib, in a block.

The superior mediastinum is now exposed and the trachea can be easily mobilized along with any palpable glands. The left innominate vein crosses the trachea and can be retracted with a tape, or divided if necessary.

Resection

If a pharyngectomy or pharyngo-oesophagectomy is being done in addition to resection of the trachea it is mobilized at this stage using the upper collar incision. When the pharynx and trachea have been mobilized, insert four catgut sutures into the peritracheal fascia, evenly spaced round the trachea, just below the level at which it will be divided; leave the sutures long with the needle attached. If the operation is being done for a stomal recurrence mobilize the involved area now with a surrounding area of normal skin and trachea. If a pharyngectomy is to be carried out do it at this stage and replace it with jejunum before creating the new stoma. Similarly, if a pharyngo-oesophagectomy is to be done transfer the stomach through the thorax to the neck prior to creating the stoma.

Repair (Fig. 9.26)

It is vital at this stage to assess the correct position of the tracheostomy. In most of these patients some of

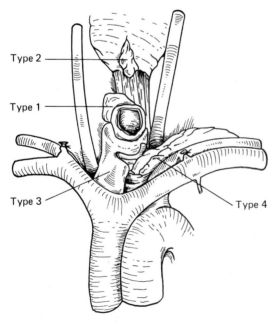

Fig. 9.24 Types of stomal recurrence.

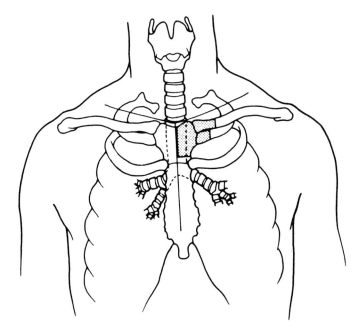

Fig. 9.25 Incision: sites of division of bone marked.

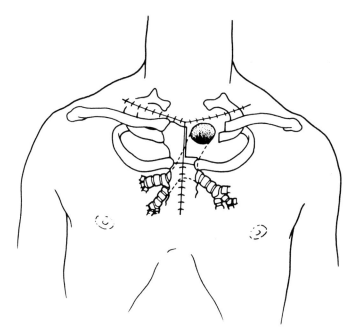

Fig. 9.26 Final division of stoma.

the skin of the neck is removed, so that a myocutaneous flap must be advanced into the defect to
protect the great vessels. The pectoralis flap is cut in
the usual fashion and the stoma is placed through it.

Lastly remove the specimen and repair the pharynx if the larynx has been removed. Suture both the
neck incisions in layers and pass a feeding tube. Use
suction drainage of the neck.

An alternative reconstruction is with a free rectus
abdominis flap.

Stomal stenosis

This may occur immediately after laryngectomy or develop years later; it must be repaired due to the danger of crusting and respiratory obstruction. Prevent stomal contracture by always making the tracheostomy through a hole in a skin flap (never in the incision) and by careful two-layer closure with meticulous skin-to-mucosa apposition (p. 118).

Stomal stenosis may also be caused by excessive scar tissue from postoperative infection or fistula, keloid formation, excessive fat around the stoma, defective or absent tracheal rings or recurrent tumour. It usually takes the form of a vertical slit or a concentric stenosis, and is very difficult to treat, as is evidenced by the multiplicity of operations to relieve it. One operation may not be satisfactory for all patients, but the first procedure to be described is suitable for most. Three other operations will be described which may all have their uses.

Procedure 1

Make two circular incisions around the tracheal opening, the outer one incising skin outside the scar tissue and the inner one incising healthy tracheal mucosa. Remove the area between the two concentric incisions and discard it, since it consists of scar tissue. Then make four radial incisions about 5 cm long at 10, 2, 4 and 8 o'clock. Undermine the skin as far as possible creating four flaps. Suture these flaps to the tracheal mucosa in two layers, one with 3/0 catgut, one with 4/0 Prolene. The contraction lines of these flaps tend to pull the tracheal mucosa upwards and outwards, thus preventing the formation of further stenosis.

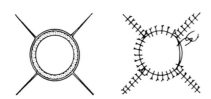

Fig. 9.27 Revision of tracheostome: procedure 1.

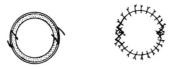

Fig. 9.28 Revision of tracheostome: procedure 2.

Procedure 2

As in the first procedure, make two concentric incisions excising the scar tissue around the mouth of the tracheostomy. The lateral part of these incisions forms one limb of a Z-plasty on each side.

Curve the limbs of the Z on each side slightly since this facilitates the creation of a circular tracheostome – when the Z-plasty is created on each side the lines of tension around the tracheostomy tend to keep it open, since they pull in the opposite direction of the original vertical scarring.

Procedure 3

This is a difficult procedure and should not be done in previously irradiated skin. Incise the scar tissue with two concentric incisions as before. Then make a swastika incision at 12, 3, 6 and 9 o'clock. Undermine the surrounding skin and rotate the flaps as shown in Figure 9.29.

Procedure 4

Make an inverted U skin flap extending from the level of the sternoclavicular joints through the middle of the stenosis. From the shoulders of the U make two 1.5 in (approx. 4 cm) incisions laterally into the neck, remove the stenosis with concentric incisions as before and elevate the lower flap down to the level of the manubrium, tying the inferior thyroid veins. Remove a section of the anterior tracheal wall and undermine a superior and lateral flap. Stitch the lower flap to the anterior tracheal wall and advance the upper flap, thereby causing a lateral pull on the revised stoma and a decrease in the width of the defect below the stoma.

All these procedures are done under local anaesthetic and there is no need for a tube to be worn after the operation.

Radiotherapy techniques

Supraglottic carcinoma

The patient lies supine, with the neck immobilized in the neutral position with the spine straight by an individually prepared Perspex beam-directing shell. This extends from the level of the upper lip to the clavicles, and prevents the patient from turning the

Fig. 9.29 Revision of tracheostome: procedure 3.

neck to either side and keeps the spine neither flexed nor extended. Two lateral opposed fields are used to encompass the supraglottis and adjacent area (Fig. 9.30). A typical field size is 8 cm high by 6 cm wide. These fields will be wedged to compensate for the contour of the neck, thereby ensuring a homogeneous dose distribution. The fields extend from the level of C2 down to the cricoid cartilage. Anteriorly they include the skin of the neck and their posterior limit is through the vertebral bodies, great care being taken not to impinge on the cervical cord. The upper anterior corner of this rectangular area is usually blocked to shield the oral mucosa.

The initial planning is done on the treatment simulator where a radiograph is taken as a permanent record of the intended field placement. Subsequently, at the first or second treatment, a double-exposure portal verification film of each field should be taken. These are for comparison with the planning film to ensure the accuracy of patient set up, and the field and block position. The treatment volume includes the whole supraglottis, irrespective of the precise location of the primary tumour, the pre-epiglottic space and the upper deep cervical (jugulo-digastric and jugulo-omohyoid) lymph nodes. Thus for the majority of patients with supraglottic tumours, those without palpable lymphadenopathy, the first echelon of nodes is treated prophylactically.

For those patients with palpable nodal involvement in whom primary surgery is not being undertaken, the whole neck should be irradiated to include the entire deep cervical chain and supraclavicular nodes on both sides. Bulky nodes which overlie the spinal cord cannot be treated adequately by lateral opposed fields, and a set-up similar to that described for pyriform fossa carcinoma should be used. Treatment is usually with 4–6 MV X-rays from a linear accelerator. A variety of dose fractionation schedules is in current use, the most common being 60 Gy in 30 fractions over 6 weeks. Many radiotherapists, however, prefer to treat over a shorter time, giving 50–55 Gy in 15–20 fractions over 3–4 weeks, or on only 3 days a week instead of 5. These various schedules are equivalent, both in terms of cure rate and late morbidity. The choice between them is largely a pragmatic one based on such factors as the workload per machine in the treatment centre and how far from the centre the patient lives. However the acute mucosal reaction is often less severe, although more prolonged, when the overall treatment time is long. Some radiotherapists, therefore, choose protracted fractionation to minimize the acute reaction when the area of mucosa to be treated is large. They are prepared to use shorter schedules for small-volume treatments where there is less risk of the patient's nutrition becoming compromised by the reaction.

Glottic carcinoma

A shell to immobilize the patient and for beam direction is prepared as described above. For early tumours (T_1 or T_2), where there is no likelihood of occult nodal involvement, very small fields are used. These are usually 5 cm × 5 cm. A perfectly fitting shell and accurate field placement are, therefore, absolutely essential to ensure that the tumour is properly covered. The fields are centred on the vocal cords, and extend up to include the thyroid cartilage and down to include the cricoid cartilage. Anteriorly the skin of the neck is included. The posterior border is at the anterior margin of the vertebral bodies (Fig. 9.31). For advanced tumours, the field is extended up or down as necessary to encompass the full extent of the disease, as revealed at examination under anaesthesia and by radiography, with a margin of about 2 cm (Fig. 9.32). For most patients a set-up using directly opposed fields, wedged to ensure homogeneity, is suitable. In squat patients with short necks, or when longer fields are needed to cover subglottic extension, two anterior oblique fields may be more appropriate. Again wedges are used to optimize the dose distribution. This set-up ensures that the patient's shoulders do not get in the way of the beam, and enables sparing of the skin at the side of the neck. Accuracy of field placement is checked by the use of planning films from the simulator, and portal verification films obtained from the treatment

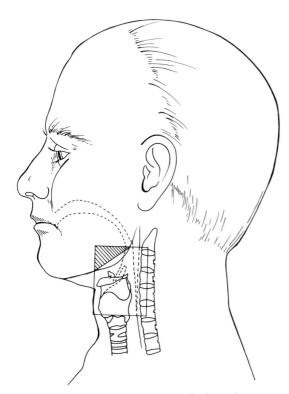

Fig. 9.30 Radiotherapy field for supraglottic carcinoma.

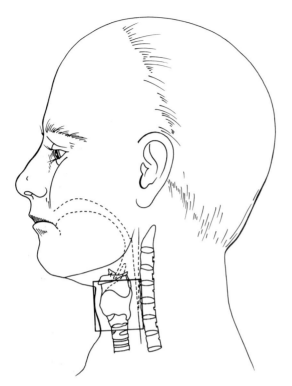

Fig. 9.31 Radiotherapy field for early glottic carcinoma.

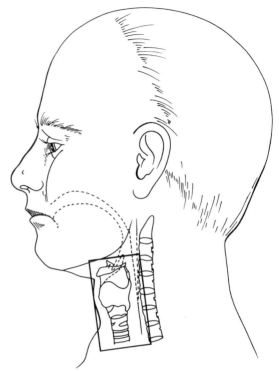

Fig. 9.32 Radiotherapy field for advanced glottic carcinoma.

machine. The prescribed dose, beam energy and fractionation schedule are the same as those used for supraglottic cancer. While surgery is the preferred treatment for the minority of patients with obvious nodal involvement, sometimes primary radical radiotherapy is used. Under these circumstances, the whole neck should also be irradiated.

Subglottic carcinoma

The treatment volume in cases of subglottic carcinoma encompasses the larynx, upper trachea and paratracheal and superior mediastinal lymph nodes. Because of the changing contour from the neck to the thorax, this is a relatively difficult area to irradiate satisfactorily. Patients are immobilized in a shell, which is also necessary for accurate alignment of treatment beams. A complex three-field technique is usually used. Left and right lateral fields have their posterior borders running through the vertebral bodies, anterior to the spinal cord and extend anteriorly to include the skin of the neck. They cover the larynx and are angled downwards to include the superior mediastinum. Wedges are used in both longitudinal and transverse directions to even out the dose distribution. Alternatively, if facilities are available, this can be achieved by the use of individually prepared tissue compensators. In addition a wedged

or compensated anterior beam is also used. This covers the width of the neck and extends from the thyroid notch down to the manubriosternal joint. Its lower corners are blocked to shield the lung apices. Dosimetry is made easier if CT planning is available. The prescribed dose fractionation schedule is the same as that used for supraglottic cancer.

Postoperative irradiation

For patients who have undergone primary surgery, postoperative radiotherapy is indicated to diminish the likelihood of local recurrence. It should be undertaken if there was histological evidence of lymph node involvement – particularly if there was any degree of extracapsular spread – or if there was direct extension of the tumour beyond the larynx into the soft tissues of the neck, oropharynx or hypopharynx. In these cases, the volume to be irradiated includes all soft tissues from the mandible to the clavicle. A full dose of 60 Gy in 30 fractions or its equivalent should be given. Treatment should be started as soon as permitted by wound healing, preferably within 3 weeks. If radiotherapy is long delayed, its chances of success are greatly diminished.

Controversies in management

Geographical and speciality variations

In different parts of the world, the management of laryngeal cancer varies. Even within one country, opinions about the best management of particular situations varies, both between the principal specialties involved and also among individual practitioners. However in some circumstances there is remarkable agreement, and the particularly controversial areas are limited. For example, a recent survey compared the policy of both otolaryngologists and radiation oncologists in Canada and the UK in the management of glottic carcinoma. For $T_1 N_0$ and $T_2 N_0$ disease there was no country or specialty difference, with radical radiotherapy recommended by more than 90% of clinicians. For $T_3 N_0$ cancer, radical radiotherapy was still the most commonly chosen treatment, although primary surgery was recommended significantly more frequently by surgeons (16%) than oncologists (4%). Radical surgery for $T_4 N_0$ cancer was chosen significantly more often by otolaryngologists (80%) and by UK doctors (73%) than by radiotherapists (53%) or Canadian practitioners (58%). For T_4 disease in Canada postoperative radiotherapy was favoured significantly more by oncologists (92%) than otolaryngologists, 47% of whom recommended surgery alone. In the UK no difference between the specialties emerged for this situation, with only 34% advising adjuvant radiotherapy.

In summary, for T_1–$T_3 N_0$ glottic carcinoma, radical radiotherapy remains the most popular treatment option. Management of $T_4 N_0$ cancer and the place of postoperative radiotherapy are more controversial.

The T_3 glottic tumour

There has been much controversy over the management of the T_3 glottic tumour; one of the causes of this controversy is that this term is used to mean two different things. Firstly, it can mean a tumour confined to one vocal cord, which is fixed, or it can mean an extensive tumour affecting two or three compartments of the larynx and which may be termed a transglottic or multiregional tumour. The latter tumour extends widely to invade the spaces within the larynx, the thyroid cartilage, and has about a 20% incidence of lymph node invasion in the neck. The former tumour can certainly be treated by irradiation with a good cure rate of about 70%. About 60% of patients will retain their larynx; the remainder will require a total laryngectomy for a later recurrence. Patients with multiregional disease often present with stridor and/or a palpable lymph node in the neck. They should virtually all be treated by total laryngectomy with radical neck dissection as indicated. Partial laryngeal procedures have been described in this circumstance, but these are dangerous brinkmanship in view of the pathological behaviour of this tumour.

Stridor

As mentioned above, some laryngeal tumours, notably the transglottic tumour, present with stridor. There are various possible ways of dealing with this situation. Firstly, a tracheostomy can be done, followed a few days later by definitive treatment either by radiation or surgery. Unfortunately this policy leads to a high incidence of recurrence of tumour within the track of the tracheostomy, even if it is excised at a subsequent total laryngectomy. For this reason, some authors have suggested the performance of an emergency laryngectomy, that is total laryngectomy carried out within about 24 h of presentation. It is doubtful if the patient can give truly informed consent in these circumstances and, furthermore, experience has shown that the mortality from this procedure is roughly the same as that from stomal recurrence if preoperative tracheostomy is done. The third alternative is to debulk the tumour as an emergency using the laser and then proceed a few days later to the appropriate definitive treatment.

Radiation necrosis

This disease should now be a thing of the past. Its main causes were inappropriate irradiation of extensive laryngeal tumours, particularly those with cartilage invasion, and more old-fashioned techniques of radiotherapy. It can be divided clinically into two types. The first type is manifest by pain in the larynx and oedema, persisting for more than 3 months after radiotherapy. Provided that the patient truly does not have a recurrence of the carcinoma this situation will usually settle down, although a tracheostomy may be needed for a few months to tide the patient over periods of respiratory obstruction. The second and more frequent form is that in which there is ulceration of the mucosa. The resulting infection usually leads to the typical foetor. This circumstance can be very difficult to distinguish from recurrent tumour; furthermore in itself it is dangerous because it can lead to a spreading infection or lung abscesses.

If the condition does not settle rapidly with antibiotics (which are usually ineffective because the larynx is relatively avascular) a total laryngectomy is needed. It should be done through a *vertical* midline incision. At the end of the operation, repair the pharynx in the usual way; sew the sternomastoid muscles over the carotid arteries to protect them, but leave the neck wound open. It is a basic surgical

principle that a heavily infected wound should not be
closed: pack the wound with a simple antiseptic such
as Acriflavine and leave it open. Once the infection
settles you should then close the neck wound a week
or so later. If a vertical incision was used this
secondary closure is easy, whereas if a horizontal
incision was used the edges retract and a flap will
then be needed to repair the defect.

Diagnosis of recurrence

Occasionally a patient's larynx may remain oedematous for more than 3 months. If the oedema does not
settle after 6 months it is wiser to assume that there is
a recurrence present, and to advise the patient to
undergo a total laryngectomy. You must, of course,
tell the patient your motive for this advice, and
emphasize that the larynx might be removed when it
does not harbour tumour.

The place of partial laryngectomy

There has been much controversy over the last 30
years as to the relative place for partial laryngectomy. The policy in southern Europe and North
America tends towards the widespread use of these
partial techniques, whereas the policy in northern
Europe and the UK tends towards irradiation of
most patients, with total laryngectomy being
reserved for a recurrence. It is true that the unusual
patient who suffers a recurrence of T_1 carcinoma can
be managed successfully by a vertical hemilaryngectomy, provided that the surgeon saw the patient
initially, and that the tumour satisfied the criteria for
this hemilaryngectomy both initially and when it
recurs – an unusual event. However, supraglottic
laryngectomy should only rarely be used for recurrence after radiotherapy, and certainly not by a
beginner. Most patients with recurrence must be
treated by total laryngectomy. Partial laryngectomy
and radiotherapy are thus in direct competition for
patients with small tumours. Despite the exagger-
ated claims made by the proponents of both sides,
the fact is that the cure rates for tumours amenable to
partial laryngectomy are similar whether the patient
is treated by radiotherapy or by partial laryngectomy. The choice of the procedure is therefore not
based on pathology or the likely outcome in terms of
survival, but on financial and political considerations.

Carcinoma-*in-situ*

Carcinoma-*in-situ* comes in three very distinct clinical types. The first is the small white patch on a cord
which, when removed, may be reported as carci-
noma-*in-situ*. These patients can be safely reviewed
and told to stop smoking. Any further recurrence can
again be stripped or fulgurated by laser and even in

the presence of continued reports of carcinoma-*in-
situ*, it seldom progresses to involve more of the
larynx.

The second type is a widespread, white/grey
change in laryngeal epithelium. The third type is the
same change, only with a reddish tinge to it. Erythroplakia can occur in the larynx as well as in the
mouth. In the experience of the authors, these
tumours behave badly. They have a worse prognosis
than a small T_1 glottic carcinoma. It may be that this
is a disease *sui generis*. It very seldom goes on to
frank carcinoma and if it does so, it takes a very long
time. Stripping is probably a waste of time in these
patients and they should be treated aggressively with
radiation.

Carcinoma-*in-situ* usually occurs in smokers but if
it occurs in a non-smoker then it is probably of a
different biological entity and, again, should be
treated more aggressively with radiation.

References and further reading

Pathology

Ackermann L V (1959) The indications for and limitations of frozen section diagnosis. *Br J Surg* **46**:336–50.
Barney P L (1970) Histopathologic problems and frozen section diagnosis in diseases of the larynx. *Otolaryngol Clin North Am* **3**:493–515.
Bauer W C (1974) The use of frozen sections in otolaryngology. *Trans Am Acad Ophthalmol Otolaryngol* **78**:88–97.
Bichler E, Mikuz G, Zingerle N (1985) A comment on laryngeal cytology. *Arch Otorhinolaryngol* **241**:209–11.
Browning G G, Busuttil A, McLay A (1976) An improved method of reporting on laryngectomy specimens. *J Pathol Bacteriol* **119**:101–3.
Byers R M, Bland K L, Borlase B, Luna M (1978) The prognostic and therapeutic value of frozen section determinations in the surgical treatment of squamous carcinoma of the head and neck. *Am J Surg* **136**:525–8.
Carbone A, Micheau C, Caillaud J M, Bosq J, Vandenbrouck C (1983) Superficial extending carcinoma of the hypopharynx: report of 26 cases of an underestimated carcinoma. *Laryngoscope* **93**:1600–6.
Davidson T M, Nahum A M, Haghighi P, Astarita R, Saltzstein S L, Seagren S (1984) The biology of head and neck cancer. Detection and control by parallel histologic sections. *Arch Otolaryngol* **110**: 193–6.
Davis G L, Sessions D G (1967) Silverman needle biopsy in the diagnosis of head and neck lesions. *Laryngoscope* **77**:376–85.
Ekem J K (1972) Improved histological technique for the study of laryngeal carcinoma. *Can J Med Technol* **34**:228–34.
Engzell U, Jakobson P A, Sigurdson A, Zajicek J (1971) Aspiration biopsy of metastatic carcinoma in lymph nodes of the neck. *Arch Otolaryngol* **72**:138–47.
Feldman Ph S, Kaplan M J, Johns M E, Cantrell R W (1983) Fine needle aspiration in squamous cell carcinoma of the head and neck. *Arch Otolaryngol* **109**:735–42.
Frable W J, Frable M A (1968) Cytologic diagnosis of carcinoma of the larynx by direct smear. *Acta cytol* **12**:318–24.

Goldman J L, Bloom B S, Zak F G, Friedman W H, Gunsberg M J, Silverstone S M (1969) Serial microscopic studies of radical neck dissections. Studies in a combined radiation and surgery program for advanced cancer of the larynx. *Arch Otolaryngol* **89**:620–8.

Hommerich K W (1982) The micromorphology of the spread tendency of larynx and hypopharynx tumors and their importance for operative indications. *Excerpta Med Int Congr Ser* **582**:67–74.

Hommerich K W (1984) Histomorphological behaviour of the tumour growth in the glottic region. In: Wigand M E, Steiner W, Stell P M (eds) *Functional Partial Laryngectomy: Conservation Surgery for Carcinoma of the Larynx*. Springer, Berlin, pp. 134–8.

Kleinsasser O, Glanz H (1982) Microcarcinoma and microinvasive carcinoma of the vocal cords. *Clin Oncol* **1**:479–87.

Kirchner J A (1977) Two hundred laryngeal cancers: patterns of growth and spread as seen in serial sections. *Laryngoscope* **87**:474–82.

Lindgren J, Olofsson J, Hellquist H B, Strandh J (1981) Exfoliative cytology in laryngology: comparison of cytologic and histologic diagnoses in 350 microlaryngoscopic examinations – a prospective study. *Cancer* **47**: 1336–43.

McDonald T J, Weiland L H, Desanto L W. (1977) A method for processing and sectioning whole laryngeal specimens. *J Laryngol* **91**:379–82.

McKelvie P (1976) Metastatic routes in the neck. In: Alberti W P, Bryce D P (eds) *Workshops from the Centennial Conference on Laryngeal Cancer*. New York, Appleton-Century-Crofts.

Michaels L (1982) Pitfalls in the histological diagnosis of premalignant lesions and carcinoma in situ of the larynx. *Excerpta Med Int Congr Ser* **582**:99–102.

Serafini I (1984) Histological examination of the excised specimen after supraglottic laryngectomy. In: Wigand M E, Steiner W, Stell P M (eds) *Functional Partial Laryngectomy: Conservation Surgery for Carcinoma of the Larynx*. Springer, Berlin, pp. 214–18.

Staging

Chandler J R, Guillamondegui O M, Sisson G A, Strong E W, Baker H W (1976) Clinical staging of cancer of the head and neck: A new "new" system. *Am J Surg* **132**:525–8.

Feinstein A R, Schimpff C R, Andrews J F, Wells C K (1977) Cancer of the larynx: a new staging system and a reappraisal of prognosis and treatment. *J Chron Dis* **30**:277–305.

Glanz H (1984) Growth, p-classification and grading of vocal cord carcinomas. *Adv Otorhinolaryngol* **32**:1–123.

Harrison D F (1979) Intrinsic weakness of the TNM system for classification of laryngeal cancers. *J Otorhinolaryngol Relat Spec* **41**:241–51.

Harwood A R, Deboer G (1980) Prognostic factors in T_2 glottic cancer. *Cancer* **45**:991–5.

Hommerich K W (1984) The TNM-classification with regard to surgical planning of partial resections of the larynx. In: Wigand M E, Steiner W, Stell P M (eds) *Functional Partial Laryngectomy: Conservation Surgery for Carcinoma of the Larynx*. Berlin, Springer, pp. 82–5.

Johns M F, Farrior E, Boyd J C, Cantrell R W (1982) Staging of supraglottic cancer. *Arch Otolaryngol* **108**:700–2.

Olofsson J, Lord I J, van Nostrand A W P (1973) Vocal cord fixation in laryngeal carcinoma. *Acta Oto-laryngol (Stockh)* **75**:496–510.

Pilsbury H R, Kirchner J A (1979) Clinical versus histopathologic staging in laryngeal cancer. *Arch Oto-laryngol* **105**:157–9.

Rare tumours

Abemayor E, Calcaterra T C (1983) Kaposi's sarcoma and community-acquired immune deficiency syndrome. An update with emphasis on its head and neck manifestations. *Arch Otolaryngol* **109**:536–42.

Abramson A L, Simons R L (1970) Kaposi's sarcoma of the head and neck. *Arch Otolaryngol* **92**:505–7.

Andrews A H (1955) Glomus tumors (non chromaffin paragangliomas) of the larynx: case report. *Ann Otol* **64**:1034–6.

Benjamin B, Carter P (1983) Congenital laryngeal hemangioma. *Ann Otol* **92**:448–55.

Calcaterra T C (1968) An evaluation of the treatment of subglottic hemangioma. *Laryngoscope* **78**:1956–64.

Canalis R F, Platz C E, Cohn A M (1976) Laryngeal rhabdomyosarcoma. *Arch Otolaryngol* **102**:104–7.

Cantrell R W, Reibel J F, Jahrsdoerfer R A, Johns M E (1980) Conservative surgical treatment of chondrosarcoma of the larynx. *Ann Otol* **89**:567–71.

Chambers R G, Friedel W (1976) Chondrosarcoma of the larynx. **86**:713–17.

DeLozier H L (1982) Intrinsic malignant schwannoma of the larynx. A case report. *Ann Otol* **91**:336–8.

Duvall E, Johnston A, McLay K, Piris J (1983) Carcinoid tumour of the larynx. *J Laryngol* **97**:1073–80.

El-Ghazali A M S, El-Ghazali S M (1982) Granular cell myoblastoma of the larynx. *J Laryngol* **96**:1177–80.

Finn D G, Goepfert H, Batsakis J G (1984) Chondrosarcoma of the head and neck. *Laryngoscope* **94**:1539–44.

Fisher E R, Wechsler H (1962) Granular cell myoblastoma – a misnomer. Electron microscopic and histochemical evidence concerning its schwann cell derivation and nature (granular cell Schwannoma), *Cancer* **15**:936–54.

Gapany-Gapanavicius B, Kenan S (1981) Carcinoid tumor of the larynx. *Ann Otol* **90**:42–7.

Garancis J C, Komorowski R H, Kuzma J F (1970) Granular cell myoblastoma. *Cancer* **25**:542–50.

Gatti W M, Strom C G, Orfei E (1975) Synovial sarcoma of the laryngopharynx. *Arch Otolaryngol* **101**:633–6.

Goldman N C, Hood C I, Singleton G T (1969) Carcinoid of the larynx. *Arch Otolaryngol* **90**:64–7.

Harrison E G, Black B M, Devine K D (1961) Synovial sarcoma primary in the neck. *Arch Pathol* **71**:137–41.

Hall-Jones J (1975) Rhabdomyosarcoma of the larynx. *J Laryngol* **89**:969–76.

Huizenga C, Balogh K (1970) Cartilaginous tumors of the larynx. A clinicopathologic study of 10 new cases and a review of the literature. *Cancer* **26**:201–10.

Hyams V J, Rabuzzi D O (1970) Cartilaginous tumors of the larynx. *Laryngoscope* **80**:755–67.

Johns M E, Batsakis J G, Short C D (1973) Oncocytic and oncocytoid tumors of the salivary glands. *Laryngoscope* **83**:1940–52.

Jokinen K, Sepalla A, Palva A (1974) Laryngeal pleomorphic adenoma. *J Laryngol* **88**:1131–4.

Kaznelson D J, Schindel J (1979) Mucoepidermoid carcinoma of the air passages: report of three cases. *Laryngoscope* **89**:115–21.

Liebner E J (1976) Embryonal rhabdomyosarcoma of head and neck in children. Correlation of stage, radiation dose, local control and survival. *Cancer* **37**:2777–86.

Liew S H, Leong A S Y, Tang H M K (1981) Tracheal paraganglioma: a case report with review of the literature. *Cancer* **47**:1387–93.

Mallonee M S, Maniglia A J, Goodwin W J Jr (1979) Adenocarcinoma of the larynx. *Ear Nose Throat* **58**:115–18.

Markel S F, Magielski J E, Beals T F (1980) Carcinoid tumor of the larynx. *Arch Otolaryngol* **106**:777–8.

Martinson F D (1967) Chemodectoma of the "glomus laryngicum inferior". *Arch Otolaryngol* **86**:70–3.

Olofsson J, Groentoft O, Soekjer H, Risberg B (1984) Paraganglioma involving the larynx. *ORL J Otorhinolaryngol Relat Spec* **46**:57–65.

Palva T, Jokinen K, Kavja J (1975) Neurilemoma (Schwannoma) of the larynx. *J Laryngol* **89**:203.

Sakakura Y, Ohi M, Yamada S, Miyoshi Y (1980) A case of subglottic hemangioma: a new technique of surgical removal. *Auris Nasus Larynx* **7**:81–88.

Sweetser T H (1921) Hemangioma of the larynx. *Laryngoscope* **3**:797–806.

Tewfik T L, Novick W H, Schipper H M (1983) Adenoid cystic carcinoma of the larynx. *J Otolaryngol* **12**:151–4.

Thomas K (1971) Mucoepidermoid carcinoma of the larynx. *J Laryngol* **85**:261–7.

Radiotherapy

Catterall M (1977) First randomized clinical trial of fast neutrons compared with photons in advanced carcinoma of the head and neck. *Clin Otolaryngol* **2**:359–72.

Croll G A, Gerritsen G J, Tiwari R M, Snow G B (1989) Primary radiotherapy with surgery in reserve for advanced laryngeal carcinoma. *Eur J Surg Oncol* **15**:350–6.

Fernberg J-O, Ringborg U, Silfversward C et al. (1989) Radiation therapy in early glottic cancer: analysis of 177 consecutive cases. *Acta Otolaryngol* **108**:478–81.

Fisher A J, Calderelli D D, Chacko D C, Holinger L D (1986) Glottic cancer: surgical salvage for radiation failure. *Arch Otolaryngol Head Neck Surg* **112**:519–21.

Fu K K, Woodhouse R J, Quivey J M, Phillips T L, Dedo H H (1982) The significance of laryngeal edema following radiotherapy of carcinoma of the vocal cord. *Cancer* **49**:655–8.

Griffin T W, Laramore G E, Parker R G et al. (1978) An evaluation of fast neutron beam teletherapy of metastatic cervical adenopathy from squamous cell carcinoma of the head and neck region. *Cancer* **42**:2517–20.

Harwood A R, Beale F A, Cummings B J, Hawkins N V, Keane T J, Rider W D (1980) T$_3$ glottic cancer: an analysis of dose time-volume factors. *Int J Radiat Oncol Biol Phys* **6**:675–80.

Hawkins N V (1975) A three fraction treatment for carcinoma of the larynx. *Can J Otolaryngol* **4**:937–8.

Howell-Burke D, Peters L J, Goepfert H, Oswald M J (1990) T$_2$ glottic cancer: recurrence, salvage and survival after definitive radiotherapy. *Arch Otolaryngol Head Neck Surg* **116**:830–5.

Jose B, Mohammed A, Calhoun D L, Tobin D A, Scott R M (1981) Management of stage II glottic cancer. *Int J Radiat Oncol Biol Phys* **7**:1021–4.

Kaplan M J, Johns M E, McLean W C et al. (1983) Stage II glottic carcinoma: prognostic factors and management. *Laryngoscope* **93**:725–8.

Kardell W D, Kearsley J H, Donovan J K (1982) Radiotherapy in the treatment of carcinoma of the vocal cords. Results of a 10-year experience. *Med J Aust* **1**:381–3.

Karim A B, Snow G B, Hasman A, Chang S C, Keilholtz A, Hockstra F (1978) Dose response in radiotherapy for glottic carcinoma. *Cancer* **41**:1728–32.

Kazem J, van den Broel P (1984) Planned preoperative radiation-therapy vs. definitive radiotherapy for advanced laryngeal carcinoma. *Laryngoscope* **94**:1355–8.

Keene M, Harwood A R, Bryce D P, Nostrand A W P (1982) Histopathological study of radionecrosis in laryngeal carcinoma. *Laryngoscope* **92**:173–80.

Lee N K, Goepfert H, Wendt C D (1990) Supraglottic laryngectomy for intermediate-stage cancer: UTMD Anderson Cancer Center experience with combined therapy. *Layrngoscope* **100**:831–6.

Levendag P C, Hoekstra C J M, Eukenboom W M H, Reichgelt B A, Putten W L J (1988) Supraglottic larynx cancer, T$_{1-4}$N$_0$, treated by radical radiation therapy: problem of neck relapse. *Acta Oncolog* **27**:253–60.

Lundgren J A V, Gilbert R W, Nostrand A W P, Harwood A R, Keane T J, Briant T D R (1988) T$_3$ N$_0$M$_0$ glottic carcinoma – a failure analysis. *Clin Otolaryngol* **13**:455–65.

McLean M (1989) Primary management of limited laryngeal cancer by radiotherapy and surgical salvage: results of 164 cases treated in a district hospital. *Clin Oncol* **1**:97–100.

Nadol J B (1981) Treatment of carcinoma of the epiglottis. *Ann Otol Rhinol Laryngol* **90**:442–8.

Nass J M, Brady L W, Glassburn J R, Prasasvinichai S, Schatanoff D (1976) Radiation therapy of glottic carcinoma. *Int J Radiat Oncol Biol* **1**:867–72.

Olofsson J, Lord I J, van Nostrand A W P (1973) Vocal cord fixation in laryngeal carcinoma. *Acta Oto-laryngol* **75**:496–510.

Olofsson J, Williams G T, Rider W D, Bryce D P (1972) Anterior commissure carcinoma. Primary treatment with radiotherapy in 57 patients. *Arch Otolaryngol* **95**:230–3.

Parsons J T, Bova F J, Million R R (1980) A reevaluation of split course technique for squamous cell carcinoma of the head and neck. *Int J Radiat Oncol* **6**:1645–52.

Pellitteri P K, Kennedy T L, Vrabec D P, Beiler D, Hellstrom M (1991) Radiotherapy: the mainstay in the treatment of early glottic carcinoma. *Arch Otolaryngol Head Neck Surg* **117**:297–301.

Sinha P P (1987) Radiation therapy in early carcinoma of the true vocal cords (stage I and II). *Int J Radiat Oncol Biol Phys* **13**:1635–40.

Viani L, Stell P M, Dalby J E (1991) Recurrence after radiotherapy for glottic carcinoma. *Cancer* **67**:577–84.

Wang C C (1973) Megavoltage radiation therapy for supraglottic carcinoma. Results of treatment. *Radiology* **109**:183–6.

Wang C C (1974) Treatment of glottic carcinoma by megavoltage radiation therapy and results. *Am J Roentgenol* **120**:157–63.

Wang C C (1984) Supraglottic carcinomas: selection of therapy and results. *Am J Clin Oncol* **7**:109.

Wang C C, Blitzer P H, Suit H D (1985) Twice-a-day

radiation therapy for cancer of the head and neck. *Cancer* **55**: 2100–4.

Wiernik G, Bates T D, Bleehen N M *et al.* (1990) Final report of the general clinical results of the British Institute of Radiology fractionation study of 3F/wk versus 5F/wk in radiotherapy of carcinoma of the laryngo-pharynx. *Br J Radiol* **63**:169–80.

Surgery

Alonso J M (1947) Conservative surgery of cancer of the larynx. *Trans Am Acad Ophthalmol Otolaryngol* **51**:633–42.

Alonso J M (1966) Partial horizontal laryngectomy. Functional or physiological operation for supraglottic cancer. *Laryngoscope* **76**:161–9.

Asai R (1972) Laryngoplasty after total laryngectomy. *Arch Otolaryngol* **95**:114–19.

Bailey B J (1975) Glottic reconstruction after hemilaryngectomy: bipedicle muscle flap laryngoplasty. *Laryngoscope* **85**:960–77.

Bailey B J, Calcaterra T C (1971) Vertical, subtotal laryngectomy and laryngoplasty. Review of experience. *Arch Otolaryngol* **93**:232–7.

Ballantyne A J, Fletcher G H (1974) Surgical management of irradiation failures of nonfixed cancers of the glottic region. *Am J Roentgenol* **120**:164–8.

Biller H F, Bernhill F R, Ogura J H, Perez C A (1970) Hemilaryngectomy following radiation failure for carcinoma of the vocal cords. *Laryngoscope* **80**:249–53.

Biller H F, Ogura J H, Pratt L L (1971) Hemilaryngectomy for T_2 glottic cancers. *Arch Otolaryngol* **93**:238–43.

Burgess L P A, Quilligan J J, Yim D W S (1985) Thyroid cartilage flap reconstruction of the larynx following vertical partial laryngectomy: a preliminary report in two patients. *Laryngoscope* **95**:1258–61.

Coates H L, Desanto L W, Devine K D, Elveback L R (1976) Carcinoma of the supraglottic larynx. A review of 221 cases. *Arch Otolaryngol* **102**:686–9.

Conley J J (1975) Regional skin flaps in partial laryngectomy. *Laryngoscope* **85**:942–9.

Croll G, Can den Broek P, Tiwari R M, Mann J J, Snow G B (1985) Vertical partial laryngectomy for recurrent glottic carcinoma after irradiation. *Head Neck Surg* **7**:390–3.

Dedo H H (1975) A technique for vertical hemilaryngectomy to prevent stenosis and aspiration. *Laryngoscope* **85**:978–84.

Hamaker R C, Singer M I, Blom E D, Daniels H A (1985) Primary voice restoration at laryngectomy. *Arch Otolaryngol* **111**:182–6.

Harrison D F (1975) Laryngectomy for subglottic lesions. *Laryngoscope* **85**:1208–10.

Isshiki N, Tanabe M (1980) A simple technique to prevent stenosis of the tracheostoma after total laryngectomy. *J Laryngol* **94**:637–42.

Kaneko T (1972) Reconstruction surgery after the partial laryngotomy. *J Japn Broncho-Esophag Soc* **23**:63–71.

Kennedy J T, Krause C J (1974) Survival rates in conservation surgery of the larynx. *Arch Otolaryngol* **99**:274–8.

Kirchner J A, Som M L (1971) Clinical significance of fixed vocal cord. *Laryngoscope* **81**:1029–44.

Kirchner J A (1979) Closure after supraglottic laryngectomy. *Laryngoscope* **89**:1343–4.

Kirchner J A (1984) Pathways and pitfalls in partial laryngectomy. *Ann Otol* **93**:301–5.

Lam K H, Wei W I, Wong J, Ong G B (1983) Tracheostoma construction during laryngectomy. A method to prevent stenosis. *Laryngoscope* **93**:212–15.

Laurian N, Zohar Y (1981) Laryngeal reconstruction by composite nasal mucoseptal graft after partial layrngectomy, three years follow-up. *Laryngoscope* **91**:609–16.

Leonard J R, Litton W R (1971) Selection of the patient for conservation surgery of the larynx. *Laryngoscope* **81**:232–52.

Lesinski S G, Bauer W C, Ogura J H (1976) Hemilaryngectomy for T_3 (fixed cord) epidermoid carcinoma of larynx. *Laryngoscope* **86**:1563–71.

Maceri D R, Lampe H B, Makielski H, Passamani P P, Krause Ch J (1985) Conservation laryngeal surgery. *Arch Otolaryngol* **111**:361–5.

McDonald T J, Desanto L W, Weiland L H (1976) Supraglottic larynx and its pathology as studied by whole laryngeal sections. *Laryngoscope* **86**:635–48.

Maran A G D, Murray J A M, Johnson A P (1982) Management techniques in the use of the Blom-Singer valve. *Clin Otolaryngol* **7**:201–3.

Marks J E, Freeman R B, Lee F, Ogura J H (1979) Carcinoma of the supraglottic larynx. *Am J Radiol* **132**:255–60.

Marshall H F, Mark A, Bryce D P, Rider W D (1972) The management of advanced laryngeal cancer. *J Larnygol* **86**:309–15.

Maves M D, Lingeman R E (1982) Primary vocal rehabilitation using the Blom-Singer and Panje voice prosthesis. *Ann Otol* **91**:458–60.

Maw A R, Lavelle R J (1972) The management of postoperative pharyngo-cutaneous pharyngeal fistulae. *J Laryngol* **86**:795–805.

Mittal B, Marks J E, Ogura J H (1984) Transglottic carcinoma. *Cancer* **53**:151–61.

Myers E M, Ogura J H (1979) Completion laryngectomy. *Ann Otol* **88**:172–7.

Myers E N (1972) Management of pharyngocutaneous fistula. *Arch Otolaryngol* **95**:10–17.

Myers E N, Gallia L J (1982) Tracheostomal stenosis following total laryngectomy. *Ann Otol* **91**:450–2.

Nichols R D, Stine P H, Greenwald K J (1980) Partial laryngectomy after radiation failure. *Laryngoscope* **90**:571–5.

Norris C M, Peale A R (1966) Partial laryngectomy for irradiation failure. *Arch Otolaryngol* **84**:558–62.

Ogura J H, Biller H F (1969) Glottic reconstruction following extended frontolateral hemilaryngectomy. *Laryngoscope* **79**:2181–4.

Ogura J H, Sessions D G, Ciralsky R H (1975) Glottic cancer with extension to the arytenoid. *Laryngoscope* **85**:1825–55.

Olofsson J, Lord I J, van Nostrand A W (1973) Vocal cord fixation in laryngeal carcinoma. *Acta Oto-laryngol (Stockh)* **75**:496–510.

Panje W R (1981) Prosthetic vocal rehabilitation following laryngectomy. The voice button. *Ann Otol* **90**:116–20.

Park N H, Major J W, Sauers P L (1982) Hemilaryngectomy and vocal cord reconstruction with digastric tendon graft. *Surg Gynecol Obstet* **155**:253–6.

Pearson B W, Woods R D, Hartman D E (1980) Extended hemilaryngectomy for T_3 glottic carcinoma with preservation of speech and swallowing. *Laryngoscope* **90**:1950–61.

Quinn H J (1984) Synovial sarcoma of the larynx treated by partial laryngectomy. *Laryngoscope* **94**:1158–61.

Quinn H J (1978) Ten years' experience with free tissue graft for glottic reconstruction. *Otolaryngology* **86**:372–9.

Radcliffe G, Shaw H J (1978) Partial laryngectomy for recurrent cancer after irradiation. *Clin Otolaryngol* **3**:49–62.

Schoenrock L, King Y, Everts E C, Schneider H J, Shumrick A (1972) Hemilaryngectomy deglutition evaluation and rehabilitation. *Trans Am Acad Opthalmol Otolaryngol* **76**:752–7.

Sedláček K (1965) Reconstructive anterior and lateral laryngectomy using the epiglottis as a pedunculated graft. *Čsl Otolaryngol* **14**:328–34.

Sessions D G, Ogura J H, Fried M P (1975) Carcinoma of the subglottic area. *Laryngoscope* **85**:1417–23.

Singer M I, Blom E D (1980) An endoscopic technique for restoration of voice after laryngectomy. *Ann Otol* **89**:529–33.

Singer M I, Blom E D, Hamaker R C (1983) Voice rehabilitation after total laryngectomy. *J Otolaryngol* **12**:329–34.

Som M I (1970) Conservation surgery for carcinoma of the supraglottis. *J Laryngol* **84**:655–78.

Som M L (1975) Cordal cancer with extension to vocal process. *Laryngoscope* **85**:1298–1307.

Som M L, Nussbaum M (1974) Surgical management of recurrent head and neck cancer. *Otolaryngol Clin North Am* **7**:163–74.

Stell P M (1975) The first laryngectomy. *J Laryngol* **89**:353–8.

Stuart D W (1966) Surgery in cancer of the cervical oesophagus plastic tube replacement. *J Laryngol* **80**:382.

Tucker H M, Wood B G, Levine H, Katz R (1979) Glottic reconstruction after near total laryngectomy. *Laryngoscope* **89**:609–18.

Weaver A W, Fleming S M (1978) Partial laryngectomy: analysis of associated swallowing disorders. *Am J Surg* **136**: 486–9.

Tiwari R M, Snow G B, Lecluse F L E, Greven A J, Bloothooft G (1982) Observations on surgical rehabilitation of the voice after laryngectomy with Staffieri's method. *J Laryngol* **96**:241–50.

Thoracotracheostomy

Aryian S, Cuono C B (1980) Myocutaneous flaps for head and neck reconstruction. *Plast Reconstr Surg* **2**:321–45.

Baek S, Biller H F, Krespi Y P *et al.* (1979) The pectoralis major myocutaneous island flap for reconstruction of the head and neck. *Head Neck Surg* **1**:293–300.

Biller H, Krespi Y, Lawson W *et al.* (1980) A one stage flap reconstruction following resection for stoma recurrence. *Head Neck Surg* **88**:357–60.

Ogura J H, Meyers E M (1979) Stomal recurrences: a clinicopathological analysis and protocol for future management. *Laryngoscope* **88**:1121–8.

Sisson G A (1969) Extended radical surgery for cancer of head and neck. *Otolaryngol Clin North Am.* 617–30.

Sisson G A (1970) Mediastinal dissection for recurrent cancer after laryngectomy. *Trans Am Acad Ophthalmol Otolaryngol* **74**:767–77.

Sisson G A, Straehley C J Jr (1962) Mediastinal dissection for recurrent cancer after laryngectomy. *Laryngoscope* **73**:1069–77.

Sisson G A, Edison B D, Bytell D E (1975) Transternal radical neck dissection: Postoperative complications and management. *Arch Otolaryngol* **101**:46–9.

Sisson G A, Bytell D E, Edison B D *et al.* (1975) Transsternal radical neck dissection for control of stomal recurrences: end results. *Laryngoscope* **85**:1504–10.

Sisson G A, Bytell D E, Edison B D (1975) Transsternal radical neck dissection (mediastinal approach) in: Anderson R, Hoopes J (eds) *Symposium on Malignancies of the Head and Neck*, vol. 11 St Louis, CV Mosby, pp. 27–30.

Sisson G A, Bytell D E, Becker S P (1977) Mediastinal dissection – 1976: Indications and newer techniques. *Laryngoscope* **87**:751–9.

10

Vocal cord paralysis

Surgical anatomy

Phonation is initiated by area 4 in the Sylvian fissure of the cerebrum. Fibres pass down the internal capsule and, in the lower pons, some fibres decussate to the opposite side before entering the medulla, terminating in the nucleus ambiguus. The vagal nuclei are thus bilaterally innervated.

The peripheral vagal trunk forms from roots emerging from the lower pons and upper medulla. It passes through the jugular foramen beside the jugular vein, posterior to the ninth cranial nerve and anterior to the 11th cranial nerve. High in the neck the vagus produces the superior laryngeal nerve that is motor to the cricothyroid muscle and sensory to the laryngeal mucosa above the vocal cords. The vagus nerve then passes through the neck in the carotid sheath between the carotid artery and the jugular vein. It enters the chest and gives off the recurrent laryngeal nerves.

On the left side, the recurrent laryngeal nerve passes anteriorly, under and then behind the aorta, beside the ligamentum arteriosum. It then passes in the tracheo-oesophageal groove and enters the larynx near the cricothyroid joint. It is thus in close proximity to the aorta, the oesophagus, the left mainstem bronchus, the mediastinal lymph nodes and the left atrium.

The right recurrent laryngeal nerve passes into the chest anterior to the subclavian artery, loops around it and returns to the neck in the tracheo-oesophageal groove. It is in close proximity to the right subclavian artery, the apex of the right upper lobe of the lung and the associated supraclavicular lymph nodes.

The recurrent laryngeal nerves are motor to all the intrinsic laryngeal muscles and sensory to the mucosa below the level of the vocal cords.

The glottis consists approximately of 60% membranous vocal cord and 40% vocal process and medial border of the arytenoid body. There is thus a mobile soft portion and a hard cartilaginous portion to the glottis. These behave in different ways when the recurrent laryngeal nerve is paralysed, and they rehabilitate in different ways.

Surgical pathology

Vocal cord paralysis may be unilateral or bilateral, abductor or adductor. This latter expression relates to the movement that the cord cannot make when paralysed.

The cord is often described as being either in the median position or in the lateral or cadaveric position. It is impossible to record accurately the position of a paralysed vocal cord. No theory fully explains the position of the paralysed cord.

Semon's theory depends on the observation that abductor fibres are more susceptible to pressure than adductor fibres. Although this is difficult to refute, it is also very hard to believe. It does, however, have the distinct advantage of having stood the test of time. Perhaps it has not been questioned because of the difficulty of questioning it.

The more acceptable theory is that put forward by Wagner and Grossman, which implies that the superior laryngeal nerve has an adductive effect through the cricothyroid muscle. This means that if there is a low lesion of the recurrent laryngeal nerve, the cricothyroid muscle will keep the cord in the mid-position, whereas if the vagus is paralysed high in the neck then the adductive effect will be lost and the cord will be in the cadaveric position.

Surgeons who deal with a large number of cases of vocal cord paralysis secondary to lung cancer, however, realize that this theory is incorrect because nearly every such patient has a vocal cord in the cadaveric position.

The exact mechanism of paralysis of the nerve is also difficult to understand. It is very rare for metastatic nodes or primary malignant tumours in the neck to paralyse the vagus nerve, even if the tumour escapes from its capsule. In the chest, however, mediastinal nodes from a lung cancer can cause a recurrent laryngeal paralysis, as can tumour extruding from the thyroid or the oesophagus. What is more difficult to believe, however, is the oft-reported Ortner's syndrome, which implies that cardiomegaly causes pressure on the recurrent laryngeal nerve, thus causing a paralysis. In order to do this, the left atrium would have to rise up to the level of the arch of the aorta and thus pass completely behind the pulmonary arteries. While not impossible, it cannot be a very frequent occurrence.

The effect of a vocal cord paralysis is dual. If the laryngeal sphincter is incompetent then phonation will be poor and aspiration will be possible. Furthermore, loss of sensation, either in the upper or the lower laryngeal compartment will result in this aspiration being undetected and aspiration pneumonia will be the result. Inability to obtain a positive subglottic pressure disorganizes the swallowing reflex and also makes it difficult to get an adequate cough to clear the lower respiratory tract.

Because of its longer course, the left recurrent laryngeal nerve is paralysed more often than the right. The ratio is about 4 : 1 and bilateral paralysis occurs in about 6% of cases. Men are affected eight times more than women, but this sex incidence will probably change as the incidence of lung cancer rises in women.

The causes of vocal cord paralysis are as follows.

1 *Malignant disease (25%)*. This is due to bronchial carcinoma (50%); oesophageal carcinoma (20%); thyroid carcinoma (10%) and nasopharyngeal carcinoma, glomus tumours and lymphomas (20%).
2 *Surgical trauma (20%)*. This can occur in oesophageal and lung surgery for carcinoma, in carotid artery surgery, congenital heart surgery, thyroid surgery, partial laryngectomy, radical neck dissection, removal of pharyngeal pouch, and anterior approaches for cervical spine fusion.
3 *Non-surgical trauma (15%)*. This is an increasing cause of vocal cord paralysis because of road traffic accidents and increasing violence in society and on the sports field. Orton's syndrome from cardiomegaly can be considered part of this. It is seen more often in horses than in humans!
4 *Idiopathic causes (15%)*. If a viral neuritis affects the nerves, it is usually on the right side. The influenza virus is often incriminated, especially because of the A2 Hong Kong 1 68 virus that affected Europe in the early 1970s. Paralysis can also occur in infectious mononucleosis.
5 *Neurological causes (15%)*. Not only can the well-known neurological diseases, such as multiple sclerosis, amyotrophic lateral sclerosis, syringomyelia and Parkinson's disease paralyse the vocal cords but small-vessel disease can also affect the brainstem causing vocal cord paralysis. It is seen as the result of head injury and neuropathies that occur in alcoholism, diabetes and the Guillain–Barré syndrome.
6 *Inflammatory causes (5%)*. This used to be a much more common cause of vocal cord paralysis but as the incidence of pulmonary tuberculosis and syphilitic aortitis has decreased, so has the incidence of paralysis due to these causes.
7 *Miscellaneous causes (5%)*. These include haemolytic anaemia, thrombosis of the subclavian vein and various collagen diseases.

Investigations

History

First of all, listen to the patient's voice as you speak to him or her. A forced whisper suggests an organic adductor paralysis whereas a faint whisper is often a sign of functional adductor paralysis. A voice which is normal in the morning and tires as the day goes on occurs in a unilateral abductor paralysis. Stridor occurs in bilateral abductor paralysis and aspiration in bilateral adductor paralysis.

Paralysis due to surgical trauma is usually seen shortly after the operation, but is often diagnosed later. For example, it is possible for a bilateral abductor paralysis to be caused by a thyroidectomy and the patient to have few or no symptoms immediately afterwards. Only several years later, when the cricoarytenoid joint becomes fixed or the vocal cords become oedematous due to an upper respiratory infection, does the patient develop stridor.

Ask about symptoms such as hoarseness, dysphagia, sore throat, pain in the ears, cough, haemoptysis and any newly noted neck lumps. Note the patient's smoking habits and also any recent illnesses, especially of the viral type.

In the case of a patient with a vocal cord paralysis secondary to an operation such as thyroidectomy, the most important thing to know is the patient's occupation, and particularly what use he or she makes of the voice.

Examination

Consideration of the causes gives an indication of what to look for in general examination of the patient. Do a full head and neck examination on every patient.

Note the position of the vocal cord and remember how difficult it is to report paramedian or cadaveric positions reliably. The best indication is the width of the membranous glottic chink on phonation. In the paramedian position it will only be about 1–2 mm. In the cadaveric position not only will the gap be greater but the tip of the vocal process will be directed medially as a definite prominence. A paralysed cord becomes bowed and atrophic and lies at a lower level than the normal cord with anterior rotation of the arytenoid.

Examine the neck and thyroid gland carefully, paying particular attention to the tracheo-oesophageal groove because of the possibility of small thyroid cancers paralysing the nerve.

Radiology

Always do a chest radiograph, both as part of the general examination and to demonstrate any lung disease, particularly carcinoma. Tomograms will almost always be needed, particularly of the left upper lobe and left hilum. A chest radiograph may also show paralysis of the diaphragm, which should be confirmed by screening.

Always do a barium swallow if the cause remains undetected after a chest radiograph. Not only will oesophageal neoplasms by noted but compression by thyroid masses and an enlarged left atrium may also be seen.

If the cord is in the cadaveric position the cause will probably be above the larynx so X-ray the base of the skull, petrous bones and nasopharynx.

If a mass is palpable in the thyroid do a thyroid scan but if nothing is palpable it is unlikely that anything will be demonstrated by a scan.

Laryngograms have limited value in this condition but may show arytenoid rotation, change in level of the cord and cord atrophy, giving it a sharper medial edge.

Laboratory investigations

A basic investigation would be a complete blood count, a differential white count, a film and erythrocyte sedimentation rate. The monospot test should probably be done; it is doubtful if screening for viruses ever has a harvest worth the cost. Routine tests for syphilis are useful. Such a multitude of medical illnesses can cause a vocal cord paralysis that it would be meaningless to list the tests here; the physician has to apply the appropriate tests to the suspected conditions.

Routine respiratory function tests will probably show loss of glottic competence, but the most important tests in a bilateral paralysis are respiratory loop tests, which will show the difference between upper and lower respiratory obstruction.

As it is so difficult to tell the position of the vocal cord, or even if the cord is paralysed and the arytenoid fixed, then if 'voice lab' facilities exist, videos of the vocal cord movement should be watched and studied. Stroboscopy does not have any place to play in the investigation of vocal cord paralysis.

Endoscopy

Most patients require a panendoscopy, comprising nasopharyngoscopy and biopsy, oesophagoscopy,

direct laryngoscopy with mobility tests of the arytenoid to see if the immobility is due to muscle paralysis or to joint fixation, and a bronchoscopy. If a mediastinal cause is suspected mediastinoscopy should be done.

If diagnosis is made clinically or radiologically, endoscopy will usually be required to confirm it. If the diagnosis remains obscure then endoscopy is mandatory.

If the patient is anaesthetized it will be impossible to assess the position of the cords but the mobility may be checked if the cords are observed while the patient is in the process of waking up without a tube.

Treatment policy

Four separate clinical problems can occur, which will be discussed separately here. In addition to the operations described, all these patients may be helped by speech therapy, particularly the patient with a unilateral abductor paralysis. Speech therapy should also be used after any of the operations described.

Unilateral abductor paralysis

This paralysis, in which one vocal cord is fixed in the paramedian position, may cause no symptoms at all, or only slight hoarseness; with the passage of time any hoarseness usually disappears spontaneously as the mobile vocal cord compensates. Such a paralysis, if on the left side, is often due to a carcinoma of the left lung. The most important point in the management of such a paralysis is to exclude, or otherwise, the presence of such a carcinoma. If a patient has a carcinoma of the left lung with a paralysed vocal cord, the carcinoma is inoperable.

Bilateral abductor paralysis

This lesion is not common: it may be caused by a peripheral neuritis or by damage to the recurrent laryngeal nerves at thyroidectomy; other treatable causes are rare. The patient generally has stridor, although not always. Particularly in a slightly built woman who is relatively inactive, there may be little or no stridor, at least for the first few months or years after the paralysis is caused. Also, because the vocal cords are in the paramedian position, the voice is usually good. Sooner or later, however, all patients with this problem will have stridor, which may be precipitated by an upper respiratory tract infection. The immediate problem is to provide a satisfactory airway, so that a tracheostomy is needed.

A patient with a tracheostomy has a choice. He or she can either keep the speaking tracheostomy tube, in which case he or she has a good voice but a hole in the neck, or he or she can opt to have an operation to have the tracheostomy removed. The most usually performed operation is that described by Woodman of lateralization of the paralysed cord.

In performing this operation, the surgeon drives a fine line between improving the airway and keeping a serviceable voice. What is certain is that the patient cannot have a good airway and a good voice. The 30% failure rate that this operation carries is probably due to the surgeon trying to keep the vocal cords too close together, or not fixing the cord laterally enough or firmly enough.

Other options that have been described in the last few years are the neuromuscular pedicle operation which, in the hands of Dr Tucker, has given 80% success in removal of the tracheostomy tube. These results, however, have not been repeated in other hands.

The authors do not have experience in laser excision of the cord because they feel that the other options are preferable.

Lateralization of a cord with a Downie's operation is effective provided the arytenoid is removed. It involves passing a 26-gauge wire around the vocal process and tightening it on the outside of the thyroid ala. If the arytenoid is not removed then Downie's operation will fail because the arytenoid tends to pull the cord back.

If the arytenoid is to be kept then the procedure can be performed endoscopically by excising a portion of the thyroarytenoid muscle and holding the mucosa of the cord back into the gap, hoping that in a 6-week period it will heal – a procedure which mimics laser excision of the posterior part of the cord.

Tucker has described a procedure for vocal fold reinnervation using a nerve–muscle pedicle. Nerve–muscle pedicle reinnervation restores not only gross movement of the vocal cord but also the ability to tense the muscles and therefore to control pitch. Theoretically at least it therefore offers a return to normal function, although with a built-in delay of 2–6 months before any improvement may be noted postoperatively. Histochemical and excitability studies following nerve–muscle pedicle implantation have demonstrated the feasibility of laryngeal reinnervation, although there is residual controversy about the clinical success.

For example, the use of the ansa hypoglossi with an omohyoid neuromuscular pedicle appears to have very varying results. The principle variable in the outcome appears to be the surgeon who performs the procedure – Tucker's group and others claim a high success rate, while other workers have had no success at all in laryngeal reinnervation with this method.

Unilateral adductor paralysis

A unilateral adductor paralysis causes not only dysphonia due to air wastage but also, because the laryngeal sphincter is incompetent and part of the larynx is insensitive, aspiration of food.

If unilateral failure of adduction is due to bronchial carcinoma then the distress of altered voice and inefficient cough can be alleviated almost immediately by an injection of the vocal cord. The substance injected was formerly Teflon but this is now available only on a named-patient basis as the substance from time to time produces a brisk granulomatous reaction associated with stridor and collagen is now preferred.

Injectable bovine collagen was introduced for the treatment of glottic insufficiency in 1983 and appears to have superior bioimplant qualities, particularly in cords which are atrophic, scarred or vocally defective. The host response is a gradual assimilation starting with ingrowth of vessels and progressive invasion of fibroblasts into the implanted collagen. In particular some of the resorbed implant is replaced by deposition of new host collagen from the metabolically active invading host fibroblasts, while the existing scar tissue softens, probably due to collagenase production by fibroblasts. A form called ZCI (Zyderm collagen 11: Collagen Corp, Palo Alto, CA) was the first injectable preparation used for clinical work. This is a highly purified suspension (65 mg/ml of bovine dermal collagen in a buffered physiological saline solution incorporating 0.3% lignocaine). The results have been shown to remain stable for at least 3 years but ZCI does have some disadvantages as it is not cross-linked and its sensitivity to collagenase could lead to long-term resorption. Also at least 60% of the volume injected is water and is therefore eliminated, requiring initial overinjection. Finally 3–4% of patients injected are hypersensitive. An alternative preparation from the same manufacturers, GAX collagen, contains a 0.0075% glutaraldehyde cross-linked collagen which is almost insensitive to collagenase. The use of GAX collagen seems to obviate the need for overcorrection and to be associated with a lower instance of hypersensitivity reaction.

Injection with alloplastic or bioimplant material remains the quickest and least expensive method of medializing a paretic vocal cord and is associated with a useful improvement in glottic efficiency, particularly in the prevention of aspiration and allied complications. None the less there is some stroboscopic and voice analysis evidence that the results of more complex procedures may produce a superior phonatory quality. The two principal alternatives to cord injection are thyroplasty and nerve transfer or other reinnervation procedures. The Isshiki type 1 thyroplasty was introduced in 1974 and involved the insertion of a block of Silastic through a window in the thyroid cartilage. The basic principle therefore is similar to the mechanism of cord injections but it requires an external approach. Proponents favour the greater degree of control over the vocal cord position by adjusting the thickness and position of the block, and also a greater degree of reversibility in the event of airway insufficiency. As with cord injection the procedure medializes only the membranous vocal cord, however, and can only partially resolve the problem of chronic aspiration because of the persistence of a posterior glottic chink. Histologically there is no evidence of intralaryngeal scarring when dissection is kept lateral to the inner perichondrium of the thyroid cartilage.

Postoperative findings include an increase in fundamental frequency and intensity of the voice and a significantly longer maximum phonation time. The procedure has the advantage of preserving normal relationships between the vocal fold mucosa and its substance, together with the associated potential for allowing recovery of normal motor function in the event of later neuromuscular regeneration. Laryngeal framework medialization not only tends to leave a posterior glottic chink, however, but also fails to allow for changes in tension in the vocal cord.

Early studies in the 1960s and 70s of reanastomosis of the severed ends of the recurrent laryngeal nerve or transposition of an extrinsic nerve to its main trunk were found to result in misdirected reinnervation with synkinesis of the laryngeal muscles, which rendered the organ functionally useless. Later attempts were made to reinnervate the posterior cricoarytenoid muscle selectively, thus restoring abductor function to a larynx with bilateral abductor paralysis. In order to achieve the normal cyclical inspiratory abductor movement of the vocal cords the ideal nerve for reinnervation should have a spontaneous inspiratory signal. The best signal is present in the phrenic nerve which in animal experiments produces good abduction. The technique has never become popular in humans because of the obvious risk of respiratory catastrophe if there is pre-existing damage to the contralateral phrenic nerve. Recently the preganglionic sympathetic neurons have been used in dog posterior cricoarytenoid muscle reinnervation, confirmed by direct laryngoscopy, electromyography and histological studies. The ansa hypoglossi is also said to demonstrate inspiratory activity and its sacrifice leaves very little deficit.

The direct reanastomosis of the ansa hypoglossi to the recurrent laryngeal nerve has the advantages of being entirely reversible and not interfering with the structure of the vocal cord. On the other hand it requires a cervical incision and is somewhat more costly to perform than other abduction procedures such as injection or thyroplasty. The most recent development in laryngeal reinnervation has been the development of pacing by electrical stimulation. Such electrical pacing of implanted nerve pedicles allows selective dynamic control of cord abduction and elongation. These techniques seem in future more likely to restore simple laryngeal functions (respiratory or deglutitive) than the more complex phonatory function.

Bilateral adductor paralysis

This paralysis if organic is fortunately the least common. It causes severe dysphonia and nearly all patients with this phenomenon suffer aspiration leading to bronchopneumonia. If this is the case it may be necessary to carry out a total laryngectomy to protect the patient from this eventuality, provided the neurological condition is not progressive.

Technique of operations for vocal cord paralysis

Woodman's operation

The patient will have a tracheostomy and so anaesthesia is applied through this route. The head is slightly extended and turned away from the paralysed side. The surgeon wants access to the cricothyroid joint and so a horizontal skin-crease incision is used at the level of the cricoid cartilage. Skin flaps are raised and the sternomastoid is retracted. Cut through the constrictor muscles on the back of the thyroid lamina and, with a finger behind the thyroid lamina, rotate the larynx. This will allow you to work directly on the cricothyroid joint, which should then be disarticulated. With a Langenbeck retractor, pull the thyroid cartilage forwards and rotate the cricoid so that the posterior cricoarytenoid muscle can be well seen. This gives access to the arytenoid, which should be disarticulated from the cricoid by entering the cricoarytenoid joint. This is done submucosally. Do not take the whole arytenoid out at this point. Dissect it submucosally and identify the vocal process. Before removing the arytenoid, put a 3/0 Nurolon suture through the vocal process and tie it round the inferior horn of the thyroid. You can then remove the body of the arytenoid. If you remove the arytenoid body too early then it is very difficult to identify the vocal process and very difficult to get a good bite with any stitch. Put another two sutures in to lateralize the cord.

It is described that at this point someone should do a laryngoscopy and estimate whether the vocal cord has been abducted to make a gap of 4 mm, but the authors find that this is an unrealistic step. The wound is drained and closed in the usual fashion.

The patient is allowed to recover from the procedure for a few days and then the tracheostomy tube is corked to see if there is an adequate airway; then it is removed.

Downie's arytenoidoplasty (Figs. 10.1–10.3)

Use a collar incision placed at the level of the thyroid cartilage. After making an incision and raising the upper and lower skin flaps, expose the thyroid cartilage vertically in the midline and then cut through the thyroid cartilage exactly in the midline, either with a dental fissure burr or with a Stryker saw. Finally, open into the laryngeal lumen with a knife and retract each half of the thyroid lamina. Remove one arytenoid by incising from the apex to the vocal process and dissecting out the cartilage using a Freer's elevator.

Expose the outer surface of the thyroid cartilage on one side by elevating the strap muscles from it. Then take a no. 26 gauge wire, threaded on a cutting needle, either curved or straight, and pass the needle through the cartilage to emerge in the laryngeal lumen immediately inferior to the posterior end of the vocal cord. Then pass the needle out through the ventricle immediately superior to the posterior edge of the vocal cord so that the wire now emerges again outside the thyroid cartilage. Tighten the ends of the wire so that the vocal cord is drawn laterally, cut the long ends off the wire and bury the remaining sharp end in the strap muscles. Close the larynx by suturing the edges of the cartilage together and close the wound in the usual way.

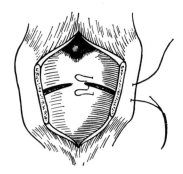

Fig. 10.1 Arytenoidoplasty via laryngofissure.

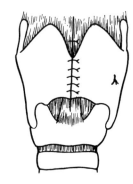

Fig. 10.2 Laryngofissure closed.

Injection technique

This operation can be done under local anaesthetic, so that the vocal cords can be seen moving when the patient attempts to speak. The larynx is therefore anaesthetized with Xylocaine.

Charge a Brüning-Arnold syringe with collagen or Teflon. The syringe has a very long needle and is controlled by a pistol grip with a ratchet handle, so designed that closure of one notch on the handle delivers 0.1 ml collagen paste. After charging the syringe, expose the larynx by direct laryngoscopy. On the paralysed side expose the upper surface of the vocal cord by retracting the false cord laterally with the end of the needle. Then push the needle into the soft tissues immediately lateral to the vocal cord, and close the handle one notch. Wait several seconds as the paste only extrudes slowly; during this period of time the vocal cord will be seen to move slowly towards the midline. Once the position becomes stationary ask the patient to say 'E' and, if the mobile cord does not approximate to the paralysed cord, inject another 0.1 ml and again wait. It should only be necessary to repeat the procedure at the most three times. Once the cords approximate the procedure is finished (Fig. 10.4).

The two most important points about this procedure are, firstly, to appreciate how slowly the paste extrudes from the needle, so that it must be kept in place after the handle has been closed for several

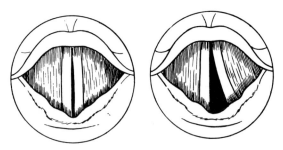

Fig. 10.3 Position of vocal cords before and after cordopexy.

seconds to allow the paste to enter the tissues; secondly, the injection must be put in exactly the right place, that is immediately lateral to the vocal cords. An injection should not be put into the subglottic space or into the edge of the vocal cord or too far laterally, as shown in Figure 10.4.

Collagen may be injected submucosally but Teflon must always be injected deeply.

Postoperative care

There is usually little special care required after this operation. The patient can eat and talk on the same

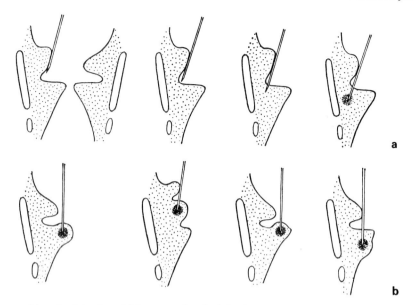

Fig. 10.4 (a) Correct positions for injection; (b) incorrect sites for injection.

day and can leave hospital the following day. No antibiotics are necessary and the procedure is usually uncomplicated.

Complications

1 Pain is usual but is mild and should be treated by simple analgesics.
2 Infection occurs occasionally and should be treated by antibiotics.
3 Laryngeal obstruction can occur if too much collagen has been injected, particularly if infection supervenes. Treat the obstruction by antibiotics and steroids and humidification, and if necessary a temporary tracheostomy. Because of the danger of laryngeal obstruction, and because it is impossible to remove the collagen once it has been injected, it is better to inject too little than too much, because it is always possible to come back later and give a further injection.

Isshiki thyroplasty

The patient will not have a tracheostomy and will be anaesthetized with an endotracheal tube. Because the larynx is being operated on, handling must be as gentle as possible to avoid laryngeal oedema, necessitating a postoperative tracheostomy.

A horizontal incision is made over the thyroid ala on the paralysed side. The strap muscles are retracted and partially dissected off the oblique line. A window is cut out of the thyroid ala. It should measure 5 × 3 mm and its upper border should be no higher than the midpoint of the thyroid ala (cord level). The anterior edge is 5 mm posterior to the

thyroid prominence. This can usually be done with a knife, but in a calcified larynx it may require a puncture wound and excision of cartilage with a sphenoidal punch forcep. Care should be taken to stay outside the internal perichondrium of the thyroid ala. The perichondrium is then dissected off the remaining ala as far posteriorly as possible.

A block of Silastic is cut in a wedge and inserted through the window in the thyroid ala, turned at right angles and locked in position. It should be placed as far posteriorly as possible in order to move the vocal process of the arytenoid. As the body of the arytenoid is not accessible from a lateral thyroid approach, and as it is a medial relation of the pyriform fossa, it is impossible to move it medially with an Isshiki operation or an injection.

Ansa hypoglossi – recurrent laryngeal nerve anastomosis

Neural anastomosis allows reinnervation of the whole hemilarynx rather than just selective reinnervation of a muscle implanted with a neuromuscular pedicle. The technique medializes the ipsilateral thyroid lamina due to loss of the lateral pull of the sternothyroid on the thyroid ala, giving an initial slight voice improvement. After complete neural regeneration of the motor axons from the ansa into the recurrent laryngeal nerve there is a low-level, tonic, non-cyclical innervation of the ipsilateral hemilarynx. A collar incision is made from the midline at the level of the cricoid cartilage across the sternomastoid muscle. Platysma is divided, the sternomastoid retracted laterally and a nerve stimulator used around the internal jugular vein. The ansa is identified when strong twitches of the strap muscles occur. The most inferior branch is used in anastomosis and is transected immediately proximal to its entry into the sternothyroid muscle. The great vessels are retracted laterally and the injured recurrent laryngeal nerve identified. The stimulator can be used to confirm its position if there is any doubt. The integrity of the distal recurrent laryngeal nerve should be confirmed. If it has been damaged then an alternative method, e.g. thyroplasty or collagen injection, should be considered. Neuroanastomosis is carried out with 10/0 nylon and the wound is closed in layers. As the procedure induces a paramedian cord without abduction it is contraindicated in any patient with reduced abduction of the contralateral cord.

Controversies in management

How do you know where the cord is?

Although some patients present with the cord definitely in the mid-position or definitely in the cadaveric position, in at least half of cases it is difficult to say exactly where the cord lies. We have found that the best way of studying this is with video films; the difficulty of actually identifying the whereabouts of the cord is accentuated by studying video films repeatedly. One's opinion on the cord position can change two or three times during the review of one video.

In late cord paralysis, one can see how far the arytenoid is dipped forward and how far the vocal process has come to lie below the glottic line. One can see how much atrophy there has been in the thyroarytenoid muscle and, with a study of these videos, it is possible to design perhaps the best rehabilitative measure.

How do you know if the arytenoid is fixed?

It is sometimes difficult to tell whether the cord is paralysed or whether the arytenoid is fixed. The apparent simplicity of the arytenoid mobilization test we feel has been overemphasized. It is difficult to move the arytenoid when the patient is asleep. Certainly gross degrees of fixation can be identified but it cannot be said that an arytenoid is fixed or mobile in every case.

How much should you investigate?

It is the authors' experience that if the cause of a vocal cord paralysis does not come to light with simple routine investigations and clinical examination then the cost-effectiveness of multiple investigations is low. The most likely things to be missed on initial examination are small lung cancers and small posterior thyroid tumours. It is doubtful if any extension of initial investigation is going to identify these small tumours, and it may just be that keeping the patient under review and keeping an open mind as to the possibility of these is the preferred option. Fifteen per cent of this group will ultimately develop a bronchial carcinoma.

How long do you wait to operate?

Although 6 months is taken as an arbitrary time for recovery of vocal cord function, there is no good reason for this. In the dog it takes about 60 days for a crushed recurrent laryngeal nerve to recover function. If this is extrapolated to the human, estimates have been made that the equivalent is about 6 months, but there seems to be no other hard evidence for this.

Certainly if somebody has a lung cancer and loses their voice and their power of coughing then there is nothing to be gained by delay, and a collagen operation ought to be performed immediately.

Why is there a 30% failure rate with a Woodman operation?

This is an intriguing question because the operation is a simple one with very few variables. The authors feel that perhaps the most important technical point in doing a Woodman's operation is to get the stitch into the cartilage of the vocal process prior to removing the arytenoid. If the arytenoid is removed before a stitch is put into place then the soft tissues of the larynx fall medially and the stitch may be placed too laterally to get decent traction. Furthermore, the stitch may well cut out and allow the cord to drift back into the mid-position. Scarring may also drag the cord back into that position, and there should be a commitment on the part of the surgeon to get the airway right in this operation rather than to preserve voice.

What do you do when a collagen injection goes wrong?

If a collagen operation goes wrong then too much has been inserted, in which case a tracheostomy is required; or the collagen has been put into the wrong place and a curious diplophonia arises. In either case, the collagen has to be removed, perhaps preceded by a tracheostomy. There is no good way to remove it other than to perform a laryngofissure and to enter the thyroarytenoid muscle. This will, of course, cause gross scarring and worse dysphonia.

References and further reading

Surgical anatomy and pathology

Brondbok Hall C, Dahl H A, Teig E, Gujord K M (1986) A histochemical evaluation of experimentally reinnervated canine laryngeal muscles. *J Otolaryngol* 15:265–72.

Fink B R, Demarest R J (1978) *Laryngeal Biomechanics*. Cambridge, Massachusetts, Harvard University Press.

Isaacson G, Kim J H, Kirchner J C, Kirchner J A (1990) Histology of Isshiki thyroplasty type I. *Ann Otol Rhinol Laryngol* **90**:42–5.

Jacobs I N, Saunders I, Wu B-L, Biller H F (1990) Reinnervation of the canine posterior cricoarytenoid muscle with sympathetic preganglionic neurons. *Ann Otol Rhinol Laryngol* **99**:167–74.

Negus V E (1947) Certain anatomical and physiological considerations in the paralysis of the larynx. *Proc R Soc Med* **40**:849–53.

Walsh F, Castelli J (1975) Polytef granuloma clinically simulating carcinoma of the thyroid. *Arch Otolaryngol* **101**:262–3.

Woodson G E (1989) Effects of recurrent laryngeal nerve transection and vagotomy on the respiratory contraction of the cricothyroid muscle. *Ann Otol Rhinol Laryngol* **98**:373–8.

Investigations

Sasaki C T, Horiuchi M, Ikari T, Kirchner J A (1980) Vocal cord positioning by selective denervation. Old territory revisited. *Ann Otol* **89**:541–6.

Slavit D H, Maragos N E, Lipton R J (1990) Physiologic assessment of Isshiki type III thyroplasty. *Laryngoscope* **100**:844–8.

Tucker H M (1986) Vocal cord paralysis in small children: principles in management. *Ann Otol Rhinol Laryngol* **95**:618–21.

Tucker H M (1980) Vocal cord paralysis – 1979: etiology and management. *Laryngoscope* **90**:585–90.

Ward P H, Berci G (1982) Observations on so-called idiopathic vocal cord paralysis. *Ann Otol Rhinol Laryngol* **91**:558–63.

Treatment

Broniatowski M, Kaneko S, Jacobs G, Nose Y, Tucker H M (1985) Laryngeal pacemaker II. Electronic pacing of reinnervated posterior cricoarytenoid muscles in the canine. *Laryngoscope* **95**:1194–8.

Broniatowski M, Davies C R, Jacobs G B et al. (1990) Artificial restoration of voice. I: Experiments in phonatory control of the reinnervated canine larynx. *Laryngoscope* **100**:1219–24.

Crumley R L (1990) Teflon versus thyroplasty nerve transfer: a comparison. *Ann Otol Rhinol Laryngol* **99**:759–63.

Crumley R L, Izdebski K, McMicken B (1988) Nerve transfer versus Teflon injection for vocal cord paralysis: a comparison. *Laryngoscope* **98**:1200–4.

Dedo H H (1971) Electromyographic and visual evaluation of recurrent laryngeal nerve anastomosis in dogs. *Ann Otol Rhinol Laryngol* **80**:664–8.

Isshiki N, Morita H, Okamura H et al. (1974) Thyroplasty as a new phonosurgical technique. *Acta Otolaryngol* **78**:451–7.

Isshiki N, Tanabe M, Sawada M (1978) Arytenoid adduction for unilateral vocal cord paralysis. *Arch Otolaryngol* **104**:555–8.

Isshiki N, Taira T, Kojima H, Shoji K (1989) Recent modifications in thyroplasty type I. *Ann Otol Rhinol Laryngol* **98**:777–9.

Koufman J A (1986) Laryngoplasty for vocal cord medialization: an alternative to Teflon. *Laryngoscope* **96**:726–31.

Lewy R B (1983) Teflon injection of the vocal cord: complications, errors and precautions. *Ann Otol Rhinol Laryngol* **92**:473–4.

Maran A G D, Hardcastle P F, Hamid A, Mackenzie I J (1986) An analysis of 102 cases of Polytef injection of the vocal cord. *J Laryngol Otol* **100**:47–51.

Maves M D, McCabe B F, Gray S (1989) Phonosurgery: indications and pitfalls. *Ann Otol Rhinol Laryngol* **98**:577–80.

Mu L, Yang S (1990) Electromyographic study on end-to-end anastomosis of the recurrent laryngeal nerve in dogs. *Laryngoscope* **100**:1009–17.

Remacle M, Marbaix E, Hamoir M, Bertrand B, Eeckhaut J (1990) Correction of glottic insufficiency by collagen injection. *Ann Otol Rhinol Laryngol* **99**:438–44.

Rontal E, Rontal M, Morse G, Brown E M (1976) Vocal cord injection in the treatment of acute and chronic aspiration. *Laryngoscope* **86**:625–34.

Sasaki C T, Leder S B, Petcu L, Friedman C D (1990) Longitudinal voice quality changes following Isshiki thyroplasty type I: the Yale experience. *Laryngoscope* **100**:849–52.

Tucker H M (1976) Human laryngeal reinnervation. *Laryngoscope* **86**:769–79.

Tucker H M (1987) Neurologic disorders. In: *The Larynx*. New York, Thieme Medical, pp. 235–58.

Tucker H M (1990) Combined laryngeal framework medialisation and reinnervation for unilateral vocal fold paralysis. *Ann Otol Rhinol Laryngol* **99**:778–81.

Ward P H, Hanson D G, Abemayor E (1985) Transcutaneous Teflon injection of the paralysed vocal cord: a new techique. *Laryngoscope* **95**:644–9.

Woodson G E, Miller R H (1981) The timing of surgical intervention in vocal cord paralysis. *Otolaryngol Head Neck Surg* **89**:264–7.

11

Trauma and stenosis of the larynx and cervical trachea

Acute laryngeal trauma

Causes of laryngeal injury

Epidemiology

There are basically two types of laryngeal trauma – penetrating wounds and blunt injuries. The blunt injuries can be high-velocity or low-velocity injuries. Penetrating wounds are caused by knives, bullets, wires and agricultural implements. High-velocity blunt injuries are usually caused by road traffic accidents or injuries at work. The velocity, however, may be so high that the wound becomes compound. Low-velocity blunt injuries rarely become compound and are due to blows with fists and as a result of sports injuries. The sports that are particularly associated with laryngeal injury are snow mobile racing, motor cycle racing, basketball and karate; injuries have even been reported due to contact with golf balls and cricket balls. Reports have also come from the sport of ice hockey where garrotting with the hockey stick is evidently practised in the professional game.

The type of individual who suffers from laryngeal trauma is usually a young male who indulges in sport, is involved in fights, or who drives cars fast and dangerously.

In North America and Western Europe, the condition of laryngeal trauma was first associated with road traffic accidents. This was when no seat belts were used or lap-type seat belts were in vogue (Fig. 11.1). Nowadays, the incidence in these countries of laryngeal damage from road traffic accidents is only a fraction of what it was. This is due to the crossover seat belt and the institution of speed limits and other safety features in cars, such as collapsible steering wheels, and air bags. In developing countries, however, when driving by a large number of people is a relatively new feature, laryngeal injuries as a result of road traffic accidents present a significant problem to practising otolaryngologists. Furthermore, in these countries there is an improving delivery of medical care and more patients are rescued from

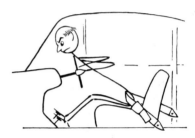

Fig. 11.1 Effect of an automobile accident with a lap-type seat belt.

road traffic accidents and removed from the site of the accident to the hospital, where previously they may have died at the roadside.

Mechanics of injury

Any classification of types of laryngeal injury is an unhelpful exercise unless it is confined to injuries of the supraglottis, the glottis, the subglottis or mixed injuries. Basically, one must consider injuries to the surrounding skeleton of the larynx, i.e. the hyoid, thyroid, cricoid and tracheal rings, and injuries to the internal soft tissues. Damage to both the skeleton and the soft tissues creates different problems and requires different modes of management.

Penetrating wounds tend to bounce off the more solid pieces of the larynx, i.e. the supporting skeleton. It would be usual for a penetrating instrument to slide off the thyroid cartilage and penetrate the thyrohyoid membrane superiorly, or to go between the cricoid and the thyroid inferiorly to penetrate the cricothyroid membrane. Each of these presents different functional problems.

Penetration of the thyrohyoid membrane causes bleeding in the paraglottic space and thus airway obstruction. It does not affect the voice in any way. A little bleeding or oedema will resolve with the normal scavenging macrophage process of the body but, if there is any significant amount of bleeding,

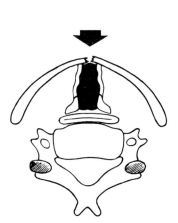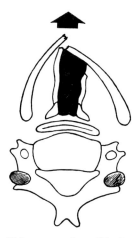

Fig. 11.2 Compression of an uncalcified cartilage leads to a linear thyroid fracture and possible detachment of a vocal cord and/or epiglottis.

then it will not all resorb and will be organized to cause some degree of stenosis of the supraglottis.

This does not happen to such an extent if the cricothyroid membrane is penetrated. The most immediate effect of this will be that air will leave the respiratory tract and will cause some surgical emphysema in the neck. The penetrating wound, however, may be covered with thyroid tissue. The bleeding may fill the subglottic space causing respiratory obstruction, but it is more likely to run down the trachea through a clean cut and cause coughing.

Low-velocity blunt injuries are unlikely to fracture the thyroid or the cricoid, but fractured hyoids are not uncommon in karate and basketball. Again there will be bleeding into the soft tissues of the paraglottic space and, if the ends of the fractured hyoid are in close apposition, then movement during swallowing will cause pain that may require treatment. The patient may have swelling also of the base of the tongue and some dysphagia.

Even though the thyroid and cricoid are not fractured, there may well be bleeding within the paraglottic space and bleeding within Reinke's space on the vocal cords. The interarytenoid space, which must be present to allow gliding and separation of the arytenoids, can fill with blood causing ultimate stenosis, but the problem is usually one of oedema and minimal bleeding rather than obliterative bleeding causing airway damage or later stenosis.

High-velocity blunt injuries will fracture the skeleton of the larynx. The fate of the thyroid cartilage depends on its degree of calcification and, thus, on the age of the patient. If the thyroid cartilage is pushed backwards over the cervical spine, then it splays apart (Fig. 11.2). A minimal injury like this with an elastic thyroid cartilage will result in no fracture, but if there is any rigidity in the thyroid cartilage or if the force is great enough, then the cartilage will usually split down the front or down the thyroid prominence. The inherent elasticity of the uncalcified cartilage will allow it to spring back into place, and there may be little damage or there may be disruption of the anterior commissure. The classically described situation of detachment of the tendon of the anterior commissure and the petiole of the epiglottis is hardly ever seen, but is so dramatic that it demands inclusion in any text on laryngeal injury. In this case, the epiglottis falls backwards and the vocal cords literally roll up on themselves towards the arytenoid. However, in an elastic thyroid with a linear fracture down the prominence, there is little in the way of disruption of the anterior commissure, but there will be bleeding into the pre-epiglottic space and posterior displacement of the epiglottis. More important is the fate of the arytenoids. As the thyroid becomes compressed against the cervical spine, the arytenoids are sandwiched. This can result in them being displaced at worst, but at best there will be bleeding into the interarytenoid space and consequent swelling.

If the thyroid is calcified and is then compressed against the cervical spine, it is unlikely to have enough inherent elasticity to return to its original position (Fig. 11.3). It will therefore shatter rather like an egg and there will be loss of the thyroid prominence. There will be similar arytenoid injury to that described above.

The cricoid is the most important part of the laryngeal skeleton. It is the only complete ring in the upper or lower respiratory tract. The thyroid and the hyoid and tracheal rings are all U-shaped with soft tissue attachments posteriorly. If the cricoid is disrupted then it will constrict. Even a linear fracture in the cricoid will cause some resorption of cartilage and reduction of the calibre of the airway at the level of the cricoid. This has severe effects on airflow as a

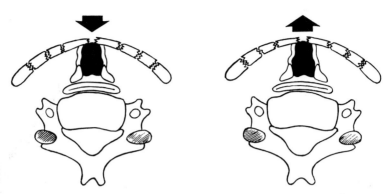

Fig. 11.3 Compression of a calcified cartilage causes flattening of the neck due to shattering of the cartilage.

consequence of Poiseuille's law relating the airflow to the fourth power of the radius of the airway. This is probably why high tracheostomies have such a deleterious effect on the airway. There is nothing magic about the first ring, but a tracheostomy tube put through an opening made by excision of the first ring will be contiguous with the cricoid cartilage and may result in enough resorption of that cartilage for the cricoid to stenose. It is rare that acute injuries damage the soft tissue within the cricoid but if a high-velocity acute injury damages the integrity of the cricoid cartilage, then there will be a very difficult defect to repair.

The final soft tissue injury from high-velocity blunt injuries takes the form of separation of the trachea from the cricoid. This usually results in death at the roadside, but it is quite possible for enough lumen to remain for the patient to breathe long enough to come into hospital. Several tracheal rings can be damaged with this sort of injury and the cricotracheal membrane may be sheared off.

Types of injury

Soft tissue

Any injury to the larynx will result in some oedema of soft tissue. This usually has no permanent effects other than in Reinke's space, where permanent oedema of the vocal cord can result, or resolve into a laryngeal polyp.

Far more important is the effect of organized haematoma. This is most marked in the supraglottic space, where there is the most scope for expansion of soft tissue and obliteration of the airway.

The interarytenoid area is also a very large potential space with debilitating consequences if organization occurs within the area.

The anterior parts of the vocal cords at the anterior commissure may be detached but, more commonly, abrasions of the mucosa here can result in anterior web formation.

The subglottic space in children is very much more important than it is in the adult, in whom subglottic space obliteration narrowing the airway is rare. It is usually the result of disorganization of the surrounding skeleton, especially the cricoid.

Glottic competence can be lost for several reasons. The most common cause is fixation of an arytenoid in an unsatisfactory position, but it can also be made incompetent by resorption of the thyroarytenoid muscle and atrophy of the cord, and also by vocal cord paralysis due to damage to the recurrent laryngeal nerve in subglottic injuries.

Skeletal injuries

The hyoid, the only bone in the respiratory tract, may be fractured and may well heal without the patient knowing anything has happened apart from a few days of discomfort. On rare occasions, the fractured ends form a bursa, which results in continual movement of the fractured edges together and this requires excision.

The thyroid cartilage, if fractured, will heal using fibrous tissue; provided it is in a good position, this is just as satisfactory as wiring or stitching it together. If, however, it is compressed, as in a calcified thyroid cartilage, then it has to be reconstituted and held outwards with a stent.

The effects of disruption of the cricoid cartilage have already been described, and any rehabilitation of this area must involve widening the cricoid cartilage and keeping the edges apart with some material that does not resorb.

At this point, it is pertinent to point out the effect of blood on cartilage. If cartilage is allowed to stay in contact with blood for any length of time, then the blood is absorbed by the cartilage. This is especially important in the trachea, where loss of the U-shaped rings perhaps causes no observable abnormality in the airway until the patient takes exercise or a deep breath. The increased velocity of airflow pulls in the weakened tracheal walls and the patient will have dyspnoea on exercise due to tracheomalacia.

If cartilage is left denuded of mucosa and is in contact with secretions, then the surface of the cartilage will become inflamed. This will result in the formation of granulations, and is most frequently seen in intubation injuries where the vocal process of the arytenoid is sometimes damaged and an intubation granuloma results. Similarly, if too large an intubation tube is used, then the anterior commissure is split and cartilage becomes bared in that area, resulting in an anterior intubation granuloma.

Investigations

History

The most important step in diagnosing an acute laryngeal injury is to be aware of the possibility in every patient who has had trauma to the upper half of the body. Dyspnoea and dysphonia are the main features leading to suspicion, with dysphagia and pain as lesser indicators.

Examination

Marks on the neck may or may not be present and their absence does not rule out a fractured larynx, but it makes such a diagnosis unlikely.

Surgical emphysema confined to the neck is almost pathognomonic of a breach in the airway. Loss of landmarks such as a thyroid prominence is also diagnostic. It should be borne in mind that any neck wound carries with it the associated possibilities of damage to the great vessels and to the cervical spine.

Radiology

Plain X-rays of the neck are helpful in confirming the presence or absence of air in the soft tissues. Tomography and laryngography are usually impractical in acute injuries. Computed tomography should be done where a fracture is suspected and not clinically obvious.

Laryngoscopy

This should be performed in all patients. If ordinary mirror examination is impossible, flexible laryngoscopy may yield valuable information.

Treatment policy

Treatment principles

Protection of the airway

This is obviously the most important feature and is probably the reason why most victims of road traffic accidents are now saved. If there is merely oedema present, with no suggestion of intraluminal bleeding or tracheal damage, then the patient can be kept at bed rest with or without steroids or steam inhalations.

More likely, however, the airway will be at risk and, rather than performing an immediate tracheostomy, the patient should be intubated. In any review of chronic laryngeal stenoses, there is always a hint of criticism in publications that anaesthetists at this point missed an acute laryngeal injury. If anyone has had a neck injury, there will be contusion and perhaps bleeding in the throat and it is quite impossible, with the equipment available to an anaesthetist and in the time available, to recognize intraluminal or skeletal damage to the larynx. Even though an endotracheal tube is not much smaller than many of the stents that are used in the later reconstruction of a larynx, neither they nor stents do anything to stop intraluminal bleeding, especially in the supraglottic area, or to prevent webs in either the posterior or anterior glottis.

In the first-aid situation, a tracheostomy may be needed but this is very much less favoured than immediate intubation.

Protection of laryngeal function

Although the larynx has functions related to swallowing closure and effort closure, by far its most important functions are in relation to breathing and speaking. It is these functions that should be protected as far as possible in the management of laryngeal injury. In the assessment of results of treatment, a success with regard to breathing is a patient who does not have to wear a permanent tracheostomy tube and who is able to lead a normal life with no or minimal dyspnoea. On the other hand, if the vocal cord had been damaged, a normal speaking voice is unlikely. Success in this function, therefore, can range from normal voice to audible phonation as opposed to a whisper.

Emphasis has been laid on the importance of preventing bleeding in the laryngeal spaces in the treatment of acute injury in the larynx. In this regard it is apposite to mention the use of stents. Many stents have been described for use in laryngeal injury, but their role should be isolated to the scaffolding of a reconstituted skeletal structure. They have no part to play in stopping bleeding and the prevention of fibrosis in the laryngeal spaces. A much better technique for this is to open the spaces and obliterate them with quilting sutures. If there is any significant degree of bleeding within the larynx, then it should be opened by way of a midline approach (laryngofissure) and the spaces evacuated and quilted with 3/0 Vicryl sutures. Inserting drains into the spaces is quite useless.

If there has been damage to the skeletal structure

then a principle of minimal debridement should be practised. There is not very much cartilage in the larynx; excision of any tracheal rings, and certainly of the cricoid cartilage, carries with it grave consequences. Although much of this cartilage may resorb, it is better to cover it with mucosa and see if it forms a scaffold for firm fibrous tissue. The worst that can happen is what one would achieve with debridement.

In general terms, the arytenoid will be swollen in nearly every moderately severe laryngeal trauma, and so the patient should be fed with a nasogastric tube to stop inhalation from glottic incompetence, certainly for a few days.

Treatment

Penetrating injuries

Injuries such as those due to knife wounds, wire wounds and wounds from agricultural or industrial implements will require treatment if there is bleeding into the supraglottic area. Nearly every such case will require to have the larynx opened and the supraglottic area drained and quilted.

Bullet wounds most certainly require exploration and debridement of cartilage, which will probably also be fractured, and exploration of the neck vessels and nerves. Reconstruction will follow the same principles as outlined previously. On occasion the injuries as the result of bullet wounds are so severe that total laryngectomy is necessary.

It is usual for patients with supraglottic injury to end up with a reasonably good voice and no permanent tracheostomy.

Low-velocity blunt injuries

The majority of these patients do not require open exploration of the larynx, but most will require observation in hospital at least overnight in case of laryngeal oedema and airway obstruction. As well as sports injuries, similar pathological consequences can follow attempted strangulation and the inhalation of fumes during a conflagration. Provided both the airway and the voice are reasonable then these patients can be observed. If either of these functions is disturbed, however, then the larynx should be intubated and perhaps later explored and reconstructed.

Many of these patients will end up with a poor voice if the glottis has been damaged, because there may well be later minor web formation or arthrodesis of an arytenoid, but it is unusual for these patients to require a permanent tracheostomy.

High-velocity blunt injuries

About half the patients who have laryngeal injuries as a result of road traffic accidents will require laryngeal exploration and reconstruction. Skeletal damage is repaired by reconstitution, usually using stents; soft-tissue injuries are dealt with by reducing bleeding, evacuating spaces and using quilting sutures.

If the cricoid is injured, then primary repair should be attempted. Only when primary repair has failed should one of the many techniques applied to chronic cricoid stenosis be applied.

Separation of the cricotracheal membrane is a fairly unusual injury and one which is dealt with reasonably by dropping the larynx in the neck and freeing the trachea down to the carina, and pulling it upwards for an end-to-end anastomosis, excising any damaged tracheal rings.

Most high-velocity blunt injuries will result in combined injuries to the glottis and subglottis. If only the glottis is involved then the results with regard to breathing should be good, but if the subglottis is involved, then the patient faces future surgery for chronic subglottic stenosis.

Technique of operations for laryngeal trauma

Fractured thyroid cartilage and internal soft tissue injuries

Make a collar incision and elevate skin flaps. Retract the strap muscles and display the thyroid prominence. A fracture line extending obliquely down the front of the thyroid cartilage will probably be seen; examine the cricoid cartilage carefully to make sure that the fracture line has not extended lower. Do a laryngofissure by separating the thyroid cartilages through the fracture line with scissors. Resuture the vocal cords to the vocal processes or the anterior commissure, depending from where they are detached; also suture the mucosal lacerations. Use 3/0 chromic catgut to repair all soft tissue lacerations. Fix the epiglottis in position by two sutures of silk, which are placed so as to hold the epiglottis forwards by anchoring it to the hyoid bone as in Fig. 11.4.

If the anterior commissure has been damaged, simple wiring of the thyroid cartilage will not suffice to prevent the formation of an anterior web. Fashion a McNaught keel using 0.18 mm-thick tantalum sheeting, cut to the appropriate size with Mayo scissors, and placed in the laryngofissure with the external flanges sutured to the thyroid perichondrium with 3/0 chromic catgut (Fig. 11.5).

An alternative to this is to put a sheet of rolled-up Silastic in the lumen of the larynx and to hold it with two transfixion sutures, fastened on the outside with Silastic buttons. These can be cut and the Silastic withdrawn after 4–6 weeks. Close the wound in layers without drainage and put the patient on penicillin.

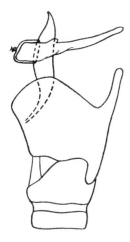

Fig. 11.4 Fixation of the epiglottis with a suture around the hyoid.

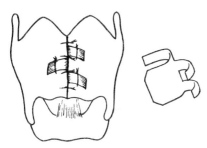

Fig. 11.5 On the right, a McNaught keel: on the left, the keel in position between the vocal cords with the flanges sutured to the thyroid cartilage.

After 4–6 weeks reopen the neck and remove the McNaught keel. There will almost inevitably be some exposed bare cartilage at the anterior commissure, and granulation tissue will form over this, which may need to be removed several times via an endoscope before the larynx is quite healed. Withdraw the tracheostomy tube when the patient can breathe normally again.

Shattered thyroid cartilage with internal soft-tissue injuries

In this case, when the thyroid cartilage is exposed instead of a single fracture line, multiple stellate fracture lines are seen with a marked flattening of the thyroid prominence. The external perichondrium is usually intact but the internal perichondrium is invariably breached with pieces of cartilage lying in the laryngeal cavity.

Do a laryngofissure and suture the internal derangements as before.

In this case a more solid splinting is required with an internal laryngeal stent. There is no ideal laryngeal stent available, as is evidenced by the multiplicity of designs that have been tried in the past. Laryngeal stents ought to be available in the theatre for children, women and men but, in an emergency, use a finger-cot filled with sponge as a temporary measure. Within a short time this must be replaced with a more permanent stent.

Laryngeal stents are either solid or hollow. The advantage of a hollow stent is that the patient can whisper through it on closing off the tracheostomy tube; its disadvantage, however, is that it causes difficulty in swallowing, as aspiration of saliva almost invariably occurs. It is better to use a solid laryngeal stent made of some inert material, such as one of the various silicone rubbers.

Fix the stent with two no. 26 stainless-steel wires passed through the neck from side to side, passing, in order, through skin, thyroid cartilage, stent, thyroid cartilage and skin (Fig. 11.6). Thread the two free ends on either side of the neck through buttons and tighten them. Further tightening at daily intervals will be required as the swelling settles. Leave the stent in the larynx for at least 3 months; when the time comes to remove it, cut the wires flush with the skin on one side and pull them through from the other side of the neck. A thread ought to be attached to the laryngeal stent so that it can be removed endoscopically. It is better if such a thread is attached to a piece of stainless-steel wire inside the laryngeal stent, as shown in Figure 11.7, to stop the thread separating from the stent at endoscopic removal.

To summarize: a laryngeal stent is required to maintain the shape of the cartilaginous framework – a keel to separate mucosal lacerations.

Fractured cricoid

This injury is invariably associated with a fracture or shattering of the thyroid cartilage with internal injury. The only reason why it is separated here, in

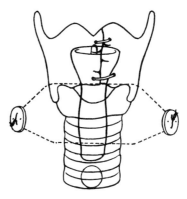

Fig. 11.6 Method of fixation of a solid laryngeal stent.

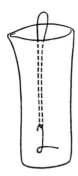

Fig. 11.7 Thread loop attached to a steel wire inside a solid laryngeal stent.

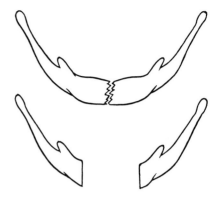

Fig. 11.8 Removal of the body in a fractured hyoid.

the description, is to emphasize the importance of its recognition when the thyroid cartilage is fractured. Chevalier Jackson once stated that 'loss of the cricoid cartilage practically always precludes the possibility of eliminating the wearing of a tracheal cannula'. This is not completely true, but any loss of cricoid cartilage must be very skilfully repaired, as will be seen later. Make every effort to retain as much cricoid cartilage as possible, and always use a laryngeal stent for 3 months.

Tracheal avulsion

In a severe injury the trachea may be avulsed from the larynx by a tear through the cricotracheal membrane. Most of these patients die immediately at the site of the accident from respiratory obstruction, but one may occasionally arrive in hospital.

Do an immediate tracheostomy and explore the larynx. It is usually possible to suture the first tracheal ring to the cricoid cartilage using 2/0 nylon sutures. Put all the sutures in place before tying them, as it is very difficult to insert extra sutures once any are tied. There is no need to use a stent, which may cause infection and breakdown of the anastomosis.

Fractured hyoid

This injury is more usual after a karate blow or a basketball accident. It never causes respiratory obstruction but there is exquisite pain every time the patient swallows. There is no point in trying to reduce and fix this fracture, as no disability occurs from removal of bone on either side of this fracture line (Fig. 11.8). Do this so that the jagged ends do not rub against each other, causing pain.

Chronic laryngeal stenosis

Chronic stenosis may be said to be established if the airway is unsatisfactory 4 weeks after the injury. It is

an important lesion which interferes with speech, breathing and the ability to clear secretions from the lower respiratory tract.

Causes

This section will be confined to chronic laryngeal stenosis in the adult. The condition, if it manifests itself in childhood, is quite different.

Common causes of chronic laryngeal stenosis in Western Europe and the USA are failed treatment or non-recognition of acute trauma, but stenosis is also seen as a complication of tracheostomy, intubation and partial laryngectomy. In Egypt, and other parts of the Middle East, scleroma is probably the most common cause of laryngeal stenosis. Tracheostomy is an operation performed well by nearly every medical practitioner involved in the care of trauma patients in Western Europe and North America, but there are still places in the world where tracheostomies can be performed badly, leading to laryngotracheal stenosis. Other systemic diseases, such as Wegener's granuloma, polychondritis and various types of autoimmune thyroiditis can also damage the subglottic area resulting in stenosis, but they are rare.

While supraglottic and glottic stenosis do occur, the most common site is the subglottic area. The main cause of this is, therefore, disruption of the supporting skeleton of the cricoid and the tracheal rings. The associated soft tissue narrowing usually reflects the lack of integrity of the supporting structures.

Effects

Much the same pathological considerations apply to chronic laryngeal stenosis as to the acute injury. The soft tissue damage is due to mucosal loss and mucosal adhesions, but above all to organization of haematoma within the paraglottic, the pre-epiglottic and the interarytenoid space.

Glottic competence is affected by web formation anteriorly, and posteriorly an arthrodesis of the arytenoid can result in an unsatisfactory position. Furthermore, the recurrent laryngeal nerves, if they are not injured in the initial trauma, stand a very high chance of injury in the ensuing treatment of chronic laryngeal stenosis. Arytenoidectomy or cordopexy almost always form part of the treatment of chronic laryngeal stenosis.

A factor in chronic laryngeal stenosis that does not, however, apply in the acute injury is that of tissue memory. If a cartilaginous framework has been disrupted, it heals with fibrous tissue whose fibrocytes have a directional memory. Thus, merely incising and separating scar tissue will lead to the tissue attempting to replace itself in its original scarred state. Reconstruction must be more sophisticated than incision and replacement. As much scarred tissue as possible should be excised, but the danger of repositioning will be ever-present. This is most important in the cricoid, where the interruption of the ring causes narrowing. The forces within the cricoid are altered, probably permanently, from this narrowing, and excision of the scarred area and separation of the cricoid ends, with support from intervening tissue, is probably the single most difficult problem in the management of chronic stenosis.

Excision of scarred soft tissue is not nearly so difficult. Wide excision of scarred tissue is, of course, necessary but grafting with split skin or mucosa usually gives good results. It must be re-emphasized, however, that no amount of satisfactory soft tissue healing will take place if the skeletal framework is disrupted or resumes its scarred altered position.

Stents are useful in supporting a reconstituted laryngeal framework and, to an extent, in separating mucosal surfaces that have been adherent. It bears repetition that stents are of little value in preventing haematoma formation within soft tissue.

Investigations

History

The cause of the chronic stenosis is obviously important. If it is a result of an excessively zealous partial laryngectomy, then it is unlikely that enough tissue will be found to augment the lumen of the larynx. Again, if it is a systemic disease that has caused the laryngeal stenosis, it is unlikely that surgery has any place to play in the management. Exceptions to this might be confined segments of scleroma in the advanced fibrotic stage, but this would be a very rare occurrence.

Perhaps the most important communication to establish between the surgeon and the patient is a mutual sense of realism. Both should realize what is and what is not possible with surgery. Both should realize that the dynamics of tissue healing can alter

any result and this should be taken into account in timing the operation. No attempts should be made to increase the laryngeal lumen until 18 months have passed from the time of the initial injury. Finally, the patient must be quite clear as to what his or her objectives from surgery will be. He or she must evaluate how much a good voice means and similarly whether he or she wants to be rid of the tracheostomy tube so much that he or she is willing to undergo surgery. More minor cases should also realize that the additional scarring of surgery could, in rare instances, result in them having a tracheostomy for the rest of their life.

Examination

The surgeon should establish with mirror or flexible endoscopy the extent of the laryngeal or subglottic stenosis, but this is not always possible and is probably the least important part of the examination. Perhaps the most important part is in the assessment of the length of the neck and, therefore, how much trachea is available for mobilization in the neck without having to go into the mediastinum.

Radiography

The first investigation should be tomography and, in cases where the subglottis cannot be visualized, then laryngography should be used. This is perhaps the only role that laryngography has now to play in the investigation of laryngeal disease. Both laryngography and tomography will give a good idea of soft-tissue scarring and distortion, but computed tomography scanning will give a very much better idea of the state of the laryngeal cartilages and should, if possible, be carried out in all instances.

Endoscopy

This is necessary to establish, as accurately as possible, the extent of laryngeal damage, but it is also useful to ascertain the lower extent of subglottic stenosis and to test for the state of the tracheal cartilages. These have to be examined from as high as possible without creating any splinting and with the anaesthetist blowing high airflows into the lungs using a Venturi system. In this way, tracheomalacia can be assessed.

The state of the arytenoids must be ascertained to see if they are fixed or not, and oesophagoscopy should be carried out in every case.

Treatment Policy

Most patients presenting for the treatment of chronic laryngeal stenosis will already have a tracheostomy. They should be warned that the results of treatment of chronic laryngeal stenosis are at best unrewarding and their tracheostomy may be permanent. In the postoperative period with resultant swelling, the patient will almost certainly have to be fed with a nasogastric tube, at least for some days. They should also be warned that it is unlikely that they will regain a normal voice, especially if the glottis has been damaged.

There is almost universal dissatisfaction with the surgical treatment of the systemic conditions that cause laryngotracheal stenosis, such as a scleroma, Wegener's granuloma and polychondritis. It is debatable whether these patients should be treated with any surgery other than occasional dilatations.

Supraglottic stenosis

There are three choices in the treatment of this condition: first, there is supraglottic laryngectomy; second, a laryngeal widening procedure; and third, laser excision. The authors do not think there is any place now for supraglottic laryngectomy in the treatment of this condition. It defies all the basic tenets of the surgery of laryngeal trauma – namely, maximal excision, there is usually nothing wrong with the supraglottic skeletal framework, and the lesion is nearly always of soft tissue. The choice lies between serial excisions of the soft tissue with the laser and the laryngeal widening operation. Laser excision allows the patient to keep the tracheostomy tube and to evaluate the effect of serial excisions. An alternative is the laryngeal widening procedure, where the larynx is opened in the midline and as much as possible of the submucosal scarred tissue removed. The remaining mucosa is stitched back against the laryngeal framework with quilting sutures, or areas of scarred tissue are grafted either with skin or buccal mucosa.

Glottic stenosis

The anterior glottic web can be dealt with by laser excision, by repeated endoscopic excision, or by external excision and separation of the anterior glottis with a Silastic or tantalum keel (McNaught keel). If an external approach is used, then the keel is kept in place for at least 5 weeks. It can then be removed with minimal reopening of the neck wound. The external approach is probably the preferred one when there is also a stenosis of the anterior parts of the false cord but, if the webbing is limited to the glottis, then laser excision or endoscopic removal is probably best in the first instance.

Posterior stenosis of the glottis is more difficult to treat. The glottis consists of roughly 40% cartilage from the medial processes and vocal processes of the arytenoids, and 60% membranous vocal cord from the vocal ligament and the attached mucosa and thyroarytenoid muscle. Posterior glottic stenosis means a stenosis between the cartilaginous aryten-

oids. This is usually accompanied by fixation of at least one arytenoid. The stenosis may be excised and the arytenoid separated by a modified keel with Silastic stenting on the end of it to keep the posterior glottis open. For this to succeed, both arytenoids must be mobile and capable of achieving glottic competence when the keel is removed. If the arytenoids are not mobile then one should be removed by a laryngofissure and the cord stitched laterally with stenting applied to stop further adhesions.

Cricoid stenosis

Enough has already been written about the biomechanics of cricoid stenosis to make it clear how a free graft in this area must work. It must keep the cricoid ring open and, to do this on a permanent basis, it must adhere to the cartilaginous ends. It is unlikely that free bone or cartilage grafts, taken from ribs, can ever achieve this objective in a satisfactory and regulated manner. Furthermore, it is certain than allografts have no place.

Perhaps the best method is to swing down the body of the hyoid bone on a muscle pedicle of sternohyoid and hope that this, wired into the arch of the cricoid, can keep it open. When this is done, the soft tissue scarring must also be removed and replaced with a skin graft and a stent applied either in the form of rolled-up Silastic above a tracheostomy tube, or in a modified tracheostomy tube. If a Montgomery T-tube is used for this, then the greatest care must be taken to see that it does not crust.

For greater degrees of cricoid stenosis, where the ring cannot realistically be reconstituted, then it is best to remove the cricoid leaving part of the posterior lamina on which sit the arytenoids. The larynx is then dropped and the trachea pulled up and joined to the lower end of the thyroid lamina anteriorly and to the arch of the cricoid posteriorly. This tends to give something of a lump in the back of the immediate subglottic space, but it is a fairly reliable procedure and can usually allow the patient to be extubated.

Tracheal stenosis

The more minor degrees of tracheal stenosis are best treated with dilatations. Very often the problem is one of tracheomalacia, rather than true stenosis, and the true stenosis cannot be seen on endoscopy or X-ray. Very often these patients are frustrated by the lack of a medical diagnosis when they know full well that they are dyspnoeic on exertion. If they are only dyspnoeic on exertion, however, they must consider very carefully whether or not to have surgery just because an operation exists to excise that weak area of trachea. This operation will almost certainly damage one or both of the recurrent laryngeal nerves and result in further surgery for vocal cord paralysis.

Attempts to strengthen the tracheal wall with Marlex mesh or other external devices, although intuitively attractive, are not often successful.

If a tracheal stenosis is severe enough to warrant the wearing of a tracheostomy tube, then it is a relatively easy matter to excise up to 4–5 cm of trachea to drop the larynx and to join the trachea on the cricoid or first tracheal ring.

If this manoeuvre is not enough to close the gap of an extensive stenosis, then a procedure, described over 20 years ago by a Dr Grillo of Boston, can be utilized. In the UK, it is often called Barclay's procedure and consists of carrying out a right thoracotomy and removing the right mainstem bronchus from the carina, closing the hole at the carina and joining the right mainstem bronchus on the left mainstem bronchus at a lower level. This gives several more centimetres of length to the trachea and does not result in stenosis further down.

If localized stenosis occurs further down the trachea, then laser excision can be used.

Results

The results from supraglottic stenoses are usually good. It is usually possible to remove the tracheostomy tube and leave the patient with a reasonable voice. Similarly, the results from the treatment of glottic stenosis should also be good, and it should be a rare event for the patient to have a permanent tracheostomy.

The results of the treatment of subglottic stenosis, however, are universally poor. Although isolated claims are made by the occasional surgeon of remarkably good results in the treatment of this lesion, they cannot be reproduced consistently by experienced laryngologists of long-standing merit. The key to the subglottis is the cricoid, and it does

appear that we have not yet found a satisfactory solution to restoring the dynamic elastic forces necessary to preserve the integrity of the only complete ring in the respiratory tract.

Technique of operations for chronic laryngeal stenosis

Laryngeal widening operation

The patient will almost certainly have a tracheostomy; anaesthesia is continued via this route. The neck is opened with a horizontal collar incision and skin flaps elevated. The scarred strap muscles are retracted so that the thyroid cartilage and cricoid are seen. The larynx is opened in the midline up to the hyoid. The lumen is entered and the thickened scar tissue between the remaining mucosa and the thyroid cartilage is excised. This is done on the paraglottic space and also in the pre-epiglottic space.

Using 3/0 Vicryl sutures, multiple quilting sutures are put in place, pulling the remaining mucosa against the external skeleton of the larynx (Fig. 11.9).

The danger from this operation on the larynx is incompetence as a sphincter mechanism but, as sensation is usually preserved, the patient is not in as much risk from aspiration pneumonia as he or she may be from other lesions causing an incompetent larynx. There is no need to remove the sutures; revision procedures may be required at later dates.

Closure is in two layers and there is no need for internal stenting.

Tracheal resection and end-to-end anastomosis

The patient will almost certainly have a tracheostomy below the tracheal stenosis; anaesthesia is

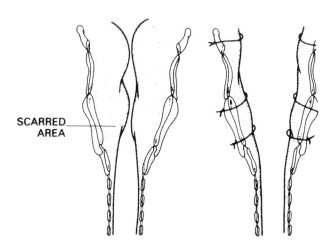

SCARRED AREA

Fig. 11.9 In the laryngeal-widening operation, a laryngofissure gives access to the laryngeal interior. The scarred submucosal tissue is removed and the mucosa quilted.

continued via this route (Fig. 11.10). A horizontal incision is made and skin flaps elevated to above the level of the hyoid and down to the suprasternal notch. The skin flaps are then held apart with a Joll's retractor. The larynx is freed as in a narrow-field laryngectomy and the entire hyoid is dissected free so that a finger can be placed behind the greater horn on each side. The posterior lamina of the thyroid cartilage is also freed so that a finger can be placed behind it.

Every attempt should be made to find the recurrent laryngeal nerves in the tracheo-oesophageal grooves, but this will probably not be possible in view of the injury that damaged the trachea.

It is important to find the normal trachea. Get under the pretracheal fascia and dissect on the tracheal wall down to the carina (Fig. 11.11). Although this operation is known as a tracheal pull-up operation, the pull-up is not as important as the laryngeal-drop part. The trachea acts as a concertina and, although it will apparently come well up into the neck, its normal tension will pull it back down into the thorax.

The most important part of this operation is thus to drop the larynx. This is done by cutting off the superior cornu of the thyroid cartilage on both sides, thus releasing the pull of the stylopharyngeus, salpingopharyngeus and palatopharyngeus muscles. The thyrohyoid membrane should be divided and the pre-epiglottic space entered. This allows the thyroid cartilage to be distracted from the hyoid. The middle constrictor should also be removed from the posterior lamina of the thyroid cartilage. There is enough slack in the soft tissue of the supraglottis on the interior part of the larynx to allow several centimetres of downward displacement.

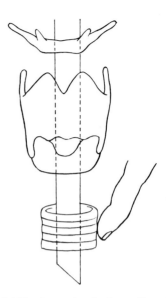

Fig. 11.11 Mobilize the trachea by finger dissection.

If the recurrent laryngeal nerves have not been found, or if it is strongly suspected that the nerve is divided on one side, then it is probably advisable to carry out a Woodman's operation on the affected side during this operation.

The trachea should be joined together or to the cricoid with 2/0 Vicryl sutures. It is important that these sutures do not enter the mucosa of the trachea. Place all the sutures before tying any, in order to distribute the tension correctly. Start trying on the posterior wall first and gradually come forward to the anterior part of the anastomosis (Fig. 11.12).

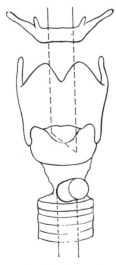

Fig. 11.10 If the anaesthetic is given via a tracheostomy, place an endotracheal tube into the upper trachea.

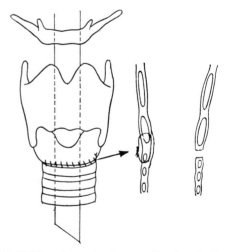

Fig. 11.12 When the trachea is sutured to the cricoid care must be taken to keep the sutures extramucosal.

It is probably better not to use a stent but to leave the tracheostomy tube in place for the immediate postoperative period. It should, however, be removed at the earliest opportunity.

Microtrapdoor flap repair

The CO_2 laser can be used to develop a microtrapdoor flap which preserves mucosa in the posterior glottis, subglottis and trachea. The stenotic scar is removed and following completion of the procedure the microtrapdoor flap can provide mucosal coverage to prevent recurrent stenosis. The flap requires to be thin enough to manipulate but not such that the blood supply is compromised. An alternative is to perform endoscopic radial laser incisions and dilation using both CO_2 and Nd:YAG lasers.

Cricoid expansion

If the stenosis involves the anterior glottis, as is commonly encountered in post-tracheostomy stenosis, then the hyoid bone can be used for grafting. A segment of the hyoid can be inserted as a free graft or as a pedicled flap. In the latter procedure the larynx and trachea are exposed through a midline vertical incision and the central part of the hyoid bone freed up as a pedicle attached to the sternohyoid muscle. The stenosed segment of the cricoid is wedged open by the pedicled flap whose attached soft tissues are sutured into place. This technique may not be adequate however for posterior subglottic or circumferential subglottic stenosis, when a tracheoplasty is indicated.

Tracheoplasty

Cartilage for grafting is obtained from the fifth or sixth costal cartilage together with its perichondrium attached. The cartilage is shaped into an anterior and a posterior graft. The posterior graft is T-shaped with phlanges which fit under the body of the cricoid cartilage. The anterior graft is spindle-shaped and bevelled towards the interior of the larynx to prevent interior displacement. The posterior cricoid lamina is split and an anterior incision is made from the midpoint of the thyroid notch down to the inferior margin of the first tracheal ring to receive the spindle-shaped wedge.

Controversies in management

How do you evaluate the results of surgery for trauma and stenosis?

The results of any procedure for these conditions can only be evaluated in terms of the difficulty the patient has in speaking or in breathing.

Speaking is such a complicated physiological manoeuvre that any scarring of the thyroarytenoid muscle, or any interference with the movement of the arytenoids, is unlikely to result in a normal voice. Most patients with laryngeal trauma that results in anything other than a little submuscosal bleeding will not recover a normal voice. The best they can hope for is the ability to phonate rather than to speak in a whisper.

The results with regard to breathing are easier to assess. If the patient does not require a permanent tracheostomy then the result is good; if he or she does require a permanent tracheostomy then the results of treatment have failed.

Is there any evidence to show that operating on an acute laryngeal trauma does any better than watching and waiting?

The authors have described a large series of acute injury and a large series of chronic laryngeal stenosis. From their results, it appears that by recognizing and treating the severe injuries early they have a 40% better chance of a good voice and three times less chance of having to wear a tracheostomy tube permanently.

Should a patient with chronic laryngeal stenosis be advised to have an operation?

A patient with chronic laryngeal stenosis and no tracheostomy is probably best advised to do without surgery if at all possible. This may result in a restriction of energetic activity but any surgery on a previously injured area can stimulate more scarred tissue and the patient may well end up with a tracheostomy that he or she did not have prior to surgery.

A patient with chronic laryngeal stenosis and a tracheostomy has little to lose from surgery. Because the surgery will be confined to the neck, there is a minimal mortality and about a 50% chance of patients being able to discard their tracheostomy tube.

If the chronic laryngeal stenosis is due to a systemic condition, such as Wegener's granuloma, lethal midline granuloma, postdiphtheritic scarring, perichondritis, scleroma, tuberculous scarring or amyloidosis, then the chance of permanent rehabilitation is small. Certainly there should be no surgery performed during the active phases of a Wegener's granuloma or scleroma.

How do you manage a patient with persistent re-stenosis?

A number of patients have aberrations of healing that result in the production of profuse amounts of scar tissue. One can operate on these patients, remove the scar tissue, and get an initial good result, but very often the surgeon takes one step forward only to go two steps back.

Patients who have persistent and increasing scarring are best advised not to have more surgery. Even laser excision seems to be ineffective in these patients, and the scarring is usually too advanced for any amount of steroid therapy.

References and further reading

Acute laryngeal trauma

Gussack G S, Jurkovich G J, Luterman A *et al.* (1986) Laryngotracheal trauma: a protocol approach to a rare injury. *Laryngoscope* **96**:660–5.

Harrison D F N (1984) Bullet wounds of the larynx and trachea. *Arch Otolaryngol* **110**:203–5.

Olson N R (1978) Surgical treatment of acute blunt laryngeal injuries. *Ann Otol Rhinol Laryngol* **87**:716–21.

Schaefer S D (1991) The treatment of acute external laryngeal injuries: 'state of the art'. *Arch Otolaryngol Head Neck Surg* **117**:35–40.

Schaefer S D, Brown O E (1983) Selective application of CT in the management of laryngeal trauma. *Laryngoscope* **93**:73–5.

Chronic laryngeal stenosis

Abedi E, Frable M A S (1983) Severe laryngeal stenosis repair: long-term follow-up using conjoint hyoid bone segments. *Laryngoscope* **93**:745–8.

Lusk R P, Gray S, Muntz H R (1991) Single-stage laryngotracheal reconstruction. *Arch Otolaryngol Head Neck Surg* **117**:171–3.

Schuller D E, Parrish R T (1988) Reconstruction of the larynx and trachea. *Arch Otolaryngol Head Neck Surg* **114**:278–86.

Simpson G T, Strong M S, Healy G B, Shapshay S M, Vaughan C W (1982) Predictive factors of success or failure in the endoscopic management of laryngeal and tracheal stenosis. *Ann Otol Rhinol Laryngol* **91**:384–8.

Strong M S, Healy G B, Vaughan C W, Fried M P,

Shapshay S (1979) Endoscopic management of laryngeal stenosis. *Otolaryngol Clin North Am* **12**:797–805.

Subglottic stenosis

Beste D J, Toohill R J (1991) Microtrapdoor flap repair of laryngeal and tracheal stenosis. *Ann Otol Rhinol Laryngol* **100**:420–3.

Cotton R T (1985) Prevention and management of laryngeal stenosis in infants and children. *J Pediatr Surg* **20**:845–51.

Cotton R T, Evans J N (1981) Laryngotracheal reconstruction in children. Five year follow-up. *Ann Otol Rhinol Laryngol* **90**:516–20.

Drake A F, Babyak J W, Niparko J K, Koopmann C F (1988) The anterior cricoid split: clinical experience with extended indications. *Arch Otolaryngol Head Neck Surg* **114**:1404–6.

Evans J N, Todd G B (1974) Laryngo-tracheoplasty. *J Laryngol Otol* **88**:589–97.

Freeland A P (1986) The long-term results of hyoid-sternohyoid grafts in the correction of subglottic stenosis. *J Laryngol Otol* **100**:665–74.

Friedman E M, Healy G B, McGill T J (1983) Carbon dioxide laser management of subglottic and tracheal stenosis. *Otolaryngol Clin North Am* **16**:871–7.

Grillo H C, Mathisen D J (1988) Surgical management of tracheal strictures. *Surg Clin North Am* **68**:511–24.

Healy G B (1982) An experimental model for endoscopic correction of subglottic stenosis with clinical applications. *Laryngoscope* **92**:1103–15.

McCaffrey T V (1991) Management of subglottic stenosis in the adult. *Ann Otol Rhinol Laryngol* **100**:90–4.

Muntz H R, Lusk R P (1990) A comparison of the cartilaginous nib graft and Evans-Todd laryngotracheoplasties for subglottic stenosis. *Laryngoscope* **100**:415–16.

Rita L, Seleny F, Holinger L D (1983) Anesthetic management and gas scavenging for laser surgery of infant subglottic stenosis. *Anesthesiology* **58**:191–3.

Shapshay S M, Beamis J F, Hybels R L, Bohigian R K (1987) Endoscopic treatment of subglottic and tracheal stenosis by radial laser incision and dilation. *Ann Otol Rhinol Laryngol* **96**:661–4.

Stolovitzky J P, Todd N W (1990) Autoimmune hypothesis of acquired subglottic stenosis in premature infants. *Laryngoscope* **100**:227–30.

12

Tumours of the hypopharynx

Surgical anatomy

The hypopharynx is divided into three sites: the posterior pharyngeal wall, the pyriform sinus and the postcricoid space.

The International Union against Cancer (UICC) and American Joint Committee (AJC) definition of these sites is shown in Table 12.1. One criticism of this definition is that the lateral limits of the posterior pharyngeal wall where it merges with the pyriform sinus are not defined. A useful working rule is to extend a line from the vocal cords in the cadaveric position backwards until they meet the posterior pharyngeal wall. This point can be regarded as the junction between the posterior pharyngeal wall and the pyriform sinus.

Surgical Pathology

Squamous carcinoma

The overall site incidence varies a little in different series according to the interests of the author, but there seems little doubt that tumours on the posterior wall of the hypopharynx are the least common variant, forming approximately one-tenth of all these

Table 12.1 The International Union against Cancer (UICC) and American Joint Committee (AJC) definitions of sites in the hypopharynx

1 Pharyngo-oesophageal junction (postcricoid area): extends from the level of the arytenoid cartilages and connecting folds to the inferior border of the cricoid cartilage
2 Pyriform sinus: extends from the pharyngoepiglottic fold to the upper end of the oesophagus. It is bounded laterally by the thyroid cartilage and medially by the surface of the aryepiglottic fold and the arytenoid and cricoid cartilages
3 Posterior pharyngeal wall: extends from the level of the floor of the vallecula to the level of the cricoarytenoid joints

tumours. The most common tumour is that of the pyriform fossa, which forms between half and two-thirds of the total; postcricoid tumours make up the remaining 40% or so. Almost all carcinomas of the hypopharynx are squamous cell in type.

Thus tumours of the pyriform fossa or sinus form the largest group of hypopharyngeal tumours. They can be divided into those primarily involving the lateral wall, or those primarily involving the medial wall, although when first seen these tumours are often extensive and there is then no practical value in subdividing them.

Tumours arising on the medial wall extend through the aryepiglottic fold to invade the paraglottic space. They thus fix the glottis on the same side. They also usually extend to the pre-epiglottic space and occasionally backwards into the postcricoid area.

Tumours arising laterally extend through the thyroid cartilage and through the thyrohyoid membrane producing a palpable mass, which should be differentiated from a lymph node by its movement on deglutition. Invasion in this direction often involves the carotid sheath and the thyroid gland in about 1 patient in 4.

Any large tumour in the pyriform fossa can extend superiorly across the pharyngoepiglottic ligament into the base of the tongue, often infiltrating beneath the mucosa (Fig. 12.1); this figure also shows other routes of spread.

Approximately 3 patients in 4 have a palpable lymph node in the neck, usually affecting the upper deep cervical group; 5% have bilaterally enlarged lymph glands (Fig. 12.2).

Tumours of the postcricoid space are the next most common hypopharyngeal tumour.

When first seen these tumours are seldom confined to the postcricoid space and extension down the cervical oesophagus to a greater or lesser extent is the rule. As in oesophageal tumours, submucosal extension is important and measures 10 mm on average. When first seen, 1 patient in 5 with this disease has an enlarged gland in the neck, virtually

161

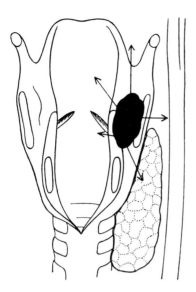

Fig. 12.1 Routes of spread of tumours of the pyriform fossa.

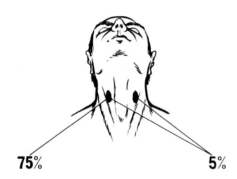

75%   **5%**

Fig. 12.2 Lymph node metastases in carcinoma of the pyriform fossa.

always of the upper deep cervical group; 1 patient in 20 has bilateral nodes (Fig. 12.3).

About 1 patient in 6 with this disease will also develop an involved lymph node in the mediastinum involving the paratracheal chain of nodes. Extension also obviously occurs readily in an anterior direction to involve the party wall between the oesphagus and trachea, and laterally to involve the thyroid gland.

About 10% of patients with a postcricoid carcinoma have an immobile vocal cord. The causes of this include invasion of the tumour out of the pharynx into the tracheo-oesophageal groove, invasion of the cricoarytenoid joint and, very rarely, extension of the tumour into the larynx itself.

Tumours of the cervical oesophagus behave in

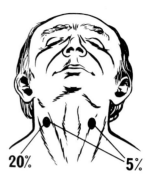

20%   **5%**

Fig. 12.3 Incidence of cervical nodes in postcricoid carcinoma.

exactly the same way as postcricoid tumours, and indeed it is very often impossible to tell whether a tumour arose primarily in the postcricoid space or in the cervical oesophagus. In the remainder of this discussion the term 'postcricoid carcinoma' will be used to include tumours of the cervical oesophagus because their management follows the same principles.

Carcinomas of the posterior hypopharyngeal wall are usually symmetrical, and are exophytic in nature rather than infiltrative. They do not usually invade anteriorly into the larynx and their lower limit is usually just above the arytenoid cartilages. About half these patients have a palpable lymph node in the neck, usually involving the upper deep cervical chain, and 5% of patients with this disease have bilaterally enlarged glands in the neck.

The UICC and AJC definition of the T stage is shown in Table 12.2. Unfortunately this staging has been drawn up without reference to reality. This is particularly true of postcricoid tumours, in which the most important prognostic factors are the vertical length of the tumour and the presence or absence of vocal cord paralysis. A much more realistic staging system for tumours of the postcricoid space would be that which is used by the AJC for tumours of the cervical oesophagus, based on the length of the tumour. The system proposed by the UICC for the cervical oesophagus is completely impracticable and indeed incomprehensible.

Table 12.2 The UICC and AJC definition of the T stage

T_1 Tumour limited to one subsite of hypopharynx
T_2 Tumour invades more than one subsite of hypopharynx or an adjacent site, *without* fixation of hemilarynx
T_3 Tumour invades more than one subsite of hypopharynx or an adjacent site, *with* fixation of hemilarynx
T_4 Tumour invades adjacent structure, e.g. cartilage or soft tissues of neck

Rare tumours

Benign

Leiomyomas are probably the commonest benign mesenchymal tumour of the hypopharynx and upper oesophagus, although they usually affect the lower third of the oesophagus. These tumours are more common in men than in women, with an estimated ratio of 2 : 1, and have a maximum incidence in the third, fourth and fifth decades. They are usually rubbery and firm in consistency and, when small, present as an intramural swelling. As they grow, however, they tend to be dragged down into the oesophagus by the normal process of swallowing and then form a polypoid swelling, which may reach considerable size. These tumours can usually be removed by dividing their pedicle through a pharyngotomy or oesophagotomy.

Lipomas and fibrolipomas occur occasionally in the hypopharynx but present a well-defined clinical entity. They are virtually always polypoidal and can arise from any site in the pharynx or upper oesophagus. They tend to be dragged downwards by the normal process of swallowing and thus can form a large pedunculated mass hanging down the oesophagus. A typical presenting symptom is dysphagia, although they may produce choking sensations, and if the tumour is extravasated upwards it can fall into the larynx and cause dyspnoea. These tumours have a very small pedicle and, as they are not malignant, can often be removed endoscopically using a snare to divide the pedicle. If there is any difficulty in this manoeuvre they can be removed through a lateral pharyngotomy.

Malignant

Leiomyosarcoma is the malignant variant of the leiomyoma. It also usually presents as a polypoid swelling hanging down the oesophagus by a pedicle, arising in the region of the arytenoid. The presenting symptoms are usually dysphagia or a feeling of choking. This tumour is usually completely radioresistant, but is not aggressively malignant and often responds well to removal, with an area of normal mucosa surrounding its pedicle, through a lateral pharyngotomy.

The carcinosarcoma, which may also occasionally be called pseudosarcoma or a spindle cell carcinoma, is a polypoid tumour occurring predominantly in men. It occurs in the elderly, being seldom recorded before the age of 45. Histologically, the stroma consists of spindle cells; scattered through this stroma or on its surface are small islands of squamous carcinoma. There is considerable controversy as to the importance and origin of the stromal element: some think that it is a reaction to the squamous carcinoma, others think that it is a true sarcoma. Whatever the truth, and despite its histologically bizarre appearance, this sarcomatous element is relatively unimportant, and metastases bearing a resemblance to this part of the tumour do not occur. Indeed, distant metastases from this type of tumour occur uncommonly. They are slowly growing tumours that are relatively benign, but late in the disease the squamous element metastasizes to the lymph nodes in the neck in approximately half of these patients.

These tumours usually arise in the region of the pyriform fossa or from the mouth of the oesophagus, are always polypoidal and are usually radioresistant. They should be treated surgically but not radically – removal of the tumour, its pedicle and an area of surrounding normal mucosa is usually all that is needed.

Investigations

History

Ask particularly about difficulty in swallowing foods, hoarseness, sore throat and pain in the ears. The clinical picture caused by a large tumour is usually unmistakable, but in the early stages the symptoms may be indefinite. Whilst a feeling of a lump in the throat, which is worse on swallowing saliva, is rarely of serious significance, vague symptoms, such as a feeling of a crumb in the throat or of persistent sore throat should be treated with suspicion. As it is impossible to examine the postcricoid space by indirect laryngoscopy, all patients with persistent throat symptoms, however non-specific, should have a barium swallow and an oesophagoscopy. This will inevitably mean that a lot of endoscopies are done with normal findings. The proportion of endoscopies with positive findings should be small, however. If every oesophagoscopy shows a tumour not enough are being done.

Ask also about the general health, but particularly about weight loss and chest symptoms, due to overspill.

A few patients with hypopharyngeal carcinoma have a history of the Paterson–Brown Kelly syndrome (anaemia, either microcytic or macrocytic, glossitis, oesophageal web, splenomegaly, koilonychia, achlorhydria). Some also have a history of irradiation to the neck, usually for thyrotoxicosis, with a long latent interval of 25–30 years. These two conditions should be asked about, as they can influence the subsequent treatment.

Examination

Carry out a routine head and neck and general examination. When examining the pharynx and larynx pay particular attention not only to obvious ulceration, but also to pooling in the pyriform fossa, and oedema of the arytenoids. Pooling in the pyriform fossa indicates failure of passage of secretions down the oesophagus, whereas oedema of the arytenoids may be the only obvious evidence on indirect laryngoscopy of a tumour either of the medial wall of the pyriform fossa or of the postcricoid space.

Also, while examining the larynx, look for paralysis of one or both vocal cords, and for direct extension of a tumour of the pyriform fossa through the aryepiglottic fold into the supraglottic area.

When feeling the neck pay particular attention to a mass close to the larynx. This may be an enlarged lymph node, or it may be a direct extension of the tumour through the thyrohyoid membrane. In the latter case the mass moves on swallowing.

In addition to the history and clinical examination of these patients, valuable information is obtained from radiology, endoscopy and biopsy, and from certain haematological investigations.

Radiology

A plain X-ray film of the soft tissues of the neck often gives much useful information in these patients. A tumour on the posterior pharyngeal wall is usually well-outlined on plain films: in postcricoid tumours there is widening of the space between the trachea and vertebral column: in tumours of the pyriform fossa destruction of the thyroid cartilage may be seen.

A barium swallow usually defines these tumours accurately. It is, however, well-known that tumours of the cervical oesophagus and postcricoid space may not be demonstrated by this technique, and investigation of a patient with dysphagia must always include oesophagoscopy. If the tumour is demonstrated by a barium swallow, the information obtained is of great value, as the lower limit of the tumour is usually well-seen; this is usually difficult or impossible to access by endoscopy because of the bulk of the tumour.

A chest radiograph should be obtained, as in all patients with head and neck cancer. Many of these patients, because of their pharyngeal and oesophageal obstruction, have spill-over of food and saliva into the trachea causing pulmonary infection. This often resembles secondary deposits.

A computed tomography scan can add a little to the investigation of these patients, notably in demonstrating the lower limit of a postcricoid tumour, the presence of mediastinal and cervical nodes, and any extraoesophageal extension at the thoracic outlet.

Endoscopy

Examination of these patients under anaesthetic is mandatory: firstly, to allow examination of the larynx, pharynx, trachea and oesophagus; secondly, to allow palpation of the pharynx; and thirdly, to obtain a biopsy specimen.

When examining a patient with one of these tumours under anaesthetic the following points are of importance. In a patient with a tumour of the posterior pharyngeal wall it is particularly important to assess the lower and lateral limits of the tumour as encroachment below the level of the arytenoid cartilages or laterally into the pyriform fossa indicates that a total pharyngolaryngectomy will be required. Also in such patients assess the mobility of the posterior pharyngeal wall on the prevertebral fascia by palpation.

Whilst examining a patient with a tumour in the pyriform fossa the main point is to establish whether the tumour can be removed leaving enough normal pharyngeal mucosa to close the pharyngeal defect. Thus not only should the exact extent of the tumour be assessed, including the presence of invasion of the larynx, but particular care should be paid to the area close to the oesophageal mouth posterior to the arytenoid cartilages. Extension beyond this point usually indicates that a total pharyngolaryngectomy will be required, because removal of the tumour at this point will necessitate removal of the entire pharyngeal lumen. At the same time, feel for extension into the base of the tongue, which is often more easily felt than seen.

Finally, in patients with a tumour in the postcricoid space or cervical oesophagus, accurate assessment by endoscopy is often difficult. Thus, while it is easy to see the top end of the tumour, it is often difficult, and frequently impossible, to pass an oesophagoscope through the tumour to assess its lower limit. This difficulty can often be overcome by dilating the tumour with bougies. A filiform bougie is left in the oesophageal lumen and it is then usually possible to pass the narrowest bronchoscope over this down the oesophagus. It is essential to examine the posterior wall of the trachea with a bronchoscope to exclude invasion of the party wall between the trachea and the oesophagus. Whilst the patient is under anaesthetic try moving the oesophagus and pharynx over the prevertebral fascia to detect any degree of fixation.

Laboratory investigations

In all patients with hypopharyngeal cancer, haematological investigation is extremely important. Many of these patients, particularly if they previously have suffered from the Paterson–Brown Kelly syndrome, are anaemic; about a third of them are deficient in electrolytes, particularly potassium; and most of them have a deficiency of the serum proteins. It is extremely important that these deficiencies should be assessed before operation and if possible made good before treatment, and certainly as soon after as possible.

Treatment policy

Twenty-five per cent of patients with a carcinoma of the hypopharynx are untreatable when they are first seen. The most important causes of untreatability are advanced age, poor general condition, an inoperable local tumour or massive neck nodes. Distant metastases are also, of course, a contraindication, but a much less common one.

Advanced age and general condition are difficult to define, but patients over the age of 75, or those with some generalized disease that has rendered them incapable of working or running a household, should not be offered surgery, both because of its morbidity and because of the rather poor chances of long-term survival. Tumours of the pyriform fossa extending into the base of the tongue are rarely cured by surgery. A postcricoid tumour fixed to the prevertebral fascia is obviously inoperable but this is a very uncommon event. A more common event indicating inoperability is a vocal cord paralysis. If this is due to extension of the tumour outside the oesophagus to invade the recurrent laryngeal nerve in the tracheo-oesophageal groove it will be found to be irremovable.

Patients with massive (fixed) nodes are very rarely cured of their disease. It used to be thought that bilateral neck nodes indicated incurability. More careful studies, however, have shown that this is not true if the nodes are small on both sides of the neck, that is less than 3 cm in diameter. Bilateral nodes larger than this, or multiple bilateral nodes, do indeed indicate incurability.

The long-term results for treatment either by surgery or by radiotherapy are not good. A small proportion of postcricoid tumours can be treated successfully with irradiation, producing a 5-year survival rate of about 30%, provided that certain criteria are rigidly observed. These are that the vertical length of the tumour must not exceed 5 cm; the vocal cords must not be immobile; and there must be no palpable nodes in the neck. If the tumour does not fulfil any one of these three criteria, the patient should be submitted to surgery. A patient who undergoes radiotherapy and who suffers a recurrence should also be considered for surgery. One of the great difficulties in this disease is a patient who has been irradiated and who has ulceration of the postcriciod space, but a biopsy does not show tumour. In the authors' experience virtually all of these patients die if they are not treated, and postmortem examination does indeed show a recurrent tumour. The presence of ulceration in the postcricoid space after radiotherapy therefore must be assumed to represent recurrent disease irrespective of the biopsy findings, and the appropriate action should be taken.

Because the pyriform fossa is a distensible space, tumours in this area are almost always large before they produce symptoms, and although the space is poor in sensory nerves, it is rich in lymphatics so that tumours in this are not only large when they first present, but they are also usually associated with enlarged lymph nodes. Therefore, most of these patients do not do well with radiotherapy, and surgery should be advised as the primary form of treatment. In most patients it is possible to resect the involved part of the pharynx, together with the larynx, preserving enough pharyngeal mucosa to repair the pharyngeal defect by first intention. In 1 patient in 3, however, where there is extension of the tumour behind the arytenoid cartilages into the oesophageal mouth, it is necessary to remove the entire pharynx, which then must be reconstructed by one of the types of skin repair to be described later. As these tumours do not extend for any appreciable distance down the oesophagus, reconstitution with a viscus is not required. Tumours in the pyriform fossa have also sometimes been managed by a supraglottic laryngectomy preserving the cords. In the authors' experience, the size of these tumours, at least as they present in UK, is such that partial surgery is not to be contemplated.

Tumours on the posterior pharyngeal wall do well with a resection through a lateral pharyngotomy, preserving the larynx. This operation is only feasible if the larynx is completely uninvolved, and if there is no extension of the tumour below the level of the arytenoid cartilages. However, if the larynx is involved, or if the tumour extends laterally into the pyriform fossa, or inferior to the arytenoid cartilages, this operation cannot be done, and a total pharyngolaryngectomy must be performed, followed by repair of the pharynx.

It has already been indicated above that two-thirds of patients with a pyriform fossa tumour only require a partial pharyngectomy (with total laryngectomy) and that some tumours on the posterior pharyngeal wall can also be treated by partial pharyngectomy. The mainstay of surgical treatment, is however, total pharyngolaryngectomy, which must on occasion be combined with total oesophagectomy. An operation restricted to the neck, that is total pharyngolaryngectomy, is indicated for tumours of the pyriform fossa extending into the postcricoid space, *small* postcricoid tumours, and tumours arising in the pharyngeal remnant after total laryngectomy carried out for laryngeal carcinoma many years previously. However, a total pharyngolaryngo-oesophagectomy is required for extensive postcricoid tumours and for tumours arising primarily in the cervical oesophagus. It is often safer also to do this operation for patients who suffer a recurrence after the treatment of a postcricoid tumour by irradiation or for those who have an irradiation-induced tumour. The reason for this is that in the latter two circumstances the most satisfactory and safest method of replacing the pharynx is by a gastric transposition. On occasion, total pharyngolaryngo-oesophagectomy is also required for invasion of the pharynx or upper oesophagus by tumours of the neighbouring organs, mainly the thyroid gland.

Total pharyngolaryngectomy with or without oesophagectomy carries the problem of replacement of the pharynx. Earlier techniques such as those using cervical skin flaps, or that using the deltopectoral flap, although they made great contributions to the surgery of this area in decades past, have now been abandoned. There are now two techniques in common use for replacement of the pharynx in the patient who has undergone a total pharyngolaryngectomy preserving the thoracic oesophagus. These are the use of the pectoralis major musculocutaneous flap, and the use of jejunal loop. If the oesophagus is removed in addition, two techniques are available for replacing it, and these are gastric or colonic transposition. The latter is less popular and will not be described here because the authors have little experience of this technique.

Radical neck dissection

This operation will often be needed since the hallmark of pyriform fossa tumours is their high incidence of lymph node involvement. In patients with a tumour on the posterior pharyngeal wall, if lymph nodes are palpable on one or both sides of the neck, do a unilateral or bilateral neck dissection. The experience of all surgeons in this uncommon tumour is so limited that it is impossible to be dogmatic about the place of prophylactic neck dissection.

In the minority of patients with pyriform fossa tumour with no palpable nodes in the neck, a functional neck dissection is indicated because of the high incidence of occult nodes in this situation.

Technique and complications of operations on the hypopharynx

Partial pharyngectomy and total laryngectomy

Mobilization of the pharynx and larynx

Mobilize the larynx and pharynx as described under the technique of total laryngectomy by dissection medial to the sternomastoid muscles and the carotid sheath; preserve the lobe of the thyroid gland on the non-involved side.

Removal of tumour

The subsequent operation is made much easier if the tracheostome is made before removing the tumour; do this as in total laryngectomy.

To remove the tumour enter the pharynx through the vallecula and divide the pharyngeal mucosa from side to side immediately above the hyoid bone externally, and immediately anterior to the epiglottis internally. At this point do not enter the pre-epiglottic space. Be careful to take a sufficiently wide margin round the superior edge of the tumour and excise widely into the base of the tongue if necessary. In order to obtain maximum exposure of the tumour, divide the lateral pharyngeal wall on the non-involved side, carrying the incision down through the opposite pyriform fossa immediately posterior to the superior cornu of the thyroid cartilage; take great care at this point to preserve as much pharyngeal mucosa as possible. Rotate the larynx laterally, with a hook round the posterior edge of the thyroid lamina, so that the tumour in the pyriform fossa can now be readily seen – carry the incision round it, down the posterior pharyngeal wall, with a margin of at least 2 cm of normal pharyngeal mucosa. Externally make the incision posterior to the superior cornu of the thyroid cartilage. Finally join the incisions across the anterior oesophageal wall immediately posterior to the arytenoid cartilages, provided this area is not involved by tumour, taking care to preserve continuity of the oesophageal lumen. Remove the specimen, in continuity with the radical neck dissection, by dividing the few fibres remaining which attach the trachea to the oesophagus.

Repair

Close the pharyngeal mucosa in a vertical line in three layers as described under the technique of total laryngectomy. Finally close the skin with suction drainage in the usual way.

Complications

1 *General complications.*
2 *Stricture formation* is more common after this operation than after total laryngectomy for laryngeal cancer because the pharyngeal remnant is much smaller. A common site is at the upper end of the pharyngeal repair, where it meets the base of the tongue. This will usually respond to a few dilatations at monthly intervals but if not it will be necessary to carry out a skin reconstruction of the pharynx.
3 *Recurrence* in the pharynx should be managed, if the tumour is still operable, by total pharyngectomy followed by repair with a jejunal loop.

Total pharyngolaryngectomy

As already outlined, this operation is required for patients with carcinoma of the pyriform fossa or of the posterior pharyngeal wall extending to the mouth of the oesophagus, and for smaller postcricoid tumours and neck nodes that are not suitable for radiotherapy.

Resection

The technique is similar to that of a laryngectomy. Make the incisions and elevate the flaps. Carry out a radical neck dissection, if necessary, leaving it attached by a large pedicle including the superior and inferior laryngeal neurovascular bundles.

Mobilize the larynx and pharynx by dissection medial to the carotid sheath on each side. Divide the superior thyroid artery and vein on each side, and the inferior thyroid artery on the side of the tumour. Both lobes of the thyroid gland must be removed in continuity in postcricoid tumours, but in pyriform fossa tumours it is usually justifiable to preserve one lobe of the thyroid gland.

After warning the anaesthetist, divide the trachea at the level of the fourth ring, bring out the distal segment through the hole in the skin flap and fashion the permanent stoma.

Now palpate the upper end of the oesophagus to feel the lower end of the tumour. Three centimetres below this point place a stay suture of 2/0 black silk through the oesophageal wall, and divide the oesophagus immediately above it, bevelling the line of section to increase the area of the oesophageal opening. Finally divide the pharynx across its entire lumen at the level of the hyoid bone.

Wash the wound, secure haemostasis and change gowns and gloves.

Repair of the pharynx

Two methods are in current use for repairing the pharynx in this situation – the pectoralis major flap or a jejunal loop. The loop is almost certainly the better in terms of morbidity because stricture formation after its use is very uncommon, whereas it occurs in about 20% of patients who have a skin flap repair.

If you have elected to use a pectoralis major flap, raise this once the excision is complete. The skin island should have a vertical length at least equal to that between the oesophageal stump and the base of the tongue, and the flap should be at least 7.5 cm wide. Raise the flap in the usual way and pass it up beneath the skin of the upper chest into the neck so that the skin island comes to face inwards. Turn the skin island into a tube and anastomose its upper end to the cut surface of the oropharynx, and the lower end of the oesophageal stump. Close the lateral seam similarly in two layers using a suture material, such as

Dexon, that is not absorbed for a period of several weeks. Use 3/0 chromic catgut on a cutting needle for the subcutaneous layers. This procedure restores pharyngeal continuity in one stage.

A repair with jejunal loop is to be preferred. Take a jejunal loop as described in Chapter 4 and reanastomose its artery and vein in the neck. The artery can usually be anastomosed end-to-end on to the superior thyroid artery or the facial artery but, if necessary, it can be anastomosed end-to-side on to the external carotid artery. Better results are probably obtained by putting a large bulldog type of clamp round the origin of the external carotid artery during the anastomosis rather than placing an arterial clamp across the smaller branch that is actually to be anastomosed. This step produces less damage to the intima of the smaller vessels. If a radical neck dissection has not been carried out, the vein is most conveniently anastomosed end-to-side to the internal jugular vein. However, if the neck had been dissected, it will usually be necessary to use an interpositional graft from the jejunal vein to a vein low in the neck, such as to the stump of the internal jugular vein or to the anterior jugular vein on the opposite side. The external jugular vein is suitable material for this interpositional graft. Once the vascular anastomoses are complete, anastomose the jejunal loop above and below to the oropharyngeal and oesophageal stumps using 2/0 or 3/0 chromic catgut for the outer layer and a running suture of Dexon (or similar material) for the inner layer. It may be difficult to make an end-to-end anastomosis above because of the disparity of size between the jejunum and the oropharynx. In this case, leave the upper end of the jejunal loop closed, make a long incision in the antimesenteric border of the upper end of the loop and anastomose this to the base of the tongue. The loop should be under slight tension to avoid a redundant loop, which causes dysphagia.

Only about 5% of these patients develop satisfactory oesophageal speech. The remainder require some type of electronic vibrator. Experience so far has shown that the tracheopharyngeal shunts are not usually effective after this procedure.

Complications

1 *General complications.*
2 *Fistulae* can occur after this operation but are generally small and virtually always close spontaneously.
3 *Stricture formation* occurs in about 20% of patients undergoing skin flap repair, but is very unusual in patients having jejunal loop repair. Periodic dilatation may be required, but if it is required too frequently it is worthwhile training the patient to dilate the oesophagus with a Hurst mercury bougie.
4 *Flap necrosis.* Between 5 and 10% of free flaps fail

due to occlusion of either the arterial or venous anastomosis. Unfortunately a flap in this situation is difficult to monitor, and also it may be difficult to see the flap with ordinary routine indirect laryngoscopy. Occasionally it may be appreciated that the flap is congested within the first 24 h after operation, and in that case the anastomoses should be re-explored. On occasion this will save the day. More commonly, flap failure is detected by established necrosis. In this circumstance the necrosed flap should be removed. Subsequent management of these cases is difficult: probably the best solution is to leave the neck widely open, and when it is cleaned to replace the pharynx by gastric transposition. Alternatively, an attempt may be made to reconstruct the pharynx in stages with a pectoralis major flap covered by a deltopectoral flap, but this is less successful.

Total pharyngolaryngo-osteophagectomy and replacement with the transposed stomach

The technique, briefly, consists of resection of the pharynx, larynx and oesophagus; the oesophagus and pharynx are then replaced by the stomach, which is mobilized through an abdominal incision, and is drawn up through the oesophageal bed, in the posterior mediastinum, and anastomosed to the pharynx.

Anaesthetic and preparation

Use a general endotracheal anaesthetic as already described.

Clean and towel the patient from the chin above to the umbilicus below.

Neck incision

The patient will often have been irradiated, so use two horizontal incisions. Mobilize the pharynx and larynx in the ususal way, including all of the thyroid gland on the specimen; carry out a radical neck dissection on one or both sides if indicated. Do not remove the specimen at this stage.

Abdominal incision

The stomach and oesophagus can be mobilized through a left thoracoabdominal incision, which gives good access to the fundus of the stomach but the thoracotomy adds to the morbidity of the operation. Also, because the patient is lying on the side during the thoracoabdominal operation, the neck part of the procedure must be carried out after the chest has been closed and the patient turned on his or her back. A left upper paramedian incision is, therefore, preferable: besides reducing the morbi-

dity this allows the pharynx and larynx to be mobilized at the same time as the stomach.

Make a left paramedian incision extended well up on the rib margin and open the peritoneal cavity. The stomach is most easily mobilized by working from above downwards so that the abdominal oesophagus must first be exposed. To achieve this, divide the left triangular ligament of the liver to mobilize the left lobe of the liver, and retract the latter to the right until the abdominal oesophagus is clearly seen (Fig. 12.4). Mobilize the abdominal oesophagus by blunt dissection and retract it with a tape. This clearly displays the gastrosplenic ligament with the vasa brevia on the left side, and the lesser omentum with the oesophageal branches of the left gastric artery on the right side. Now divide the gastrosplenic ligament (Fig. 12.5) with the vasa brevia, and tie the vessels. Divide the greater omentum away from the stomach, preserving the marginal vessel orginating from the right gastroepiploic artery (Fig. 12.6). As the omentum is divided, stitch the omental vessels on the stomach side to prevent the suture being pulled off as

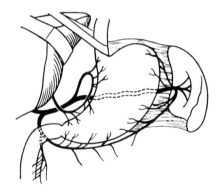

Fig. 12.4 Left triangular ligament of liver divided, and left lobe retracted to show abdominal oesophagus.

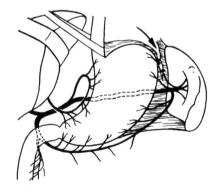

Fig. 12.5 Upper end of gastrosplenic omentum divided.

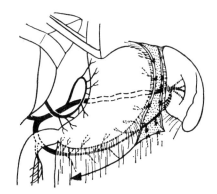

Fig. 12.6 Greater omentum divided.

the stomach is later drawn up through the mediastinum. Continue mobilization down to the first inch of the first part of the duodenum and mobilize the second part of the duodenum by Kocher's manoeuvre.

Now divide the lesser omentum and divide and transfix the left gastric artery; an anomalous hepatic artery may arise from the left gastric artery – look for it before dividing the vessel.

Now do a pyloromyotomy by invaginating the pylorus between finger and thumb, rupturing its fibres. This allows adequate drainage of the stomach – a formal pyloroplasty is usually unnecessary.

The stomach is now fully mobile. Next mobilize the oesophagus by passing the hand up through the hiatus, and dissecting carefully with the finger in the plane next to the oesophageal wall; rupture the fibres of the vagus nerve whilst doing this by digital dissection (Fig. 12.7).

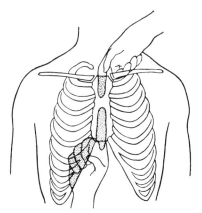

Fig. 12.7 Digital mobilization of entire oesophagus.

At the same time mobilize the oesophagus from above through the neck incision. Take great care while doing this, again by keeping strictly next to the oesophagus. The posterior wall of the trachea, in particular, must be carefully preserved during this manoeuvre, and it is important during this part of the operation to deflate the cuff of the anaesthetist's endotracheal tube to avoid stretching of, and damage to, the tracheal wall.

Once the oesophagus has been mobilized, introduce a long rubber tube drain into the mediastinum through the hiatus. Do this before the stomach is drawn up into the chest, because it is difficult to place the drain afterwards. Bring this drain out through a stab wound on the left flank.

By traction on the pharynx and oesophagus above, draw the stomach up into the mediastinum to lie in the oesophageal bed, at the same time also guiding it from below. The bulk of the stomach acts as a plug to stop any bleeding vessels in the mediastinum, so that there is little bleeding. Now close the abdominal incision with deep tension sutures.

The fundus of the stomach will now be lying in the neck. Divide the oesophagus at the oesophageal opening into the stomach and close it. Remove the pharynx, larynx and entire oesophagus. Fashion the tracheostomy at this stage.

After washing the wound and changing gowns and gloves make a separate horizontal incision in the fundus of the stomach and fashion a pharyngogastric anastomosis using two layers of interrupted sutures of 2/0 black silk. Make the outer posterior layer first, then the inner, next the inner anterior layer, and finally the outer anterior layer. Close the skin incision with suction drainage in the customary fashion.

Postoperative care

1 *General care.*
2 *Radiography.* A chest radiograph is taken immediately after the operation to exclude pneumothorax.
3 *Feeding.* These patients have an ileus lasting about 4 days so that full tube feeding cannot be started for 5 or 6 days. Because of this and because of their poor general condition feed them intravenously (See Chapter 3). Start tube feeds when bowel sounds return, and if the neck wound has healed, start feeding by mouth after 1 week.
4 *Sutures.* Abdominal tension sutures are removed after 2 weeks.
5 *Drains.* Abdominal drain – continue suction drainage on this until it is dry, and remove it, usually after about 5 days.
6 *Thyroid and parathyroid replacement.*
7 *Speech therapy.* These patients rarely develop oesophageal speech and should be given the opportunity of developing valve speech. The insertion of a valve presents no special difficulty and hypertonicity is never a problem.

Complications

1 *General complications.*
2 *Pneumothorax.* A chest radiograph should, therefore, be taken immediately at the end of the operation; if a pneumothorax is present, introduce an underwater drain into the pleural cavity.
3 *Bleeding.* It might be expected that as the oesophagus is mobilized by blind dissection, which does not allow bleeding points to be found and tied, excessive bleeding might take place after this operation. This does not appear to be so, probably because the torn vessels retract and are plugged by the bulk of the stomach lying in the posterior mediastinum.

   Haematoma formation in the mediastinum should be prevented, however, by use of a long suction drain passing through the stomach bed, through the hiatus and into the mediastinum.
4 *Fistula.* Occasionally a small fistula forms which heals spontaneously but, in view of the high vascularity of the stomach, large areas of necrotic breakdown causing large fistulae are not seen after this operation. Strictures do not occur.
5 *Regurgitation.* Most of these patients swallow well, but a few suffer regurgitation due to minor hold-up at the pylorus. This can be overcome by instructing the patient to eat small meals every 2 h, taking the food slowly. Regurgitation of acid does not occur because of the vagotomy which, of necessity, is undertaken during dissection of the oesophagus.

Lateral pharyngotomy for tumours of the posterior pharyngeal wall

Because of their size and frequent association with an enlarged lymph node, tumours on the posterior pharyngeal wall often do not do well with radiotherapy. This method of treatment has often been preferred in the past, however, because the only surgical treatment in common use was resection of the pharynx and larynx. However, if the tumour has not extended below the arytenoid cartilage into the cervical oesophagus, or laterally into the pyriform fossa, these tumours can be resected through a lateral pharyngotomy, so preserving the larynx.

For the very occasional tumour of the posterior pharyngeal wall with extension into the pyriform fossa or downwards into the oesophagus, a total pharyngolaryngectomy will be required with reconstruction of the pharynx, as described earlier in this chapter.

Anaesthesia

General endotracheal anaesthesia is induced and the patient's neck skin cleaned and towelled. Make a tracheostomy through a small vertical incision, sited so that it will not interfere with the proposed skin incision. Put a cuffed tube through the tracheostomy and continue general anaesthesia through this. Then clean the patient's skin again and replace the towels, excluding the tracheostomy from the operation field by stitching the towels to the skin.

Incision

The skin incision varies, depending on whether a radical neck dissection is to be done and whether the patient has previously been irradiated. In the non-irradiated patient, if a radical neck dissection is to be carried out, do the operation through a Y-type of incision. If a neck dissection is not being done, then the operation can be carried out through a skin-crease incision on one side of the neck, extending from the midline to the posterior border of the sternomastoid muscle at the level of the superior border of the thyroid cartilage. If the patient has been irradiated and no neck dissection is contemplated, then the operation can again be carried out through a single collar incision, as just described.

Radical neck dissection

Do a radical neck dissection if appropriate and leave the specimen attached by a pedicle extending from the hyoid bone above to the lower border of the tumour below.

Pharyngotomy

If a radical neck dissection is not being done, mobilize the larynx and pharynx by retracting the sternomastoid muscle laterally and dissecting medial to the carotid sheath. Using cutting diathermy divide the muscles attached to the upper border of the hyoid bone just above its lateral end; divide the mucosa with scissors and enter the pharynx through the vallecula. Exposure of the pharynx can be improved if required by resecting part of the hyoid bone. Insert a retractor through this incision into the pharynx and retract the epiglottis anteriorly. Continue the incision downwards to open up the lateral wall of the pharynx, the incision running immediately posterior to the superior cornu of the thyroid cartilage.

Once the lateral pharyngotomy incision has been completed and the epiglottis retracted forwards, the tumour of the posterior wall of the pharynx can be easily seen and resected (Fig. 12.8), with a 2 cm margin of normal pharyngeal mucosa, still in continuity with the neck dissection, if this has been done.

Repair

The most satisfactory repair is that achieved by a revascularized forearm flap. Take a forearm flap of sufficient size, as described in Chapter 4. This can be harvested during the excisional phase using the

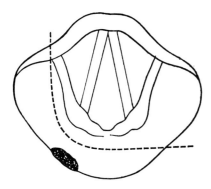

Fig. 12.8 Area of resection of tumour on the posterior pharyngeal wall.

forearm on the opposite side to that on which the surgeon is standing.

At the end of the excisional phase take very great care to ensure that the bleeding points in the edge of the pharyngeal mucosa have been dealt with. This can be tedious. Then introduce the skin flap. It is probably easier to suture the skin flap in place first, or at least to put it into its final position and tack it temporarily in place with a few sutures, to ensure that there will be no tension on the vascular pedicle once the microvascular anastomosis has been completed.

Now carry out the microvascular anastomosis. The remarks made above (see Total pharyngolaryngectomy) for finding vessels for anastomosis to a jejunal loop apply equally well to this situation.

Postoperative care

1 *Routine care.*
2 *Tracheostomy.* Remove the tracheostomy as soon as possible – usually after about 1 week.
3 *Tube feeding.* In order to allow the skin graft on the posterior pharyngeal wall to take properly, do not begin feeding by mouth for 2 weeks after the operation.

Complications

1 *General complications.*
2 *Sloughing of the graft can occur.* This is often not catastrophic, and the denuded posterior pharyngeal wall will heal slowly by granulation tissue over many weeks.

Radiotherapy techniques

Pyriform fossa carcinoma

A beam-directing shell, similar to that used for patients with supraglottic carcinoma, is prepared with the patient lying supine and the neck straight. In the rather unusual case of T_1 or T_2 N_0 disease, a single-phase technique using relatively small parallel opposed wedged fields is possible. The fields extend from the level of the second cervical vertebra down to 1 cm or so below the cricoid cartilage. Anteriorly they cover the skin of the neck and their posterior limit lies over the vertebral bodies, great care being taken to ensure that the spinal cord is not included. The upper anterior corners of these fields are blocked to shield the submandibular gland and oral cavity. The treatment volume is therefore slightly larger than that required for supraglottic tumours. By including the entire larynx and laryngopharynx, the upper deep cervical nodes at the angle of the jaw and the upper oesophagus, both the primary tumour and possible areas of occult extension are covered. Check that films are taken on the treatment machine to verify the accuracy of set-up and field placement. Treatment is with 4–6 MV X-rays; a dose of 55 Gy in 20 daily fractions or its equivalent is prescribed.

In the more common case of locally advanced tumours and where there is lymph node involvement, a two-phase technique is preferred. This is designed for patients with unilateral nodal disease, but can be modified to treat those with minor bilateral nodes. Patients with extensive, fixed bilateral nodes are probably incurable by any means, and should receive symptomatic care only. A similar two-phase technique is also used for supraglottic tumours with bulky nodes. The shell for the first phase holds the patient with the neck extended; this tilts the oral cavity up and largely out of the treatment field. The position of any palpable nodes is marked with wire on the shell. Initially large parallel opposed fields are used to treat the whole neck, including the primary tumour and involved nodes (Fig. 12.9). Check radiographs are used to ensure that all nodal disease, as indicated by the wire markers, is included in the target volume. The dose which may safely be given to such a large field is limited by the tolerance of the spinal cord. A dose of 40 Gy in 20 fractions over 4 weeks is within safe limits and is adequate to eradicate subclinical disease.

The second phase follows immediately the first phase is finished. It gives additional irradiation to a smaller volume, including the primary tumour and initially palpable nodes. For this phase, a fresh shell with the neck straight may be required. This is particularly important if the patient's neck has become thinner during the first phase of treatment due to regression of nodal disease or general weight loss. As nodes may overlie the cord, a parallel pair of fields is not suitable, and a more complex set-up is necessary. A large lateral field which covers the hypopharynx and node mass on the affected side is combined with a smaller contralateral anterior oblique field. This arrangement gives an anterolateral

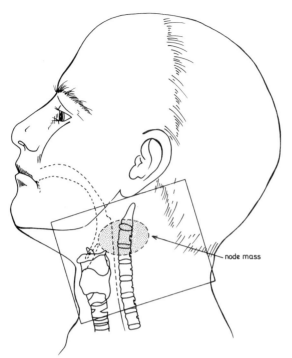

Fig. 12.9 Phase 1 radiotherapy field for an advanced pyriform fossa carcinoma with nodal metastasis.

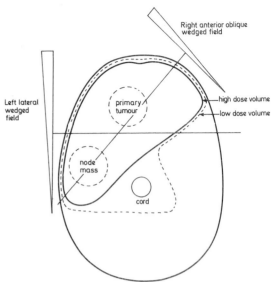

Fig. 12.10 Plan of radiotherapy field arrangement in the second phase of treatment of an advanced pyriform fossa carcinoma with nodal metastasis.

kidney-shaped high dose volume which covers the primary tumour and nodes, but avoids the cord (Fig. 12.10). A further 25 Gy in 22 fractions over 2½ weeks is given. In those patients with bilateral nodal disease, the second phase of treatment as described above will be given from the worst affected side, and the nodes on the opposite side will not be covered. These may be treated concomitantly by giving a similar dose with electrons to small fields. The rationale for using electons in this situation is that their limited penetration prevents cord tolerance being exceeded. In addition, a further small volume boost using electrons may be given to any residual palpable nodes, to bring the total dose to 70 Gy in 35 fractions over 7 weeks.

The principal acute adverse effect of this treatment is mucositis, and great care must be taken to ensure that the patient is adequately nourished throughout. One should resist the temptation to allow a break in treatment to allow the acute reaction to settle, as this significantly compromises the already slim chances of cure. Smoking exacerbates the mucosal reaction and so, for this reason as well as others, should be discouraged.

Postcricoid carcinoma

Accurate delineation of disease extent is necessary for the radical radiotherapy of all head and neck cancers, and postcricoid carcinoma is no exception. Of particular importance here is the lower limit. The treatment volume encompasses the primary tumour and extends 3 cm below this point to cover any occult submucosal spread. The lower cervical nodes are also included, but because of the large area which would need to be covered, no attempt is made to treat prophylactically all possible areas of lymphatic spread. Several field arrangements may be used to irradiate this volume satisfactorily. The choice depends on the length of the tumour and the build of the patient. In a thinner patient with a long neck or short tumour, two lateral fields extending from the level of the hyoid bone to 3 cm beyond the macroscopic limits of the tumour are used. These are angled downwards to avoid the shoulders and ensure adequate coverage of the lower part of the volume. In squatter patients or if the tumour is more extensive, a third field may be added anteriorly, using a similar arrangement to that recommended for subglottic tumours. Alternatively, a pair of appropriately wedged anterior oblique fields may be used. The prescribed dose with any of these arrangements is as described for supraglottic carcinoma.

Carcinoma of the posterior pharyngeal wall

As is the case for postcricoid carcinoma, the patient is treated lying supine, with the neck fixed in a shell with the spine straight. The treatment volume for carcinoma of the posterior pharyngeal wall includes the primary tumour with a margin of 2–3 cm, and the first echelon of nodes in the deep cervical chain. Usually a parallel pair of lateral fields is adequate, but sometimes they may need to be angled inferiorly, as described for postcricoid carcinoma. Again, no attempt is made to treat the whole neck. The dose fractionation schedule is selected as for supraglottic carcinoma.

Postoperative radiotherapy

It has been indicated that the preferred treatment for many patients with carcinoma of the hypopharynx is with primary surgery. For the majority of patients, adjuvant radiotherapy is appropriate. It has been shown that postoperative irradiation results in significantly better local control than preoperative radiotherapy. Whether this is translated into better survival is not clear, but improved local control is a worthwhile achievement on its own. In addition, there are fewer surgical complications in patients receiving postoperative irradiation. Probably all but those exceptionally few patients who have undergone surgery for a $T_1 N_0$ carcinoma, for whom the chances of cure by surgery alone are excellent, should receive postoperative radiotherapy.

Controversies

What is the best method of pharyngeal replacement?

The various situations and the best ways of dealing with them have been outlined above. Controversy continues, however, about which is the best way of replacing the pharynx. There is, in fact, no answer to this question. The surgery should be tailored to the individual patient, to the pathology, and to the available skills. Pharyngeal replacement can be assessed by various criteria, including the mortality of the procedure, the length of the patient's stay in hospital, and the quality of the patient's swallow. Pharyngeal replacement is the head and neck procedure *par excellence* that can lead to the death of the patient. Various criteria are used for operative mortality, but most authors do not state the time interval after the procedure that they include in the period of operative mortality. Some include deaths occurring during the operation, some those occurring in the first 24 h, some within the first week; many do not define the period at all.

In a recent confidential review by the Royal College of Surgeons, the definition of a surgical death was one that occured within the first 30 days after the operation. Under this criterion the mortality from gastric transposition is about 20% while that for skin flap repair or jejunal loop repair is about 5%. The median length of stay in hospital in previous

times, using the deltopectoral flap repair, was 3 months. This fell to about 40 days for pectoralis major flap repair, and to 20 days for repair with the jejunal loop. A reasonable figure for gastric transposition would be 30 days.

As regards the quality of the swallow, gastric transposition is much the best procedure, as the swallow is normal after it. The ability to swallow is good after a jejunal loop repair, although a very small proportion of patients do occasionally require dilatation. The main disadvantage of repair with skin flaps is stenosis, usually at the lower junction between the oesophageal stump and the skin flap. This was very common in deltopectoral flap repairs, but still occurs in about 20% of patients undergoing a repair with a pectoralis major flap.

The Paterson–Brown Kelly syndrome

Known in North America as the Plummer–Vinson syndrome, this has in times past been thought to be important in the genesis of postcricoid carcinoma. However, in the authors' experience a clear preceding history of this syndrome is only obtained in about 5% of patients with postcricoid carcinoma, and its importance in this disease does appear to have been vastly over-rated.

Choice of treatment

In general terms in the UK the choice of treatment depends on how many patients with carcinoma of the hypopharynx the surgeon sees in a year. The standard of surgery required for the treatment of hypopharyngeal cancer is very much higher than that for other head and neck tumours. If a surgeon has the experience, the expertise, the facilities and the team structure, then surgery would seem to be the modality of choice. If, however, these facilities are not available then the occasional surgeon has the choice of sending the patient for radiation therapy which is an inferior method of treatment or else the patient should be referred to a major centre that performs a lot of this sort of surgery.

The overall survival rate after surgery for carcinoma of the hypopharynx regardless of site is 25–30%. It is difficult to get figures to estimate the survival after irradiation but it would seem reasonable to estimate that around 10% will survive.

Salvage surgery

If a laryngeal tumour shows ulceration a few months after irradiation then, in spite of a negative biopsy, a recurrence should be presumed to be present and treated accordingly. The same applies to hypopharyngeal cancer. If after a good initial radiotherapy result the area becomes ulcerated, then recurrent disease should be presumed to be present and treatment carried out. Surgery after radiotherapy in the postcricoid region is difficult. It is probably better to treat all of these patients by gastric transposition.

Radiological assessment

The authors feel that a soft tissue lateral film of the neck gives more information than a barium X-ray. The only value of a barium X-ray is to show the lower extent of the tumour and even then the surgeon really only needs to know one thing. Is it above or below the clavicle?

Neither radiology nor endoscopy is 100% certain of diagnosing the tumour if it is small. It is estimated that there is a 94% chance that a tumour less than 3 cm will be missed by a radiologist. Fifty per cent of false-negative reports from radiology have also been missed at previous endoscopy – and endoscopy is only 90% accurate.

Globus syndrome

This is probably one of the most common presenting symptoms at an ear, nose and throat clinic. A number of small hypopharyngeal tumours present in this manner and it is the authors' practice to examine these patients and to take a plain lateral film of the neck. If it is clear, then the patient should be reassured and another appointment made for 1 month later. If patients still have symptoms, then they should be endoscoped. If symptoms persist, despite negative endoscopic findings, the patient should not be discharged from the clinic follow-up until all possibilities of development of a carcinoma have gone.

Nutritional factors

The average weight loss of a person presenting with a hypopharyngeal cancer is 10 kg. In response to weight loss, a normal person mobilizes peripheral protein to the liver. Tumours alter normal metabolic response and it is possible that the lean body mass is preserved by insulin.

Although hyperalimentation was formerly a popular method of stopping the patient losing weight and even perhaps increasing the patient's weight slightly before surgery, it is now not so popular. It has been realized that hyperalimentation may benefit the tumour and not the host and thus it is now limited to 5 days.

References and further reading

Surgical anatomy and pathology

Elwood P C, Jacobs A, Pitman R G, Entwhistle C C (1964) Epidemiology of the Paterson–Kelly syndrome. *Lancet* 2:716–20.
Hahn S S, Spaulding C A, Kim J A, Constable W C (1987) The prognostic significance of lymph node involvement in pyriform sinus and supraglottic cancers. *Int J Radiat Oncol Biol Phys* 13:1143–7.
Jacobs A (1962) Post-cricoid carcinoma in patients with pernicious anaemia. *Br Med J* 2:91–2.
Larsson L G, Sandstrom A, Westling P (1975) Relationship of Plummer–Vinson disease to cancer of the upper alimentary tract in Sweden. *Cancer Res* 35:3308–16.
Tani M, Amatsu M (1987) discrepancies between clinical and histopathological diagnoses in T$_3$ pyriform sinus cancer. *Laryngoscope* 97:93–6.
Weber R S, Goepfert H (1989) Cancer of the hypopharynx and cervical oesophagus. In: Myers E N, Suen J Y (eds) *Cancer of the Head and Neck*. New York, Churchill Livingstone, pp. 509–31.
Willatt D J, Jackson S R, McCormick M S, Lubsen H, Michaels L, Stell P M (1987) Vocal cord paralysis and tumour length in staging postcricoid cancer. *Eur J Surg Oncol* 13:131–7.

Investigations

Larsson S, Mancuso A, Hoover L, Hanafee W (1981) Differentiation of pyriform sinus cancer from supraglottic laryngeal cancer by computed tomography. *Radiology* 141:427–32.
Lufkin R B, Hanafee W N, Wortham D, Hoover L (1986) Larynx and hypopharynx: MR imaging with surface coils. *Radiology* 158:747–54.

Surgery of the hypopharynx

Coleman J J, Searles J M, Hester R *et al.* (1987) Ten years' experience with the free jejunal autograft. *Am J Surg* 154:394–8.
Driscoll W G, Nagorsky M J, Cantrell R W, Johns M E (1983) Carcinoma of the pyriform sinus: analysis of 102 cases. *Laryngoscope* 92:556–60.
Krespi Y P, Sisson G A (1984) Voice preservation in pyriform sinus carcinoma by hemicricolaryngopharyngectomy. *Ann Otol Rhinol Laryngol* 93:306–10.
O'Dwyer T P, Gullane P J, Awerbuch D, Ho C-S (1990) Percutaneous feeding gastrostomy in patients with head and neck tumors: a 5 year review. *Laryngoscope* 100:29–32.
Rees R S, Ivey G L, Shack R B, Franklin J D, Lynch J B (1986) Pectoralis major musculocutaneous flaps: long-term follow-up of hypopharyngeal rconstruction. *Plast Reconstr Surg* 77:586–91.
Silver C E, Cusumano R J, Fell S C, Strauch B (1989) Replacement of upper esophagus: results with myocutaneous flap and with gastric transposition. 99:819–21.
Stein D W, Schuller D E (1989) Advantages of pectoralis musculocutaneous flap in pharyngeal reconstruction. *Laryngoscope* 99:691–6.

Stell P M (1984) Replacement of the pharynx after pharyngolaryngectomy. *Ann R Coll Surg Engl* **66**:388–90.

Stell P M (1988) The present status of surgery in the treatment of carcinoma of the hypopharynx and cervical oesophagus. *Adv Otorhinolaryngol* **39**:120–34.

Vries E J de, Stein D W, Johnson J T *et al.* (1989) Hypopharyngal reconstruction: a comparison of two alternatives. *Laryngoscope* **99**:614–17.

Radiotherapy

Bataini P, Brugere J, Bernier J, Jaulerry C H, Picot C, Ghossein N A (1982) Results of radical radiotherapeutic treatment of carcinoma of the pyriform sinus. *Int J Radiol Oncol Biol Phys* **8**:1277–86.

Fletcher G H (1977) Place of irradiation in the management of head and neck cancer. *Semin Oncol* **4**:375–85.

Marks J E, Freeman R B, Lee F, Ogura J H (1978) Pharyngeal wall cancer: an analysis of treatment results, complications and patterns of failure. *Int J Radiat Oncol Biol Phys* **4**:587–93.

Snow J B, Gelber R D, Kramer S, Davis L W, Marcial V A, Lowry L D (1981) Comparison of preoperative and postoperative radiation therapy for patients with carcinoma of the head and neck: Interim report. *Acta Otolaryngol* **91**:611–26.

Strong M S, Vaughan C W, Kayne H L *et al.* (1978) A randomised trial of preoperative radiotherapy in cancer of the oropharynx and hypopharynx. *Am J Surg* **136**:494–500.

13

Tumours of the nose and sinuses

Surgical anatomy

The maxillary sinus is a box bounded by the eye, the nose, the mouth, the pterygoid space and the nasopharynx. It has outlets to the ethmoid sinuses, the nose and the roots of the teeth if the floor is dehiscent.

The nasofrontal suture line is the surface marking of the level of the cribriform plate. The cribriform plate lies about 2.5 cm posterior to the nasofrontal suture line, and in between the two is the upward extension of the anterior ethmoid cells (Fig. 13.1). Laterally, the cribriform plate is bounded by the superior extension of the ethmoid cells, called the fovea. Removal of the entire ethmomaxillary block takes out the three nasal turbinates, whereas removal of the lateral wall, as in a lateral rhinotomy, only removes the middle and inferior turbinates (Fig. 13.2).

The ethmoid sinus is a labyrinth of anything from three to 17 cells, extending posteriorly to be contiguous with the sphenoid sinus. It is superior to the level of the cribriform plate in the anterior fossa. It is penetrated by the anterior and posterior ethmoidal

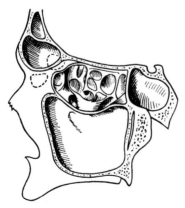

Fig. 13.1 Extension of anterior ethmoidal cells above level of cribriform plate.

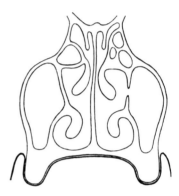

Fig. 13.2 Relations of the floor of the nose and maxilla.

arteries. The anterior artery enters the sinus 4 cm behind the medial ligament of the orbit and the posterior ethmoidal artery 2.5 cm behind this. Just a few millimetres behind the posterior ethmoidal artery is the optic nerve, but it is frequently protected from the ethmoid block by a stout bar of bone. In 10% of cases, however, this bar of bone is missing and the optic nerve is contiguous with the ethmoid sinuses. It is enclosed in a sheath of dura and forms the site of entry into the brain of ethmoidal tumours.

The orbit is the key to the management of ethmomaxillary tumours. The eye is held in position by the medial ligament of the orbit and also the lateral ligament. The superior oblique and the inferior rectus are attached to the periosteum of the orbit and so, if the eye is to be of any use after surgery in this area, it is important always to work under the periosteum so as not to disturb these muscles. The lacrimal sac lies between the lacrimal bone and the frontal process of the maxillary bone, and behind the medial ligament of the eye. It is always damaged in any form of maxillectomy but the resulting defect into the nasal cavity acts as a large dacrocystorhinostomy and the patient does not have symptoms.

The superior and inferior orbital fissures offer

routes of entry and exit of tumour, to and from the orbit. The periosteum of the orbit also seems resistant to the spread of carcinoma; the advantage of any craniofacial approach is that the periosteum can be dealt with more accurately from above than it can be from below.

The floor of the nasal cavity is formed by the hard palate; the floor of the maxillary antrum is the alveolus. The premolar and molar teeth are in intimate relationship to the floor of the maxillary sinus.

Attached to the posterior wall of the maxillary antrum are the pterygoid plates. The space between the pterygoid plates and the maxillary sinus is the pterygomaxillary fissure, through which travels the maxillary artery.

The infratemporal fossa is the space behind the maxillary antrum, bounded medially by the pterygoid plates and laterally by the zygomatic arch, coronoid process and ascending ramus of the mandible. Inferoposteriorly it connects to the parapharyngeal space and superiorly lies the sphenoid bone, the foramen ovale and the foramen spinosum. It contains the mandibular branch of the fifth cranial nerve, the pterygoid muscles, the maxillary artery and the venous plexus. Tumours can spread into this space from contiguous structures; primary and metastatic tumours can also occur here.

The lymphatic drainage of the maxillary antrum is not fully understood. It is probably scanty and possibly drains posteriorly to the retropharyngeal nodes. Occasionally lymphatics go directly from the antrum to the jugulodigastric node. The anterior part of the nasal cavity drains to the submandibular nodes. An enlarged neck node at first presentation probably means tumour has broken out of the maxillary antrum to involve the rich lymphatic areas of the cheek.

The nasal septum consists of the quadrilateral cartilage, the vomer and the perpendicular plate of the ethmoid. Anteriorly it is contiguous with the medial crura of the lower lateral cartilages. Tumours in the anterior part of the nose not only involve the nasal septum but very quickly go through into the gingivobuccal sulcus and, thus, involve the muscles of the upper lip and the mouth.

The anatomy of the cribriform plate has to be known in order to perform craniofacial surgery. It lies at the level of the nasofrontal suture line and laterally is the raised fovea on either side. Anterior to the crista galli is a foramen for an emissary vein to come from the sagittal sinus. About 2.5 cm behind the posterior extent of the cribriform plate lies the optic chiasma; the optic nerves have to be visualized during craniofacial surgery so that ethmoidal resection can take place, preserving vision. The olfactory nerves, ensheathed in dura, pass through the perforations in the cribriform plate. The dura is so closely applied to this area that it is impossible to elevate and expose the roof of the ethmoids without tearing the dura to such an extent that grafting is required.

Surgical pathology

Epidemiology of carcinoma

In the USA and the UK, the incidence of nasal tumours is about 10 per million population per year. In Japan and in parts of Africa, the rates are more than twice that. The best recognized aetiological factor in the UK is the wood industry. People working with hardwoods run the same risk of developing adenocarcinomas of the ethmoids as do smokers of developing lung cancer.

Retrospective cohort studies of nickel-refining workers in Wales, Norway and Canada show that the risk is 100 times greater than in people not involved in this occupation. The risk increases with the length of exposure and the age at first exposure. The risk only involves those who work in the refining process and not those in the manufacturing process.

There is also epidemiological evidence that there is an increased risk in boot and shoe workers. It has been reported in people working with mustard gas, isopropyl oil and hydrocarbon gas, as well as in people who have had thorium dioxide injected into the sinus. Snuff is a well-recognized aetiological factor in the Bantu.

The male : female ratio is 2 : 1, and the average age at first diagnosis is 55 years. Figure 13.3 shows the site incidence of cancer of the nose and sinuses. There are no true precancerous conditions and early diagnosis is the exception rather than the rule.

Classification of carcinoma

Harrison has said that attempts at classifying this tumour finitely are both impractical and unrealistic.

Ohngren (in 1933) had divided them into anteroinferior and posterosuperior by means of an imaginary line extending from medial canthus to the angle of the jaw. The American Joint Committee (AJC) suggests the classification given in Table 13.1.

To differentiate between T_1 and T_2 is, in daily practice terms, totally unrealistic.

Other systems have been proposed by experienced surgeons but, as there is no universally accepted classification, they are at the moment best ignored.

Benign tumours

Osteomas

An osteoma is a benign osteogenic tumour of slow growth containing mature bone. They are found most frequently in the mandible but, when they occur in the upper jaw, they are commonest in the

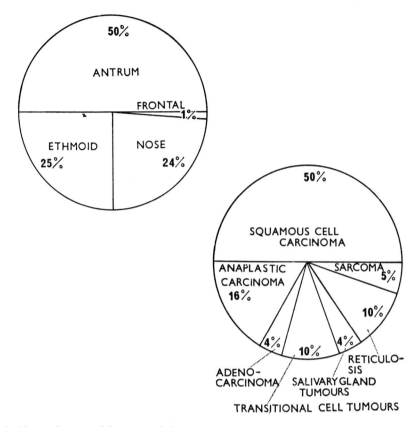

Fig. 13.3 Site incidence of cancer of the nose and sinuses.

Table 13.1 American Joint Committee (AJC) classification of nasal carcinoma

T_1	Tumour confined to antral mucosa of infrastructure
T_2	Tumour confined to suprastructure mucosa without bone destruction or to infrastructure with destruction of medial or inferior bony walls only
T_3	More extensive tumour invading skin of cheek, orbit, anterior ethmoid sinus or pterygoid muscle
T_4	Mass of tumour with invasion of cribriform plate, posterior ethmoid sinus, sphenoid sinus, nasopharynx, pterygoid plate or base of skull.

frontoethmoid region. When they fill the entire frontal sinus they extend into the ethmoid labyrinth through the inferior portion of the frontal sinus. When located away from the sinus ostium they are silent and are only discovered incidentally during radiographic examination. When they block the sinus drainage, a mucocele can develop, requiring removal of the osteoma with an osteoplastic flap or external frontoethmoidectomy.

Osteomas in the ethmoid sinuses present a very different problem. They most usually present with proptosis and have almost always invaded the orbit. If they extend posteriorly they can be contiguous with the sphenoid bone through which the optic nerve travels. They are unlike frontal sinus osteomas in that they cannot be removed easily by knocking off a stalk. They require a full frontoethmoidectomy, preferably under direct vision. The very large compacted ones are better removed via a craniofacial approach.

Osteomas occurring together with other soft tissue tumours and intestinal polyposis comprise Gardner's syndrome. It is an autosomal dominant and 50% of the offspring will be affected. The incidence of malignant degeneration of the intestinal polyps is 40%.

Chondromas

These can develop anywhere in the nose and sinuses. The difference between the benign and malignant varieties is difficult to predict histologically, but in general, cartilaginous tumours eventually have a malignant potential. In the final analysis, those that metastasize are malignant and those that do not probably are not. They do have an aggressive nature and do tend to recur; for the reason, resection ought to be more aggressive than with osteoma.

Ossifying fibroma

This is a variant of fibrous dysplasia. It belongs to a range of benign fibro-osseous lesions that occurs in the jaws, and is closely related to cementifying fibroma, benign cementoblastoma, periapical fibrous dysplasia and true fibrous dysplasia. Both ossifying and cementifying fibromas occur in the mandible and maxilla, and present as painless swellings. There is an equal sex incidence and the greatest incidence of occurrence is in the third and fourth decade.

Fibrous dysplasia

Fibrous dysplasia is often first diagnosed in infancy or childhood. It shows a predilection for the maxilla; females are more affected than males. It presents as a painless slow-growing swelling of the maxilla and progresses to deformity. It is said that growth may slow or cease after puberty. It has a fairly characteristic radiographic appearance.

Haemangioma

This very often occurs on the nasal septum. It is a cavernous haemangioma with a propensity to recur if resection is not adequate. It presents as epistaxis.

Haemangiomas elsewhere in the upper jaw are extremely rare. They have been reported in the frontal bone, the nasal bones and the maxilla. They seem to occur between the ages of 20 and 50 and females predominate. If the teeth are associated with the haemangioma, copious bleeding ensues on their removal. Haemangiomas are nearly always benign so a policy of non-intervention is probably the best one.

They have a characteristic radiographic appearance. The soap-bubble appearance may represent a giant cell tumour of the jaws but in haemangiomas the lacunae are smaller and interspersed with a fine fibrillar network which may show a sunray or sunburst appearance in profile.

Intermediate tumours

Inverted papilloma

This forms 1–4% of all nasal neoplasms and has an incidence of 4 per million population. The male : female ratio varies from 3 : 1 to 10 : 1. Less than 10 cases have been described in children and the maximum age incidence is in the sixth decade. It is very rare in blacks.

The papillomas present as firm, bulky, red and vascular masses, usually on one side of the nose. In 60% of patients, the symptoms have been present for less than a year, but in 20% the patient has had the symptoms for more than 5 years. One in four has a wrong diagnosis made at the initial consultation.

Histologically they show patterns of inversion or papilliferous outgrowths, and are covered with squamous or transitional epithelium. There is an intact basement membrane and microcysts are present. There is cellular atypia in 10%.

There is a lot of confusion regarding their place in the biological spectrum of neoplasia. Their association with malignancy has been described by various authors as anything from 1.5 to 56%. It is probably best to regard inverted papillomas as an intermediate tumour and, when it turns into transitional cell carcinoma, this can be regarded as a nonkeratinizing squamous cell carcinoma.

Another source of confusion is the failure to separate synchronous from metachronous lesions. Most cases presenting with malignancy do so as synchronous lesions. The incidence of metachronous lesions is around 1% in the literature.

Three categories have been suggested:

1 That the carcinoma and inverted papilloma occupy the same anatomical region without histological evidence that one gives rise to the other.
2 That inverted papilloma does not recur after treatment but is succeeded by invasive carcinoma.
3 Inverted papilloma showing transition into a focus of in situ or invasive carcinoma.

There have only been a handful of cases described that fulfil the criteria of category 3.

The risk of synchronous malignancy is unknown but may be up to 15%, so every case of inverted papilloma should have complete excision and multiple sections should be examined to rule out the existence of a synchronous carcinoma.

Haemangioperiocytoma

This was first described in 1942, its place in the biological spectrum of neoplasia has not been established. It shows a great lack of uniformity in appearance, growth and biological behaviour. the lesion presents as a painless mass that sometimes grows quickly and causes facial swelling and/or nasal obstruction. It is found wherever there are capillaries.

Meningioma

Extracranial meningiomas arise from ectopic arachnoid tissue but can also spread to the frontal sinuses. They are locally recurrent and difficult to eradicate surgically, which is the only modality to which they are sensitive.

Basal cell carcinoma

The skin of the nose is the most common site for basal carcinoma in the head and neck. It is 30 times more common than squamous carcinoma. The peak incidence is in the sixth to the eighth decade and there is no sex difference. The commonest areas affected are the side, the dorsum and the tip of the nose. Although several histological types have been described, it is preferable to define them either as circumscribed or infiltrative. The clinical appearance can vary from small nodular growths to chronic ulcers or ulceronodular lesions. The border of an ulcer may be rolled or it may be flat. Four out of 10 will recur and, although distant metastases are rare, recurrent morbidity and possible gross destruction of the face give high priority to successful first-attempt therapy.

Malignant tumours

Squamous carcinoma

Because the lateral wall of the nose, the maxillary antrum and the ethmoid sinuses are contiguous, it is usually impossible to say where a squamous carcinoma has begun. It is commonly accepted, however, that about 50% begin in the maxillary antrum and that about 50% are squamous cell carcinomas. Almost every patient has signs of bony destruction when first seen because this is the only way that symptoms can occur. The tumour can leave the maxillary antrum by going into the nasal cavity, the ethmoid, the orbit via the inferior orbital fissure, the soft tissues of the cheek by erosion of

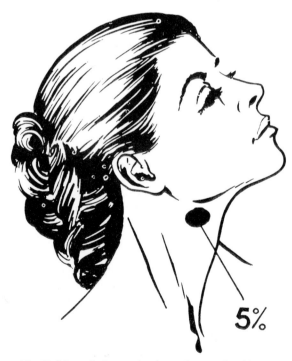

Fig. 13.4 Spread of antroalveolar and antroethmoidal tumours

the anterior wall, or on to the palate or alveolar ridge through the dental foramina. Finally it can go into the buccal sulcus.

A carcinoma of the ethmoid can exit into the orbit, the nose and the sphenoid by direct spread, and most importantly, into the anterior fossa through the fovea or the cribriform plate. Before invading these other structures, however, they usually fill the maxillary antrum. Five per cent of patients with antroalveolar or antroethmoidal tumours will have a metastatic lymph node (Fig. 13.4). Not all of these lymph nodes, however, will contain tumour, because if the soft tissues of the face are affected, some may be inflammatory. If an ethmoidal tumour has metastasized to the neck nodes then the patient is incurable, but if tumour of the lower part of the maxillary antrum has metastasized then the patient does have some small chance of cure.

One in 3 patients ultimately dies of metastases, the commonest sites being the abdominal viscera, the lungs and the bones. One patient in 5 will develop a second primary tumour, usually in the bronchus.

Adenocarcinoma

These are uncommon except in people working in the hardwood industry. They are also related to isopropyl alcohol and chrome inhalation. Inhaled dust particles will travel along the middle turbinate and larger particles will be deposited there, resulting in delayed mucociliary transport.

Adenocarcinoma has the same bone erosive properties as squamous carcinoma and presents in the same way. The metastatic rate to lymph nodes is identical. Histologically adenocarcinomas are best classified into high-grade and low-grade and of these the high grade seems to have the worst prognosis.

Tumours of minor salivary glands

The adenoid cystic carcinoma and the mucoepidermoid carcinoma can present in the nasal sinuses. Adenoid cystic carcinomas showing solid areas of malignant cells, rather than the classic Swiss-cheese pattern, are more malignant. Vascular invasion is commoner, distant metastases more frequent and death more likely. Perineural invasion is said to occur and there is ample scope for this in the nasal sinuses via the infraorbital nerve, the maxillary nerve, the greater palatine nerve and the sphenopalatine foramen. They can also spread intracranially through the olfactory nerves and in the pterygoid space through the posterior dental nerves.

Malignant melanoma

Malignant melanomas comprise about 1% of nasal and paranasal sinus cancers. They are more likely to arise from the mucous membrane of the septum and the lateral nasal wall than from the maxillary or ethmoid sinuses. This is probably just as well because the survival of patients with melanoma of the sinuses is almost zero whereas a reasonable response rate can be expected from treating melanoma of the septum or lateral nasal wall.

The sex ratio of the incidence is equal and the peak is in the fourth to sixth decade. Histologically there is no relationship to Clark's skin classification. Fifty per cent survive 3 years but since more will die over a 10-year period, a 5-year survival figure is meaningless.

Melanomas often present as polypoidal swellings that may be slate grey, blue or black. There are often regional satellites and about 4 out of 10 will have a neck node at some stage in the disease. The fact that amelanotic melanomas quite frequently present as unilateral polyps emphasizes the fact that all polypoidal material must be sent for pathological examination.

Their biological behaviour is totally unpredictable. Some can be removed never to reappear, while others progress relentlessly to widespread disseminated disease and death in a few months. Another group of melanomas responds to initial therapy and appears to be held in check by a competent immune system for many years until they also recur.

Esthesioneuroblastoma

This is also known as an olfactory neuroblastoma or neuroendocrine tumour and until recently was rarely described. It resembles an anaplastic carcinoma and so was formerly underreported. They may remain undiagnosed unless the pathologist uses special tumour markers.

The tumour arises in the upper part of the nasal cavity from stem cells of neural crest origin but differentiate into olfactory sensory cells. When the biopsy shows large nests of characteristic cells separated into compartments with rosette formation the histological diagnosis is easy but sometimes the tissue provides only sheets of densely packed uniform round cells and it is these that are mistaken for undifferentiated carcinoma.

The tumour differs clinically from sympathetic neuroblastoma in that all ages are affected and urinary vanillylmandelic acid and homovanillic acid are usually not detectable. The tumour seems to occur within two age peaks, around 20 and 50 years, and neuroendocrine tumour is the name proposed for those found in the older age group. At the 20-year peak there is a lower incidence of local recurrence and a higher incidence of metastasis and at the 50-year peak there is a higher incidence of local recurrence and a lower incidence of metastasis.

It is a slow-growing tumour which may become very large and destructive and by its very nature must be regarded as involving the cribriform plate.

A clinical staging has been proposed for these tumours. Group A tumours are confined to the nasal cavity, group B to the nasal cavity and one or more paranasal sinuses and group C tumours extend beyond these limits. It is however difficult to estimate the spread of these tumours and to apply this system of staging.

Osteogenic sarcoma

This presents as an enlarging firm mass that is rock-hard on palpation. It is well-seen radiologically; surgical excision may be made difficult by extension to the skull base. The 5-year survival is in the range of 10–20%.

Malignant fibrous histiocytoma

This can arise in areas of previous bone disorders, such as Paget's disease and fibrous dysplasia. It has also been reported in patients who have undergone irradiation to the area. It presents as a gradually expanding mass that is hard on palpation and often difficult to differentiate from an osteogenic sarcoma. If it invades the skull base it becomes non-resectable.

Lymphoreticular neoplasms

These come in three varieties: midline malignant reticulosis, extramedullary plasmacytomas, and non-Hodgkin's lymphoma.

Midline malignant reticulosis is different clinically from Wegener's granuloma. The patients are not ill and start with very mild symptoms of a lesion in the centre part of the face. However, it rapidly goes on to ulceration and then to destruction. Histologically there are indications of histiocytic malignancy plus necrosis and vasculitis. It is best regarded as a lymphoma and treated as such.

Extramedullary plasmacytoma occurs usually in the head and neck. Most are solitary and should be regarded as a tumour of well-differentiated B lymphocytes. It replaces rather than invades tissue. Most do not go on to generalized multiple myelomatosis.

Non-Hodgkin's lymphoma can arise in the nose and paranasal sinuses. When lymphoma occurs in a facial bone one of three clinical states may prevail:

1 The lesion may be considered to be primary in the involved bone.
2 Similar lesions may be found in regional or distant lymph nodes.
3 The osseous lesion may be a secondary deposit in a patient with a known diffuse malignant lymphoma.

Investigations

History (Fig. 13.5)

A patient with a tumour in the maxillary antrum may present with facial swelling, facial pain, or anaesthesia in the area of the infraorbital nerve. He or she may also have nasal obstruction, epistaxis, dental signs and symptoms, such as toothache, loose teeth and ill-fitting dentures, or a persistent oroantral fistula. Proptosis or diplopia is rare.

Patients with ethmoidal tumours, however, will very often complain of proptosis or diplopia, and usually have a nasal obstruction and epistaxis. Facial swelling is less common and dental symptoms are very unusual.

Examination

Examine the face for fullness of one cheek, numbness and ptosis due to a Horner's syndrome. Inspect the nose, nasopharynx and mouth for evidence of tumour and for numbness of the hard palate, indicating involvement of the greater palatine nerve. Examine the pharynx and the larynx for evidence of ninth and 10th cranial nerve palsies; finally, palpate the hard palate, the buccal sulcus and the anterior surface of the antrum.

Examine the eyes for proptosis and for ophthal-moplegia. Since diplopia is a very difficult sign to pick up in its early stages, the patient should be referred to an ophthalmologist. Palpate the neck for enlarged nodes and see if the patient has trismus.

Radiology

Radiology is vital to define the site and extent of the disease in order to plan treatment. Every patient should have a computed tomography (CT) scan but it should be realized that this overestimates tumour spread because of surrounding oedema; this error may be as high as 30%. Nearly every patient will show bone destruction on X-ray examination. The most important areas to see are the cribriform plate, the fovea, the posterior wall of the maxillary sinus, the optic foramen, the medial part of the orbit and the sphenoid sinus. This is best delineated with coronal rather than axial scanning.

Retained secretions in the frontal and sphenoid sinuses can simulate tumour; magnetic resonance imaging is useful in making the differentiation.

Chest radiographs should not be forgotten in order to exclude secondary spread.

Laboratory investigations

If myeloma is suspected, estimate the plasma proteins and examine the urine for Bence Jones protein. If there is a watery nasal discharge, examine it to see if it is cerebrospinal fluid using either Clinistix, injecting fluorescein or with a radioisotope test. With olfactory neuroblastoma, it is important to remember that some tumours are secretors, so catecholamines should be estimated before giving the patient a general anaesthetic.

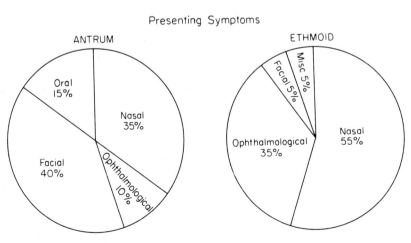

Fig. 13.5 Presenting symptoms.

Biopsy

This is best done intranasally. It is not a good oncological principle to open the cheek tissues and do a Caldwell–Luc approach. Use should be made of sinus endoscopes. If there is any suggestion that the frontal sinus is affected by tumour it is easy to pass an endoscope into the sinus and obtain an appropriate sample.

Any enlarged node in the neck should be aspirated for cytology or biopsied. A metastatic node may indicate that the patient is incurable but, on the other hand, every enlarged node is not metastatic. It may be inflammatory and it is important to know this before starting treatment.

Treatment policy

Benign tumours

Osteomas of the frontal bone are removed with either a frontoethmoidectomy or preferably an osteoplastic frontal flap. Osteomas of the ethmoids are more difficult to treat and may cause blindness if treated inappropriately. They are best approached with a lateral rhinotomy or, if they are very close to the optic foramen, consideration should be given to a craniofacial resection.

Chondromas should be treated with local excision but it should be wide because of the aggressive, recurrent nature of these tumours.

Ossifying fibromas and cementomas are easily shelled out and fibro-osseous dysplasia should be treated cosmetically by drilling away the excess tissue.

Intermediate tumours

Transitional cell papillomas tend to recur: after intranasal removal, the recurrence rate is 80%, after Caldwell–Luc 60% and after medial maxillectomy 30%. They are, therefore, best treated aggressively in the first instance with a lateral rhinotomy after the initial diagnostic polypectomy. There is a definite propensity to malignancy, even though it is not as frequent as was formerly thought.

Lymphomas are treated by grading and assessment of spread, and then by radiotherapy and chemotherapy. Midline reticuloses are treated with radiotherapy and perhaps immunosuppressive drugs such as azothioprine and steroids.

Basal cell tumours of the nasal skin can be irradiated or treated surgically. If surgical treatment is undertaken then every effort should be made to clear the tumour at the first attempt. What should not be done is minor local treatment by dermatologists because this scars the area and makes the detection of recurrence very difficult.

Haemangioperiocytomas are locally aggressive and should be widely excised, as should meningiomas.

Malignant tumours

Before treating any patient with a malignant sinus tumour you should realize that about half are incurable. This must not, however, lead to a policy of despair because if the tumour is not removed it will fungate into the mouth or orbit, causing a far worse deformity than any operation. Of those who are incurable, about 1 in 5 is inoperable due to involvement of the nasopharynx and widespread intracranial and pterygoid involvement; or the patient may be a poor surgical risk, may have distant metastases or may even refuse to have a disfiguring operation.

Three out of 10 patients eventually lose their eye, a subject of much emotion. Too often the cure is compromised by leaving the eye, which is understandable as both surgeon and patient are loathe to sacrifice an eye that still functions normally. The dangers of keeping the eye, however, must be realized because the tumour will almost certainly recur and the eye will then be useless.

Involvement of the pterygoids is difficult to treat. Tumour there cannot be eradicated according to oncological principles. Attempts have been made to enlarge the surgical access to this area with infratemporal fossa approaches but it is still not an oncological operation. It is, however, better to make the attempt to clear the pterygoids than to leave the tumour to grow uncontrolled in this site.

Young people with undifferentiated tumours of the maxillary sinus are a special problem. If it is truly an undifferentiated carcinoma then they are never cured by surgery and the treatment may be worse than the disease. They should, therefore, only be treated with radiotherapy.

Before deciding on a treatment policy, you need to talk to the patient and the family. It is impossible to treat the nose or sinuses without severe disfigurement. This disfigurement may be coped with by the patient but if it is not, then you have not carried out a successful treatment. It is usually impossible for the patient to perceive what he or she will look like after one of these operations or what it will entail. The surgeon, however, must do the utmost to make sure that he or she has informed consent from the patient and family.

The surgeon then involves colleagues. It is important to give the prosthodontist at least 1 week to do any work necessary for the initial operation. The radiotherapist should meet the patient before the operation so that the transition to radiotherapy after surgery can be smooth. The patient should be examined by an opthalmologist to determine any clinical involvement of the orbit and, if a craniofacial operation is to be done, then the neurosurgeon should at least be consulted.

For no very good reason, the fashion with regard to radiotherapy has changed. Until a few years ago, radiotherapy was traditionally used first, followed by surgery, but now it is the other way round. There are now basically only three operations that are carried out for cancer of the maxillary and ethmoid sinuses – lateral rhinotomy, partial maxillectomy and craniofacial resection.

For squamous carcinoma, it is sometimes possible to do a partial maxillectomy leaving the floor of the orbit and the orbit. It is never possible to do this for an adenocarcinoma because it involves the ethmoids. A squamous or an adenocarcinoma involving the ethmoids should be subject to a craniofacial approach, and the resection should be widened if an adenocarcinoma is in the area. The resection may be less wide for an olfactory neuroblastoma.

The periosteum of the orbit is frequently resistant to tumour growth and, although the patient should always give permission for an orbital exenteration before a craniofacial approach, it is sometimes possible to keep the orbit and merely remove the orbital periosteum in one area.

The treatment of malignant melanoma should be tailored to the tumour. If it lies discretely on a turbinate, a wide local excision should be performed and, if the periphery is clear of tumour, then a wait-and-see policy should be adopted. If it presents as polyps a lateral rhinotomy should be the original approach with permission to proceed to whatever resection seems appropriate in the light of the findings.

If it is decided to treat a patient with metastatic neck nodes, a radical neck dissection should be carried out, together with the primary excision, realizing that there is no possibility of an incontinuity resection.

Adjuvant therapy

Every patient who has a maxillectomy should have postoperative radiotherapy. If the eye has been preserved, appropriate steps should be taken to protect it. After 4 weeks, the cavity should be in good enough condition for the radiotherapist to apply a full dose to the area. The advantage of doing the operation first is that special attention can be given to areas where tumour clearance was minimal.

Chemotherapy has little place to play in the management of squamous or adenocarcinoma. It may be used for melanoma but its main place is in the management of lymphoma.

The Japanese and the Dutch have described the use of 5-fluorouracil cream as an adjuvant therapy. They do a debulking tumour operation and follow it by radiotherapy. The cavity is then packed with 5-fluorouracil on a weekly basis. Very careful debridement is done and this packing is continued for several weeks.

Technique of operations on the nose and sinuses

Operations on the skin around the nose

The nasal skin is so fixed and inelastic that primary closure, after removal of tumours in this area, is usually impossible; either local flaps or full-thickness skin grafts must be used. Local rotation flaps are best, as they contain adipose tissue, which supplies the missing thickness, and they have the added advantage of a good colour match.

Full-thickness skin grafts have a much better colour than split-thickness grafts, but they are never as good as adjacent skin.

All the operations described here are for small basal cell or squamous cell carcinomas of the skin around the nose. The principles of these operations can also be applied to other facial sites. Several points are common to all these operations, as outlined next.

Anaesthesia

In the UK most of these operations are done under general anaesthetic with added infiltration of local anaesthetic (2% Xylocaine and 1:80 000 adrenaline). In the USA they are usually done using local anaesthetic only.

Preparation

The area should be carefully shaved and in men, rotation flaps should be planned so as not to rotate hair bearing skin on to the nose. This applies especially when removing tumours from the area of the medial canthus, when no non-hair-bearing skin may be available in someone with bushy eyebrows, which meet in the midline.

Clean the skin with Cetavlon, as any solution containing spirit may be harmful to the eyes. It is also advisable to use Steridrapes. Protect the eyes by closing the lids with a piece of adhesive tape, but it may be necessary, on occasion, to do a temporary tarsorrhaphy.

Technique

Accurate planning of rotation flaps is essential, so outline them in methylene blue before cutting them. Make all incisions with a knife held at right-angles to the skin edge as any bevelling produces an ugly scar. Use sharp pointed scissors to undermine the surrounding areas and while this must be done widely, care must be taken not to go too deep because the facial nerve may be damaged in this way. The most important point of the technique is that absolute haemostasis must be secured before moving the flaps. On no account use diathermy, and tie any large vessels with 3/0 chromic catgut ties. Use pressure with adrenaline swabs for the general ooze that occurs. The flaps should move into position easily and the donor site should also close easily. If this situation exists then only a one-layer closure is needed using 3/0 dermalene on a cutting needle. Dog ears will be present in almost every case and they must be excised. If the flaps do not move easily or the donor site does not close easily then there is abnormal tension and more undermining is needed.

Aftercare

Once the wound is closed, cover it with *tulle gras* and mould a piece of dental stent to the area in order to keep some pressure on it; the stent is kept on with adhesive tape. Take this off after 3 days and apply antibiotic cream to the edges of the wound. There is never any need for drainage, and the stitches are removed in 5 days.

Complications

The worst thing that can happen is that bleeding may occur under the flap which will lift the flap so that the wound breaks down. It may also break down if there is too much tension due to insufficient undermining. Rotation flaps should generally be made in a one-to-one length : breadth ratio. If the length is greater than the breadth then there is slight danger of ischaemic necrosis but this is uncommon in the face.

Sites suitable for primary closure

1 *Tumour of the nasolabial crease.* Excise the tumour in an ellipse and continue the incision down along the nasolabial crease (Fig. 13.6). Widely undercut the lateral side of the incision and move it medially for closure. If there is a lot of tension, as there may well be, the wound should be closed in two layers.
2 *Tumours of the bridge of the nose.* Tumours in the centre of the bridge of the nose are rather rare, but they can be removed by making an incision shaped like the head of an arrow, as shown in Figure 13.7. By undercutting this almost down to the medial canthi on both sides it can be closed primarily without any tension or dog ears.

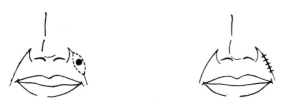

Fig. 13.6 Excision of tumour of the nasolabial fold.

Sites requiring the use of a local rotation flap

1 *Tumours of the medial canthus.* The tumour is excised with an ovoid incision, which is continued upwards on to the upper lid as a rotation flap, as shown in Figure 13.8. The area is widely undercut as usual and the flap turned down into the defect. This is a rather difficult site in which to get complete haemostasis but this must be secured, as it is very important to apply a dental stent at this site. If the tumour is higher up the nose then use a similar incision with the rotation flap taken from the forehead.
2 *Tumours on the lateral surface of the nose.* If the tumour is more than halfway up the nose, excise it in a circular fashion and plan a rotation flap with its base downwards (Fig. 13.9). Undercut the lateral margin widely and move the rotation flap in towards the defect, excising the dog ear which will inevitably form at the rounded end of the rotation flap site.
   If the tumour is in the lower half of the nose then excise it in the usual fashion and plan a rotation flap in the reverse direction with its base pointing upwards (Fig. 13.10). In this case the dog ear will form at the lower part, i.e. the rounded end of the rotation flap.

Sites suitable for grafting

1 *Tumours of the tip of the nose.* Tumours which are in the centre of the tip of the nose are either grafted with a full-thickness skin graft (taken postauricularly; Fig. 13.11) or closed primarily by shortening the septum. Rotation flaps cannot be used because the skin of the nose is too inelastic.
   Excise the tumour and stitch the skin graft in place, then cut the ends of alternate sutures short and leave the others long. Tie these over a bolster of Flavine wool to hold the graft in place, and finally place a dental stent over the nose and fix it with 12 mm adhesive tapes.
2 *Tumour of the ala.* It is possible to remove a notch out of the ala of the nose and sew it up primarily, but this leaves a very ugly deformity.
   It is possible to cut an adjacent rotation flap running in the nasolabial groove and to rotate this in, turning the end round to form a new ala (Fig. 13.12). This can be rather difficult and can produce on occasion a bulky ala. It is therefore better to take a composite graft from the helix of the ear in a triangular form and stitch it into the defect.

Through-and-through defects

If a tumour of the lateral surface of the nose has invaded deeply then it will have to be excised causing a through-and-through defect – a hole in the side of the nose. This can be covered by a prosthesis but it

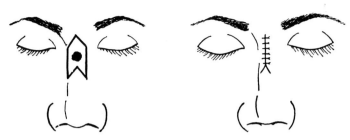

Fig. 13.7 Excision of tumour of the bridge of the nose.

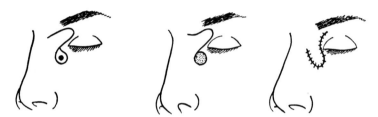

Fig. 13.8 Excision of tumour of the medial canthus.

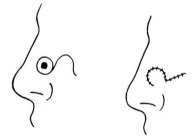

Fig. 13.9 Excision of tumour of the lateral surface of nose.

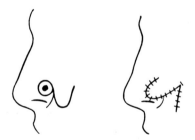

Fig. 13.10 Excision of tumour of the lateral surface of nose with rotation flap.

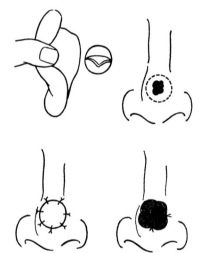

Fig. 13.11 Excision and grafting of tumour of tip of nose.

may fall off. These defects can be closed by using the type of forehead flap shown in Figure 13.13.

On the side of the forehead matching the side of the nose that has the hole in it, a rotation flap is marked with methylene blue so that its length when turned downwards on itself will fill the gap. It is important to overestimate this by about 25%. Using the border of this flap that is nearer the midline of the forehead, another rotation flap is marked – this time slightly longer than the previous one, as this one will turn down to form the outer skin cover. When these are marked the flap is cut and turned down into the defect. It is stitched with the skin surface towards the inside of the nose. The second and larger flap is then cut and rotated downwards to form the outer skin cover and it is stitched to the skin of the external nose. The forehead is widely undercut and can easily be brought together for primary closure. After 3

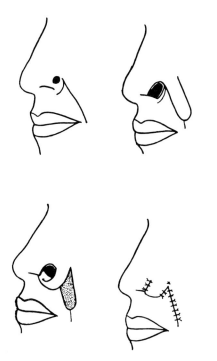

Fig. 13.12 Creation of new ala from local flap.

weeks the pedicles of the rotation flap are cut and the lower part of the forehead is resutured because it will have dog ears on it.

Total rhinectomy

This operation is performed for squamous carcinoma that affects the vestibule or the skin of the nose. The operation itself is not complicated; as wide a margin as possible is taken round the tumour and the whole external nose and septum is cut off flush with the face. The mucosa is stitched to the skin edge.

Reconstruction can be performed with a forehead flap and, if this technique is used, it is better to use a tissue expander in the forehead for some months to get sufficient skin to do a satisfactory closure and reconstruction.

Probably the best method of reconstructing the loss of a whole nose is with an external nasal prosthesis fixed on to spectacles.

Radiotherapy technique for tumours of the skin of the nose

Basal cell carcinomas and the occasional squamous carcinoma which arise on the skin of the nose can usually be dealt with swiftly and effectively with radiotherapy. Because of their position, they tend to present early for treatment, although one does rarely see a patient with a very advanced tumour which has

been neglected for years. The limited penetration of these tumours allows superficial X-rays (100 kV), which treat a depth of less than 1 cm, to be used in most cases. Larger tumours are better treated with electrons which have deeper, but still limited, penetration. For example, 10 MeV electrons will effectively treat a depth of 3 cm, but there is a rapid fall-off of dose beyond this.

The area to be treated must be clearly defined. This will include the tumour with a margin of at least 5 mm all around. An appropriately sized lead cut-out is selected to allow irradiation of this area and to shield the surrounding skin. For irregularly shaped lesions, and for those situated on an uneven contour such as the bridge of the nose or where adjacent structures such as the eye need to be meticulously shielded, the lead cut-out should be prepared individually for each patient. Otherwise a standard cut-out may be used.

The dose and fractionation prescribed depend principally on the size of the tumour. Those smaller than 2–3 cm diameter should receive 35 Gy in five fractions over 1 week and larger ones 45 Gy in 10 fractions over a fortnight. To avoid the need for multiple attendances, frail elderly patients may be given a single 20 Gy treatment, but the control rates and cosmetic results are less good. If there is involvement of the nasal cartilage, and for bulky or deeply penetrating tumours, for example at the columella, more protracted treatment, e.g. 55 Gy in 20 fractions over 4 weeks with electrons, is recommended.

A skin reaction proceeding to moist desquamation will inevitably follow. This can be soothed with zinc and castor oil or 1% hydrocortisone cream. If the ala nasi is treated, there will in addition be a mucosal reaction within the vestibule. A fillet of lead inserted into the nasal cavity will prevent a reaction on the nasal septum. When the area is healed, the patient should be advised to avoid exposing it to direct sunshine, either by wearing a hat with a brim or using a sunblock cream.

Lateral rhinotomy (medial maxillectomy)

Anaesthetic

The patient should be anaesthetized with an oro-endotracheal tube and the head is flexed during the operation. Protect the eyes during the operation by a temporary tarsorrhaphy.

Incision

The incision, usually ascribed to Moure, but actually first described by Michaux in 1848, begins midway between the medial canthus and the bridge of the nose, at the level of the upper border of the pupil; it then continues downwards on the lateral edge of the nose and curves medially below the lower ala to the

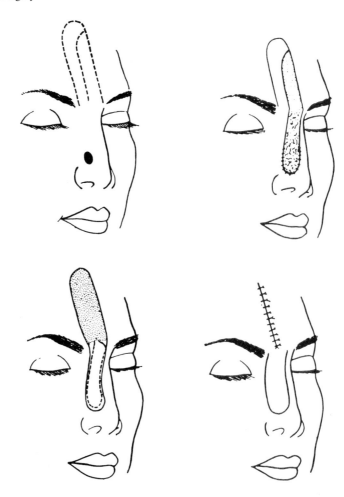

Fig. 13.13 Repair of full thickness defect of nose.

midline at the columella; it does not continue through the upper lip (Fig. 13.14). Make the incision with a knife down to bone, and then elevate the soft tissues from the anterior wall of the antrum laterally, and from the nasal bones medially, with a large periosteal elevator; hold the two flaps apart with a self-retaining retractor (Fig. 13.15).

An alternative incision that is becoming increasingly acceptable is the degloving approach. An incision is made in the gingivolabial sulcus from tuberosity to tuberosity. By combining this with intercartilaginous and full transfixion incisions in the nose it is possible to elevate the facial tissues from the underlying bone up to the frontoethmoid suture line. The access is good, a facial scar is avoided and healing is good.

Excision

Using a 9 mm osteotome, make a cut along the floor of the nose entering the maxillary antrum to the pterygoid plates. Then with a fissure burr, make a cut in the anterior wall of the antrum to just below the orbital floor. With the osteotome, cut up the nasal maxillary suture line to the frontonasal suture (Fig. 13.15). With the 7 mm osteotome, make a cut along the frontoethmoidal suture, having ligated and divided the ethmoidal arteries. Go as far back as the posterior ethmoidal artery in order to stay away from the optic nerve. Complete the excision by dividing

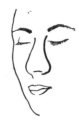

Fig. 13.14 Lateral rhinotomy: Moure's incision.

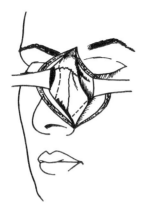

Fig. 13.15 Lateral rhinotomy: flaps elevated.

the orbital floor and freeing the ethmoids from the orbital periosteum. The lateral wall of the nose can now be removed with Mayo scissors, completing the dissection.

Pack the nose with BIPP and close the incisions with 3/0 chormic catgut and 5/0 Nurolon. Remove the pack in 7 days and keep the crests moist in order to ease removal.

Complications

1 General complications.
2 Crusting – this is treated by frequent removal and loosening with 5% propylene glycol nasal drops.
3 Because the nasolacrimal duct has been divided there may be some temporary lacrimation but, as an effective dacrocystorhinostomy has been made, this stops quite quickly.

Partial maxillectomy

Preparation

Prepare the patient's face in the usual way but never shave the eyebrows because they regrow in an irregular fashion. The patient is laid supine on the table with the head extended and a temporary tarsorrhaphy (Fig. 13.17) is done with 5/0 silk. The two sutures are put in in the following way – take a bite of the lower lid and then a bite of the upper lid opposite to the initial stitch; then thread the needle through a piece of thin red rubber catheter to stop the stich cutting into the upper lid. Insert the needle next into the upper lid, then the lower lid, pass it through another red rubber catheter and tie it. Put two such sutures in place.

Do a tracheostomy in the usual way and continue general anaesthesia via this route.

Incision

Mark out a Weber–Fergusson skin incision (Fig. 13.17), starting at the philtrum of the lip on the operative side, and go up to the columella. Then continue round the margin of the ala of the nose and up the lateral border of the nose to the medial corner of the eye. Turn laterally in a rounded fashion to go 5 mm below the lid margin on the lower lid. If you go too near the margin of the lower lid, the patient may get ectropion and if you go too far away he or she may get lymphoedema. The incision is continued to just past the lateral canthus.

Critical suture points are marked, taking great care to mark the vermilion border. Incise with a knife right down to the bone taking the incision inside the mouth and in the gingivobuccal sulcus as far back as the tuberosity of the maxilla. Elevate the cheek flap, including the buccinator muscle, with cutting diathermy but leave the orbicularis oculi muscle intact around the eye.

In some patients it may not be necessary to do the complete Weber–Fergusson incision. If you leave out the part of the incision below the eye, the rest of the incision is known as a Fergusson incision.

An alternative is the degloving approach (see pp. 188 and 265).

Excision

If the patient has upper teeth, remove the upper central incisor on the side of the operation. With a knife, make a stab wound into the nasopharynx at the junction of the hard and soft palate in the midline and pass a pair of right-angled forceps through this. Pass a Gigli saw blade through the nostril on the involved side, pick it up with the forceps and bring it out through the mouth (Fig. 13.18). Now divide the hard palate longitudinally through the floor of the nasal cavity, just lateral to the nasal septum, with the Gigli saw. Then incise across the soft tissues of the posterior edge of the hard palate to the tuberosity of the maxilla, meeting the incision you originally made in the gingivobuccal sulcus. This detaches the soft palate from the hard palate. With a Stryker saw or a fissure burr, divide the nasal process of the maxilla starting in the pyriform aperture and continue to cut just below the orbital rim around to the pterygomaxillary fissure (Fig. 13.19). Mobilize the lateral wall of the nose by dividing, with stout scissors, between the superior and inferior turbinates. In order to gain access to the pterygoid space, divide the temporalis muscle from its attachment to the coronoid process of the mandible, and transect the process at its origin from the ramus of the mandible. Put an osteotome into the pterygomaxillary fissure and divide the pterygoids from the maxilla, which can then be removed, cutting the soft tissue attachments with Mayo scissors (Figs. 13.20 and 13.21).

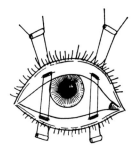

Fig. 13.16 Temporary tarsorrhaphy.

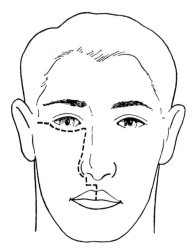

Fig. 13.17 Weber–Fergusson incision.

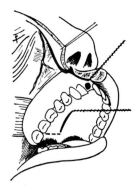

Fig. 13.18 Maxillectomy: division of hard palate.

When the specimen is removed, pack the cavity with warm saline and leave it in place for some time.

Then check the mucosal edges for clearance of tumour by taking a frozen section.

If the patient does not have dentures, pack the

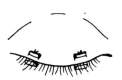

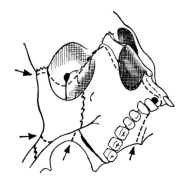

Fig. 13.19 Maxillectomy: sites of division of bony struts.

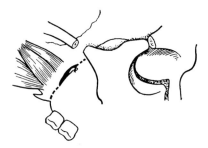

Fig. 13.20 Maxillectomy: separation of pterygoid plates.

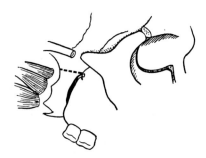

Fig. 13.21 Maxillectomy: division of pterygoid plates.

cavity with Whitehead's varnish and put stay sutures from the palate remnant to the buccal mucosa to keep the pack in place. If he or she has an upper denture, or if a partial upper denture has been made prior to the operation, the pack can be kept in place with this.

Aftercare

1 General care.
2 Remove the pack in 10–14 days. Have a prosthodontist take a provisional impression to make a temporary denture with an obturator. Thereafter the patient is seen by the prosthodontist until a final prosthesis is made.

The prosthesis can be a one-piece or a two-piece model. If it is a two-piece model then the obturator portion is kept in place either with a pivot fixation or with magnets. If it is one-piece, then the obturator portion should be hollow for lightness.

Complications

1 General complications.
2 Notching of the lip. This is caused by an improper closure and atrophy of the orbicularis oris muscle. If it occurs then it can be corrected with a Z-plasty.
3 Granulomas. If the obturator is too large it can create granulomas on originally bare areas in the cavity. These can look like recurrences and should always be removed for biopsy. If they are granulomas, then the obturator needs to be adjusted.

Craniofacial resection

Anaesthesia

It is important to maintain cerebral circulation and to cause shrinkage of the brain for easy manipulation. The patient is given 200 ml of 20% mannitol in 20 min, and also 150 mg hydrocortisone. The arterial pressure is kept at normal or slightly elevated levels. Shrinkage of the brain is also assisted by deliberate hyperventilation.

Incision

The craniotomy can be performed from a bicoronal incision, which gives good access and allows the preparation of a good galeal flap for closure of the defect; but it does tend to get in the way of the facial incision and it takes time to do.

The preferred way is to do the facial incision with a Fergusson approach and to continue this up through the medial canthus on to the forehead up to the hairline (Fig. 13.22). This allows retraction of the frontal bone. It is easier and quicker but it is more difficult to create a satisfactory galeal flap.

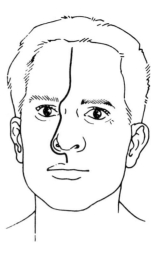

Fig. 13.22 Incision of craniofacial resection: midline forehead incision combined with lateral rhinotomy incision.

Craniotomy

Whichever incision is made, a shield-shaped segment is removed from the frontal bone (Fig. 13.23). Care is taken to make this segment come right down to the floor of the anterior fossa so that one is not working over a ledge. Care is also taken not to cut the dura or to tear it, especially in older patients. It is better not to tear the sagittal sinus at this point or else the bleeding can be very troublesome. The dura is lifted off the cribriform plate and fovea back to the optic foramen, and the optic nerves are visualized. The frontal lobe is then retracted and operability assessed (Fig. 13.24).

Contraindications to further surgery are:

1 Extension of the tumour into the frontal lobes.
2 Extension of the tumour beyond the posterior margin of the cribriform plate.
3 Extension of the tumour to involve both optic nerves.
4 Extension of the tumour laterally outside the boundaries of the fovea.

Maxillectomy

If the operation is to proceed then a maxillectomy is done in keeping with the extent of the tumour. Although it may be possible to retain the palate and even the orbital floor, we will describe here the complete maxillectomy.

Proceed as described in the first part of the partial maxillectomy. With an osteotome, cut up to the frontonasal suture line and then along the frontoethmoidal suture. With a Gigli saw, the zygomatic arch is divided, as is the orbital floor through the inferior orbital fissure. The maxilla is disarticulated from the

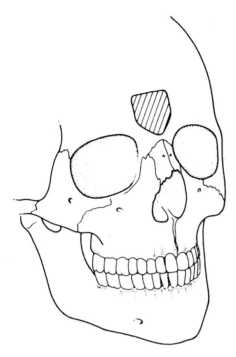

Fig. 13.23 Shield-shaped window cut in frontal bone for access.

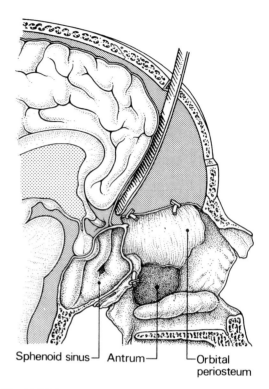

Sphenoid sinus┘ Antrum┘ └Orbital periosteum

Fig. 13.24 Retraction of the frontal lobe to give access to the fovea and cribriform plate.

pterygoid plates or the pterygoid plates can be removed along with the maxilla.

Attention is then turned to the anterior fossa again and cuts are made through the fovea on each side and through the posterior part of the cribriform plate. Cutting through the anterior ethmoid cells allows the whole segment to be removed in a block (Figs. 13.25 and 13.26).

Eye removal or preservation

The decision as to what to do with the eye is made at two points in the operation. If obvious tumour extension through the periosteum is seen in the early part of the maxillectomy, then the eye is included in the resection at this point. If the periosteum is clear, however, along the floor and along the ethmoids, wait until the specimen has been removed and then take frozen sections from the posterior ethmoid in the area of the optic foramina. If these are clear, and if sufficient support remains laterally for the eye, then it can be preserved; but if the support of the eye is damaged, of if there is tumour in the posterior ethmoids, then the eye is removed at this point.

Closure

The dural defect is closed with the fascia lata graft using 5/0 Nurolon for the repair. The repair is

strengthened by cutting a flap of frontalis and galeal aponeurosis, and slipping it under the dura in the anterior fossa. This can be further protected by putting in a cartilage graft from the nasal septum or a bone graft from the iliac crest.

The facial wound is sutured meticulously or else

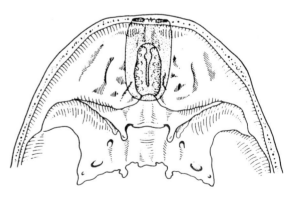

Fig. 13.25 Horizontal section of skull from above to show portion of osteotomy in anterior cranial fossa. Excision line runs through fovea on each side and the posterior wall of the frontal sinus.

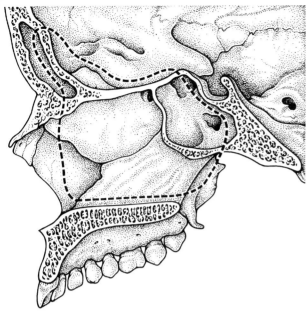

Fig. 13.26 Area of sinus tissue usually removed in a craniofacial excision.

there will be oedema around the inferior part of the orbital wound. A Whitehead's varnish pack is put in place, and the oral defect closed with the patient's own denture or a specially made partial denture.

Aftercare

1 General care – although most head and neck patients get out of bed the next day, it is important that patients who have had their cranial cavities opened remain in bed for some days in the supine position.
2 Antibiotics – because of the danger of meningitis and because the nasal cavity is connected to the anterior fossa, the patient is covered with an antibiotic mixture such as metronidazole and Augmentin (amoxycillin). The metronidazole is continued for 10 days and the Augmentin for 3 weeks.
3 The patient is put on to neurological observations and special note is taken of any change in consciousness levels.
4 Most patients benefit from being on anticonvulsants for at least 1 year after the operation.
5 Cerebrospinal fluid leak – this is expected, but if the closure has been adequate it should not be troublesome and should seal quite quickly. If it does not, consideration has to be given to inserting a lumbar drain or even regrafting.

Complications

1 Sudden death – this has been recorded if patients get up too quickly after this operation.

2 Persistent cerebrospinal fluid leak.
3 Meningitis.
4 Venous bleeding.
5 Convulsions.

Radiotherapy techniques

Tumours of the nasal cavity and sinuses

The techniques used by the radiotherapist for treatment of carcinoma of the nasal fossa, maxillary antrum and ethmoid sinuses are essentially the same whether the plan is to use radical radiotherapy alone, or to give preoperative or postoperative treatment. For radiotherapy planning and treatment the patient lies supine, with the head fixed in a neutral position by an individually prepared beam-directing Perspex shell. The mouth is held open by a block to depress the tongue and lower lip which, by, keeping them out of the treated volume, diminishes the intraoral acute mucosal reaction. The bite block has a central hole which allows the patient to breathe through the mouth during treatment.

The volume to be treated includes the primary site, areas of known tumour extension and also, because of the difficulties of accurate assessment, other routes of potential local spread. This entails treatment of a block of tissue containing the maxilla on the affected side including the alveolus, the whole nasal cavity and ethmoid complex, the pterygopalatine fossa and often the orbit. In the unusual case where there is demonstrable nodal spread, the ipsilateral neck should also be irradiated. The critical structures which must be spared are the contralateral eye, the brainstem and upper cervical cord. The treatment volume is covered by two fields – one anterior, the other lateral.

The anterior field (Fig. 13.27) extends from its upper border at the superior margin of the orbit down to include the hard palate and alveolar ridge. Medially it extends across the midline to the opposite inner canthus, and its lateral border encompasses the gingivobuccal sulcus and cheek. If there is no orbital involvement the ipsilateral cornea, lens and lacrimal gland should be shielded. If it is necessary to treat the orbit, the unpleasant acute corneal reaction can be minimized by cutting a hole in the shell, and treating with the patient's eye open. If the soft tissues of the cheek are involved, wax bolus should be applied over this area of the shell to ensure that the skin receives an adequate dose, otherwise the shell may be cut out to minimize the acute skin reaction over the cheek.

The upper and lower limits of the lateral field (Fig. 13.28) match those of the anterior field. The lateral field extends posteriorly from the lateral orbital margin, that is behind the anterior chamber of the eye, to the anterior margin of the vertebral bodies, thus including the pterygopalatine fossa and lateral

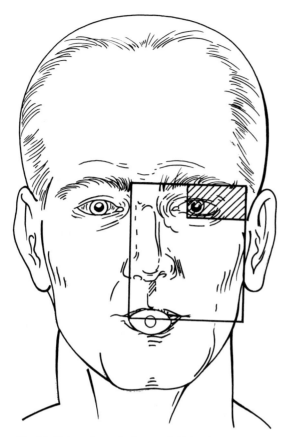

Fig. 13.27 Anterior radiotherapy field for the treatment of a carcinoma of the left maxillary antrum.

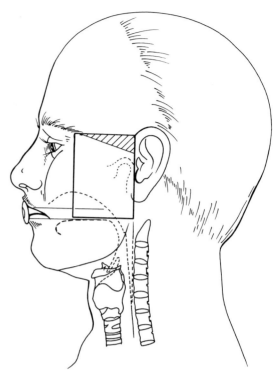

Fig. 13.28 Lateral field for the irradiation of the antrum.

pharyngeal lymph nodes. The upper posterior corner of this field should be blocked, to shield the brain-stem. The lateral field should be angled 5–10° posteriorly, to avoid irradiation of the contralateral eye. To be on the safe side, the dose received by the opposite eye should be checked by thermolumines-cent dosimetry during the first one or two fractions.

Megavoltage X-rays (4–6 MV) should be used. A variety of dose fractionation schedules is in current use, the most popular being 50–55 Gy in 16–20 fractions over 3–4 weeks or 60–65 Gy in 30–32 fractions over 6–6½ weeks.

The principal acute side-effect is mucositis affect-ing the palate and upper alveolus on the treated side. Care should be taken to maintain oral hygiene and ensure that the patient receives adequate nourish-ment. In addition, the patient should be warned that he or she will lose the hair over the back of the head where the anterior beam exits.

A variety of intracavitary techniques has been described for postoperative irradiation or treatment of small local recurrences. A cast is made of the surgical defect in the maxilla. This is loaded with a

suitable radionuclide and worn by the patient for a period calculated to give an appropriate dose. The principal limitation of this method is that there is a rapid fall-off of dose away from the surface of the mould, and so only the relatively superficial tissues are effectively treated.

Controversies in management

Is transitional cell papilloma a premalignant condition?

The problems of evaluating transitional cell papil-loma, as found in the literature, come from vari-ations in the histology, the sample size and, most importantly, in where the papers emanate from. Most of the big series come from tertiary referral centres which see transitional cell papillomas that have become malignant. Three situations can prob-ably exist. The first is that non-keratinizing squamous cell carcinoma and benign inverted papil-loma can occupy the same anatomical region with no evidence that one gives rise to the other. Second, benign inverted papilloma can be treated success-fully and may be followed many years later (up to 20) by carcinoma. Third, there is no doubt that a small proportion (1%) who have inverted papilloma do show a focus of transition into carcinoma.

The pathologist reports an undifferentiated carcinoma

Undifferentiated carcinomas are rare. A similar histological picture is produced by lymphomas, amelanotic melanomas, olfactory neuroblastomas and rhabdomyosarcomas. If you get a report of undifferentiated carcinoma, make sure the pathologist has used tumour markers to see if epidermis really is the origin of the tumour. In this way some apparently untreatable tumours will become treatable.

How do you react when the CT scan shows widespread infiltration of the tumour?

The most important thing is to ask for coronal views of the CT scan as well as axial views. Some patients find it difficult to stay in position long enough to have coronal scanning but only in this way can all the information be available. Blockage of the ostia will often lead to fluid accumulation in the sinuses and this cannot be differentiated from tumour by a CT scan. Similarly, extension of tumours through the bony margins will cause surrounding oedema, which again is indistinguishable from tumour. The authors believe that a CT scan overestimates tumour spread by 30%.

Is there any place for doing a radical maxillectomy with orbital exenteration instead of a craniofacial approach?

In the view of the authors, far more control can be exerted over the management of the eye from above than from below. Coming from below to go to the posterior ethmoids is inherently a very dangerous procedure; with modern anaesthesia and postoperative care, there is very little morbidity in a craniofacial approach.

What do you do if a prosthodontist is not available?

This is a situation that occurs in many parts of the world. There is usually no problem about the oral rehabilitation because there is always somebody in the district who can make an upper denture. At worst, a piece of gutta percha can be moulded into an obturator to sit on top of an ordinary denture. If no eye prosthesis is reconstructed, then the patient should merely wear a black patch over the eye or a pair of dark glasses.

Is it ever worthwhile rehabilitating the orbit with skin flaps?

A smaller cavity can be created by putting in a forehead flap, a sternomastoid flap or a free latissimus dorsi flap. A similar result, however, can be obtained by leaving the eyelids and suturing them together and grafting the underside. There is thus very little place for flap reconstruction of the orbit to make a prosthesis sit better.

Preoperative or postoperative radiotherapy?

If either surgery or radiotherapy alone were able to achieve local control in the majority of patients, then there would be little reason to combine these treatments. However single modality treatment for sinus tumours has an unacceptable failure rate, so radiotherapy and surgery are often combined. Irradiation is capable of eradicating microscopic residual disease which cannot be detected at operation, and surgery can remove bulky tumour which cannot be sterilized by the maximum tolerated radiation dose.

There are several possible advantages of using radiotherapy prior to surgery. Principally, by shrinking the tumour, inoperable cancers may sometimes be rendered operable, or the magnitude of operation necessary may be reduced. Secondly, by sterilizing most tumour cells before opration, it reduces the chance that surgical manipulation may lead to either distant metastasis or local seeding in the operative field. Lastly, radiotherapy is likely to be more effective without the hypoxia which may be caused by tissue disruption during surgery. A policy of preoperative irradiation has been shown in laboratory animals to be superior to one of postoperative treatment. The claimed disadvantage of preoperative radiotherapy that surgical complications may be increased, either directly or because the patient has been allowed to become malnourished, has perhaps been overstated. Another disadvantage of giving preoperative treatment is that a patient who has a good initial response to irradiation (or one who finds the morbidity unacceptable) may refuse to undergo the preplanned surgery, and therefore lose the best chance of successful treatment.

One important benefit of initial surgery is that tumour extent will be more precisely known than is otherwise possible. Also, wound healing will not be impaired by prior irradiation. In addition, there should be only microscopic residual disease, which is more easily eradicated by irradiation than gross disease. A major problem is that if the start of postoperative radiotherapy is delayed by prolonged wound healing, the chances of achieving local control are diminished.

While local control of sinonasal tumours is improved by the use of combined modality treatment, there is little hard clinical evidence to show that preoperative radiotherapy gives better results than postoperative treatment, or vice versa. A pragmatic policy is to use preoperative irradiation where there is doubt about the resectability of the tumour, surgery first for patients with clearly operable lesions and radical radiotherapy alone for patients whose general condition precludes major surgery. Once a treatment policy has been determined for an individual patient, it is usually better to stick with it. For example, to cancel an operation because of an unusually good response to preoperative radiotherapy is to court disaster.

Management of tumours of the septum and vestibule

These tumours can be described as bad actors. They present as small indolent ulcers and there is a long diagnostic delay. The septum and the vestibule are lined by cartilage and thin squamous epithelium, and have a rich lymphatic drainage. Thirty per cent of these tumours have metastatic nodes, and invasion of cartilage and of cervical nodes. Thus the prognosis is below 10%. All histological types of tumour can occur in the area and there is no best treatment. Most series have been small, and there seems to be no difference in survival between primary surgery, primary radiotherapy or a combined treatment. The overall survival rate is between 20 and 30%. Surgical excision of the area presents a horrendous defect because it usually involves the upper lip. The basic reconstruction is of the external nose and the upper lip with an Abbe flap, and an external prosthesis or forehead flap.

Sinus tumours in children

Most sinus tumours in children are benign. Rhabdomyosarcomas are the most common malignant neoplasm and are treated with wide excision, radiotherapy and chemotherapy. Those with parameningeal involvement have the worst prognosis and are treated with intrathecal chemotherapy and craniospinal irradiation.

Prosthetic problems

Immediately after the excision a temporary obturator made of stent or gutta percha attached to a previously prepared upper denture is placed in the defect. The obturator material can be encouraged to stick to the upper denture by wires set in the upper surface of the denture. Grafting of the cavity is rarely necessary. The obturator should be left for 2 weeks and the denture and obturator should be removed under general anaesthesia. Care should be taken at this point not to split the lip if a Weber–Fergusson incision has been used. An impression is taken of the cavity and thereafter further fittings are done in the prosthodontist's office. The prosthodontist should try to create as large a prosthesis as possible to keep the facial contour, but small enough for the patient to be able to remove and clean it. It is better if the obturator is hollow for lightness. It can be fixed on to the denture either by studs or by magnets or may form an integral part of it.

The eye presents a greater difficulty to the prosthodontist. If the orbit is exenterated and no facial skin is removed then it is preferred practice to sew the lids together after excising the eyelashes and to graft the undersurface with a split-thickness skin graft. In this way a shallow depression is created in the area over which the patient can wear a black patch. Alternatively, the prosthodontist can create a shallow prosthesis containing an artificial eye held on by spectacle frames.

If the eyelids are removed a sternomastoid myocutaneous flap can be used to close the defect. Recent advances with osseointegrated systems have considerably improved prosthetic attachments.

References and further reading

Acheson E D, Cowdell R H, Hadfield E, Macbeth R G (1968) Nasal cancer in woodworkers in the furniture industry. *Br Med J* ii:587–96.

Allen A C, Spitz S (1953) Malignant melanoma. *Cancer* 1–45.

Ash J E, Old J W (1950) Hemangiomas of the nasal septum. *Trans Am Acad Ophthalmol Otolaryngol* 54:350–6.

Atallah N, Jay M M (1981) Osteomas of the paranasal sinuses. *J Laryngol Otol* 95:291–304.

Bailey B J, Barton S (1975) Olfactory neuroblastoma. Management and progress. *Arch Otolaryngol* 101:1–5.

Bankaci M, Myers E N, Du Bois P (1979) Angiosarcoma of maxillary sinus. *Head Neck Surg* 1:274–80.

Barton R T H, Hogetveit A C H (1980) Nickel-related cancers of the respiratory tract. *Cancer* 45:3061–4.

Batsakis J G (1970) Mucous gland tumors of the nose and paranasal sinuses. *Ann Otolaryngol* 79:557–62.

Bernstein J M, Montgomery W W, Balogh K (1966) Metastatic tumors to the maxilla, nose, and paranasal sinuses. *Laryngoscope* 76:621–50.

Bloch D M, Bragoli A J, Collins D N, Batsakis J G (1979) Mesenchymal chondrosarcomas of the head and neck. *J Laryngol Otol* 93:405–12.

Calcaterra T A, Thompson J H, Pagha D E (1980) Inverting papillomas of the nose and paranasal sinuses. *Laryngoscope* 90:53–60.

Compagno J, Hyams V J (1976) Hemangiopericytoma-like intranasal tumors; a clinicopathological study of 23 cases. *Am J Clin Pathol* 66:672–83.

Compagno J, Wong RT (1977) Intranasal mixed tumors (pleomorphic adenomas): a clinicopathologic study of 40 cases. *Am J Clin Pathol* 68:213–18.

Conley J (1966) Cancer of the skin of the nose. *Arch Otolaryngol* 84:55–60.

Conley J, Dingman D L (1974) Adenoid cystic carcinoma in the head and neck (cylindroma). *Arch Otolaryngol* 100:81–90.

Damjanov I, Maenza R M, Snyder G G, Ruiz J W, Toomay J M (1978) Juvenile ossifying fibroma. *Cancer* 42:2668–74.

Dodd G D, Jing B S (1972) Radiographic findings in adenoid cystic carcinoma of the head and neck. *Ann Otol Rhinol Laryngol* 81:591–8.

Eichel B S, Harrison E G, Devine K D, Scanline P, Brown H (1966) Primary lymphoma of the nose, including a relationship to lethal midline granuloma. *Am J Surg* **112**:597–605.

Enzinger F M, Weiss S H (1983) Soft tissue tumors. St Louis, CV Mosby.

Friedmann I, Osborn DA (1965) Metastatic tumours in the ear, nose and throat region. *J Laryngol Otol* 576–87.

Friedmann I, Osborn D A (1982) *Pathology of Granulomas and Neoplasms of the Nose and Paranasal Sinuses* London, Churchill Livingstone.

Fu Y S, Perzin K H (1974) Non-epithelial tumors of the nasal cavity, paranasal sinuses and nasopharynx: a clinico-pathologic study, I: general features and vascular tumors. *Cancer* **33**, 1275–88.

Fu Y S, Perzin K H (1974) Non-epithelial tumors of the nasal cavity, paranasal sinuses and nasopharynx: a clinico-pathologic study, II: osseous and fibro-osseous lesions, including osteomas, fibrous dysplasia, ossifying fibromas, osteoblastoma, giant cell tumor and osteosarcoma. *Cancer* **33**:1289–1305.

Fu Y S, Perzin K H (1974) Non-epithelial tumors of the nasal cavity, paranasal sinuses and nasopharynx: a clinico-pathologic study, III: cartilaginous tumors (chondroma, chrondrosarcoma). *Cancer* **34**:453–63.

Fu Y S, Perzin K H (1975) Non-epithelial tumors of the nasal cavity, paranasal sinuses and nasopharynx: a clinico-pathologic study, IV: smooth muscle tumors. *Cancer* **35**:1300–8.

Fu Y S, Perzin K H (1976) Non-epithelial tumors of the nasal cavity, paranasal sinuses and nasopharynx: a clinico-pathologic study, V; skeletal muscle tumors (rhabdomyoma and rhabdomysarcoma). *Cancer* **37**:364–76.

Fu Y S, Perzin K H (1976) Non-epithelial tumors of the nasal cavity, paranasal sinuses and nasopharynx: a clinico-pathologic study, VI: fibrous tissue tumors. *Cancer* **37**:2912–28.

Fu Y S, Perzin K H (1977) Non-epithelial tumors of the nasal cavity, paranasal sinuses and nasopharynx: a clinico-pathologic study, VII: myxomas. *Cancer* **39**:195–203.

Games-Araujo J J, Ayala A G, Guillamondevi O (1975) Mucinous adenocarcinomas of nose and paranasal sinuses. *Cancer* **36**:1100–5.

Gaze M N, Kerr G R, Smyth J F (1990) Mucosal melanomas of the head and neck: The Scottish experience. *Clin Oncol* **2**: 277–83.

Garrington G E, Scofield H H, Cornyn J, Hooker S P (1967) Osteosarcoma of the jaws. *Cancer* **20**:377–91.

Gibson T, Walker F M (1951) Large osteoma of the frontal sinus. *Br J Plast Surg* **4**:210–17.

Goepfert H, Guillamondegni O M, Jesse R H, Lindberg R D (1974) Squamous cell carcinoma of nasal vestibule. *Arch Otolaryngol* **100**:8–10.

Goepfert H, Luna M A, Lindberg R D, White A K (1983) Malignant salivary gland tumors of the paranasal sinuses and nasal cavity. *Arch Otolaryngol* **109**:662–8.

Hallberg O E , Begley J W (1950) Origin and treatment of osteomas of the paranasal sinuses. *Arch Otolaryngol* **51**:750–60.

Hardwood A R, Knowling M A, Bergsagez D E (1981) Radiotherapy of extra-medullary plasmacytoma of the head and neck. *Clin Radiol* **32**:31–6.

Harrison D F N (1977) Lateral rhinotomy: a neglected operation. *Ann Otol Rhinol Laryngol* **86**:756–9.

Harrison D F N (1978) Critical look at the classification of maxillary sinus carcinomata. *Ann Otol Rhinol Laryngol* **87**:1–7.

Harrison D F N (1984) Osseous and fibro-osseous conditions affecting the cranio-facial bones. *Ann Otol Rhinol Laryngol* **93**:199–203.

Harrison D F N (1984) Surgical pathology of olfactory neuroblastoma. *Head Neck Surg* **7**:60–4.

Harrison D F N (1987) Some thoughts on the natural history, pathogenesis and management of juvenile angio-fibroma. *Arch Otolaryngol* **113**:936–42.

Holdcraft J, Gallagher J C (1969) Malignant melanomas of the nasal and paranasal sinus mucosae. *Ann Otol Rhinol Laryngol* **78**:1–20.

Howard D J, Lund V J (1985) Ewing's sarcoma of the ethmoid sinuses. *J Laryngol Otol* **99**:1019–23.

Howard D J, Lund V J (1985) Reflections on adenoid cystic carcinoma of the nose and sinuses. *Otolaryngol Head Neck Surg* 338–40.

Hyams V J (1971) Papillomas of the nasal cavity and paranasal sinuses: a clinicopathological study of 315 cases. *Ann Otol Rhinol Laryngol* **80**:192–206.

Hyams V J, Batsakis J G, Michaels L (1988) Tumors of the upper respiratory tract and ear. (Atlas of tumor pathology, 2nd ser, fasc 25) Washington, Armed Forces Institute of Pathology.

Iwamura S, Sugiura S, Nora Y (1972) Schwannoma of the nasal cavity. *Arch Otolaryngol* **96**:176–7.

Kapadia S B, Desai U, Chen V S (1982) Extramedullary plasmacytoma of the head and neck: a clinicopathologic study of 26 cases. *Medicine* **61**:317–29.

Karma P, Rasanen O, Karja J (1977) Nasal gliomas: a review and report of 2 cases. *Laryngoscope* **87**:1169–70.

Katz A, Lewis J S (1971) Nasal gliomas. *Arch Otolaryngol* **94**:351–5.

Kilby D, Ambegoakar A G (1977) The nasal chondroma. *J Laryngol Otol* **91**:415–26.

Kjeldsberg C R, Minckler J (1972) Meningiomas presenting as nasal polyps. *Cancer* **29**:153–6.

Lederman M (1970) Tumours of the upper jaw: natural history and treatment. *J Laryngol Otol* **84**:369–401.

Lewis J S, Hutter R V P, Tollefsen H R, Foote F W Jr (1965) Nasal tumors of olfactory origin. *Arch Otolaryngol* **81**:169–73.

Lund V J (1983) Tumours of the nasal cavity and the paranasal sinuses. *Otorhinolaryngology* **45**:1–12.

Michaels L (1987) *Ear, Nose and Throat Histopathology*. London, Springer.

Michaels L, Hyams V I (1975) Objectivity in the classification of tumours of the nasal epithelium. *Postgrad Med J* **51**:655–707.

Oberman H A, Rice D H (1976) Olfactory neuroblastoma. *Cancer* **38**:2494–502.

Ohngren L G (1933) Malignant tumours of the maxillo-ethmoidal region: a clinical study with special reference to the treatment with electrosurgery and irradiation. *Acta Otolaryngol* **19**(suppl):1–112.

Osborn D A (1970) Nature and behavior of transitional tumors in the upper respiratory tract. *Cancer* **25**:50–60.

Osborn D A (1977) Morphology and the natural history of cribriform adenocarcinoma (adenoid cystic carcinoma). *J Clin Pathol* **30**:195–205.

Perzin K H, Fu Y S (1980) Non-epithelial tumors of the nasal cavity, paranasal sinuses and nasopharynx: a clinico-pathologic study, XI: fibrous histiocytomas. *Cancer* **45**:2616–26.

Perzin J H, Gullane P, Clairmont A C (1978) Adenoid cystic carcinomas arising in salivary glands: a correlation of histological features and clinical course. *Cancer* **42**:265–82.

Perzin K H, Cantor J O, Johannessen J V (1981) Acinic cell carcinoma arising in the nasal cavity: report of a case with ultrastructural observations. *Cancer* **47**:1818–22.

Rice D H, Batsakis J G, Headington J T, Boles R (1974) Fibrous histiocytomas of the nose and paranasal sinuses. *Arch Otolaryngol* **100**:398–401.

Ringertz N (1938) Pathology of malignant tumors arising in the nasal and paranasal cavities and maxilla. *Acta Otolaryngol* (suppl) **17**:1–405.

Robin P E, Powell D J (1980) Regional node involvement and distant metastases in carcinoma of the nasal cavity and paranasal sinuses. *J Laryngol Otol* **94**:301–9.

Robin P E, Powell D J, Stansbie J M (1979) Carcinoma of the nasal cavity and paranasal sinuses: incidence and presentation of different histological types. *Clin Otolaryngol* **4**:431–56.

Robitaille Y, Seemayer T A, El Deiry A (1975) Peripheral nerve tumors involving paransasal sinuses: a case report and review of literature. *Cancer* **35**:1254–8.

Sehdev M K, Huvos A G, Strong E W, Gerold F P, Willis G W (1974) Ameloblastoma of maxilla and mandible. **33**:324–33.

Shah J P, Huvos A G, Strong E W (1977) Mucosal melanomas of the head and neck. *Am J Surg* **134**:531–5.

Spiro R H, Koss L G, Hajdu S I, Strong E W (1973) Tumors of minor salivary origin: a clinicopathologic study of 492 cases. *Cancer* **31**:117–29.

Tabb H G, Barranco S J (1971) Cancer of the maxillary sinus: an analysis of 108 cases. *Laryngoscope* **81**:818–27.

Weiss S W, Enzinger F M (1978) Malignant fibrous histiocytoma. *Cancer* **41**:2250–66.

Wilhelmsson B, Hellquist H, Olofsson J, Klintenberg C (1985) Nasal cuboidal metaplasia and dysplasia: precursor to adenocarcinoma in wood-dust exposed workers? *Acta Otolaryngol* **99**:641–8.

Woodson G E, Robbins K T, Michaels L (1985) Inverted papilloma: considerations in treatment. *Arch Otolaryngol* **111**:806–11.

Radiology

Lloyd G A S (1988) Diagnostic imaging of the nose and paranasal sinuses. London, Springer.

Lund V J, Howard D J, Lloyd G (1983) CT evaluation of paranasal sinus tumours for craniofacial resection. *Br J Radiol* **56**:439–46.

Lund V J, Howard D J, Lloyd G A S, Cheesman A D (1989) Magnetic resonance imaging of paransasal sinus tumors for craniofacial resection. *Head Neck Surg* **11**:279–83.

Lund V J, Lloyd G (1984) Radiological changes associated with inverted papilloma of the nose and paranasal sinuses. *Br J Radiol* **57**:455–61.

Management

Barbosa J F (1961) Surgery of extensive cancer of paranasal sinuses. *Arch Otolaryngol* **73**:129–38.

Chung C T, Rabuzzi D D, Sagerman R H et al. (1980) Radiotherapy for carcinoma of the nasal cavity. *Arch Otol* **106**:763–6.

Frazell E (1955) The surgical treatment of cancer of the paranasal sinuses. *Laryngoscope* **65**:557.

Kagan A R, Nassbaum H, Rao A (1981) The management of carcinoma of the nasal vestibule. *Head Neck Surg* **4**:125–8.

Ketcham A S, Wilkins J M, Van Buren J M et al (1963) A combined intracranial facial approach to the paranasal sinuses. *Am J Surg* **106**:698.

Ketcham A S, Hoye R C, Van Buren J M et al. (1966) Complications of intracranial facial resection for tumors of the paranasal sinuses. *Am J Surg* **112**:591.

Ketcham A S, Chretien P B, Van Buren J M, Hoye R C, Beazley R M, Herdt J R (1973) The ethmoid sinuses: a re-evaluation of surgical excision. *Am J Surg* **126**:469–76.

Lund V J, Harrison D F N (1988) Craniofacial resection for tumors of the nasal cavity and paranasal sinuses. *Am J Surg* **156**: 187–90.

Manson P W, Carmella M, Clifford M A, Iliff N T, Morgan R (1985) Mechanisms of global support and post traumatic enophthalmos, I: the anatomy of the ligament sling and its relation to intramuscular cone orbital fat. *Plast Reconst Surg* **77**:193–202.

Myers E N, Schramm V L, Barnes E L (1981) Management of inverted papilloma of the nose and paranasal sinuses. *Laryngoscope* **91**:2071–84.

McCarten A B (1963) The combined transzygomatic approach in resection of maxilla. *Am J Surg* **106**:696–7.

New S B (1918) The use of heat and radium in the treatment of cancer of the jaws and cheeks. *JAMA* **71**:1369.

Schall L A (1951) Malignant neoplasms of the nase, paranasal sinuses and nasopharynx: evaluation of surgical treatment. *Trans Am Acad Ophthalmol Otolaryngol* **55**:209–13.

Schram V L, Myers E N (1978) Lateral rhinotomy. *Laryngoscope* **88**:1042–5.

Shaw H J (1966) Combined therapy for cancer of the upper jaw and paranasal sinuses. *J Laryngol Otol* **80**:105.

Sisson G A (1970) Symposium treatment of malignancies of the paranasal sinuses. *Laryngoscope* **80**:945.

Smith R R, Klopp C T, Williams J M (1954) Surgical treatment of cancer of the frontal sinus and adjacent areas. *Cancer* **7**:991.

Tabb H G (1959) Maxillectomy in carcinoma of the antrum. *Laryngoscope* **69**:119.

Urban C, Rosen G, Huvos A G et al. (1983) Chemotherapy of malignant fibrous histiocytoma of bone. *Cancer* **51**:795–802.

Walker E H, Snow J B (1969) Management of melanoma of nose and paranasal sinuses. *Arch Otolaryngol* **89**:652–70.

14

Tumours of the ear

Surgical anatomy

Auricle

The skin of the lateral surface of the auricle is tightly bound down to the yellow elastic cartilaginous framework, whereas the skin on the medial surface is much looser, due to the subcutaneous layer. The skin immediately behind the postaural crease is free from large hair follicles and so is useful for full-thickness skin grafts. A wedge of the helix of the auricle can be removed either for a composite graft or for tumour excision, with easy primary closure involving little alteration in the shape of the ear. As the skin is so closely applied to the perichondrium, excision of part of the auricle must involve a marginally greater removal of cartilage than skin, in order to secure an accurate repair.

External auditory meatus (Fig. 14.1)

The eternal auditory canal can be subdivided into two parts:

1 A cartilaginous portion: tumours arising here spread easily because the cartilaginous walls present little resistance; spread may be anteriorly into the parotid gland or posteriorly into the postauricular sulcus. The cartilage of the external auditory canal is an inward prolongation of the cartilage of the pinna, so that tumours may readily spread in this cartilaginous layer outwards into the concha.
2 The bony portion of the canal: this is surrounded by dense bone, which provides an effective barrier to spread of the tumour that is then deflected along the canal into the middle ear.

Middle ear and mastoid (Fig. 14.2)

The middle ear and mastoid may be divided into two parts: petromastoid and tubotympanic.

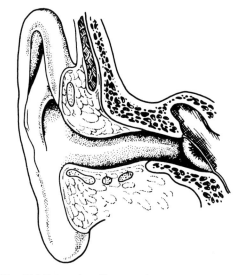

Fig. 14.1 External auditory meatus.

Petromastoid tumours

The petromastoid unit includes the tympanic cavity and the mastoid antrum. Tumours arising here may include those:

1 limited to the tympanic cavity;
2 limited to the mastoid antrum;
3 involving the tympanic cavity and mastoid antrum;
4 involving the tympanic cavity and external auditory canal.

Descriptions of the pathological anatomy in these cases rest on the descriptions of normal anatomy. Almost all carcinomas of the middle ear arise in patients with long-standing chronic otitis media who have usually undergone previous mastoidectomy. The anatomy is then very different from the normal state and this factor contributes largely to the poor prognosis in these patients. Superiorly, the mastoid

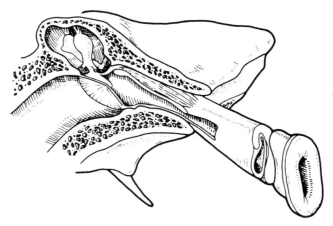

Fig. 14.2 Middle ear and eustachian tube.

cavity is bounded by the thin tegmen tympani, which may have been breached at previous surgery. Medially, the promontory of the middle ear is usually exposed, with two important practical results: first, the facial nerve is either exposed or covered only by a thin layer of bone in its intratympanic course so that facial paralysis is a frequent accompaniment of disease in this area; second, there are several pathways readily available for medial spread of the tumour into the petrous apex. The oval and round windows are theoretical pathways, but more important is the track of cells leading above, below and behind the labyrinth into the petrous apex. The tumour thus gains access to the petrous pyramid lying medial to the bend of the internal carotid artery.

In the patient who has undergone a mastoidectomy, the tumour has ready access to the base of the skull, particularly the jugular foramen, and this fact is one explanation for the paralysis of the lower cranial nerves. An alternative explanation is metastasis to the node situated over the transverse process of the atlas in the lateral compartment of the parapharyngeal space.

Postmortem examinations of patients who died of middle ear carcinoma have shown the possible pathways of spread of middle ear carcinoma. In addition to local invasion of the remnants of the ossicles, the stapedius muscle and the facial canal, there are two important directions of spread. The first is within the eustachian tube; the medial bony wall of the eustachian tube and the associated bony wall of the middle ear cavity are separated from the carotid canal by a thin layer of bone, and this appears to be a frequent route of spread of tumours to the carotid canal. Second, the tumour spreads into the mastoid air cells, penetrates the thin bony wall of the posterior group of air spaces and thus reaches the internal auditory meatus. The structures in the labyrinth are remarkably resistant to the tumour.

Tubotympanic tumours

These tumours either arise in the middle ear and spread into the bony eustachian tube or may even arise within the tube itself. The bony portion of the eustachian tube is anatomically part of the tympanic cavity and has been termed the protympanum. Tumour probably spreads within the surrounding fascial space rather than along the tube. Invasion of these fascial spaces gives the tumour access to the trigeminal or occulomotor nerves in the lateral wall of the cavernous sinus.

Lymphatic drainage

The lymphatic drainage of the external auditory meatus follows the same course as that of the auricle, that is, it may go in one of three directions:

1 anteriorly to the parotid lymph glands, especially to the gland in front of the tragus;
2 inferiorly to the lymph glands that lie along the external jugular vein and those under the sternomastoid muscle;
3 posteriorly to the mastoid lymph nodes.

The lymphatics of the middle ear and mastoid are less well-defined. Anatomical texts state that the lymph vessels are arranged, like the blood vessels, in two sets on the medial and lateral surface of the tympanic membrane. However, in virtually all patients with carcinoma of the middle ear, the tympanic membrane has been destroyed. The lymphatic pathways in such patients do not appear to have been defined, but are probably sparse, as is shown by the paucity of lymph node metastases in this disease.

Pathology

A classification of primary and secondary tumours of the ear is given in Table 14.1.

The commonest tumour of the auricle is carcinoma, which may be either squamous cell or basal cell, their respective incidences varying from country to country. Both are commoner in adult men and present as a warty lesion or an ulcer, usually on the helix. They must be distinguished from the benign tumours such as epithelioma adenoides cysticum, molluscum contagiosum and naevus, and this is done by biopsy. Basal cell tumours do not metastasize, but squamous cell tumours metastasize to the pre- and postauricular nodes.

Only epithelial tumours of the external and middle ear will be discussed in this chapter; the mesodermal tumours, notably the glomus tumour, are no longer the province of the head and neck surgeon but are dealt with by an otologist. However, some of the techniques described under petrosectomy may be applicable to this tumour.

External auditory canal

Squamous carcinoma

Squamous carcinoma constitutes about 90% of all malignant tumours. It can originate in any portion of

Table 14.1 Primary and secondary tumours of the ear

Benign tumours	Malignant tumours
Epithelial	Epithelial
Primary cholesteatoma (primary cholesteatoma, choristoma, adenoma)	Squamous cell carcinoma Adenocarcinoma (hidradenocarcinoma)
Mesenchymal	
Jugulotympanic paraganglioma (glomus jugulare tumour, chemodectoma)	Melanoma Basal cell carcinoma Sebaceous cell carcinoma
Osteoma	Mesenchymal
Haemangioma	Sarcoma
Neurogenic tumours	Multiple myeloma
Xanthoma	Haemangioendothelioma
Giant cell tumour	Malignant xanthoma
Benign osteoblastoma	

Secondary tumours	
Direct extension from:	Distant metastases from:
Nasopharynx	Kidney
External ear	Lung
Parotid	Prostate
Meningioma	Breast
	Thyroid

the external auditory meatus but most often arises in the bony rather than in the cartilaginous portion. Most tumours develop slowly, although occasionally rapid growth is seen.

Invasion of the cartilage of the membranous portion is usually a late development. As the cartilage provides a barrier, extension is usually along the perichondrium. The tympanic membrane limits spread of the disease, but eventually weakens and breaks down, allowing invasion of the middle ear. Facial nerve paralysis develops when the middle ear and mastoid have been involved. Squamous cell carcinoma extends through the cartilaginous and bony walls of the canal late in the disease, invading the surrounding parotid gland anteriorly or the sternomastoid muscle insertion inferiorly and posteriorly.

Metastasis to cervical lymph nodes from squamous cell carcinoma in this area is a late manifestation of the disease, occurring in about 20% of patients. Lesions in the posterior wall of the canal usually metastasize to the nodes in the subcutaneous tissue overlying the insertion of the sternomastoid muscle. Tumours originating in the inferior portion of the canal generally metastasize directly into the subdigastric (jugulodigastric) lymph nodes, while those originating in the anterior portion of the canal metastasize to the preauricular lymph nodes lying in the parotid gland.

Adenocarcinoma

The so-called ceruminous glands of the external auditory meatus are typical apocrine sweat glands. Their secretion is a watery fluid devoid of lipids. These glands do not secrete the wax of the meatus, which is produced by sebaceous glands, and their title is therefore not justified. Tumours arising from these ceruminous glands may be divided into adenomata, mucoepidermoid carcinoma, adenoid cystic carcinoma and adenocarcinoma.

The term hidradenoma and ceruminoma are synonymous, and either may be used as a blanket term for all these benign and malignant tumours. Hidradenoma is a better term; ceruminoma is a misnomer because the ceruminous glands are modified sweat glands.

Hydradenomata have two histological features of diagnostic significance: first, a two-layered epithelial structure, analogous to that of a normal sweat gland, consisting of an inner oxyphilic columnar layer and an outer myoepithelial layer. The second is a variable degree of interglandular stroma. They may also have a papillary or a cystic pattern. They cause obstruction but seldom pain. An adenoma which is clearly benign requires local excision.

For *mucoepidermoid carcinoma* wide excision of the entire external auditory canal, radical mastoidectomy, excision of the mandibular condyle and total parotidectomy with preservation of the facial nerve are recommended.

Adenoid cystic carcinoma is by far the most common ceruminous tumour and resembles the tumour found elsewhere. It causes pain, and has a long natural history ranging from 10 to 30 years, terminating in death from local invasion or distant metastases. Radiotherapy has little to offer these patients and the recommended treatment is wide excision of the external auditory canal and surrounding bone, part of the pinna, extended radical mastoidectomy, excision of the dura, total parotidectomy, and excision of the mandibular condyle and any involved surrounding structures.

Finally, simple *adenocarcinoma* may occur; it has a wide histological spectrum of glandular adenoid tubular and adenoid cystic patterns. The basic pattern is that of adenocarcinoma with two-layered eosinophilic glands. This tumour infiltrates widely into the middle ear, mastoid, etc. It is a very aggressive disease, often presenting with facial paralysis, and usually proving fatal within 4 years.

Malignant melanoma

Malignant melanoma is exceedingly rare; only one authentic tumour arising primarily in the meatus has been recorded.

Basal cell carcinoma

Basal cell carcinoma arising primarily in the external auditory meatus is rare. It tends to affect the sexes equally and occurs in late middle life. Good results can be obtained by sleeve resection. The prognosis is favourable.

Sebaceous tumours

Sebaceous cell carcinoma is extremely uncommon; fewer than 100 cases affecting any part of the body have been described. These tumours may arise anywhere but their greatest concentration is in the head and neck, mainly on the concha and nose. There are three types:

1 sebaceous adenoma;
2 basal cell carcinoma with sebaceous differentiation;
3 true sebaceous carcinoma.

One case has been reported affecting the ear.

Middle ear

Choristoma

A choristoma is a mass of normal tissue at an abnormal site. Seven salivary gland choristomata of the middle ear have been reported – six were in

females. The tumours all presented with deafness, usually lifelong, and many patients showed other anomalies of the middle ear, such as absence of the stapes and an abnormal course of the facial nerve. Attempts to remove the tumour were abandoned in most cases because it was attached to the facial nerve, and because other middle ear structures could not be identified.

Benign adenoma

Benign adenomata of the middle ear have recently been reported. The tumour incidence is divided equally between the sexes with a maximum age incidence between 40 and 50 years. The main symptom is unilateral progressive deafness, and the principal clinical finding is a conductive hearing loss. The external canal is usually normal, and the tympanic membrane intact in 75% of patients; 25% have a perforation through which the middle ear tumour can often be seen. Preoperative radiology shows a mass in the middle ear or mastoid, but no bone destruction.

Some adenocarcinomata of the middle ear, previously described, may have been benign adenomata, which would explain the unusually good prognosis reported for adenocarcinoma in some series.

Adenocarcinoma

If glandular tumours of the external ear are rare, such tumours of the middle ear are even rarer. This is interesting as the middle ear is lined by glandular epithelium. Thirteen patients have been reported in the literature, with a female predominance and a median age of onset of about 40 years. Deafness, pain and facial paralysis were the presenting symptoms in decreasing order of frequency. Most were treated by mastoidectomy followed by radiotherapy. The prognosis was quite good: 6 out of 8 patients were alive at 2 years.

Squamous carcinoma

Virtually all malignant epithelial tumours of the middle ear are squamous in type. As the tumour grows it cases extensive bony destruction. The petrous pyramid and especially the labyrinth resist invasion longer than other structures. The pathway of least resistance is through the thin roof of the middle ear into the middle cranial fossa. The dura itself provides a strong barrier and the most common pathway of transdural invasion is along the seventh and eighth nerves in the internal auditory canal, and the petrosal nerve. The temporomandibular joint and the parotid gland may be involved relatively early. Involvement of the 9th, 10th, 11th and 12th cranial nerves indicates extension into the neck and along the base of the skull. The tumour may also extend along the eustachian tube to the nasopharynx. These clearly preclude resection *en bloc*.

Lymph node metastases occur in 10–15% of cases and about 10% develop a node metastasis later. Distant metastases are rare but have been reported in the liver, brain, lung and bones.

The cause of death in most cases is cachexia due to a combination of intolerable pain, opiates and cranial nerve involvement. Occasionally, invasion of the meninges leads to fatal intracranial complications; erosion of the jugular bulb or carotid artery may cause terminal haemorrhage.

Staging

Neither the International Union against Cancer (UICC) nor the American Joint Committee (AJC) has developed a staging system for carcinoma of the ear. Based on the criteria used for other sites, the classification given in Table 14.2 seems to be a reasonable suggestion. This staging system significantly predicts survival in carcinoma of the ear.

Epidemiology

Incidence

Incidence figures for the UK only became available in 1967. The age-adjusted incidence (registration of new cases) rate has remained steady at about 1/million per year for women and 0.8/million per year for men. The male:female sex ratio is also stable, at about 1:1.2.

Mortality

The age-adjusted mortality rates are similar for each sex but there is a falling trend for men which has resulted in a decrease in the male:female sex ratio between 1960 and 1980 from 1.2:1 to about 1:2.

Mortality from cancer of the middle ear for the 10-year cohorts born around 1881–1921 reveals a marked difference between men and women. Each

male cohort has experienced a lower age-specific mortality than the preceding cohort, while there has been no apparent change in the age-specific death rates for successive female cohorts. In men, the mortality decreases after 70–75 years of age, whereas the mortality continues to rise for women. The falling trend in mortality for men but not for women may be due to exposure to an occupational carcinogen, which was the cause of the relatively high rate in men in the 19th century. Also, these men were involved in the 1914–18 war and it has been shown that mustard gas is associated with a higher risk of death from neoplasm of the respiratory tract (including paranasal sinuses) than expected.

Aetiology

External auditory meatus

The most commonly discussed aetiological factor is chronic inflammation. Irradiation injury in the form of repeated treatment of external otitis has also been mentioned. Highly speculative uninvestigated causes include carcinogens produced by the indigenous microbial flora. Aflatoxin B, a potent hepatic carcinogen, is produced by *Aspergillus flavus*, an occasional transient contaminant of the ear canal. Equally speculative is the production of carcinogens within cerumen. If chronic inflammation and infection are important it is curious that carcinomata arising in patients with long-standing chronic otitis media always do so in the remnants of the middle ear cleft and never in the external auditory canal over which the discharge also flows.

Tumours of the ear can be chemically induced in animals. One dose of azoxymethane (a derivative of dimethylhydrazine) injected into rats induces squamous cell carcinoma of the sebaceous glands of the external auditory meatus in about 15% of animals. Epidermoid carcinomas develop spontaneously in the external canal and middle ear of elderly female gerbils.

Middle ear

Pre-existing chronic otitis media is commonly believed to be the main predisposing cause of carcinoma of the middle ear.

The progression from chronic otitis media to squamous carcinoma was certainly well-known a century ago and was reported by Politzer in his textbook of 1883: a frequent history of chronic otitis media in patients with carcinoma of the middle ear has been reported over a long period. As many as 85% of all cases of malignancy have chronically discharging ears.

Irradiation-induced carcinomas have been recorded after irradiation therapy to the head and

---

Table 14.2 Staging of carcinoma of the ear

T_1 Tumour limited to the site of origin, that is with no facial nerve paralysis and no bone destruction.

T_2 Tumour extending beyond the site of origin, indicated by facial paralysis or radiological evidence of bone destruction, but no extension beyond the organ of origin

T_3 Clinical or radiological evidence of extension to surrounding structures (dura, base of the skull, parotid gland, temporomandibular joint, etc.)

T_x Patients with insufficient data for classification, including patients previously seen and treated elsewhere.

neck, and exposure to radium has also been implicated.

Assessment

Clinical

Local assessment is designed to identify the extent of the tumour, and particularly those factors which render the patient incurable.

A history of chronic otitis media suggests a tumour arising in the middle ear, and absence of this history suggests origin in the external canal. Rarely, the history may also indicate aetiological factors such as previous irradiation. Most patients complain of discharge and deafness, but vertigo is rarely seen. Pain, particularly if deep and boring, indicates dural invasion. Clinical examination of the meatus and middle ear and mastoid cavity (if present) demonstrates the tumour.

Facial paralysis, trismus (indicating invasion of the pterygoids or temporomandibular joint), fullness of the parotid gland (indicating spread through the cartilaginous meatus), fullness of the infratemporal fossa, and perichondritis of the auricle are all important physical signs. Cervical nodes should be felt for, especially in the upper deep cervical and pre- and postauricular groups. Lesions of the lower cranial nerves indicate extension of the tumour to the base of the skull.

Laboratory tests

In addition to the usual general laboratory tests, the aural discharge should be tested for glucose to exclude a cerebrospinal fluid leak.

Radiology

Radiological techniques include plain mastoid and temporal bone radiographs, hypocycloidal tomograms in the coronal and sagittal plane, and computed tomography (CT) scans. Plain views and tomograms are used to look for erosion of the petromastoid and tympanic bones, whereas CT scans are used to assess soft tissue extension of the tumour upwards and backwards to the cranial cavity and downwards and forwards into the infratemporal fossa.

Most patients give a history of chronic ear infection, so that sclerosis of the mastoid and clouding of the cells are to be expected and are of no diagnostic value. Ragged erosion, often extensive or in an unusual site, suggests tumour. An important sign on the lateral mastoid view is erosion of the articular fossa of the temporomandibular joint, and this is present in 30% of patients. Erosion of the bone of the external auditory meatus is best shown by lateral tomograms.

The avascular bone of the labyrinth is relatively unaffected by carcinoma, and erosion of this area with direct invasion of the inner ear is a late radiological feature.

Extension of the tumour anteriorly to penetrate the bony septum separating the middle ear cavity from the carotid artery is of great pathological importance. This is followed by spread around the artery and extension around the eustachian tube towards the postnasal space. Erosion of the carotid septum and the margins of the bony eustachian tube, and even soft tissue extention of the tumour anteriorly, can be demonstrated by tomography and high-resolution CT scanning. Enlargement of the retropharyngeal lymph nodes may also be demonstrated by CT scan.

Other routes of spread of the tumour are upwards through the tegmen tympani, backwards through the mastoid air cells and then through the thin plate of bone forming the posterior wall of the pyramid and underlying the lateral sinus. Erosion of these areas may also be demonstrated radiologically. Once the tumour reaches the cranial cavity, the dura is infiltrated and this is rapidly followed by death. It is thus unlikely that any significant extension into the middle or external cranial fossa would be shown on a conventional CT brain scan. A carotid angiogram is thus of no value except to demonstrate a blocked lateral sinus. When the carotid artery itself is infiltrated death soon follows. Retrograde jugular venography may be useful to assess the extent of the disease by demonstrating obstruction of the lateral sinus by tumour.

The differential radiological diagnosis of squamous carcinoma of the middle ear includes tuberculosis otitis media, malignant otitis externa and glomous jugulare tumour.

The gold standard in imaging is the CT scan. The spine of the sphenoid is readily seen and is a convenient landmark serving the following purposes:

1 Radiological evidence of invasion of the petrosphenoidal region medial to the spine of the sphenoid may indicate a tubotympanic rather than a petromastoid tumour, particularly if symptoms such as ophthalmoplegia, obscure facial pain or trigeminal sensory loss are present.
2 Bone destruction medial to the sphenoidal spine also indicates that cure by any method of treatment is unlikely. The presence of such an extension is an absolute contraindication to radical surgery as the disease is no longer contained within the temporal bone.
3 A submentovertical view occasionally shows destruction of the arch of the atlas due to metastases to the lateral retropharyngeal node with paralysis of the last four cranial nerves.

A CT scan is useful in showing invasion superiorly, which is one of the most critical areas. A CT scan is not capable of showing invasion of the inferior surface of the dura, but this is not too important because it is possible to resect the dura if only its inferior surface is invaded. If the invasion passes through the entire thickness of the dura, the overlying brain will be abnormal because it is either infected or indeed invaded by tumour. In that case it can be demonstrated by enhancement. Such invasion indicates inoperability.

Treatment policy

Untreatable patients

Very few papers comment on the patients who are impossible to treat, and those who are perhaps better left alone. In the authors' series, 10% of patients were untreatable because of extensive disease, poor general condition or distant metastases.

Radiotherapy

The most favoured role for radiotherapy is in conjunction with surgery, and the usual routine is to carry out a radical mastoidectomy and to follow this by postoperative radiotherapy (see below). The advantages are:

1 reactions are lessened and the patients are made more comfortable; and
2 higher doses can be given with less risk of complications.

This treatment produces a crude 5-year survival of about 35%. In most series, results for tumours of the external auditory meatus are about 10% better than those for tumours of the middle ear and mastoid. Little attention has been paid to the problem of primary recurrence after failed radiotherapy. This is surprising because the chance of failure of treatment at the primary site has been high in almost all reported cases. In the authors' experience, surgery has been of no value for recurrence of a middle ear tumour after radiotherapy, but is occasionally of value for recurrent tumours of the external meatus, particularly of the non-squamous variety.

Radiotherapy techniques

Carcinoma of the external auditory meatus and carcinoma of the middle ear and mastoid

One radiotherapeutic technique is used for carcinoma of the ear, whether it has arisen in the external auditory meatus, the middle ear cleft or mastoid air cells. The same technique is used for postoperative irradiation as for radical radiotherapy after a biopsy only.

The treatment is planned and executed with the patient lying supine, immobilized in a Perspex beam-directing shell. The neck is well extended so that the treatment plane, which runs parallel to a line joining the top of the pinna to the floor of the orbit, is vertical. Clinical and radiological assessment defines the extent of disease to be treated, which as a minimum includes the petrous temporal bone, mastoid and adjacent lymph nodes. These are encompassed in a wedge-shaped volume, with its apex just anterior to the brainstem. The anterior border includes the preauricular lymph nodes, and the posterior limit takes in the mastoid process. The upper margin runs along a line from the floor of the orbit to the top of the pinna. The lower margin includes the tip of the mastoid process, and the submastoid lymph nodes (Fig. 14.3). This volume is designed to cover the tumour and possible extensions adequately, while sparing the eyes, brainstem and upper cervical cord from excessive dose. It is covered by anterior and posterior oblique fields, which are wedged to ensure dose homogeneity (Fig. 14.4). A dose of 55–65 Gy in 20–32 daily fractions over 4–6½ weeks is given using megavoltage equipment.

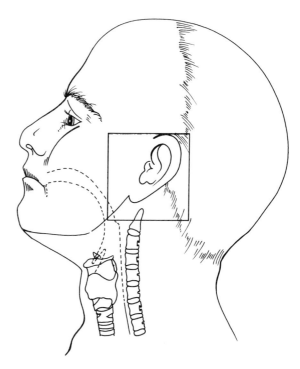

Fig. 14.3 Volume to be irradiated in carcinoma of the middle ear and mastoid.

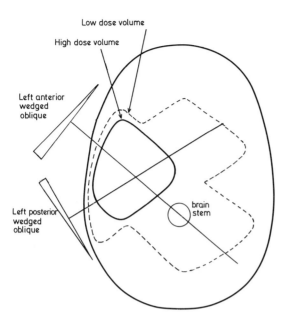

Low dose volume

High dose volume

Left anterior
wedged
oblique

Left posterior
wedged
oblique

brain
stem

Fig. 14.4 Plan of field arrangements for the irradiation of the middle ear and mastoid.

Carcinoma of the pinna

While small tumours of the helix may best be dealt with by surgery, small lesions at the entrance of the auditory canal and more extensive carcinomas may be treated satisfactorily with electron beam therapy to preserve the structure of the auricle. An appropriately shaped lead cut-out, allowing treatment of the tumour with a 1 cm margin, should be made. The external meatus should be plugged with wax to prevent deep penetration of the electrons through the air space. The surface of the tumour should be covered with an appropriate thickness of wax bolus, selected for the energy of electrons to be used, to give the required depth of penetration and a full surface dose. Using 8–10 MeV electrons, 45 Gy in 10 fractions over 2 weeks to 55 Gy in 20 fractions over 4 weeks should be given, depending on the size of the area treated.

Complications of radiotherapy

The external auditory canal

Osteonecrosis of the bony portion of the canal and stenosis are two possible complications. The osteoradionecrosis is usually seen as an exposed area of bone that ultimately forms a scale-like sequestrum. The process is painful and tedious, but healing ultimately occurs. Stenosis of the canal can occur if radiation is given after a sleeve resection or if local radium is inserted into the canal.

The middle ear and mastoid

The possible complications are osteonecrosis and damage to the brain, brainstem or eyes.

Osteonecrosis

Osteonecrosis after radiotherapy usually means persistent disease unless the dosage given has been excessive.

Damage to the brain, brainstem or eyes

Damage to the eyes should be avoided, but it is impossible to irradiate the petrous temporal bone and much of the middle cranial fossa without irradiating cerebral tissue. Providing that large volumes of tissue are not irradiated to high doses the risk of damage seems to be small. Brain necrosis is more likely to follow radiotherapy in elderly patients whose vasculature is already the seat of arteriosclerotic changes.

The facial or auditory nerves in their extracranial course are never damaged by therapeutic radiation, and any impairment of their function is due either to involvement by cancer or to a postoperative complication if radical surgery has been employed.

Conductive deafness after radiotherapy

The loss of hearing following radical mastoidectomy for petromastoid carcinoma is not influenced in any way by radiation. Postradiation conductive deafness may occur in patients who have been successfully irradiated for carcinoma of the external auditory meatus. If the middle ear was normal to start with and the patient is free of recurrence, the possible causes include:

1 thick mucus in the nasopharynx blocking the eustachian opening;
2 atresia of the eustachian orifice, which is rare and is the result of necrosis of the eustachian cartilage, characterized by severe earache and trismus;
3 fibrosis of the fascial space surrounding the levator palati muscle.

Surgery

Surgery to the primary tumour may be used in the following ways:

1 as a preliminary measure, usually a radical mastoidectomy, before radiotherapy;
2 as a primary form of treatment;
3 for salvage after failed radiotherapy.

Due to the close proximity and possible involvement of cartilage, tumours of the auricle are best treated by surgical removal, which also has the advantage of a short stay in hospital. Many will do equally well, however, with radiotherapy, particularly a radium mould.

Tumours on the helix may be removed either in an ellipse- or a wedge-shaped excision. After removal of tumours in the concha or antihelix the resultant defect is impossible to close primarily and a postauricular flap is used. With larger tumours, involving removal of the whole auricle or a large part of the auricle, there is no point in trying to rebuild it; a prosthesis is the best replacement. If part of the ear is left then this can be used to hold the prosthesis, but if the whole auricle is removed and the defect closed with a skin graft, then some form of adhesive can be used to apply the artificial ear to the side of the head.

Carcinomas of the external auditory meatus are uncommon and probably no one surgeon has sufficient experience of them to be dogmatic about treatment. As radiotherapy does not interfere with the subsequent operation, and as the operation is mutilating, a patient with a squamous carcinoma of the external auditory meatus should almost certainly be given a course of radiotherapy. He or she should be followed up closely thereafter to detect a recurrence of the primary tumour. This is quite likely because the original tumour almost certainly invaded bone and was therefore relatively radioresistant.

Adenoid cystic carcinomas are said to be radioresistant and require radical surgery. For these tumours and for recurrent squamous carcinomas after radiotherapy the operation required usually entails removal of the auricle, the external auditory meatus, most of the mastoid process, the posterior meatal wall including the facial nerve, the anterior meatal wall with the temporomandibular joint and usually the parotid gland. If the neck glands are involved a radical neck dissection should of course be carried out in continuity.

Combined surgery and postoperative radiotherapy

This is the routine used most often and consists of a radical mastoidectomy (extended if necessary), followed as soon as healing is complete by radiotherapy for the following reasons.

1 The temporal bone is one of the densest bones in the skull, and its invasion by tumour is inevitably associated with sepsis, which militates against the use of radiotherapy.
2 It is very difficult to assess by clinical or radiological means the full extent of the petromastoid tumour. Preliminary surgical exploration is therefore necessary because this helps to remove necrotic or invaded bone and determine the extent of the tumour.
3 The patient is usually made more comfortable by the operation and loses many of the symptoms.
4 A cavity is provided for drainage and inspection.

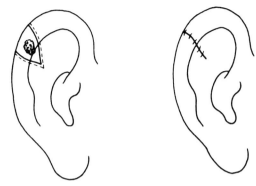

Fig. 14.5 V-excision of helical tumour; dashed line shows amount of cartilage to be removed.

Technique of operations on the auricle

Excision of helical tumours

Up to 2–3 cm of the helix can be removed in a V (Fig. 14.5), as a full-thickness excision, without deforming the appearance of the ear. In doing this, excise marginally more cartilage than skin, in order to secure good skin apposition. Use 3/0 silk to close the skin – there is no need to use any sutures in the cartilaginous layer.

If more than 2–3 cm is to be removed then a deformed auricle is inevitable. Rather than extending the V and closing the defect primarily, it is better to excise the tumour in a rectangular fashion; reconstruct the defect by using a postauricular full-thickness skin flap (Fig. 14.6). After 3 weeks cut the flap, leaving sufficient length to roll the end on itself to form a new helix and to provide cover for the medial part of the flap. Close the donor site by advancing the edges.

Excision of a conchal tumour

If a conchal tumour is excised in a ellipse and the defect is closed primarily, the deformity is very

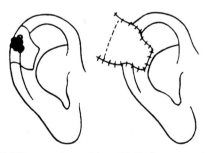

Fig. 14.6 Rectangular excision of helical tumour with reconstruction by a postaural flap. After 3 weeks the flap is divided along the dashed line and rolled over to form the new helix.

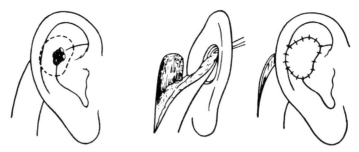

Fig. 14.7 Through-and-through excision of a conchal tumour with repair by an inferiorly based postaural flap. The medial side of the flap is skin-grafted and, after 3 weeks, the pedicle is divided and returned to the donor site.

noticeable. A satisfactory result can usually be obtained by repairing the defect with a postaural flap as in Figure 14.7, or more simply by a full-thickness skin graft. Excise the tumour with a margin of normal tissue, and the subjacent cartilage, in one block. Trim the edges of the cartilage back beneath the skin edges, and secure haemostasis, leaving a bed consisting of the skin and subcutaneous tissue of the posterior part of the auricle.

Take a full-thickness graft from behind the opposite ear, and stitch it in place. Hold it in place with Acriflavine wool, which fits snugly into the depression of the concha. Cover this for a few days with a mastoidectomy dressing. Remove the dressing and stitches after 5 days.

Excision of large tumours of the auricle

Tumours that require excision of all or most of the auricle present special problems. The actual excision is relatively easy but attempts should be made to preserve at least a small portion of the upper helical rim (Fig. 14.8), if it is compatible with tumour removal; this remnant makes the fitting of an artificial ear easier.

If the whole auricle is removed keep some skin on the medial side of the auricle (Fig. 14.9), and this, attached to the skin behind the postaural crease, can be used to close the defect. This is preferable to using

split-thickness skin. In this case an artifical ear must be fitted by skin adhesives.

Technique of petrosectomy

Preparation

One of the main technical difficulties with this operation is bleeding from the major venous sinuses. The lateral sinus should therefore be obliterated about 10 days before the main operation. Expose the mastoid process through a postaural incision and then expose the lateral sinus with a cutting burr as in mastoid surgery. Pack off the sinus with a BIPP pack and close the wound loosely.

As part of the preoperative preparation of the patient, warn him or her that he or she will almost inevitably have a facial paralysis after the operation, although this blow can be softened to some extent by explaining that the disease will in any case ultimately cause a facial paralysis and that nerve grafting will be done. Warn the patient also that he or she will be deaf after the operation, although of course if the tumour has invaded the middle ear he or she will

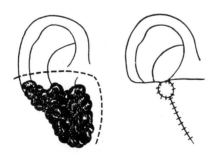

Fig. 14.8 Excision of the auricle leaving a helical rim for fitting a prosthesis.

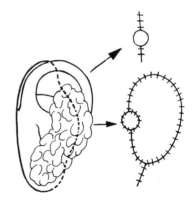

Fig. 14.9 Total excision of auricle; if some postaural skin is left, then primary closure can be done, but if not, a split-thickness skin graft is used.

already be deaf. The night before operation have the head shaved on the involved side.

Incision

The incision must encompass the entire ear, and in most cases the auricle itself will also be removed in continuity with the skin. The entire incision is shown in Figure 14.10; begin by making the superior part 2 cm above the superior attachment of the auricle. This incision is used to expose the middle cranial fossa to assess invasion of the dura. If the dura is indeed invaded, particularly if this invasion extends medially, the operation may well have to be abandoned. For this reason only the upper part of the incision is made first to save making an extensive needless incision that must then be closed. The remaining part of the incision incorporates a standard parotidectomy incision. It starts at the upper level of the helix just in front of the auricle, dips down into the anterior incisura, gently curves under the lobe of the ear and continues down the neck to the level of the hyoid bone if the auricle is not to be removed. If a neck dissection is to be done the incision is continued to the point of the chin and then an appropriate incision for a neck dissection is made in the lower part of the neck.

If the whole auricle is to be removed, continue the upper part of the incision round the ear to meet the original incision under the lobe of the ear.

Elevate the facial skin and neck skin to expose the parotid gland.

Elevate the tissues around the ear to expose as much mastoid bone as possible. The way this is done will depend on whether some auricle is to be kept or not.

Do not detach the anterior meatal wall from the parotid or else a tumour-containing area will be entered.

Excision

Carry the skin incision above the auricle straight down on to the squamous temporal bone, and elevate the soft tissues above and below. Use a cutting mastoid burr to cut through the squamous temporal bone over a distance of about 1 cm. Once the bone is opened, introduce a Pennybacker to open up the defect to allow wide exposure of the dura. Then use a blunt periosteal elevator, of which the Adson pattern is much the best, to elevate the dura from the floor of the middle cranial fossa, provided that tumour has not penetrated the dura at this point. If the dura is invaded it is possible to excise a small area, but if the dural invasion extends medially to or beyond the apex of the petrous bone, the tumour is inoperable.

If the tumour is operable, continue removing the bone in an anterior direction using the Pennybacker's forceps. The line of excision through the bone is shown in Figure 14.11. In addition divide the zygoma at the point shown in the diagram.

Now continue the soft tissue dissection down the anterior border of the parotid gland, sacrificing all the branches of the facial nerve. Continue the dissection deeply until the ascending ramus of the mandible is exposed. Now divide the ascending ramus of the mandible just below the notch to ensure that the temporomandibular joint is left on the specimen (Fig. 14.12).

Continue the dissection posteriorly, first making the skin incision over the mastoid process. Again, elevate the soft tissues off the bone and then continue cutting through the bone with Pennybacker's forceps exposing the lateral sinus, which should not bleed as it has already been obliterated.

Dissect forward through the floor of the middle ear so that the bone has now been divided on all sides. The specimen is now still attached by the firm bone of the petrous apex. This can be divided either by a cutting burr or with an osteoprobe. If an osteoprobe is used it is safer to use a curved pattern. Cut through the petrous apex in one of these two ways and remove the specimen, if possible in one piece. Very

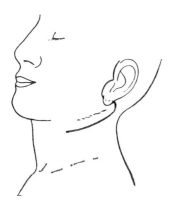

Fig. 14.10 Incision for removal of auricle and temporal bone.

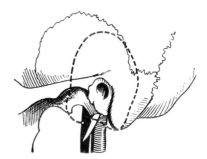

Fig. 14.11 Showing the limits of removal in temporal bone resection.

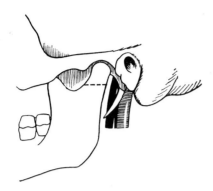

Fig. 14.12 Divide the neck of the mandible and leave it attached to the anterior meatal wall.

often, however, the main specimen becomes detached before the hard bone of the petrous apex can be removed.

Repair

There are several structures to be repaired after this procedure, including the dura, the skin and the facial nerve.

If the dura has been resected, repair it with a piece of lyophilized dura cut to the appropriate size and stitched in with 3/0 chromic catgut sutures. Small tears in the dura can be oversewn.

There are various methods of repairing the skin, but the only two reliable methods are the anteriorly based scalp flap or a free flap; much the best is the rectus abdominis free flap, which is easy to harvest. It can be taken during the excision, and it provides both muscle and skin. The muscle is very useful for filling the defect and sealing any small dural tears. The pectoralis major myocutaneous flap has the advantage of bulk but it may not always reach the upper limit of the defect. The technique of facial nerve grafting is outlined on pp. 284–6.

Reconstruction of the facial nerve is better not attempted. It is usually not possible to find the stump of the facial nerve; furthermore, if the patient already had a facial paralysis before the operation, it is a waste of time trying to graft the nerve. The theoretical possibilities are a cross-face nerve graft or a hypoglossal facial anastomosis. However, most patients have had enough after a petrosectomy and opt for accepting the defect.

The anterior scalp flap depends on its extensive vascularity and its mobility. The scalp consists of three layers: the skin, the subcutaneous fatty layer and the muscular/aponeurotic layer consisting of the occipitofrontalis muscle anteriorly and posteriorly joined in the centre by the epicranial aponeurosis. These three layers are separated from the pericranium by a layer of loose areolar tissue. The main blood vessels lie in the dense subcutaneous tissues

and are superficial to the muscle. The vessels are derived anteriorly from the internal carotid artery (from the supraoribtal and supratrochlear branches of the ophthalmic artery) and over the rest of the scalp from terminal branches of the external carotid artery, mainly the superficial temporal and occipital. These vessels anastomose freely with each other and with the corresponding vessels of the opposite side. Flap necrosis is therefore not to be feared.

The head must be shaved at the start of the procedure. The flap is marked out at the end of the exisional phase. Three points must be borne in mind: the flap must pass over a curved surface convex outwards; the flap must sink into a defect of fair size; and the pivot point is furthest from the defect. A flap 25 cm long and 12 cm wide is usually the minimum required. The flap is marked out, and tape is used to assess the adequacy of the length of the flap. Because the first and third layers of the flap are firmly united by fibrous processes passing through the second, fatty layer, this flap does not retract after it has been elevated, unlike all other flaps. There is thus no need to allow extra length for retraction.

The flap is now cut along the lines marked out, and incised down to the loose areolar layer. Great care must be taken not to damage the pericranium. The flap is now easily developed, working in the areolar layer. Bleeding is always profuse and bleeding points are grasped initially by forceps, and later coagulated or tied.

The flap is now rotated into the defect and sutured in place over a suction drain. The bare area on the pericranium is best dealt with by a split-skin graft applied 24–48 h later, using the delayed primary grafting technique.

If the pericranium is damaged, for example by the diathermy, split skin will not take on the bare bone of the skull. This problem is dealt with by allowing the graft to heal over the rest of the scalp until the denuded area demarcates. The outer table of the bare area of the skull is then removed with a mastoid drill until diploe is reached. This is then left exposed to granulate, and the wound will then heal by second intention.

Aftercare

1 *General care.*
2 *Antibiotics* – almost certainly the area was infected preoperatively so antibiotics are needed.
3 *Care of the eye.* It is probably worthwhile carrying out a lateral tarsorrhaphy. This may not be necessary, however, as eye problems can occasionally be surprisingly few after a facial nerve division.
4 *Prosthetic care.* If the patient is concerned about the paralysis of the corner of the mouth it is possible to improve the position of the face at rest, by attaching a hook to the dentures to hold up the corner of the mouth, by building up the flange of

the upper denture, or by operations involving masseteric or temporalis muscle swings. If the auricle has been removed it is possible to fit the patient with an artificial ear. The only exception to this may be in a woman with long straight hair. Such a prosthesis can be made in latex or acrylic, and attached either by skin adhesives or by osseo-integrated implants.

Complications

1 *General complications.*
2 *Intracranial complications.* The main postoperative complications of this procedure relate to the cranial cavity. A cerebrospinal fluid leak is a distinct possibilitiy, but usually closes spontaneously, particularly if a muscle-bearing free flap is used. A brain abscess is a further possible complication.

References and further reading

Aitkin M, Clayton D (1980) The fitting of exponential Weibull and extreme value distributions to complex censored data using GLIM. *Appl Stat* **29**:156–63.

Ariyan S, Sasaki C T, Spencer D (1981) Radical en bloc resection of the temporal bone. *Am J Surg* **142**:443–7.

Arthur K (1976) Radiotherapy in carcinoma of the middle ear and auditory canal. *J Laryngol.* **90**:753–62.

Aub J C, Evans R D, Hemplemann L H H, Marland H S (1952) Late effects of internally deposited radioactive materials in man. *Medicine* **31**:221–9.

Batsakis J G (ed) (1979) Epidermal carcinomas of the nose and ear. In: *Tumours of the Head and Neck*, 2nd edn. Baltimore, Williams & Wilkins.

Batsakis J G, Hardy G C, Hishiyama R H (1967) Ceruminous gland tumors. *Arch Otolaryngol* **86**:92–5.

Beal D D, Lindsay J R, Ward P H (1965) Radiation-induced carcinoma of the mastoid. *Arch Otolaryngol* **81**:9–16.

Bodenham D C (1972) The complementary roles of ENT and plastic surgery in major malignancies of the middle ear. *Proc R Soc Med* **65**:248–9.

Boland J, Paterson R (1955) Cancer of the middle ear and external auditory meatus. *J Laryngol* **69**:468–78.

Broders A C (1921) Epithelioma of the ear: a study of 63 cases. *Surg Clin North Am* **1**:1401–10.

Campbell E, Volk B M, Burklund C W (1951) Total resection of temporal bone for malignancy of the middle ear. *Ann Surg* **134**:397–404.

Cankar V, Crowley H (1964) Tumors of ceruminous glands: a clinicopathological study of 7 cases. *Cancer* **17**:67–75.

Caplinger C B, Hora J F (1967) Middle ear choristoma with absent oval window. *Arch Otolaryngol* **85**:39–40.

Chen K T K, Dehner L P (1978) Primary tumors of the external and middle ear. *Arch Otolaryngol* **104**:247–52.

Clairemont A A, Conley J J (1977) Primary carcinoma of the mastoid bone. *Ann Otol Rhinol Laryngol* **86**:306–9.

Coleman C C (1966) Removal of the temporal bone for cancer. *Am J Surg* **112**:583–90.

Conley J (1965) Cancer of the middle ear. *Ann Otol Rhinol Laryngol* **74**:555–72.

Conley J, Schuller D E (1976) Malignancies of the ear. *Laryngoscope* **86**:1147–63.

Conley J J, Novack A J (1960) The surgical treatment of malignant tumors of the ear and temporal bone. *Arch Otolaryngol* **71**:635–52.

Crabtree J A, Britton B H, Pierce M K (1976) Carcinoma of the external auditory canal. *Laryngoscope* **86**:405–15.

Dehner L P, Chen K T K (1980) Primary tumors of the external and middle ear. *Arch Otolaryngol* **106**:13–19.

Doble H P, Snyder G G, Carpenter RJ (1981) Sebaceous cell carcinoma of the external auditory canal. *Otolaryngol Head Neck Surg* **89**:685–8.

Ellis M, Pracy R (1959) Carcinoma of middle ear. *Br Med J* **1**:1413–25.

Fairman H D (1972) Radical surgery for carcinoma of the middle ear. *Proc R Soc Med* **65**:247–8.

Figi F A, Hempstead B E (1943) Malignant tumors of the middle ear and the mastoid process. *Arch Otolaryngol* **37**:149–68.

Figi F A, Weisman P A (1954) Cancer and chemodectoma in the middle ear and mastoid. *JAMA* **156**:1157–62.

Friedmann I, Radcliffe A (1954) Otosclerosis associated with malignant melanoma of the ear. *J Laryngol* **68**:114–19.

Furstenburg A C (1924) Primary adenocarcinoma of the middle ear and mastoid. *Ann Otol Rhinol Laryngol* **33**:677–89.

Gillanders D A, Worth A J, Honore L H (1974) Ceruminous adenoma of the middle ear. *Can J Otolaryngol* **3**:194–201.

Goldman N C, Hardcastle B (1973) Partial temporal bone resection for basal cell carcinoma of the external auditory canal with preservation of facial nerve and hearing. *Laryngoscope* **84**:84–9.

Goodwin W J, Jesse R H (1980) Malignant neoplasms of the external auditory canal and temporal bone. *Arch Otolaryngol* **106**:675–9.

Harrison K, Cronin J, Greenwood N (1974) Ceruminous adenocarcinoma arising in the middle ear. *J. Laryngol* **88**:363–8.

Hicks G W (1983) Tumours arising from the glandular structures of the external auditory canal. *Laryngoscope* **93**:326–40.

Holmes K S (1960) The treatment of carcinoma of the middle ear by the 4MV linear accelerator. *Proc R Soc Med* **53**:242–4.

Hociota D, Ataman T (1975) A case of salivary gland choristoma of the middle ear. *J Laryngol* **89**:1065–8.

Holmes K S (1965) Carcinoma of the middle ear. *Clin Radiol* **16**:400–4.

Hyams VJ, Michaels L (1976) Benign adenomatous neoplasm (adenoma) of the middle ear. *Clin Otolaryngol* **1**:17–26.

Jaffee I S, Page R S (1961) Adenocarcinoma of the middle ear. *Laryngoscope* **71**:392–5.

Jesse R H, Healey J E, Wiley D B (1967) External auditory canal, middle ear, and mastoid. In:*Cancer of the Head and Neck* McComb W S, Fletcher G H. Baltimore, Williams & Wilkins pp. 412–17.

Johns M E, Headington J T (1974) Squamous cell carcinoma of the external auditory canal: a clinicopathologic study of 20 cases. *Arch Otolaryngol* **100**:45–9.

Johnstone J M, Lennox B, Watson A J (1957) Five cases of hidradenoma of the external auditory meatus. *J Pathol Bacteriol* **73**:421–7.

Juby H B (1957) Tumors of the ceruminous glands – so called ceruminoma. *J Laryngol* **71**:832–7.

Kelham B H (1959) Carcinoma of the middle ear with extensive spread along the eustachian tube. *J Laryngol* **73**:124–8.

Lamont J T, O'Gorman T A (1978) Experimental colon cancer. *Gastroenterology* **75**:1157–69.

Lederman M (1965) Malignant tumours of the ear. *J Laryngol* **79**:85–119.

Levy E, Sommerfeld W S (1961) Hidradenoma of external auditory meatus (so-called ceruminoma). *Rev Laryngol* **82**:476–9.

Lewis J S (1973) Squamous carcinoma of the ear. *Arch Otolaryngol* **97**:41–2.

Lewis J S (1975) Temporal bone resection: review of 100 cases. *Arch Otolaryngol* **101**:23–5.

Lewis JS (1979) Tumours of the middle-ear cleft and temporal bone. In: *Scott Brown's Disease of the Ear* 4th edn. Ballantyne J, Groves J, London, Butterworth, pp. 385–404.

Lewis J S (1981) Cancer of the external auditory canal, middle ear, and mastoid. In: *Cancer of the Head and Neck*. Suen, Myers (eds). New York, Churchill Livingstone, pp. 557–75.

Lewis J S (1983) Surgical management of tumors of the middle ear and mastoid. *J Laryngol* **97**:299–311.

Lewis J S, Page R (1965) Radical surgery for malignant tumors of the ear. *Arch Otolaryngol* **83**:56–61.

Lewis J S, Parsons H (1958) Surgery for advanced ear cancer. *Ann Otol* **67**:364–71.

Lodge W O, Jones H M, Smith M E N (1955) Malignant tumors of the temporal bone. *Arch Otolaryngol* **61**:535–41.

MacBeth R (1960) Some thought on the Eustachian tube. *Proc R Soc Med* **53**:151.

Manning K P, Skegg D C G, Stell P M, Doll R (1981) Cancer of the larynx and other occupational hazards of mustard gas workers. *Clin Otolaryngol* **6**:165–70.

Mark I, Rothberg M (1951) Mixed tumor of skin of external auditory canal. *Arch Otolaryngol* **53**:556–9.

Michaels L, Wells M (1980) Squamous cell carcinoma of the middle ear. *Clin Otolaryngol* **5**:235–48.

Mischke R E, Brackmann D E, Gruskin P (1977) Salivary gland choristoma of the middle ear. *Arch Otolaryngol* **103**:432–4.

Morton R P, Stell P M, Pharoah P O D (1984) Epidemiology of cancer of the middle ear cleft. *Cancer* **53**:1612–17.

Nandi S P, Shaw H J (1961) Hidradenoma of external auditory meatus associated with facial palsy and choronic otitis media. *J Laryngol* **75**:922–96.

Newhart H (1917) Primary carcinoma of the middle ear: report of a case. *Laryngoscope* **27**:543–55.

Nichinsson A G (1933) Ein Fall einer Epithelgeschwulst des aeusseren Gehoerganges. *Monatschr Ohrenher* **67**:210–21.

Noguera J T, Haas F R (1969) Congenital ossicular defects with a normal auditory canal: its surgical treatment. *Eye Ear Nose Throat Monogr* **43**:37–9.

O'Neill P B, Parker R A (1957) Sweat gland tumours ('ceruminomata') of external auditory meatus. *J Laryngol* **71**:824–31.

Parsons H, Lewis J S (1954) Subtotal resection of the temporal bone for cancer of the ear. *Cancer* **7**:995–1001.

Peele J C, Hauser C H (1941) Primary carcinoma of the external auditory canal and middle ear. *Arch Otolaryngol* **34**:254–266.

Phelps P D, Lloyd G A S (1981) The radiology of carcinoma of the ear. *Br J Radiol* **54**:103–9.

Politzer A (1883) *Textbook of Diseases of the Ear*. Cassells J P transl. London, Bailliere Tindall & Cox, pp. 650–5.

Pulec J L (1977) Glandular tumours of the external auditory canal. *Laryngoscope* **87**:1601–11.

Ruben R J, Thaler S U, Holzer N (1977) Radiation induced carcinoma of the temporal bone. *Laryngoscope* **87**:1616–21.

Schall L A (1934) Neoplasms involving the middle ear. *Arch Otolaryngol* **32**:548–53.

Schewe E J, Pappalardo C (1962) Cancer of the external ear. *Am J Surg* **104**:753–5.

Siedentop K H, Jeantet C (1961) Primary adenocarcinoma of the middle ear. Report of three cases. *Ann Otol Rhinol Laryngol* **70**:719–33.

Sinha P P, Aziz H I (1978) Treatment of carcinoma of the middle ear. *Radiology* **126**:485–7.

Smith H W, Duarte I (1962) Mixed tumors of the external auditory canal. *Arch Otolaryngol* **75**:28–33.

Sorenson H (1960) Cancer of the middle ear and mastoid. *Acta Radiol* **54**:460–8.

Steffen T N, House W F (1962) Salivary gland choristoma of the middle ear. *Arch Otolaryngol* **76**:74–5.

Stell P M, McCormick M S (1984) Carcinoma of the middle ear: prognostic factors and a suggested staging system. *J Laryngol Otol*.

Stone H E, Lipa M, Bell D B (1975) Primary adenocarcinoma of the middle ear. *Arch Otolaryngol* **101**:702–5.

Tabb H G, Komer H, McLaurin J W (1964) Cancer of the external auditory canal: treatment with radical mastoidectomy and irradiation. *Laryngoscope* **74**:634–43.

Taylor G D, Martin H F (1961) Salivary gland tissue in the middle ear. *Arch Otolaryngol* **73**:49–51.

Truffert P (1922) Les aponeuroses de la trompe d'Eustache. *Ann Mal Oreil Larynx* **41**:498–507.

Tucker W N (1965) Cancer of the middle ear. *Cancer* **18**:642–50.

Wang C C (1975) Radiation therapy in the management of carcinoma of the external auditory canal, middle ear, or mastoid. *Radiology* **116**:713–15.

Ward J M (1975) Dose response to a single injection of azoxymethane in rats. *Vet Pathol* **12**:165–77.

Ward G E, Loch W E, Lawrence W (1951) Radical operation for carcinoma of the external auditory canal and middle ear. *Am J Surg* **82**:169–78.

Wetli C V, Pardo V, Millard M, Gerston K (1972) Tumors of ceruminous glands. *Cancer* **29**:1169–78.

Wilson J S P, Blake G B, Richardson A E, Westbury G (1974) Malignant tumours of the ear and their treatment. *Br J Plast Surg* **27**:77–91.

Zeroni (1899) Ueber das Carconom des Gehoerorganes *Arch Ohrenheilkunde* **8**:141–90.

15

Tumours of the lip

Surgical anatomy

The lips are the anterior boundary of the oral cavity and are covered with non-keratinizing stratified squamous epithelium. They appear red because this epithelium is transparent and contains no hairs, sebaceous glands or pigment in its substance. The mucosa of the lips covers the orbicularis oris muscle. On the vermilion border the mucosa is closely applied to the muscles but on the lingual surface there are many mucous glands and supporting tissue within the muscle and the mucosa. The distance between the surface epithelium of the lip and the orbicularis oris is only about 2 mm. An ulcerative squamous carcinoma can, therefore, fix the skin quite early to the deep substance of the lip.

The major blood supply of the lip comes from the facial artery, which gives off small submental arteries to the lower lip and gives rise to the inferior and superior labial arteries. These vessels encircle the mouth between the orbicularis oris and the submucosa of the lip.

The upper and lower lips have a cutaneous and a mucosal system of lymphatics. In the lower lip there is one medial and two lateral collecting trunks. The medial trunk drains the inner third of the lip and the lateral trunks drain the outer two-thirds. The medial trunk drains to the submental lymph nodes and the lateral trunks to the submandibular triangle lymph nodes. Numerous anastomoses account for the bilateral metastases seen in midline tumours. Collecting lymph trunks enter the mental foramen in 22% of subjects.

Drainage of the upper lip is to preauricular, infraparotid, submandibular triangle and submental lymph nodes.

The commissure of the mouth is a very delicately formed structure that is difficult to remake. For this reason it is better to keep the commissure if at all possible in any lip operation rather than attempting to remake one.

Surgical pathology

The lip is the most common site of cancer in the mouth. In the USA the incidence is 18 per million population. Ninety-three per cent of tumours present on the lower lip (Fig. 15.1); the male : female ratio is 80 : 1. In the upper lip the commonest tumour is the basal cell carcinoma: this is commoner in females and the male : female ratio is only 5 : 1.

Lip cancer is commonest in the white male smoker who has a fair or ruddy complexion and light hair, in the sixth decade.

Tumours occur on the lower lip on the exposed vermilion border just outside the line of contact with the upper lip, usually halfway between the midline and the commissure. More than 30% of patients with carcinoma of the lip have outdoor occupations. The effect of solar exposure is the loss of elastic fibres, atrophy of fat and glandular elements, and hyperkeratosis with atypica. The lower lip receives most solar irradiation and the upper lip is, by comparison, shaded. The lip is susceptible to actinic change because, in the white population, it lacks a pigment layer for protection. Lip cancer is 10 times commoner in whites than non-whites.

This cancer is traditionally associated with pipe-

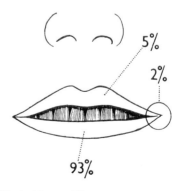

Fig. 15.1 Site incidence of lip cancer.

smoking but nowadays heavy cigarette smokers are the most frequently involved group. Syphilis plays little part in the development of lip cancer now, but the neoplasm is associated with poor dental hygiene, chronic alcoholism and chronic immunosuppression.

Ninety-eight per cent of tumours of the lower lip are squamous cell carcinoma. The remainder are basal cell tumours and minor salivary gland tumours, predominantly adenoid cystic carcinoma or muco-epidermoid carcinoma.

There are three types of squamous carcinoma – exophytic, verrucous and ulcerative. Verrucous tumours are extremely rare and exophytic tumours are probably the commonest. Exophytic lesions become necrotic and ulceration occurs late, when the tumour is over 1 cm. The ulcerative type is minimally elevated and ulceration occurs early; it is usually of a higher histological grade and fixes the muscle earlier.

Carcinoma of the upper lip and commissure grows more rapidly, ulcerates sooner and metastasizes earlier than lower lip cancer. There is an increased incidence of metastases with increasing tumour size.

Clinically apparent cervical lymph node metastases occur in fewer than 10% of patients with carcinoma of the lower lip. Approximately 20% of patients with commissure lesions will have lymph node metastases. Some 5–15% of patients will develop lymph node metastases at some time in the future. Not all lymphadenopathy represents metastasis. Infection of the tumour or poor oral hygiene may cause adenopathy.

Malignant melanomas are rare within the vermilion portion of the lip but may occur in the skin. Sarcomas of the lip are extremely rare.

Benign and malignant tumours of minor salivary gland origin are rare in a lip. They develop in the depths of the labial substance without any connection to the mucous membrane.

Myoblastomas have been reported in the lip but these remain below the mucosa. Pyogenic granuloma has a softer consistency than cancer; it can arise during pregnancy.

Keratoacanthoma can occur on the cutaneous aspect of the lip and give the appearance of a carcinoma. It is usually circular with a central crater. It may grow rapidly but then tends to regress spontaneously.

Syphilitic chancres, leprosy, sarcoidosis and Crohn's disease are other causes of granulomatous cheilitis.

The main distinction between carcinoma and other lip lesions, however, is from hyperkeratosis and cheilitis. Leukoplakia, in association with carcinoma of the lip, has been reported in from 2 to 75% of cases. The frequency with which malignant changes occur in leukoplakia of the lip is unknown but it may approach 30%. Cheilitis may be associated with chronic dermatitis and eczema, or with prolonged exposure to sunshine.

Investigations

History

Ask how long a tumour has been present and about the patient's smoking habits. The occupation is important because lip tumours are commoner in outdoor workers. Carcinoma of the lip tends to have a protracted clinical course. A history of recurrent lip crusting that bleeds readily on removal of the crust is characteristic. It is uncommon for carcinoma to arise *de novo* from an entirely normal lower lip. Three per cent of patients develop metastases very early, when the primary lesion is 1 cm or less, and this indicates very agressive biological behaviour. Pain and tenderness only occur when infection is present.

Examination

It is vital that the tumour be measured and its position accurately recorded to help in planning the operation. Also carefully note the degree of infiltration by bimanual palpation of the lip. Ascertain whether the lesion extends on to the alveolus, as this completely changes treatment policy. Look for hypoanaesthesia in the distribution of the mental nerve because the tumour may grow along that nerve into the medullary portion of the mandible. This is more likely to occur in older patients who are edentulous. Finally, feel the neck for metastatic nodes and examine the rest of the upper air and food passages for other primary tumours.

Radiology

This is of limited value in lip cancer unless mandibular invasion is suspected.

Laboratory investigations

Again, these are of no great value, although it is wise to screen for syphilis.

Biopsy

This is mandatory prior to treatment because hyperkeratosis, cheilitis, keratoacanthoma and other benign lesions can be confused with carcinoma. An incisional biopsy is to be preferred to an excisional biopsy. Biopsy of the centre of an ulcerative or exophytic tumour, however, may show only necrotic debris.

Treatment policy

The survival rates of cancer of the lip, treated with radiation therapy or surgery, are very similar. Both modalities are expected to give greater than 85% cure rate. The cure rate drops significantly as the size of the tumour increases. Curability falls to 59% for lesions 2–3 cm in diameter and to 41% for tumours larger than 3 cm. There is a close relationship also between histological grade and curability: there is a 95% 3-year cure rate for grade 1 carcinomas but only 45 and 38% respectively for grades 3 and 4.

The advantage of surgical therapy is that it immediately eradicates the disease, has no effect on adjacent normal tissue, and gives an opportunity to examine the specimen pathologically. Radiotherapy can be interstitial, contact or external beam. Care must be taken to protect the adjacent uninvolved tissue by proper shielding to limit the amount of mucositis and radiodermatitis.

Leukoplakia of the lip or actinic cheilitis is best managed with a lip shave, which constitutes both treatment and diagnosis.

Up to one-third of the lip can be resected and closed primarily. Larger defects require additional tissue from another location for a reconstruction. Most tumours can be managed by a V-shaped wedge excision.

If more than one-third of the lip is excised then tissue is borrowed from the opposite lip using an Abbe lip switch technique. Lesions near the commissure can be treated by the Estlander modification of the Abbe procedure. This does require, however, a second-stage reconstruction of the commissure.

Large tumours of the centre of the lower lip are best reconstructed with the Bernard technique, which employs lateral advancement flaps. Oral mucosa on the inside of Burrows triangle is preserved and used to restore the vermilion border.

The main complaints of patients undergoing lip reconstruction are drooling, poor speech intelligibility, cracking and fissuring of the tissues, and inadequacy of stomal size. A more pleasing functional result can be obtained in the reconstruction of large lip defects using the Karapandzic principle, which consists of mobilizing arterialized, innervated flaps of skin and orbicularis oris muscle from the surrounding network of suspensory muscles.

In very large lip defects lacking available adjacent flap tissue, a distant flap must be used. A myocutaneous flap is too thick and the preferred ones are the deltopectoral flap for the lower lip and a forehead flap for the upper lip. Both of these must be lined with split-thickness skin.

Only 50% of patients with carcinoma of the lip and regional node metastases are cured. It is impossible to achieve continuity between the primary excision and the neck dissection, so this means that cancer-containing skin lymphatics are transected. This is borne out by the high incidence of recurrence in the upper incision line of the neck dissection. Consideration must, therefore, be given to planned postoperative radiotherapy to the chin and neck region.

Technique of lip operations

Wedge excision

Preparation

Pay great attention to the patient's teeth, as it is unwise to operate in the presence of gross dental infection. It is well worth while spending time extracting the teeth, and allowing the alveolus to heal, before an operation on the lip if the condition of the teeth is bad. The patient's skin is prepared in the usual fashion and all facial hair removed by shaving. Nasal sepsis must also be dealt with before surgery.

Anaesthesia

All these patients should be anaesthetized with a nasal endotracheal tube, and the anaesthetic tubes brought out over the patient's head, so that they are out of the way of the operating field. Pack the oropharynx and remove the pack at the end of the operation, so that the anaesthetist does not disturb the lip repair.

Excision

Mark out the tumour with at least a 5 mm margin on either side. If there is any doubt as to whether more than one-third of the lip will be excised when these marks are made, put the lip on the stretch and measure the distance accurately. On no account should more than one-third of the lip be removed with this operation. Continue the marks down over the chin in the form of a V (Fig. 15.2). If the point of the V is too high, then the excision will take the form of a shield rather than a wedge, leading to an untidy repair with a dog ear at the lower end. With methylene blue, tattoo the vermilion border accurately so

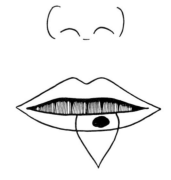

Fig. 15.2 Wedge incision – line of V-excision.

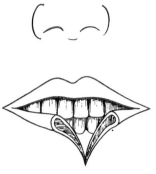

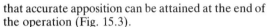

Fig. 15.3 Wedge excision – specimen removed; note the dot marking the vermilion skin junction.

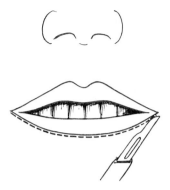

Fig. 15.5 Lip shave – incision along the vermilion skin junction.

that accurate apposition can be attained at the end of the operation (Fig. 15.3).

An assistant firmly holds the lip on either side between the finger and thumb to control arterial bleeding. With a knife held exactly at right angles to the lip, cut the tumour out in a wedge. The assistant then releases one side of the lip slowly; identify, clamp and tie the inferior labial artery with 4/0 chromic catgut. Repeat this on the opposite side. Control other small bleeding vessels with coagulation diathermy.

Repair

First suture the orbicularis oris muscle with 3/0 chromic catgut. If this layer is omitted there will be tension on the skin and mucosal suture lines, producing an ugly thinning of the repaired portion of the lip. Then match the vermilion border with 5/0 Nurolon, and use the same suture material to sew up the skin (Fig. 15.4). Finally use 3/0 chromic catgut to close the mucosa on the inner surface. It is important not to tear the red margin of the lip on the upper surface, as a necrotic area forms causing a notch.

Aftercare

1 General care.
2 The patient is not allowed to suck anything and takes a soft diet from the time he or she recovers from the anaesthetic.
3 The wound is kept clean twice a day be removing crusts and applying antibiotic cream.

Lip shave and vermilion advancement

This operation can be performed on its own if the carcinoma is very superficial, or it may be combined with a wedge excision. If it is combined, then it is easier to sew up the muscle layer of the wedge before doing the lip shave.

Make an incision, accurately, along the vermilion border (Fig. 15.5) with an assistant's finger in each corner of the mouth to keep the lip on the stretch. Elevate the mucosa off the orbicularis oris muscle, with a knife at first (Fig. 15.6) and then the blunt point of scissors. At the back of the lip is a thicker layer of mucous glands. It is important just to elevate the mucosa, which must on no account be button-holed, as this causes crusting and a dip in the final repair. Continue elevation right down into the sulcus

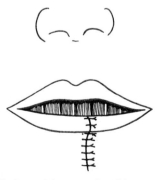

Fig. 15.4 Wedge excision – repair; taking care to get accurate apposition of vermilion edges.

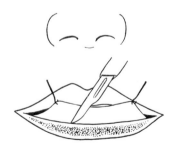

Fig. 15.6 Lip shave – vermilion elevated off orbicularis oris.

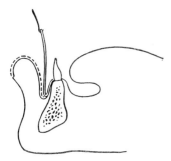

Fig. 15.7 Lip shave – mucosal elevation must be carried on down into the sulcus.

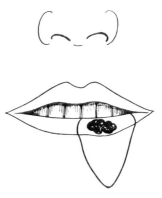

Fig. 15.9 Abbe lip switch operation – incision marked as a shield.

and on to the alveolus (Fig. 15.7). This is very important because if the mucosa is not elevated this far, retraction occurs later and after a year the lip will not be red.

After full elevation of the mucosa hold it on two skin hooks, bring it forward out of the mouth and cut off the cheilitic portion with scissors, keeping the form of the lower margin of the vermilion, i.e. a gentle curve.

Then re-attach the remaining mucosa to the skin (Fig. 15.8) with interrupted sutures of 5/0 Nurolon, after haemostasis has been secured with adrenaline swabs. It is important to make a rather larger lower lip than is ultimately desired, because of subsequent contraction of the wound.

Aftercare

1 General care, including a soft diet.
2 Keep the area free of crusting with antibiotic cream.

Abbe lip switch operation

This operation is indicated if more than one-third of the lower lip has to be removed. It uses an axial flap consisting of skin, muscle and mucous membrane, pedicled on the superior labial artery.

Outline a shield-shaped incision with dye (Fig.

15.9), as opposed to the V-incision marked for the earlier type of operation. This tumour will obviously be much larger than the earlier tumour, which the V-wedge excision is used for, so mark out a minimum of 1 cm of normal tissue on either side. Also mark the vermilion border with dye on a needle. Using a ruler and accurate measuring, outline a similar triangular area on the upper lip (Fig. 15.10), whose length is equal to that of the defect, while the base is one-half of that of the defect. This gives proportionate shortening of the upper and lower lips. The pedicle of the flap should be medial and contain the superior labial artery, which runs 5 mm above the upper margin of the red of the lip; it is better to leave a thick pedicle rather than risk damaging the artery. These flaps rarely die but if the artery is damaged then they certainly will, producing a horrendous defect.

When all the marks have been made, excise the tumour with a knife held at right angles to the skin and the lip. Then cut the upper flap and mobilize it except for its medial pedicle. It will, of course, be necessary to cut down to the muscles of the face and

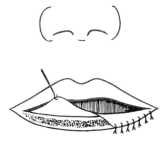

Fig. 15.8 Vermilion advancement – once the leukoplakic lip has been trimmed off, the healthy mucosa is stitched forwards to form a new lip.

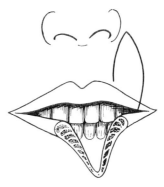

Fig. 15.10 Abbe lip switch operation – 2 : 1 flap marked out on upper lip, based on the superior labial artery, which runs above the vermilion.

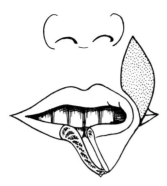

Fig. 15.11 Abbe lip switch operation – flap turned into the defect leaving the commissure intact.

to incise the mucosa of the upper buccoalveolar sulcus.

Now rotate the flap into the defect (Fig. 15.11) and place one 5/0 Nurolon suture through the needle marks at the vermilion edges. Suture the flap to the defect in three layers as before, taking great care with the muscle layer.

When the flap is sutured in position, mobilize the lateral area of the donor site widely to allow primary closure, also in three layers. The commissure should be kept at all costs, no matter how small it is. Finally, sew the cut ends of the lip at the commissure to the bare area of the flap, in three layers, so that no bare areas remain (Fig. 15.12).

Aftercare

1 General care.
2 The patient should be fed with a feeding cup.
3 Keep the wound free of crusting with an antibiotic cream.
4 Three weeks later the pedicle is transected as a second stage. Incise the previous incision for a length equal to that of the pedicle and make

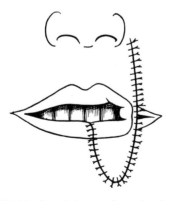

Fig. 15.12 Abbe lip switch – repair, sewing the ends of the commissure to the bare areas on the flap.

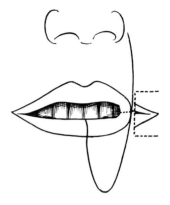

Fig. 15.13 Second-stage Abbe lip switch – solid line shown the healed initial incision. Transect the pedicle and make vertical and horizontal incisions, and lateral incisions, all the same length.

a lateral extension, again of equal length (Fig. 15.13).

Follow a similar procedure in the upper lip, forming a double Z-plasty. Reapproximate the vermilion borders, and sew up the skin extensions in the shape of a T, as in Figure 15.14. These sutures can be removed after 5 days and the patient discharged from hospital.

Bernard reconstruction

There is very rarely any need to do this operation, as tumours of the lower lip that cannot be handled by one of the preceding operations are very rare. It is done, however, when a very large amount of lower lip has to be removed. Its principles are illustrated in Figures 15.15–17.

Burrows operation for upper lip cancer

This is basically an advancement flap used for rare tumours in the middle of the upper lip, which are not

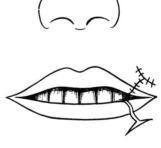

Fig. 15.14 Second-stage Abbe lip switch – when the vermilion margins are reapproximated, the incisions are closed in a T.

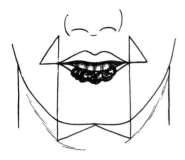

Fig. 15.15 Bernard reconstruction – incisions are made as marked.

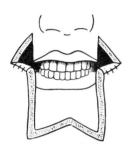

Fig. 15.16 Bernard reconstruction – the lower lip is removed together with two triangles at the commissure. The mucosa is retained in the triangular areas and swung down to form a new red surface as shown.

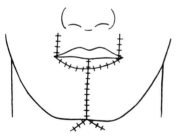

Fig. 15.17 Bernard reconstruction – when the margins are brought together the lower lip is formed of the areas covered previously by mucosa.

suitable for Abbe lip switch flaps. Its principle is shown in Figures 15.18 and 15.19.

This operation leads to ugly commissures because they are rounded, and they will require to be corrected at a later stage.

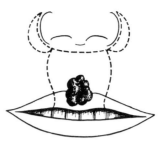

Fig. 15.18 Burrows operation – incisions are made as shown, including a through-and-through excision of an elliptical area around the alae.

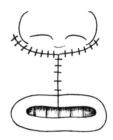

Fig. 15.19 Burrows operation – when the edges are brought together there is a rounding of the commissures.

Correction of rounded commissure

This operation is based on the double Z-plasty principle (Fig. 15.20). It is usually done 5 weeks after the initial operation.

Make an incision exactly at the middle of the rounded corner of the mouth, about 2.5 cm long. At the end of this, make two 2.5 cm incisions upwards and downwards, and then lateral extensions from these for the same distance, but angled at 60°. When the flaps are transposed and sutured, the angle of the mouth is sharpened. Further sharpening can be done using a modified vermilion advancement technique.

Estlander flap for angle tumours

Perform a through-and-through excision of the tumour, taking away the angle of the mouth; then outline an Estlander flap to lie parallel to the nasolabial groove, taking care to keep the labial artery

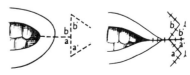

Fig. 15.20 Commissureplasty.

intact. Swing the flap down into the defect, which it should fill accurately if it has been planned properly, and close it in three layers. This leaves a rather gaping nasolabial incision, but with adequate undermining this can be closed in two layers. The usual aftercare is followed and if any reshaping of the commissure is required the previous technique can be used.

Radiotherapy techniques

External beam therapy

The lower lip is an ideal site for orthovoltage (300 kV) X-ray therapy. The patient lies supine, and the upper lip is protected by a shaped lead sheet which also enters the mouth and lies between the lower lip and the mandible, thus shielding the tongue and lower alveolus. A second sheet of lead overlies the lower lip, revealing the tumour with a 1 cm margin of healthy tissue through an appropriately sized semicircular aperture. Using a single anterior field, a fractionated course of 50 Gy in 15 fractions over 3 weeks or its equivalent is given.

Despite its suitabiity for treating carcinoma of the lip, some radiotherapy centres no longer have orthovoltage facilities. It is considered an obsolescent modality because the physical characteristics of the beam limit its usefulness in treating disease at other sites. Electron beams, generated by a linear accelerator, are increasingly being used instead of orthovoltage therapy. The set-up for treatment of lip carcinoma with an electron beam is similar to that used with orthovoltage equipment. It is, however, somewhat more cumbersome as the lead shielding needs to be thicker and the intraoral part of the posterior lead sheet has to be covered in a thick layer of wax to absorb the secondary X-rays generated when high-energy electrons strike heavy metals. In addition, because of the physical characteristics of electron beams, a wider margin of 2 cm of normal tissue around the tumour has to be included in the treatment volume. Electrons of 8–10 MeV should be used, and the prescribed dose and fractionation schedule will be the same as that used for orthovoltage treatment.

Interstitial therapy

Its accessibility, and the relatively small size of most of its cancers, make the lip a suitable site for interstitial treatment. The original technique, still in use, entails implantation with rigid needles containing caesium (which replaces the now obsolete radium). More recently, new techniques involving the use of hollow, fine flexible plastic or rigid metal tubes which are subsequently loaded with iridium wire have been developed. Whichever technique is employed, the implantation is usually performed under general anaesthesia. Both the old and new methods are effective, but better results using iridium have been reported. However as these studies were not randomized trials but retrospective comparisons with historical controls, great caution is needed in interpreting the claimed superiority of iridium – many other unidentified factors may have contributed to this apparent benefit. A genuine advantage of iridium wire afterloading is that because there is no radiation exposure to staff during the implant procedure, great care may be taken to ensure perfect geometry of the implant, and hence an optimal dose distribution. In addition the energy of the radiation emanating from iridium is lower than that from radium or caesium, making radiation protection easier. From the patient's point of view flexible tubes cause less discomfort. However iridium wire is costly, and has a half-life of only 74 days, whereas caesium needles with a half-life of 30 years can be reused almost indefinitely.

The usual dose prescription for implants with caesium needles is 60–70 Gy over 6–7 days, calculated under the Manchester rules. With iridium, a slightly shorter overall time is often used; 60 Gy, calculated according to the Paris system of dosimetry, is given over about 5 days.

A rarely used technique for irradiation of lip cancers involves the preparation of a device which sandwiches the lip between two plates of Perspex, each loaded with a suitable distribution of an appropriate radionuclide. This double mould or surface applicator is worn intermittently, for exmple for 6 hours each day for 8 days. The preparation of a good double mould requires certain technical skills, and when lip cancer can effectively be treated in simpler ways, it is not surprising that its use is limited.

Whether external beam or implant irradiation is used, it is inevitable that there will be a brisk mucosal and cutaneous reaction. This will proceed to moist desquamation on the skin, and formation of a fibrinous membrane within the mouth, both of which will take at least a couple of weeks to heal. Ultimately, however, a good functional and cosmetic result is usual. Later there may be some atrophy of the substance of the lip, and the skin will become depigmented and may show telangiectasia, but bad scarring is unusual.

Controversies

Staging of lip cancer

Various authors have used different classifications when reporting their results for carcinoma of the lip. The TNM staging system for mouth tumours does not include the lip because there is a great difference between lip cancer and mouth cancer. The

International Union against Cancer (UICC) classification takes account of the infiltration as well as the size, as both features correlate with tumour behaviour and prognosis. For example, a tumour may be less than 2 cm in its greatest dimension and still be classified as T_3 if it is deeply infiltrative. Tumour classifications that do not take account of invasion are probably invalid. This would apply to the American classification detailed by the Task Force for Head and Neck Sites in 1976.

There is a very close relationship between the prognosis for cure of lip cancer and the degree of cellular differentiation at the time of initial examination. A 5-year cure rate of 71% for grade 1 and 46% for grade 3 carcinomas has been reported.

Any classification system, therefore, must take account of the three variables – size, infiltration and tumour grade.

Management of malignant change in actinic cheilitis

It is often difficult to know if an area in a lip affected by actinic cheilitis has become malignant and has been infiltrated. If during a lip shave an area of infiltration is found, frozen sections should be called for. The lip shave can then be accompanied by a wedge excision and primary closure.

Management of upper lip tumours

Malignant tumours of the upper lip account for 1–7% of all carcinomas of the lip (see Surgical pathology, above). The 5-year survival rate for upper lip cancer is only 50–60%. Very occasionally a wedge excision can be performed but more usually Gillies advancement flaps are required for the closure of central upper lip defects. If the whole upper lip has to be removed, then the surgeon is presented with probably the most difficult reconstruction in the head and neck region. A bipedicled forehead flap has to be used for this work.

Upper lip tumours presenting with nodes are potentially incurable. The upper lip drains to the preauricular, infraparotid, submandibular and submental nodes. Thereafter, drainage goes to the deep jugular chain. If neck nodes are palpated, therefore, there must also be nodes within the facial tissue, thus rendering the patient inoperable.

Changes after radiation therapy

After radiation therapy there is permanent hypersensitivity to thermal and actinic stimuli. Patients who have outdoor occupations remain at a disadvantage, therefore, after such therapy. Local changes include atrophy of lip musculature in the irradiated field. This leads to close attachment of the vermilion to the underlying muscles and to general hardness in the area. It is very often difficult to know whether or not there has been recurrence and frequently these patients will herald recurrent disease with a neck node. In cases of deformity after irradiation or doubt as to the biological state of the tissue, a wedge excision of the irradiated area should be considered.

The place of prophylactic neck dissection

The place of prophylactic neck dissection in patients with cancer of the lip has not been prospectively studied. The cure rate from therapeutic neck dissection for a subsequently confirmed occult metastasis compares favourably with the results of elective neck dissection. Some authors have recommended aggressive treatment, including bilateral suprahyoid neck dissection if the primary lesion is greater than 1.5 cm in diameter, if the cancer is in the upper lip, if the cancer is recurrent or if it is poorly differentiated. If tumour is found in the suprahyoid specimens, a full radical neck dissection is then performed on the side of node involvement.

References and further reading

Surgical anatomy and pathology

Baker S R (1989) Cancer of the lip. In: Myers EN, Suen J Y (eds), *Cancer of the Head and Neck*. New York, Churchill Livingstone, pp. 383–415.

Baker S R, Krause C J (1980) Carcinoma of the lip. *Laryngoscope* **90**:19–27.

Batsakis J G (1991) Oral monomorphic adenomas. *Ann Otol Rhinol Laryngol* **100**:348–50.

Clark D B, Priddy R W, Swanson A E (1990) Oral inverted ductal papilloma. *Oral Surg Oral Med Oral Pathol* **69**:487–90.

Owens O T, Calcaterra T C (1982) Salivary gland tumors of the lip. *Arch Otolaryngol* **108**:45–7.

Sack J G, Ford C N (1978) Metastatic squamous cell carcinoma of the lip. *Arch Otolaryngol* **104**:282–5.

Surgery

McGregor I A (1983) Reconstruction of the lower lip. *Br J Plast Surg* **36**:40–7.

McGregor I A, McGregor F M (1986) The lips. In: *Cancer of the Face and Mouth: Pathology and Management for Surgeons*. Edinburgh, Churchill Livingstone, pp. 135–78.

Spira M, Hardy S B (1964) Vermilionectomy: review of cases with variations in technique. *Plast Reconstr Surg* **33**:39–46.

16

Tumours of the oral cavity

Surgical anatomy

The anatomical regions and sites forming the oral cavity under both the International Union against Cancer (UICC) and American Joint Committee (AJC) classifications are shown in Table 16.1.

The buccal mucosa is covered with non-keratinizing, stratified squamous epithelium. It covers the parotid duct and multiple minor salivary glands. It is fairly loose generally but is tight over the buccinator muscle. It is also rather tightly fixed in the upper and lower sulci and for this reason it is very difficult to stitch a skin graft to these sites. The mucosa also covers the alveoli, so that tumours of the buccal mucosa may well involve the upper and lower alveoli. The lymph drainage from the buccal mucosa is to the submandibular lymph nodes and from there to the lower deep cervical chain.

The rest of the mouth is covered by the same type of epithelium and there are multiple minor salivary glands in the hard palate and fewer in the floor of the mouth. There are also collections of minor salivary glands at specific sites, as shown in Table 16.2. The interlacing muscle fibres of the tongue form an easy pathway for the spread of cancer, and the constant movement of the tongue also disseminates the cancer widely. For this reason, tongue tumours must always

be assessed by palpation, and excisional margins must usually be greater than 2 cm.

Lymph from the tip of the tongue drains to the submental nodes and to nodes in the deep jugular chain (Fig. 16.1). The sublingual portion of the tongue drains to the submandibular nodes, and the rest of the anterior two-thirds of the tongue drains to the deep jugular chain from the level of the omohyoid to the posterior belly of digastric. This is important because the only gland enlarged in a tumour on the lateral border of the anterior two-thirds of the tongue may be the jugulo-omohyoid node.

It is also important to realize that lymph from the anterior part of the mouth drains to the *lower* jugular chain, making a suprahyoid neck dissection illogical.

The tip and middle of the tongue have a rich bilateral capillary lymph network but this is less on the lateral margins.

The U-shaped floor of the mouth drains mainly to the submandibular glands and the upper deep jugular chain. There is a moderate bilateral lymphatic drainage from the anterior parts of the U.

The lymph drainage of the alveolus is much the

Table 16.1 Anatomical regions and sites of the oral cavity

Buccal mucosa
    Mucosal surfaces of upper and lower lips
    Mucosal surface of cheeks
    Retromolar areas
    Buccoalveolar sulci, upper and lower
Upper alveolus and gingiva
Lower alveolus and gingiva
Hard palate
Tongue
    Dorsal surface and lateral borders anterior to vallate
    papillae (anterior two-thirds)
    Inferior surface
Floor of mouth

Table 16.2 Sites of minor salivary glands in the oral cavity

Labial glands in the submucosa of the inner surface of the lips
Retromolar glands in the vicinity of the opening of the parotid duct
Buccal glands in the mucous membrane of the cheek
Glands of the floor of the mouth
Lesser sublingual glands near the major sublingual gland
Glossopalatine glands, extending posteriorly from the lesser sublingual glands to the mucosa of the glossopalatine fold
Palatine glands, some 400 in number, distributed over the hard and soft palates and uvula, but not in the midline nor anterior to a line between the first molar teeth
Lingual glands situated close to the inferior surface of the tongue on each side of the frenulum, and at the base and lateral borders of the tongue.

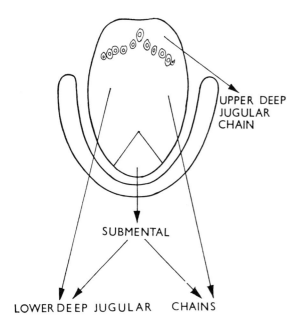

UPPER DEEP
JUGULAR
CHAIN

SUBMENTAL

LOWER DEEP JUGULAR   CHAINS

Fig. 16.1 Lymph drainage of tongue.

same as that of the floor of the mouth but the capillary network is less extensive.

In any cancer of the mouth, nodes in front of and behind the facial artery as it crosses the mandible (pre- and postfacial nodes) are often affected and must be included in the field of any radical neck dissection.

The mandible is a key structure in intraoral malignancy. The pattern of invasion by tumour and the mechanism of spread within bone determine the surgical approach to many tumours; its blood supply influences both excisional and reconstructive techniques. Loss of the teeth causes changes in the shape, structure and vascularity, as well as in patterns in tumour spread.

The body of the mandible can be divided into an upper part, which carries the teeth and is covered by mucoperiosteum (the alveolar segment), and a lower part, covered by periosteum alone. On its labial and buccal surfaces the line that separates the two runs along the lower buccal sulcus; on the lingual surface the line corresponds largely to that of the mylohyoid line on the bone.

The alveolar segment, with its covering of mucoperiosteum, is in direct contact with the oral cavity and it is the only part of the mandible which is, strictly speaking, intraoral.

These lines, along which mucous membrane and periosteum separate on each side of the bone, are approximately similar both in level and direction, running backwards and slightly upwards to meet behind the third molar where the pterygomandibular raphe is attached to the bone.

The mucosal surface behind the third molar, between it and the maxillary tuberosity, is called the retromolar trigone. There the mucosa overlies the anterior border of the ramus, separated from it by the pterygomandibular raphe where the buccinator and the superior constrictor muscles decussate.

Running through the mandible on each side, transmitting the inferior alveolar nerve with its accompanying vessels, is the mandibular canal. The site of entry of the neurovascular bundle into the canal is marked on the medial surface of the ramus by a bony spur, the lingula. The nerve leaves the outer surface of the mandible below the first premolar tooth.

The mandible has a comparatively small proportion of cancellous bone, which is concentrated in the body. Through this bone runs the mandibular canal and, as it has no lining of compact bone, the canal is in direct contact with the cancellous bone of the body. The ramus has very little cancellous bone and what there is, is largely localized just behind the third molar.

The tooth sockets are lined by a thin layer of compact bone, the lamina dura, and each is in continuity with the mandibular canal through the foramen opposite the apex of each root, which carries the vessels and nerves supplying the pulp of the teeth.

Considerable changes in the mandible occur after extraction of the teeth: the socket fills with blood clot which organizes rapidly to form cancellous bone. The overlying mucosa heals extremely rapidly. Whilst the socket fills rapidly with bone the projecting margins of the original socket are resorbed and the bone in this area is rounded down to produce the narrow ridge typical of an edentulous mandible.

When there is extreme resorption the bone is referred to as 'pipestem'. In such a mandible the floor of mouth, the occlusal surface of the alveolus, and the buccal sulcus are all virtually on the same plane. The alveolus is reduced to a strip of mucoperiosteum between the mucosal surface on each side. The mandibular canal and its contained inferior alveolar vessels and nerve comes to lie much closer to the occlusal surface.

A further anatomical effect of losing teeth is the relative change in the site of attachment of the mylohyoid to the mandible. Resorption of the alveolar segment leaves the attachment much closer to the occlusal ridge. The rise of the mylohyoid line in passing backwards brings the muscle insertion alongside the ridge in the molar region. This is of major importance as a factor in the mechanism of mandibular invasion by tumour.

In addition to the general remodelling associated with the edentulous state the tooth socket disappears, the line of teeth being converted into an occlusal ridge. All along the line of the crest the bone is imperfectly sealed by cortex and, where the cortical deficiencies are present, the mucoperiosteum is in direct continuity with the cancellous bone of the medulla. These defects are usually small but some can be as large as 2 mm in diameter. At their most frequent, virtually the entire ridge lacks a cover of cortical bone, the appearance being of a 'moth-eaten' line, 2–3 mm broad, all along the crest where the surface consists of cancellous bone.

In the mandible the absence of a protective cover of compact bone over the entire occlusal ridge means that virtually from the outset tumour is free to infiltrate through into the medullary cavity and reach the inferior alveolar nerve, with the potential thereafter for perineural spread.

Blood supply of the mandible

The intact mandible derives its blood supply from the inferior alveolar vessels, and from its soft tissue attachments.

Inferior alveolar vessels

These vessels, in addition to supplying the teeth, supply the surrounding bone also. The calibre of the artery and, presumably, the proportion of the total blood supply of the mandible it carries, alter both with age and whether or not teeth are present. It is thought that the blood flow decreases with age and loss of teeth.

Soft tissue attachments

The ramus has extensive vascular sources provided by the bony attachments of the pterygomasseteric muscle sling.

The alveolar segment of the body of the bone is covered with mucoperiosteum through which it is vascularized. This alveolar mucoperiosteum in turn derives its blood supply from the soft tissues attached to the bone, below the lower buccal sulcus laterally and the mylohyoid line medially (Fig. 16.2).

On its lingual surface the mandibular body, below the line of reflection of mucosa, has no soft tissue attachments and hence, no vascular sources other than those provided by the linear attachment of mylohyoid and the genial muscles at the symphysis. In contrast, the entire labial and buccal surface below the lower buccal sulcus is covered by soft tissue firmly attached to the bone. This attachment ends at the lower border of the body, except on each side of the symphysis where the bone broadens for the attachment of the digastric muscle.

Thus the body of the mandible receives the bulk of its blood supply from its labiobuccal aspect and not from its lingual side.

Surgical pathology

The relative incidence of different types of oral tumours is shown in Table 16.3. The incidence of tumour at various sites is shown in Table 16.4. It can be seen that squamous carcinoma forms the vast majority and it will be discussed first.

Squamous carcinoma

Many factors have been blamed for being carcinogenic, such as smoking, broken teeth, dental caries, spices, hot foods, avitaminosis, chronic glossitis, malnutrition, alcoholism, cirrhosis, chemical poisoning, the Plummer–Vinson syndrome and lichen planus. There is no evidence to show that these are at all premalignant but they are certainly associated factors.

The only true premalignant lesions in the oral cavity are leukoplakia and erythroplakia. Leukoplakia literally means a white plaque; it is used in

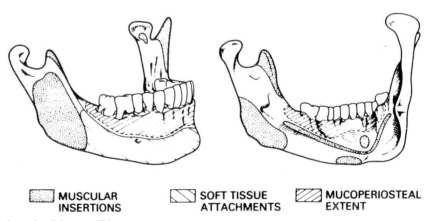

MUSCULAR INSERTIONS   SOFT TISSUE ATTACHMENTS   MUCOPERIOSTEAL EXTENT

Fig. 16.2 Blood supply of the mandible.

Table 16.3 The incidence of mouth tumours

Type of tumour	Incidence
Ectodermal	
Miscellaneous benign (mainly neural tumours)	1.0%
Benign salivary	2.0%
Squamous carcinoma	85.0%
(verrucous carcinoma	5%)
Malignant salivary	5.0%
Melanoma	0.1%
Mesodermal	
Haemangioma	1.5%
Granular cell myoblastoma	1.0%
Other benign	1.0%
Malignant	
Non-Hodgkin's lymphoma	1.0%
Hodgkin's lymphoma	0.1%
Fibrosarcoma	0.5%
Other sarcomas	1.0%
Metastatic	1.0%

Table 16.4 Site incidence of oral squamous carcinoma

Site of carcinoma		Incidence
Retromolar		2%
Buccal mucosa		10%
Tongue		35%
Lateral border	31%	
Tip	2%	
Dorsum	2%	
Floor of mouth		30%
Anterior	25%	
Lateral	15%	
Lower alveolus		15%
Upper alveolus		5%
Hard palate		3%

different ways by different authors. For example, some authors include other white lesions in the mouth, such as lichen planus, whereas most restrict the term to abnormal keratinization; the white appearance of lesions in this condition is usually due to the fact that keratin becomes white when it is wet. Furthermore, the term leukoplakia has no pathological significance. The interest of this lesion is due to the fact that a small proportion do become malignant.

There are various clinical appearances: an area of soft, white, velvety mucosa; a patch of white, resembling paint on the mucosa; an area of distinct pallor described as leukoplakia simplex; and verrucous leukoplakia combining leukoplakia with erythroplakia. Some leukoplakias show an irregular mixture of white areas and red areas. It is the erythroplakias that are the most dangerous lesions and the ones that are the most likely to become malignant.

About 80% of leukoplakias show a combination of hyperkeratosis, parakeratosis and acanthosis with no evidence of epithelial dysplasia. Moderate dysplasia is found in about 10% of specimens and severe dysplasia or carcinoma-*in-situ* in about 5%, many of which will be predominantly erythroplakia.

Leukoplakia most commonly occurs on the buccal mucosa, followed by the alveolar mucosa, the tongue, lip, palate, floor of the mouth and gingiva in that order. In the buccal mucosa the most common site is the occlusal line.

Lichen planus is a keratin-producing disease that usually affects the buccal mucosa; it is easily recognized by the multiple narrow grey but slightly elevated lines that converge towards each other forming a meshwork. The intervening mucosa looks rather oedematous. Another variety presents as elevated white spots and there is also a hypertrophic type resembling leukoplakia. Less frequent are the erosive and ulcerative varieties. If dyskeratosis is found in these lesions, they are premalignant but this is the exception rather than the rule.

Fordyce's disease consists of ectopic aggregates of sebaceous glands looking like clusters of greyish white or yellow nodules. It is not premalignant, nor is the white spongy naevus, which looks like leukoplakia and occurs in childhood.

Recent reports have shown that 80% of acquired immune deficiency syndrome (AIDS) sufferers develop hairy oral leukoplakia. This is a unilateral corrugated lesion on the posterolateral border of the tongue. However it may occur on the floor of the mouth, buccal mucosa and palate. Histological examination shows a thick epithelium with hyperkeratosis, areas of koilocytes and pyknotic nuclei.

Buccal carcinoma

Buccal carcinoma affects men more than women, occurs in the older age group and has a definite geographic incidence, being commonest in Indian communities in Africa and South East Asia (where it forms 40% of all cancers); in this region the chewing of betel nut and reverse smoking are common habits. It is also fairly common in the USA, where a percentage of the population still chew tobacco. It is, however, uncommon in the UK.

Buccal cancer is often diagnosed at a late stage, as this is the most insensitive part of the mouth.

The cheek forms the lateral wall of the mouth and consists of the buccinator muscle, external fibroadipose tissue and skin. The mucosal surface extends from the upper to the lower gingivobuccal sulci, where the mucosa is reflected over the upper and lower alveolar ridges, and forms the commissure of the lips and overlies the ascending ramus of the mandible. The most common site for buccal carcinoma is the commissure of the mouth, along the occlusal plane and in the retromolar areas.

There are three clinical types of buccal carcinoma, the exophytic, the ulceroinfiltrative and the verrucous, in that order of frequency. Most buccal carcinomas are well-differentiated in type, and carcinoma of the buccal mucosa is the commonest cancer in the mouth to be associated with pre-existing leukoplakia. Exophytic carcinomas are found most often around the buccal commissure whereas ulceroinfiltrative carcinomas invade the buccinator muscle early and present a deep excavating ulcer with diffuse peripheral extension. Lesions lying posteriorly extend easily into the pterygomaxillary fossa, and they can also invade the anterior tonsillar pillars, the alveolar ridges and the pterygoid fossa. The verrucous tumour most commonly occurs on the lower buccal sulcus and the lower alveolus. It can occur elsewhere in the mouth, but forms no more than 5% of all oral cancers. It has a characteristic papillary appearance: although it often appears relatively innocuous it invades the soft tissues of the cheek, the maxilla and the mandible. It rarely metastasizes even to lymph nodes, and almost never distantly.

Only 15% of buccal carcinomas are associated with palpable glands when first seen, and it is said that 5% have microscopically positive lymph nodes when none are palpable.

Carcinoma of the tongue

Carcinoma of the tongue is a disease of the middle-aged and elderly, with an equal sex incidence. Fifty years ago it was predominantly a disease of men, and there is no explanation for this change in the sex ratio.

Most squamous carcinomas are well-differentiated; poorly differentiated varieties are rare. Fifty per cent of carcinomas in the mouth arise in the anterior two-thirds of the tongue, and 85% of these arise from the lateral border (Fig. 16.3). Tumours arising from the dorsum, the ventral surface, or the tip are very uncommon. The incidence of lymph node metastases is shown in Table 16.5. Tongue

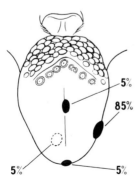

Fig. 16.3 Site of incidence of tumours of the oral tongue.

tumours may be infiltrative or exophytic. The infiltrative types may appear to be quite small on the surface, but palpation shows that they have invaded most or part of the tongue. The behaviour of the tumour becomes more aggressive the further posterior in the mouth the lesion lies: the incidence of lymph node metastases increases, and the ability of the tumour to spread from the tongue to the tonsillar pillars, the retromolar area and the floor of the mouth also increases. Large invasive carcinomas can also extend beneath intact mucosa into the muscles of the posterior third of the tongue and thence into the pre-epiglottic space. The tumour extends within the musculature of the tongue, but particularly in a posterior direction beneath an intact mucosa. Infiltration of the muscles ultimately causes immobility of the tongue. The tumour invades with ease through the midline septum of the tongue.

The incidence of lymph node metastases is proportional to the size of the tumour, and there is also correlation between certain histological grades of the tumour and lymph node metastases.

Carcinoma of the floor of the mouth

Tumours of the floor of the mouth are usually divided into those arising from the anterior part and those arising from the lateral part. The reason for this distinction is the differing surgical problems of these two sites. In many series about two-thirds of floor of the mouth tumours are said to arise in the anterior segment but that has not been our experience. A very common site in the anterior floor of the mouth is around the papilla at the point where the submandibular duct opens. Remaining tumours are distributed evenly along the floor of the mouth. These tumours spread marginally in a medial and lateral direction. Medial spread is therefore into the side of the tongue and deep spread occurs to the base of the tongue, particularly into the hyoglossus and genioglossus muscles. Lateral spread on to the alveolar periosteum is more important and more interesting. The point at which the tumour reaches the lingual surface of the mandible depends on two factors: Firstly, the level of the attachment of the mylohyoid muscle to the mandible, which rises steadily from the anterior floor backwards towards the molar region, and secondly, on whether the patient has teeth or not. In the dentate mandible the teeth form some barrier preventing spread from the lingual to the buccal surfaces.

Table 16.5 Oral squamous carcinoma: incidence of lymph node metastases

N_0	65%
N_1	15%
N_2	10%
N_3	10%

However, it is not often that a patient is seen with a carcinoma of the floor of the mouth who still has teeth. Much more often he or she is edentulous, in which case the sequence of pathological events is different. The alveolar segment of the mandible has been resorbed, and the occlusal ridge does not have a complete covering of cortical bone but is penetrated by foramina, so that the tumour can readily spread into the mandible through these, gaining access to the medullary cavity and to the inferior alveolar nerve (Fig. 16.4). This nerve provides an important pathway of spread of the tumour, and indeed the tumour can spread relatively rapidly along the nerve as far as the pterygoid fossa and the base of the skull.

Another important structure in the spread of tumour of the floor of the mouth is the muscle floor formed by the mylohyoid muscle. Anteriorly this presents a barrier to the inferior spread of tumour, but the muscle is deficient posteriorly and, in this area, the mucosa of the floor of the mouth lies very close to the overlying skin, separated only by subcutaneous tissue. Tumours here can thus spread relatively easily into the submandibular area, forming a palpable and ultimately visible lump.

Carcinoma of the lower alveolus

Carcinoma of the lower alveolus generally affects the anterolateral part; spread on to the floor of the mouth occurs readily. Thirty per cent of such patients have radiological evidence of bone destruction.

A tumour arising from any of the common primary sites (floor of mouth and tongue) can invade the mandible, but this process is most important in alveolar tumours. Tumour reaches the mandible by marginal spread in the mucosa and submucosa overlying the sublingual gland, the submandibular gland and mylohyoid. These structures appear to act as a significant barrier to deep infiltration, and initial involvement of the bone by direct spread is frequently confined above the mylohyoid line. The height of this line on the bone varies in the dentate and edentulous mandible (see Surgical anatomy, above) and this, together with a resorption of the alveolar segment that follows loss of the teeth, makes the spread pattern quite different in the two mandibles, dentate and endentulous.

In the endentulous mandible (Fig. 16.4) the proximity of the mylohyoid line to the occlusal ridge brings the tumour rapidly to this part of the bone. Once there, the absence of a cortical bone barrier along the line of the occlusal ridge allows the tumour to spread freely downwards into the medullary cavity.

In the dentate mandible the tumour spreading marginally reaches the bone at a much lower level, though still just above the mylohyoid line. There it involves the mucoperiosteum of the alveolar segment and, by infiltration deeply, the underlying cortex.

It is striking how seldom, both in the dentate and endentulous mandible, the bone is involved by direct extension below the mylohyoid line, even in the presence of extensive metastatic disease involving the submandibular nodes.

The proximity of the mucosa in the retromolar trigone to the bone, the presence of foramina behind the third molar, even in the dentate mandible, and an absence of cortex in the endentulous mandible results in early invasion with particular spread to the medullary bone that is present in the anterior part of the ramus in this region.

On its buccal aspect the level of the lower buccal sulcus corresponds largely to that of the mylohyoid line and the mechanism of spread from a buccal

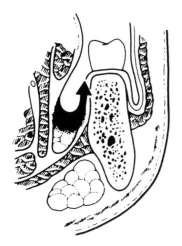 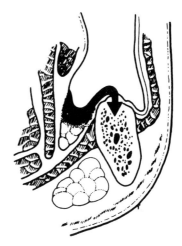

Fig. 16.4 Pathways of spread of tumour into the mandible. (a) Dentate; (b) edentulous.

carcinoma into the mandible is largely similar to that of tumour spreading from the floor of mouth, whether the bone is dentate or endentulous.

Once the tumour is within the medullary cavity the inferior alveolar nerve provides a ready pathway for perineural spread. Spread is predominantly proximal, towards the trigeminal ganglion. Perineural spread occurs in an unobtrusive manner with little involvement of the surrounding mandible. Until a relatively late stage the nerve looks clinically normal. Spread of tumour is not continuous along the nerve and this makes pathological examination of multiple samples desirable.

The site and frequency of lymph node metastases are the same as for tumours of the floor of the mouth. Carcinomas of the gingiva generally affect the premolar and molar areas, and quite often arise in an area of leukoplakia. These tumours may be ulcerating or exophytic. At least 50% of these tumours invade the underlying bone, by the same pathways as already indicated for tumours of the floor of the mouth. These tumours metastasize first to the submandibular nodes, and this metastasis is often fixed to the periosteum if not to the mandible.

Carcinoma of the upper alveolus and hard palate

Squamous carcinoma of these sites is uncommon, and tumours here are much more likely to be salivary in type. However, this statement is only true of the UK: squamous carcinomas, in certain parts of India, are very common on the hard palate due to the curious habit of smoking chuttas with the burning end inside the mouth. Squamous carcinoma of the hard palate is a disease of elderly men, usually detected in the seventh decade of life and often preceded by leukoplakia.

Second tumours

The hallmark of mouth cancer is the propensity for second tumours: mouth cancer is frequently multiple both in time and space. Up to 30% of patients with mouth cancer later develop another tumour, the commonest sites again being in the mouth, but also in the lung.

T stage

The definition of T categories of squamous carcinoma of the oral cavity is shown in Table 16.6. There is general agreement between the UICC and AJC schemes.

Node metastases

The incidence of lymph node metastases, using the UICC classification, is shown in Table 16.5. There is

Table 16.6 TNM clinical classification: T – primary tumour

T_x	Primary tumour cannot be assessed
T_0	No evidence of primary tumour
T_{is}	Carcinoma-*in-situ*
T_1	Tumour 2 cm or less in greatest dimension
T_2	Tumour more than 2 cm but not more than 4 cm in greatest dimension
T_3	Tumour more than 4 cm in greatest dimension.
T_4	Tumour invades adjacent structures, e.g. through cortical bone, into deep (intrinsic) muscle of tongue, maxillary sinus, etc.

no difference in lymph node metastatic rates between various sites, but the rate increases with increasing T stage, and decreasing differentiation of the tumour.

The level of the nodes in the neck is important in prognosis. Unlike most other head and neck sites the submandibular groups of nodes is invaded first.

Other tumours

Sarcoma

Fibrosarcoma and other soft tissue sarcomas occur in younger patients and even infants. There are very few clinical features to differentiate them from carcinoma, although sarcomas tend to grow more quickly.

Lymphoma

Both Hodgkin's and non-Hodgkin's lymphoma occur rarely in the mouth. The commonest site is the palate.

Malignant melanoma

This tumour is very rare and usually occurs on the upper alveolar ridge and palate. It often develops from a pre-existing naevus, usually in the young.

Minor salivary gland tumours

The pathology of salivary gland tumours is dealt with fully in Chapter 19. However, salivary gland tumours can occur in the mouth. The two commonest types are the pleomorphic adenoma and the adenoid cystic carcinoma.

In reported series of minor salivary gland tumours, the incidence of malignancy varies from 32 to 88%. This depends on the type of department reporting the incidence, and the difference in histological interpretation of highly cellular pleomorphic adenomas and mucoepidermoid tumours.

These tumours arise from the sites shown in Table 16.2. The commonest site is the posterior part of the hard palate. The cheeks, tongue, floor of mouth and retromolar region are rarely affected. The differential diagnosis includes mucocele, fibroma, sebaceous cyst, calculus, lipoma, haemangioma and lymphangioma.

They present as slow-growing, non-ulcerative masses in patients between the ages of 30 and 60 years, with no significant sex or race incidence. Although a smooth palatal mass should always raise the suspicion of a minor salivary gland tumour it is reported that a correct clinical diagnosis is made in only 10% of patients.

Granular cell myoblastoma

This is a smooth, sessile swelling on the tongue; the lesion arises from voluntary muscle but may not be a true tumour and may merely represent a degenerative lesion. Radical treatment is not necessary. The most important point about this tumour is that the pathologist must recognize it; the epithelium covering it often shows changes described as pseudoepitheliomatous hyperplasia, which can be misdiagnosed as being malignant.

Epidemiology

Mortality figures for cancer of the tongue in England and Wales are available from 1911 to 1988. Pronounced changes have occurred for both men and women during this period. The age-adjusted mortality rate (AMR) for men dying from cancer of the tongue has fallen from a peak of 106 per million in 1919 to less than 10 per million in recent years. The figure for women has also fallen from a peak of 12 per million in 1929 to about 5 per million in the late 1970s. The male : female ratio has changed from 9 : 1 to 1.5 : 1, reflecting the relatively greater fall in AMR for men. Cohort analysis also reveals more pronounced changes for men than women. Peak mortality from cancer of the tongue was in the 65–75-year age group in the male cohorts born in the mid 19th century, but in the later cohorts the age-specific mortality rate continued to rise with increasing age to a plateau at 80 years of age. In contrast, the female cohorts generally showed a steady rise in death rate with increasing age, with no peak or plateau effect.

Figures for alcohol and tobacco consumption over the period 1850–1950 suggest that alcohol has played a more significant role than tobacco in the changing trends in tongue cancer for England and Wales.

The decreasing frequency of cancer of the oral cavity is probably due to the decreasing incidence of syphilis, and abandoning of clay pipes and chewing tobacco, and the improved standard of dentistry throughout the population; a cancer of the mouth is now seldom seen in a patient with good dentition.

Investigations

History

The patient usually consults a doctor or dentist having noticed a mass or an ulcer in the mouth. Pain is a prominent feature especially if the ulcer is touched; the pain may be referred to the ear because of the lingual nerve. Alveolar or palatal tumours may be invasive and may interfere with the fitting of the patient's dentures. Sometimes the first sign is an enlarged neck node. Generally speaking the more anterior the tumour, the earlier the patient seeks advice.

Examination

The mouth should be examined with two tongue blades, and a certain routine should be followed in every case. First, examine the teeth and the alveolar margins. Then pull the buccal mucosa outwards with the tongue blades and examine the sulci, the buccal mucosa and the parotid duct. Next ask the patient to put out the tongue, and examine it for movement and mobility; now ask him or her to place the tip of the tongue behind the upper alveolus so that the anterior floor of the mouth can be examined. Continue the examination round the floor of the mouth on each side and, at the posterior part of this fossa, where it meets the tongue and the anterior pillar, pay special attention to the linguoalveolar sulcus ('coffin corner'). Tumours at this site can be missed if it is not properly examined with the tongue blades. Inspect the tonsil, the posterior wall of the oropharynx, and the hard and soft palates. Finally, do an indirect laryngoscopy to examine the vallecula, epiglottis and aryepiglottic folds, and examine the posterior part of the soft palate with a nasopharyngeal mirror. Make an accurate drawing of the tumour using the teeth as landmarks. Accurate measurements must be done as it is very easy to get the margins of clearance wrong in the mouth. The local examination is completed with a manual palpation of the tumour. Examination of the rest of the head and neck and other systems is then carried out.

It is sometimes helpful to paint the tumour with 2% toluidine blue for 30 s and then asks the patient to wash all the dye out of the mouth. Although this is not an established technique, it appears that most malignant tumours in the oral cavity stain with toluidine blue while other lesions, such as granulomas and papillomas, do not take up the stain and are washed clean with water.

Radiology

Plain films of each half of the mandible and orthopantomograms should be taken to show erosion of the mandible by tumour, dental conditions such as apical abscesses or retained roots, or radionecrosis if the patient has previously had radiotherapy. There are several characteristic radiological patterns of invasion of the mandible by squamous carcinoma. These include smooth pressure erosion of the superior surface of the alveolus, an irregular invasive bone defect, floating teeth, displaced bony fragments, pathological fractures and, rarely, an expanded inferior dental canal. A chest radiograph should of course always be taken.

Laboratory studies

There are no special laboratory investigations other than those required for a routine preoperative check. The appropriate tests of syphilis are occasionally worth doing but syphilis in association with oral cancer is now rare.

Biopsy

It is unwise to do a biopsy under local anaesthesia because of the risk of metastases due to a rise of tissue pressure. If the tumour is large then a biopsy can be taken in the outpatient department using punch forceps without the use of a local anaesthetic. When the lesion is less than 1.5 cm admit the patient to hospital and carry out a biopsy excision under a general anaesthetic. If it turns out to be a carcinoma and the margins are clear of tumour, then a 'wait-and-see' policy may be adopted.

Make an accurate drawing of the size and extent of the tumour using all available landmarks.

Treatment policy

Surgery has no part to play in the treatment of either sarcoma or lymphoma. The treatment for these is radiotherapy. The only issue to be discussed here, therefore, is the treatment of squamous carcinoma and the salivary tumours. Virtually all of the latter require surgery.

To manage oral cancer properly you need skills in ablative and reconstructive surgery, a command of some basic dental skills, and the help of a prosthetic specialist or oral surgeon.

Some general points will be made first.

1 T_1 and early T_2 tumours can be treated with either surgery or radiotherapy alone. The larger T_2 and smaller T_3 lesions are best treated by surgery. Massive tumours do very badly with any treatment and may best be left untreated.
2 Radiotherapy of the mouth requires that the mandible will be irradiated to a greater or lesser extent. Osteoradionecrosis of the mandible is a risk even if no further surgery is performed, but is an almost certain complication if anything other

than wide resection of the mandible is done in any salvage surgery. If a mandible has been irradiated, later excision and bone grafting will be impossible. This is important in lesions of the anterior floor of mouth, where loss of the anterior arch of the mandible is totally disabling.
3 Radiotherapy does not cause dental caries. It does however predispose to periodontal disease, which in turn causes marginal caries. This is treatable if diagnosed early but, if it goes on to cause pulpitis and root abscess, then osteoradionecrosis of the mandible will follow. Dental extraction before radiation is not mandatory if future dental care can be regular and thorough. If, however, the teeth are initially poor and the patient is not dentally conscious, then all the teeth should be extracted and the sockets stitched 10 days before irradiation.
4 Removal of soft tissue from the mouth cripples both eating and speaking, especially if the tip of the tongue is immobilized. Two methods are available for this situation. Firstly, primary closure is done and 6 weeks later the scarred area is opened up and a split-thickness skin graft applied. This is held in place with a modified denture – the epithelial inlay technique. The second method is to use immediate reconstruction with a local or distant flap.
5 Invasion of the periosteum of the mandible by tumour used to be an indication for removal of that part of the mandible. It has been general experience, however, that tumour recurrence within the bone is rare and so the principle of partial mandibulectomy is now accepted. Either the upper half or lower half of the mandible may be removed, the lingual plate or the outer surface, or any combination of these.
6 If neck nodes are palpable the patient should be treated by surgery. In the case of a small (T_1 on T_2) tumour with no palpable neck nodes, as the first echelon of nodes is usually irradiated *en bloc* with the primary tumour, elective irradiation of the lower neck is not necessary. Patients irradiated for larger tumours with no palpable nodes should however receive prophylactic neck irradiation in addition, as the risk of occult nodal involvement is greater. If no neck nodes are palpable and the primary lesion is treated surgically, then an elective neck dissection should probably be done if the primary tumour is greater than 3 cm in its greatest diameter. This is because the incidence of neck node metastases is proportional to the size of the primary tumour.
7 Carcinoma of the mouth appears to be one of those tumours where the survival can be improved by the use of postoperative radiotherapy, although this matter has not been proven by controlled trials. Preoperative radiotherapy has previously been very popular but has now been largely abandoned.

An outline of treatment policy will now be given for each site.

Leukoplakia

A biopsy should be taken in every case, and should be cut if possible from what appears to be the most active part, particularly if the lesion appears to be more an erythroplakia than a leukoplakia. If histology shows little or no dysplasia the patient probably requires no further treatment, although laser fulguration can be used. Aetiological factors such as carious teeth and heavy smoking should be eliminated if possible and the patient reassured. Such patients almost certainly do not require follow-up.

The patient with leukoerythroplakia is quite different. The histology report will usually show severe dyskeratosis or carcinoma-*in-situ*. The entire affected area should be stripped off and submitted to serial histological examination. The denuded area is covered with a split-skin graft using the quilting technique (see below) or vaporized with the laser.

Buccal carcinoma

The buccal mucosa is very elastic, but cancers arising in the mucous membrane invade fairly early so that attempts at wide but superficial removal in this area run the risk both of failure to get deep enough and, by reason of scarring, restricting the opening of the mouth. The decision regarding assessment of tumour invasion is therefore critical.

A small tumour ($<$ 2 cm) can be removed locally, with a reasonably safe margin of normal tissue and primary closure. Interstitial radiotherapy provides a satisfactory alternative to excision of small tumours at this site.

If the tumour is surrounded by a large area of leukoplakia and a wide excision of buccal mucosa is needed, then skin grafting will be required.

Tumours larger than this are generally managed by radiotherapy, with surgery being reserved for recurrence. Tumours of the buccal mucosa that involve the upper alveolar sulcus are difficult to get access to and even more difficult to graft. These tumours should be aproached with a Fergusson incision.

Large buccal cancers that require removal of facial skin can be managed in one of two ways, depending on their site. If they are near the lower alveolus they are removed together with the adjacent skin of the cheek and upper half of the adjacent alveolus. The defect is closed by suturing the mucosa of the tongue or floor of mouth, depending on the extent of the incision, to the remaining upper buccal mucosa to provide inner lining. Advancement of the neck flaps supplies the outer lining. If they are near the upper alveolus then that operation is impossible because it is too high for the tongue to stretch without crippling the mouth. A through-and-through excision is performed, and the defect is closed by two flaps. This is one of the few situations where a forehead flap may still be used, and one surface will almost certainly be provided by a microvascular flap, notably a radial forearm flap.

Carcinoma of the tip of the tongue

Excise this in a V-shaped fashion so that a new tongue tip can be made.

Carcinoma of the dorsum of the tongue

If the tumour is less than 2 cm in diameter, excise it in an ellipse and close the tongue defect primarily. Alternatively, small tumours may be treated by interstitial irradiation. Surgical treatment for larger tumours would require an extensive operation, and so radiotherapy is preferred in order to preserve the tongue. As large tumours cannot be treated by interstitial irradiation alone, external beam radiotherapy, perhaps combined with an interstitial implant, is used.

Carcinoma of the lateral border of the tongue

If no glands are palpable then the choice lies between interstitial irradiation and partial glossectomy. If the tumour is greater than 3 cm in size then either external beam irradiation is used or hemiglossectomy is performed. If glands are palpable, hemiglossectomy with radical neck dissection is preferable. This can be done without splitting the mandible (pull-through technique).

Carcinoma of the anterior floor of the mouth

If this tumour invades the alveolus then the anterior part of the mandible must be resected. This gives a horrible cosmetic deformity called the 'Andy Gump' deformity (after the character in the American strip cartoon), so that primary bone grafting must be performed to avoid this. Primary bone grafting should never be done after radiotherapy because of the high rate of failure, due usually to necrosis and infection. Radiotherapy should therfore never be used, even in the combined form; primary surgery, with removal of the floor of the mouth, the anterior segment of mandible, and a neck dissection if a gland is palpable, should be performed.

In this situation it is often possible to preserve the basal segment of the mandible, consisting of hard cortical bone that is seldom invaded by the tumour. If this is not possible the entire anterior segment must be resected and replaced by one of the techniques described below.

If no glands are palpable it is advisable to do a bilateral suprahyoid dissection. Examine all the glands histologically and, if any are positive, continue at a later stage to do a radical neck dissection on that side. This is the only site where a partial neck dissection is admissible. If the alveolus is not invaded then the tumour should be removed together with the lingual plate and the upper half of the mandible.

Carcinoma of the lateral floor of mouth and lower alveolus

If there are no glands palpable in the neck, and there is no radiological evidence of destruction of the mandible, the patient should be treated by radiotherapy. If, however, there are enlarged glands in the neck or destruction of the mandible the patient should be treated by a pelvimandibulectomy, that is removal of the floor of the mouth in continuity with a partial mandibulectomy; a radical neck dissection is carried out on the same side. The soft tissue reconstruction can either be by primary closure, in which case there will be no sulcus left on that side of the mouth with subsequent difficulties in eating and speaking, or the soft tissue defect can be filled with local or distant flaps. If the mandible is invaded then remove the horizontal ramus and replace it with a bone graft.

The salivary tumours

The salivary tumours are considered in greater detail in Chapter 19. The most common problem is the tumour on the hard palate, which may be a benign pleomorphic adenoma or a malignant adenoid cystic carcinoma. Both of these are usually treated surgically by resection of the hard palate and alveolus, as described for tumours of the nose and sinuses in Chapter 13.

Salivary tumours also occur occasionally elsewhere in the mouth, usually on the floor of the mouth and the alveolus. These are almost always of the malignant varieties, either adenoid cystic carcinomas or mucoepidermoid carcinomas. Very small tumours, 1 cm in diameter or less, may be controlled for long periods by radiotherapy, but the vast majority require surgery, which should be at least as extensive as that described for squamous carcinoma at the same site.

Repair

Many procedures have been described for repairing the soft tissue defect in the mouth. Small defects without loss of the bulk of the tongue can be covered by split-skin grafts, preferably using the quilting technique, as described below. For the other defects it is necessary to define first of all what has been removed, and therefore what would be replaced. The possibilities are: mucosal lining alone, lining plus bulk, lining plus bone, and lining plus bulk plus bone.

Mucosa alone can be replaced with the lingual flap, the nasolabial flap (which is more rarely used), a deltopectoral flap (which is now rarely used), or a free flap consisting of skin only, in particular the radial forearm flap. The use of an opened jejunal loop has been described for mucosal closure. If it is longer than 7 cm then the arterial arcade can survive interruption by opening jejunum and laying it out. Loops smaller than this however necrose and should be avoided. The radial forearm flap is the best alternative.

The forehead flap should be preserved for revision surgery, but the alternatives are so numerous that it is almost never used nowadays.

Some situations, especially subtotal glossectomy, require reconstitution of skin and muscle bulk. There are several possibilities, including a pectoralis major flap and a free rectus abdominis flap, or a free latissimus dorsi flap. The technique for the first of these flaps is described in Chapter 4.

Loss of lining and bone is usually due to resection of a carcinoma of the anterior part of the alveolus with the neighbouring floor of the mouth. This problem can be tackled in many ways, which indicates, of course, that none of them is satisfactory. Most of the attention in the literature has been devoted to techniques of transferring bone and overlying skin to the mouth, but in reality the main problem is not in the graft but in the recipient site. Several factors militate against a high success rate: the mandible has very often been irradiated; even before the development of carcinoma the mandible is usually atrophic because of loss of teeth; osteoblastic activity is low; the graft is potentially exposed to saliva and infection from the mouth; and the temporomandibular joint is probably the most mobile joint in the body after the shoulder joint.

The problem can be tackled in two ways – either the 'big bang' approach in which an attempt is made to repair all the tissues lost at one stage, or, alternatively, an efficient oral seal is achieved, the remaining mandibular stumps are fixed in the appropriate position by an arch bar, and mandibular continuity is reconstituted later. For the beginner it is better not to attempt one-stage reconstruction of a soft tissue and bone defect in the mouth, and the surgeon should be content with achieving a good water-tight seal. In most circumstances a pectoralis major flap is suitable for this purpose. Once the soft tissues have healed, that is after about 3 weeks, the site is reopened from below and the mandibular continuity is restored either by a free bone graft or a tantalum tray.

The mandible can also be reconstructed by a preformed titanium-mesh tray or a Dacron urethane perforated tray, which will support harvested cancellous bone. The titanium tray can be moulded and cut with the supplied instruments and held in place with titanium screws inserted into any remaining healthy bone fragments. The Dacron urethane tray can be cut with scissors and moulded in hot water. It is advisable to screw the tray to overlap any healthy remaining bone (if present) by at least 15 mm to obtain good stability.

A complete mandible can be reconstructed using the same technique, and mandibular condyles can be bolted to the tray for articulation with the glenoid fossae.

Intermaxillary fixation after surgery is not necessary, and early movement of the reconstructed mandible should be encouraged.

These trays can be used for primary or secondary reconstruction, although generally secondary reconstruction is favoured. The techniques can be used after radiotherapy, but delayed healing is certain in the treatment of such patients. The harvested cancellous bone should be condensed firmly into the tray to give the maximum density. Trays should be removed in 3–4 months so that muscle function can mould and stabilize the newly constructed mandible.

Methods of providing lining and bone in one stage include a forearm flap with a segment of radius, and the use of a trapezius flap with the spine of the scapula.

Finally, the replacement of two skin surfaces, for example after resection of a buccal carcinoma, needs to be considered. There are various combinations available, particularly a forehead flap and a free radial forearm flap.

Technique of operations for tongue cancer

Local excision of mouth cancers

Many mouth cancers of 1.5 cm in diameter or less can be managed successfully by local sharp or laser excision. The operation is done under general anaesthetic, and no preliminary tracheostomy is needed. Hold the mouth open with a prop placed between the teeth, and excise the area with a 1 cm margin. Mark the margins of the excised specimen so that the pathologist will later be able to orientate it and identify any resection margins that are not clear to tumour.

Change your gloves and then secure haemostasis. If the excision has been done by a laser it is said that grafting of the defect is not needed, but certainly if the defect was created either by a knife or a cutting diathermy the resected area should be grafted. Use the quilting technique as follows. Take a thin split-skin graft of appropriate size from the thigh or the upper arm, and stitch this in place with interrupted 3/0 silk sutures on a cutting needle all round the edge of the defect. Then place further interrupted sutures through the graft and through the bed about 5 mm

apart to achieve overall anchorage, thus ensuring that capillaries as they grow in are not sheared off. Finally, make small nicks in the graft between the sutures so that any serum or blood can escape. A tie-over dressing is not necessary with this type of graft.

This operation is suitable for smaller tumours provided that invasion of the substance of the tongue is minimal. Larger tumours should be treated by a subtotal glossectomy.

Hemiglossectomy

Before any operation on the tongue is contemplated, the use that the patient makes of the voice must be considered. If he or she depends on the voice for a livelihood then attempts must be made to leave a good tip to the tongue and to supply a sulcus so that the patient can wear dentures, either immediately or later.

The question of standing teeth will also have to be considered. If the patient is to have pre- or postoperative radiotherapy then all these teeth should be removed before radiation. If primary surgery is being used then only bad teeth need to be removed before it. If all the teeth are good then it is only necessary to take out the lower lateral incisor tooth on the side of the jaw that is to be split. The tooth roots go about halfway down into the mandible: if a root is cut a dental abscess can occur leading to nonunion of a split mandible. If a tooth is damaged in an irradiated jaw then the abscess will cause osteoradionecrosis and it is possible for the mandible to necrose up to both condyles.

The operation begins with a tracheotomy and the general anaesthetic is continued via this. Use electrocautery to excise the primary lesion within the mouth before beginning the resection. This is done to prevent spillage when the tongue is handled. At the time of resection the coagulated area is excised with a further margin of 1 cm of surrounding tissue.

Incision and radical neck dissection

A T on-its-side incision is suitable for most purposes.

Do a standard radical neck dissection and leave it attached at the submandibular region. The first question to answer when that dissection is completed is whether to do a lip-splitting incision or not. It is quite possible to do this operation without splitting the lip, which is preferable as it prevents oedema and a scar. Continue the upper part of the neck incision 5 cm across the midline and upwards almost to the mandible. Elevate the skin off the mandible; prevent troublesome bleeding from the mental foramen by first isolating and dividing the vessels that pass through it. Cut the mucosa in the gingivolabial sulcus, thereby entering the mouth.

Excision

Access to the tongue tumour can be obtained either by a mandibulotomy or by the pull-through procedure.

Mandibulotomy

Incise the periosteum just posterior to the mental foramen and elevate it for 1 cm on either side. This is rather difficult to do medially where the periosteum may be torn, but this does not usually matter. Mark a step with methylene blue as shown in Figure 16.5, and drill four holes as shown; it is very much easier to drill these holes before the mandibulotomy due to the stability of the mandible. Put a malleable copper retractor on the medial surface of the mandible when drilling these holes to protect the soft tissues. With a Stryker saw or dental fissure burr cut along the marks and swing the mandibular fragments apart. The mandible bleeds from its medulla and this can be stopped either with bone wax or coagulation diathermy. Never split the mandible in a straight line or in the midline because adequate fixation is not possible and non-union is likely.

Pull-through procedure

Expose the mandible in its periosteum with the first group of muscles – the anterior belly of the digastric

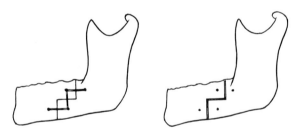

Fig. 16.5 Mandibulotomy.

muscle. Make an incision along the external surface of the inferior border of the horizontal ramus. Lift the periosteum of the inner surface of the mandible using a periosteal elevator. Divide the anterior belly of the digastric muscle close to its attachment to the digastric fossa on the lower border (Fig. 16.6a).

The second layer of muscle making up the floor of the mouth is the mylohyoid muscle. Divide this close to its attachment along the mylohyoid line on the mandible (Fig. 16.6a). The third layer of muscles is exposed – the geniohyoid muscle anteriorly and the hyoglossus muscle posteriorly. Cut the geniohyoid muscle close to its attachment to the inferior genial tubercle on the posterior aspect of the symphysis menti. Occasionally it is necessary to divide the anterior margin of the hyoglossus muscle to aid exposure and mobilization. This exposes the deepest layer of the floor of the mouth, the genioglossus muscle and intrinsic muscles of the tongue (Fig. 16.6b). Division of the genioglossus muscle and the periosteum of the mandible is carried out at the apex of the alveolar ridge. This allows the tongue, the intervening lymphatics and the periosteum to be delivered into the neck, still in continuity with the neck dissection.

Excision of the tumour

Hold the tip of the tongue in a towel clip, pull it forward, and remove the tumour with cutting diathermy along the tattoo marks. It will be necessary to stop and tie the lingual artery, but do not waste time tying the other bleeding points until the tumour has been removed. Take at least a 4 cm margin and remember that the clearance margin must be in depth as well as width. Take the cutting diathermy through the muscles of the floor of the mouth and remove the whole specimen, always keeping the diathermy at right angles to the tattoo marks. If it is

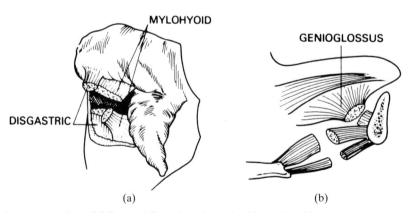

Fig. 16.6 Pull-through procedure. (a) Exposed digastric and mylohyoid muscles; (b) the genioglossus muscle divided.

angled then there will be poor tumour clearance in its deeper parts. Secure haemostasis with coagulation diathermy and 3/0 silk ties, wash the wound out and change gown and gloves.

If the tumour is greater than 3 cm in diameter or there is deep invasion of the tongue, a subtotal glossectomy is needed, sparing only a stump of tongue above the vallecula and of the base of the tongue on the side opposite the lesion.

Repair

After excision of very small tumours (less than 2 cm) it is possible to close the defect primarily. But after removal of larger segments (up to half the body of the tongue) an immediate split-skin graft should be inserted to allow mobility and so as not to cripple speech and swallowing. If more than half of the tongue has been removed it is also necessary to add bulk, and this is achieved with a distant flap either from the temporal area or a deltopectoral flap.

Close the tongue in two layers, the deeper layer being for muscles using mattress sutures of 2/0 chromic catgut. Stitch the mucosa with 3/0 silk and tie the knots inside the mouth so as to evert the suture line. Sew the tip up in order to make a new tip and then sew the lateral border of the tongue to the remaining mucosa in the floor of the mouth.

Put the ends of the jaws together and wire them as shown in Figure 16.5 with two horizontal wires. Be sure to tuck the cut ends of the wire into the drill holes so they do not stick out into the mouth. Suture the periosteum back across the split in the mandible with 3/0 chromic catgut and then put another layer of sutures under the suture line in the floor of the mouth using whatever muscle tissue is available. No external fixation is needed for the jaw. Put some water into the mouth to make sure the wound is watertight. Put suction drains in the neck and close the skin in the usual manner.

If primary closure is not possible but less than half of the tongue has been removed the remaining raw surface may be lined with split skin to preserve mobility of the tongue; as less than half of the tongue has been removed it is not necessary to replace the bulk of the tongue. The split skin can be applied with the quilting technique described above. Occasionally the inlay technique can be useful. It should only be used if a mandibulotomy has not been done. At the end of the excisional phase achieve absolute haemostasis of the tongue with diathermy. Take a thin split-thickness skin graft from the thigh and wrap it with the raw surface outwards over a tube of red rubber of diameter 1–1.5 cm and of a length equal to the sagittal length of the defect in the tongue. The skin graft is fixed on the tube either with skin glue or by suturing the graft with fine catgut sutures along the tube.

Now place the tube with the skin graft draped over it between the remnant of the tongue and the body of the mandible. Suture the remaining part of the tongue to the remaining part of the buccal mucosa in two layers in such a way as to bury the skin tube completely. Reinforce this closure and immobilize the tongue by passing two wire sutures round the mandible, through the tongue and over the graft as shown. The principle of this technique is thus that the graft is protected from the influence of saliva and is immobilized by the wire suture.

A week or 10 days after the original operation reanaesthetize the patient and cut down through the tongue on to the tube, which is removed leaving a skin-lined sulcus.

If more than half the tongue has been removed, flap repair will be required to replace lining and bulk. The possibilities include a pectoralis major flap and a rectus abdominis free flap.

Aftercare

1 General care.
2 Keep the tracheostomy in place for a week.
3 Start on a soft diet after 10 days but wait for 2–3 months before allowing chewing.
4 Dentures should not be worn for at least 3 months.
5 If there is a poor sulcus after primary closure and the patient wishes to wear dentures, then put in an epithelial inlay after 3 months. The technique for this is as described above.
6 If a patient who has undergone extensive surgery in the mouth wishes to have first-class dental rehabilitation, one suitable solution is offered by osseointegrated implants. It has been shown that titanium pegs can be implanted into the mandible and that bone will grow into the implant by direct physical apposition without any foreign body reaction or intervening fibrous layer. Some months after the implant has been introduced the overlying mucosa is divided and a further peg is attached to the implant. The peg is used to anchor a denture.

Complications

1 *Bleeding from the tongue.* This must be stopped because the whole tongue can swell and the suture line burst. It usually can be stopped by operating through the mouth, reopening the suture line and catching the bleeding points. This is the main reason why all patients having tongue operations should have a tracheostomy.
2 *Non-union of the mandible.* There are many reasons for this, the commonest being that a tooth root has been damaged, that a drill hole has gone through a tooth root, or that the mandible has been divided through a tooth root (Fig. 16.7). Never split irradiated bone because it is prone to non-union. If a fistula occurs due to breakdown of

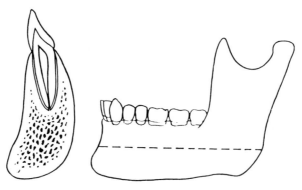

Fig. 16.7 The roots of the teeth come halfway down the mandible, so that drill holes above the dashed line in the diagram will almost certainly go through a root. This is why it is wise to consider removal of the teeth prior to any mandibular surgery.

the mouth wound, then saliva will get into the mandible and it will not heal. A common way to get a fistula in this situation is to leave the ends of the wire rather long, so that they protrude into the mouth and act as a track for saliva. If the mandible is wired as described, then it will be adequately fixed; if it is wired with fixation in only one direction, or too loosely, then it will not heal due to poor fixation.

The treatment of this depends upon the cause. If the trouble is due to a tooth then the tooth and adjacent ones should be removed under antibiotic cover. If the mandible still does not heal, it should be reopened and rewired, and cancellous bone chips packed around the split.

If non-union is due to a fistula, close it, put the patient on antibiotics, and if the mandible still does not heal, reopen it and rewire it as before.

If the patient has been irradiated, excise a wide segment of mandible and hope that the osteo-radionecrosis does not proceed up to the condyles. It is better to accept a small deformity rather than the ultimate gross deformity.

3 *Poor speech.* The speech result depends on how much of the floor of the mouth has been removed, but matters can always be improved by providing a tip to the tongue or an epithelial inlay to make a new sulcus. This allows the patient to wear dentures, which vastly improves the speech. Repairing the defect with a flap as a primary procedure allows the tongue to be freely mobile from the earliest stages.

4 *Recurrence in the primary site.* Wide excision of the tongue, hemimandibulectomy and repair with a flap might be possible.

5 *Recurrence in nodes.* If the patient had an involved gland in one side of the neck he or she has an even chance of developing one on the other side. Therefore see the patient at monthly intervals for 2 years, and longer thereafter; carry out a radical neck dissection if a node appears.

Operations for tumours of the floor of the mouth and alveolus (Pelvimandibulectomy)

Tumours of this area are dealt with in a very similar manner by the operation of pelvimandibulectomy.

Anaesthetic, incision and radical neck dissection

Use a general anaesthetic, but do a temporary tracheostomy and continue the anaesthetic through this. Make a T on-its-side type of incision. If you are a beginner it is better to give yourself good access to the mouth by splitting the lip in an S-shape (Fig. 16.8) but the cosmetic results are improved by not splitting the lip.

If the patient has an enlarged node in the neck, a radical neck dissection is done and left with its pedicle on the submandibular area.

Removal of the primary tumour

Raise the superior cervical flap well up over the mandible, with or without splitting the lower lip. Divide the oral mucosa in the gutter lateral to the mandible, well away from the tumour.

It is usually necessary to remove a segment of the mandible but it is virtually always possible to preserve either the lower border of the mandible or its outer plate, thus preserving bony continuity, which is superior to removal of the mandible and grafting.

If the tumour affects the alveolar ridge remove the superior part of the mandible (i.e. the alveolus) in the appropriate area. Divide the mandible with a Stryker saw or a fissure burr on a dental drill,

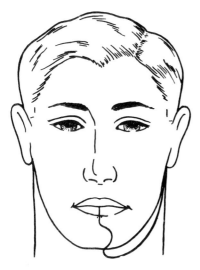

Fig. 16.8 The upper neck incision is extended to a lip-splitting incision in an S-shaped fashion.

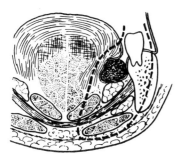

Fig. 16.9 Removal of lingual plate of mandible in continuity with the tumour.

working from outside through the access provided by elevating the cheek. Leave the segment of mandible in continuity with the primary tumour.

Alternatively, if it is thought that the lingual plate of the mandible is invaded, this can also be removed in continuity with the primary tumour as shown in Figure 16.9.

Repair

The soft tissues must be replaced after resection of a carcinoma of the floor of the mouth or of the alveolus in two circumstances.

1 When part of the mandible has been resected laterally leaving an area of raw bone, particularly if the patient has been irradiated, or if a full-thickness excision of the mandible has been carried out and a bone graft has been inserted.

2 When the anterior part of the floor of the mouth has been resected. Replacement of the soft tissues of the floor of the mouth is necessary in this case, otherwise suturing of the anterior part of the tongue remnant to the labial mucosa leads to ptosis of the lower lip and to interference with articulation.

Fortunately, the amount of tissue removed in such cases may not be such as to require replacement by a large flap. The lateral part of the floor of the mouth and the alveolus can be covered with a lingual flap, and the anterior part of the floor of the mouth can be replaced by a nasolabial flap.

Lingual flap

In order to be able to use this flap satisfactorily the greater part of the tongue must have been preserved, including its blood supply from the lingual artery. Mark out the tongue flap, using dye, with a line extending along the dorsum of the tongue to define an area consisting of half the width of the tongue, so that the lingual artery is included in the base of the flap. Open up the curled edge of the flap, transpose it laterally, and stitch it into place over the exposed alveolus and the floor of the mouth. Close the edge of the anterior two-thirds or free portion of the tongue primarily in two layers, using 3/0 chromic catgut and 3/0 black silk on a cutting needle to reconstitute the tip of the tongue. It is possible to leave the remaining part of the donor site on the central one-third of the tongue raw to granulate, but there is a danger that it will adhere to the flap. It is probably preferable, therefore, to stitch a split-skin graft over this area. This flap is extremely vascular and provides a very good result both in regard of cover of the defect in the bone and of restitution of articulation.

Nasolabial flap

The nasolabial flap for use in repair of the anterior part of the floor of the mouth is based inferiorly on the branches of the superior labial artery, which pierce the subcutaneous tissue from its bed to supply a rich dense subdermal network of vessels. The flap may be used either as a normal pedicled flap, leaving a temporary fistula that is closed after division of the pedicle, or it may be used as a subcutaneous pedicle flap so that the operation can be completed at one sitting.

Mark out a flap based inferiorly, running in the nasolabial fold. The base of the flap lies approximately 1 cm inferolateral to the angle of the mouth, and the tip of the flap lies at the point where the nasolabial groove meets the nose. Elevate the flap preserving all of the subcutaneous tissue within it and the perforating branches of the superior labial artery in its base (if a radical neck dissection has been carried out, the facial artery should be preserved if at all possible). Then develop a tunnel beneath the buccal mucosa, emerging at the alveolus. If the flap is to retain its pedicle, push it through this tunnel; it should be of sufficient length to reach to the opposite side of the defect. Sew this flap into the anterior part of the defect and then raise a similar nasolabial flap from the opposite side of the cheek; pass this through a similar tunnel and suture it into the posterior half of the defect, suturing its anterior edge to the posterior edge of the first flap and its posterior edge to the edge of the ventral surface of the tongue (Fig. 16.10).

Close the primary defect in two layers down to the point where the flap passes into the cheek, leaving a temporary fistula. Three weeks later, divide the base of the pedicle, return it to the cheek and close the defect, excising any unsightly scar.

With greater experience the flap can also be used as a subcutaneous pedicle. After the flaps have been raised, take off the epidermis from the part of the pedicle that is to be buried, using an electric dermatome set at 12/1000 of an inch (0.3 mm). Pass the flaps into the defect and suture them in place as before; close the primary defect in the nasolabial groove completely.

Bone grafts

There is almost no place now for the use of a free bone graft in the reconstruction of a mandible. The recipient site is so unhealthy that the surprising fact is not that so many failed in the past but that any took at all. Reconstruction of the mandible needs bone, muscle and overlying skin so that the lining of the oral cavity is integral to the bone graft. This means that there is only place for a myo-osseocutaneous graft. There are a number of choices, amongst which are:

1 the pectoralis major myo-osseocutaneous graft, including the sixth rib;
2 the trapezius myo-osseocutaneous graft containing the spine of the scapula;
3 the radial forearm flap containing part of the radius.

We shall now describe the technique for the use of the pectoralis major myo-osseocutaneous flap.

This flap is cut as described in Chapter 4. The periosteum of the sixth rib is elevated, taking care not to damage the pleura medial to the rib. The piece of bone that has been removed from the mandible is measured and the rib cut to this length. A Kirschner wire is passed along the medulla of the bone and left projecting about 1–2 cm at each end. If the rib needs to be bent into shape make vertical cuts 1.5 cm apart in its inner table. Drill two holes vertically above each other in either end of the rib graft and in each of the bone ends. Place the rib graft in position pushing the wire up the medulla of each of the mandibular fragments. Finally wire each end of the rib graft to the sawn ends of the mandible, as shown in Figure 16.11.

Operations on the buccal mucosa

Local excision and primary closure

This operation can be done for tumours that are no more than 2 cm at the widest point. The line of incision with a knife or laser beam should include a reasonably safe margin of at least 1 cm of normal

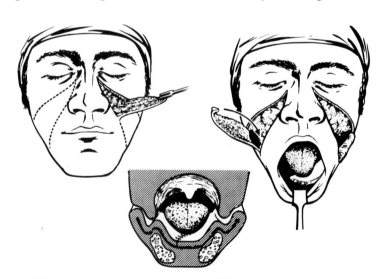

Fig. 16.10 Technique of elevation and transportation of nasolabial flap.

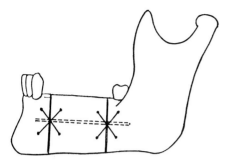

Fig. 16.11 A rib graft wired in place and fixed by a Kirschner wire.

tissue, and its edges should be horizontal to facilitate closure (Fig. 16.12).

Close the incision by interrupted sutures of 3/0 chromic catgut. If there is any tension on the suture line, use mattress sutures of 3/0 silk.

Local excision and skin grafting

This operation is needed to remove a large area of leukoplakia or for a tumour more than 3 cm in diameter.

The area is going to be closed by a skin graft so there is no need to compromise on the safety of the margins. Excise the lesion with a good margin, making certain that the lines of excision do not extend upwards or downwards into the sulci as it is very difficult to stitch a skin graft on these areas. Gauge the depth of the excision by the extent of infiltration; this operation should not be done if the subcutaneous tissues of the cheek are involved. No

attention need be paid to the position of the parotid duct, as cutting it does not lead to complications.

Take a split-thickness skin graft from the inner side of the thigh, and make a template of the size required from *tulle gras*. Place the skin on this template and cut it to size. With the *tulle gras* in place, stitch in the skin graft with interrupted sutures of 3/0 silk, using the quilting technique.

Tumour of the superior gingivobuccal sulcus

In this area surgical access is difficult, and skin grafts are almost impossible to suture into place and fix satisfactory. The best access is achieved by a Fergusson incision on the face (Fig. 16.13). The patient is prepared in the usual manner and anaesthetized with a nasal endotracheal tube, and the throat is packed. Mark a Fergusson incision from the lower border of the nasal bone in the nasobuccal sulcus, following the margin of the nose down to the ala, to the midline of the columella and then down through the lip in an S-shape. Tattoo the vermilion borders, and make the incision with a knife held at right angles to the skin. Elevate the cheek flap after cutting the mucosa in the upper sulcus.

Before making the incision it is wise to tattoo a safe margin of the intended excision on the mucosa. When this point is reached, stop elevation of the mucosal part of the cheek flap. Excise the lesion round the tattoo marks with a fairly deep margin. Secure haemostasis and close the defect by approximation of the mucosal edges with 3/0 chromic catgut, with the knots inside the mouth. If the tumour is more than 3 cm in diameter, fill the defect with a flap as described below.

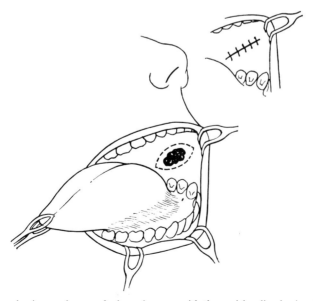

Fig. 16.12 Local excision and primary closure of a buccal cancer with the excision line horizontal.

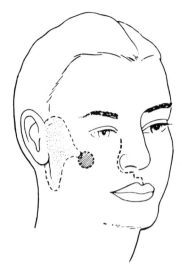

Fig. 16.13 For access to tumours in the superior gingivo-buccal sulcus, approach via a Fergusson incision.

Deeply infiltrating tumours of the buccal mucosa combined with neck dissection

As described previously there are two operations possible at this site, depending on whether the tumour is nearer the lower alveolus or the upper alveolus.

For tumours nearer the lower alveolus

First do a preliminary tracheostomy through a small horizontal incision and establish general anaesthesia via this route, so that the endotracheal tube does not get in the way.

Incision

Whether or not the patient has been irradiated, use double horizontal incisions and leave the neck dissection pedicled on the submandibular region. Secure complete haemostasis in the neck and then turn to the primary tumour.

Excision

The tumour will probably involve skin, and will almost certainly be larger on the inside of the mouth than it is on the skin of the cheek. For this reason, therefore, the amount of skin of the cheek to be removed must be marked within the mouth. Mark a safe margin around the tumour on the inside of the mouth, and stick a needle through this circle at various points so that it comes out of the skin of the cheek; paint the needle with dye and withdraw it sharply in order that the margin can be identified on the outside of the cheek. Using the marks on the outside of the cheek, incise the skin through and

through, keeping the knife at right angles, and leave the specimen attached to the lower alveolus. With a Stryker saw, divide the upper half of the adjacent alveolus. By extending the incision down the adjacent part of the floor of the mouth and through into the mandibular region, remove the specimen in continuity. This last step often results in loss of continuity but it should be maintained if at all possible.

Repair

Removal of the tumour leaves a hole in the cheek that must be closed by a lining with epithelium on the inside and on the outside. The inner lining is provided by the cut surface of the floor or mouth sutured to the remaining buccal mucosa or the superior margin of the excision. This is done in one layer using 3/0 silk. The external defect is closed with a pectoralis major myocutaneous flap so that the muscle sits next to the inner lining and the skin closes the facial defect.

This effectively cripples the oral cavity. About a month after healing has taken place the patient may want a second-stage operation so that it is possible for him or her to wear a partial or complete denture. A lingual sulcus must be made and for this the technique of epithelial inlay is used. Prior to this a temporary denture for the patient must have been made so that it can be applied at the time of the operation.

Infiltrate the intended area of the sulcus with local anaesthetic and make an incision around the alveolus. Deepen it to the lowest part of the sulcus and right back to the angle of the mandible.

From a prepared thigh take a split-thickness skin graft and place it on *tulle gras* and then drape it over a piece of gutta percha which is fixed to the dentures by screws when it is hardened. Put the denture in place and fit the gutta percha carrying the skin graft into the sulcus. Pass wires around the jaw to hold the denture firmly on to the alveolus. Do this with a no. 26 wire which is passed very close to the alveolus on the lingual side down to the lowest part of the jaw and then picked up on the outer side of the alveolus and brought back up into the mouth. Tighten the wire around the denture so that it is firmly attached to the alveolus. Cut off the ends and put a piece of bone wax on the sharp end of wire to stop it abrading the tongue.

Cut the wires after a week, pull them out through the mouth and remove the denture with the gutta percha stent, leaving the skin graft in place. Final dentures are then put in right away and are kept in permanently, as for some months after this operation the sulcus tends to disappear unless it is kept open with the specially made dentures, even though the skin graft has completely taken.

Tumours opposite the upper alveolus

For tumours in this area, the previous repair cannot be used because the inner lining cannot be provided by the tongue. The most suitable solution is a free radical flap for inner lining and a temporal flap for outer cover.

Radiotherapy techniques

External beam irradiation

Before a beam-directing shell is made, an individualized bite block or gag is prepared to hold the mouth open and depress the tongue. This has a central tube to enable the patient to breathe through the mouth if necessary. The patient is treated supine, immobilized in the shell. It can be helpful for treatment planning if the margins of the tumour have been marked at examination under anaesthesia by the insertion of inert, radiopaque metal seeds, and for the position of any palpable nodes to be marked with wire. The treatment volume embraces the primary tumour with a margin of at least 2 cm, and the first echelon of nodes. The precise arrangement of radiation fields to treat this volume is chosen to minimize the dose to oral mucosa and salivary glands. With small lateralized tumours of the tongue, floor of mouth or buccal mucosa, this will most often entail the use of an anterior and a lateral field, appropriately wedged to ensure dose homogeneity. In the case of retromolar trigone tumours, anterior and posterior oblique lateral fields, similar to those used for lateral oropharyngeal tumours (Chapter 17) can be used. For larger tumours, and those which cross the midline, parallel opposed fields may be necessary, at the expense of more mucositis and a greater likelihood of xerostomia. When lower neck irradiation is necessary, an anterior field is used, the upper margin of which abuts on to the lower margin of the fields treating the primary tumour. Irradiation of only one side of the neck is often appropriate, but if there is any likelihood of bilateral nodal involvement, both sides should be treated. This requires a split anterior field, that is one with a midline block to shield the spinal cord, larynx, hypopharynx and upper oesophagus. Treatment is with megavoltage photons from a linear accelerator, or less commonly a cobalt unit, giving 55 Gy in 20 daily fractions over 4 weeks. If large volumes are included, some prefer to give treatment over up to $6\frac{1}{2}$ weeks, prescribing a dose of 65 Gy in 32 daily fractions. A brisk mucositis is inevitable, regardless of the fractionation schedule chosen. It is therefore very important to ensure that oral hygiene is maintained, and that the patient continues to eat and drink adequately, using liquidized food and high-calorie supplements. Mucaine, Difflam, or aspirin mucilage may also help to alleviate the discomfort.

Interstitial therapy

The oral cavity is the most common site for interstitial implantation of radionuclides. There are several reasons for this. Firstly, many oral tumours are particularly suitable for this form of treatment, being small, relatively well-demarcated and also anatomically easily accessible – by no means a trivial reason. Secondly, the fact that interstitial therapy treats a small localized volume with rapid fall-off of dose remote from the implant enables a higher radiation dose to be given to tumours than would be tolerated by the larger volumes inevitably included by external beam irradiation. In addition, adjacent structures such as bone and salivary glands receive a lower dose from an implant than they would with external beam irradiation, diminishing morbidity and thereby making treatment more acceptable from the patient's point of view. Finally, clinical experience suggests that for suitable tumours control rates are better with interstitial therapy although, as in so many other settings, no comparative trials have been done to prove this.

Although radium needles were used very successfully for decades, they have now become obsolete, principally for reasons of radiation protection. Initially they were superseded by caesium needles which are used in exactly the same way, but more recently iridium wire has been introduced. This is more versatile as it is flexible and can be cut to any length, enabling its use in situations where rigid needle implants were not possible. Another advantage, from the operator's point of view, is that radiation protection is easier. Firstly, insertion of applicators into which the radioactive sources are subsequently put (afterloaded), when the accurate positioning of the tubes has been verified radiographically, means that there is no radiation exposure to staff in the operating theatre. Secondly the radiation from iridium is far less penetrating than that from radium, making the shielding of nursing staff and visitors on the ward easier. The principal disadvantage of iridium is its relatively short half-life, making re-use impracticable and therefore increasing the cost.

There are two main techniques of iridium wire implantation. The choice between them is usually dictated by the site and size of the tumour to be treated. For small tumours of the floor of mouth or lateral border of tongue, iridium wire 'hairpins' may be used (Fig. 16.14). Under a short general anaesthetic, a steel applicator with two parallel slotted legs 12 mm apart is inserted into the tumour. Further applicators are then put in parallel with the plane of the first. When the position of the applicators is satisfactory, iridium wire hairpins, with their legs cut to an appropriate length, are slid down the slots in the applicator legs and sutured in place, and then the applicators are removed. The legs of the hairpins lie

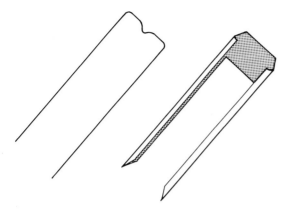

Fig. 16.14 Iridium wire hairpin and applicator.

along a double plane, and enable treatment of a slab of tissue approximately 2 cm thick. Further X-rays are then taken for dosimetric purposes, to determine the length of time the implant must remain in place for the prescribed dose to be delivered. The patient is able to eat and drink while the implant is in place, and it is removed at the end of treatment on the ward with no need for a second anaesthetic. Alternatively, flexible plastic tubes can be implanted percutaneously into the tumour using a steel introducer. Several parallel tubes about 1 cm apart will be used. For small tumours these will all lie in the same plane, but for larger tumours, a volume implant will be formed from two parallel planes. When treating small tumours of, for example, the buccal mucosa, the tubes will be more or less straight, but for larger tumours of the dorsum of the tongue or floor of mouth the tubes may be looped. The tubes are held in position by ball-shaped plastic washers and

crimped lead discs. The tubes are not radiopaque, and are therefore loaded with inert wire before X-rays are taken for dosimetric purposes. Iridium wire, cut to appropriate lengths so that it will not protrude through the skin, is sealed inside finer plastic tubes and afterloaded into the outer plastic tubes (Fig. 16.15). At the end of treatment, the implant is easily removed on the ward. The skin punctures heal well and become almost invisible. The prescribed dose, calculated according to the Paris system, is the same whether hairpins or plastic tubes are used.

For small tumours where the risk of occult nodal disease is slight, radical radiotherapy can be given by interstitial therapy alone. For larger tumours an initial course of external beam therapy to the primary tumour and first echelon of nodes is followed by an interstitial boost about 3 weeks later. Usually 60 Gy is given over 5 days when interstitial treatment alone is used. When external beam irradiation has been used first, giving a dose of 45–50 Gy in 20–25 fractions over 4 or 5 weeks, the prescribed dose from the implant will by 20–30 Gy over 2–3 days.

References and further reading

Surgical anatomy and pathology

Banoczy J, Csiba A (1976) Occurrence of epithelial dysplasia in oral leukoplakia. *Oral Surg Oral Med Oral Pathol* **42**:766–74.
Chu F W K, Silverman S, Dedo H H (1988) CO_2 laser treatment of oral leukoplakia. *Laryngoscope* **98**:125–30.
Close L G, Burns D K, Reisch J, Schaefer S D (1987) Microvascular invasion in cancer of the oral cavity and oropharynx. *Arch Otolaryngol Head Neck Surg* **113**:1191–5.
Holm L E, Lundquist P G, Silfversward C, Sobin A (1982)

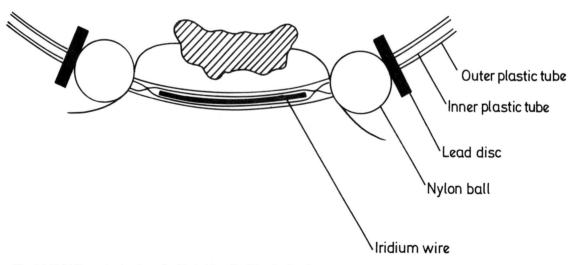

Outer plastic tube
Inner plastic tube
Lead disc
Nylon ball
Iridium wire

Fig. 16.15 Iridium wire implant afterbladed into flexible plastic tube.

Histological grading of malignancy in squamous cell carcinoma of the oral tongue. *Acta Otolaryngol* **94**:185–92.

Johnston W D, Ballantyne A J (1977) Prognostic effect of tobacco and alcohol use in patients with oral tongue cancer. *Am J Surg* **134**:444–7.

Loree T R, Strong E W (1990) Significance of positive margins in oral cavity squamous carcinoma. *Am J Surg* **160**:410–14.

McGuirt W F (1983) Snuff dipper's carcinoma. *Arch Otolaryngol* **109**:757–60.

Medina J E, Dichtel W, Luna M A (1984) Verrucous-squamous carcinomas of the oral cavity: a clinicopathological study of 104 cases. *Arch Otolaryngol* **110**:437–40.

Shafer W G, Waldron C A (1975) Oral carcinoma in situ. *Cancer* **36**:1021–8.

Shah J P (1990) Patterns of cervical lymph node metastasis from squamous carcinomas of the upper aerodigestive tract. *Am J Surg* **160**:405–9.

Shah J P, Strong E W, De Cosse J J, Itri L, Sellars P (1983) Effect of retinoids on oral leukoplakia. *Am J Surg* **146**:466–70.

Stutley J, Cook J, Parsons C (1989) Normal CT anatomy of the tongue, floor of mouth and oropharynx. *Clin Radiol* **40**:248–53.

Weber R S, Palmer J M, El-Naggar A, McNeese M D, Guillamondegui O M, Byers R M (1989) Minor salivary gland tumours of the lip and buccal mucosa. *Laryngoscope* **99**:6–9.

Williams R G (1981) The early diagnosis of carcinoma of the mouth. *Ann R Coll Surg Engl* **63**:423–5.

Investigations

Cooke J, Parsons C (1989) Computed tomographic scanning in patients with carcinoma of the tongue. *Clin Radiol* **40**:254–6.

Farrar W B, Sickle-Santanello B J, Keyhani-Rofagha S, DeCenzo J F, O'Toole R V (1989) Follow-up on flow cytometric DNA analysis of squamous cell carcinoma of the tongue. *Am J Surg* **157**:377–80.

Unger J M (1985) The oral cavity and tongue: magnetic resonance imaging. *Radiology* **155**:151–3.

Surgery of tongue cancer

Callery C D, Spiro R H, Strong E W (1984) Changing trends in the management of squamous carcinoma of the tongue. *Am J Surg* **148**:449–54.

Conley J, Sachs M E, Parke R B (1992) The new tongue. *Otolaryngol Head Neck Surg* **90**: 58–68.

Harrison D (1983) The questionable value of total glossectomy. *Head Neck Surg* **6**:632–8.

Mendenhall W M, Parsons J T, Stringer S P, Cassisi N J, Million R R (1989) Radiotherapy after excisional biopsy of carcinoma of the oral tongue/floor of the mouth *Head Neck* **11**:129–31.

Panje W R, little A G, Moran W J, Ferguson M K, Scher N (1987) Immediate free gastro-omental flap reconstruction of the mouth and throat. *Ann Otol Rhinol Laryngol* **96**:15–21.

Panje W R, Scher N, Karnell M (1989) Transoral carbon dioxide laser ablation for cancer, tumours and other diseases. *Arch Otolaryngol Head Neck Surg* **115**:681–8.

Shack R B (1986) Carcinoma of the tongue and tonsil. *Surg Clin North Am* **66**:83–96.

Weber R S, Gidley P, Morrison W H et al. (1990) Treatment selection for carcinoma of the base of the tongue. *Am J Surg* **160**:415–19.

Surgery of floor of mouth and alveolar tumours

Calteux N, Hamoir M, Eeckhaut J, Vanwijck R (1988) Reconstruction of the floor of the mouth after total glossectomy by free transfer of a gastro-omental flap. *Head Neck Surg* (suppl 11):S12–16.

Coleman J J, Wooden W A (1991) Mandibular reconstruction with composite microvascular tissue transfer. *Am J Surg* **160**:390–5.

Edelman G (1989) Speech and swallowing difficulties and their management. In: Stafford N, Waldron J (eds) *Management of Oral Cancer*, Oxford, Oxford University Press, pp. 183–95.

Klotch K W, Gump J, Kuhn L (1991) Reconstruction of mandibular defects in irradiated patients. *Am J Surg* **160**:396–8.

McConnel F M S, Teichgraeber J F, Adler R K (1987) A comparison of three methods of oral reconstruction. *Arch Otolaryngol Head Neck Surg* **113**:496–500.

Panje W R, Smith B, McCabe B F (1980) Epidermoid carcinoma of the floor of the mouth: surgical therapy vs combined therapy vs radiation therapy. *Otolaryngol Head Neck Surg* **88**:714–20.

Soutar D S, Widdowson W P (1986) Immediate reconstruction of the mandible using a vascularized segment of radius. *Head Neck Surg* **8**:232–46.

Soutar D S, Scheker L R, Tanner N S B, McGregor I A (1983) The radial forearm flap: a versatile method for intra-oral reconstruction. *Br J Plast Surg* **36**:1–8.

Steckler R M, Edgerton M T, Gogel W (1974) 'Andy Gump'. *Am J Surg* **128**:545–7.

Tucker H M (1989) Nonrigid reconstruction of the mandible. *Arch Otolaryngol Head Neck Surg* **115**:1190–2.

Urken M L (1991) Composite free flaps in oromandibular reconstruction: review of the literature. *Arch Otolaryngol Head Neck Surg* **117**:724–32.

Surgery of the buccal mucosa

Bloom N D, Spiro R H (1980) Carcinoma of the cheek mucosa: a retrospective analysis. *Am J Surg* **140**:556–9.

Bunkis J, Mulliken J B, Upton J, Murray J E (1982) The evolution of techniques for reconstruction of full-thickness cheek defects. *Plast Reconstr Surg* **70**:319–27.

McGregor I A, Reid W H (1970) Simultaneous temporal and deltopectoral flaps for full-thickness defects of the cheek. *Plast Reconstr Surg* **45**:326–31.

Magee W P, Posnick J C, Williams M, McCraw J B (1986) Cancer of the floor of mouth and buccal cavity. *Surg Clin North Am* **66**:31–58.

Narayanan M (1970) Immediate reconstruction with bipolar scalp flap after excision of huge cheek cancers. *Plast Reconstr Surg* **46**:548–53.

Vegers J W M, Snow G B, van der Waal I (1979) Squamous cell carcinoma of the buccal mucosa – a review of 85 cases. *Arch Otolaryngol* **105**:192–5.

17

Tumours of the oropharynx

Surgical anatomy

The oropharynx extends from the level of the hard palate superiorly to the level of the hyoid bone inferiorly. Its anterior limit is the anterior faucial pillar, but this is contiguous with the retromolar trigone. It is divided into the following:

1 The anterior wall, which is made up of the base of the tongue posterior to the foramen caecum, the vallecula, the lingual surface of the epiglottis; it is bounded by the pharyngoepiglottic folds.
2 The lateral wall, which is made up of the anterior pillar (palatoglossus), posterior pillar (palatopharyngeus) and the pharyngeal tonsil.
3 The roof, which is formed of the soft palate containing the two heads of palatopharyngeus, the levator palati, the tensor palati, and the palatoglossus. The oral surface of the soft palate is oropharynx and the nasopharyngeal surface is part of the nasopharynx.
4 The posterior wall, which extends from the level of the hard palate to the level of the hyoid and is anterior to the second and third cervical vertebrae. This consists of the superior and middle constrictors and the buccopharyngeal fascia, which separates it from the prevertebral fascia.

The lateral wall of the oropharynx is the medial wall of the parapharyngeal space. If a tumour extends through the lateral wall of the oropharynx, it enters the parapharyngeal space and becomes contiguous with the carotid sheath, the symphathetic chain, the styloglossus, the stylopharyngeus and the pterygoid muscles.

Tumours of the posterior wall usually extend upwards into the nasopharynx and downwards into the hypopharyngeal region, and are probably best considered as parts of the contiguous regions rather than separately as part of the oropharynx.

The most important area in the oropharynx, however, is the base of the tongue. The base of the tongue is made up of the genioglossus muscle, which is attached to the hyoid. Tumour infiltration into this muscle by definition almost involves the whole of the tongue because the distance between the genioglossus at the base of the tongue and the muscles of the anterior part of the tongue in the submental space is only about 2.5 cm. Furthermore, the base of the tongue is contiguous with the vallecula, which is the roof of the pre-epiglottic space; spread is early into the pre-epiglottic space and thus a tongue tumour becomes a laryngeal tumour.

The lymphatic drainage from the oropharynx is mainly into the jugulodigastric node. It also drains into the retropharyngeal and parapharyngeal nodes, which essentially are the upper deep jugular chain.

The area is lined with squamous epithelium and so squamous carcinoma is the commonest tumour. There is abundant lymphoid tissue, however, in the palatine tonsil and also in the lingual tonsil; the soft palate, especially, is rich in minor salivary glands.

Surgical pathology

Epidemiology

The annual incidence of carcinoma of the oropharynx in the UK is 8 per million and in the USA it is 60 per million. The maximum age incidence is in the seventh decade, and the male:female ratio for squamous carcinoma is 10:1. The classical pattern of the epidemiology, however, is changing. The age of patients at presentation is decreasing and patients in the fourth and fifth decades of life are not uncommon. The male:female ratio is also changing, and ratios as low as 4:1 have been described.

The most significant aetiological factor is tobacco, but tumours in this area are also seen in heavy drinkers. It is probable that the cause is related to the synergistic effect of alcohol and tobacco. The mixing of tobacco with lime, as in betel nut chewing, causes well-differentiated tumours of the mouth, but it also has an effect in the causation of oropharyngeal cancer.

The incidence of non-Hodgkin's lymphoma is rather different. Although the maximum age incidence is in the sixth decade, the male : female ratio is only 2 : 1.

Tumour types

Because of the three types of tissue in the oropharynx, squamous cell carcinoma, lymphoma and minor salivary gland tumours can occur. Squamous cell carcinoma is the commonest malignancy and forms 90% of the tumours in this region. Non-Hodgkin's lymphomas account for 8% and minor salivary gland tumours for 2%.

With regard to squamous carcinoma, the most common site is the lateral wall (60%), then the base of the tongue (25%), the soft palate (10%) and finally the posterior wall (5%).

Ninety per cent of lymphomas occur in the lateral wall or the base of the tongue; minor salivary gland tumours have a predilection for the soft palate, followed by the lateral wall and then the base of the tongue.

Staging is according to tumour size. The staging, as suggested by the American Joint Committee (AJC) and International Union against Cancer (UICC) is shown in Table 17.1.

Lymphatic metastasis is related to the depth of tumour invasion and the size of the tumour. The spread is in an orderly fashion from superior to inferior but the odd feature of oropharyngeal tumours is the frequency with which they affect the nodes in the posterior triangle. The drainage is down the lymph nodes and along the accessory nerve in the posterior triangle. In other head and neck tumours, nodes in the posterior triangle herald a fatal outcome but this is not the case in oropharyngeal tumours.

Bilateral lymphatic metastases are often seen in tumours of the soft palate and base of tongue, and contralateral node metastases may occur if the patient has had previous neck surgery or irradiation.

One in 3 patients with tumours of the oropharynx will, at some time in the disease, develop a second primary, so it is important to consider the presence of a synchronous second primary if contralateral nodes are found.

Again, as distinct from other head and neck

tumours, 8% of patients will have distant metastases discoverable at presentation.

Tumour spread

Lateral wall tumours

These are the commonest tumours and may spread directly to the retromolar trigone and on to the buccal mucosa, as well as into the muscles of the tongue. If they erode deeply, they will involve the pterygoid muscles producing trismus, and if they go laterally then they will involve the inferior alveolar nerve, especially in elderly patients, since in the edentulous mandible the inferior alveolar nerve is more superior than usual.

Lesions of the inferior pole of the tonsil are difficult to see and sometimes primary tumours can hide within the tonsillar crypts. It is this group of tumours that present with a metastatic lymph node with an apparent occult primary site. They can remain occult for a number of years.

Fifty per cent of these patients will have metastatic nodes on first presentation.

Base of tongue tumours

These are the next commonest. Symptoms frequently do not appear until these lesions are at an advanced stage. They spread through the genioglossus muscle and they very quickly involve the entire tongue, pushing it upwards and forwards. It is, therefore, often the case that the whole tongue needs to be removed from what appears to be a fairly small mucosal tumour at the base. Muscle contractions of the genioglossus help to propel the malignant cells not only into the lymphatic system but through the spaces between the intrinsic tongue muscles.

Approximately 60–70% of these patients will have a positive cervical node at initial presentation, and 20–30% will have bilateral nodes. Twenty per cent of patients will present with nodes and no apparent primary.

Soft palate tumours

Carcinoma of the soft palate occurs almost exclusively on the anterior surface. It may appear with leukoplakia and it is common in heavy smokers. Occasionally several small primary tumours are seen in the same patient. As the tumour enlarges, it may involve the palatine nerves and the back of the maxillary antrum. It will certainly involve the nasopharynx and may go into the superior pole of the tonsil.

About 50% of these patients will have a clinically positive node at initial examination and 15% will have bilateral nodes.

Table 17.1 Staging of tumours of the oropharynx

T_X	Tumour cannot be assessed
T_0	No evidence of primary tumour
T_{is}	Carcinoma-in-situ
T_1	Tumours 2 cm or less at largest diameter
T_2	Tumour between 2 and 4 cm
T_3	Tumour larger than 4 cm in diameter
T_4	Massive tumour, larger than 4 cm, with deep invasion into antrum, pterygoid muscles or neck skin

Posterior wall tumours

These are very rare and all described series involve only a handful of cases. No definitive statements can, therefore, be made about this tumour except that it often involves the nasopharynx or the hypopharyngeal posterior wall. The prevertebral fascia seems to act as a barrier to spread and bilateral metastases are possible.

Lymphoma

These consist almost entirely of non-Hodgkin's lymphoma. The histological classification, staging and relative site incidence of these lymphomas are described in Chapter 7.

Lymphomas affect particularly young individuals and can present with unilateral enlargement of the tonsil. Unless an adequate biopsy is taken, these are often reported as poorly differentiated tumours. Any poorly differentiated tumour reported from the oropharynx should be studied again using monoclonal markers and appropriate stains for squamous cells to exclude lymphoma.

Minor salivary gland tumours

On the soft palate, most minor salivary gland tumours are benign because of the frequency of pleomorphic adenomas at this site. Elsewhere in the oropharynx, however, malignant tumours are the rule, with adenoid cystic and mucoepidermoid tumours predominating. Adenoid cystic tumours invade perineural lymphatics and there is a rich source of tumour spread in this area along the palatine nerves and inferior alveolar nerves.

Investigations

History

The patient usually complains of a sore throat, otalgia or dysphagia. A small proportion of patients present because they have noticed an ulcer in the oropharyngeal region, and about 20% will present with a metastatic node in the neck. Patients with lymphoid enlargement from lymphoma may complain of muffled speech and difficulty in getting food out of the mouth in the first stage of swallowing. Patients with more advanced tumours will complain of more pain and perhaps trismus.

The difficult group are those with tumours of the base of the tongue. Nothing may be seen and they may visit a number of specialists for diagnosis of their symptom of referred ear pain or deep throat pain with no radiological or clinical signs.

Examination

Examine the mouth and the oropharynx in the usual way, and look into the nasopharynx to see if this area is involved. The most important examination is palpation, and this is applied especially to the base of the tongue. Masses due to lymphoma are firm and rubbery to palpation; salivary gland tumours are very often not ulcerated and have a firmer consistency than lymphomas. Palpation is of vital importance to assess the extent of tumour spread into the tongue or the palate.

Examine the neck and assess the nodes; if lymphoma is suspected, examine the other node-bearing areas for nodal enlargement.

Radiology

The most important assessment of spread of an oropharyngeal tumour concerns the parapharyngeal space. This is well shown with a computed tomography (CT) scan in an axial plane. Very often the swelling in the area will lead to overassessment of tumour spread, especially in the area of the nasopharynx. Nodal enlargement in the retropharyngeal area and subdigastric area can be assessed by a CT scan.

It is important to know whether or not the mandible has been invaded, but this is very rare in oropharyngeal tumours. Far more sinister is the perineural spread down the inferior alveolar nerve. Magnetic resonance imaging is not yet at a stage where this can be detected reliably but it is forecast that this form of imaging will allow the detection of perineural spread.

Also take radiographs of the chest because of the high incidence of distant metastases and second primary tumours.

If a lymphoma is suspected then it is staged by scanning.

Laboratory investigations

The usual blood count, erythrocyte sedimentation rate and urine analysis will, of course, be required. If the patient suffers from a lymphoma, estimation of liver function, plasma proteins and immunoglobulins will also be required.

Biopsy

All patients with oropharyngeal masses should be given a general anaesthetic and a panendoscopy carried out. This is to assess the extent of the oropharyngeal tumour and also to look for metastatic disease or synchronous second primaries.

Incisional biopsy of all tumour masses should be performed but, if there is smooth regular enlargement of one tonsil, then a tonsillectomy should be done because lymphoma is the likely diagnosis and a pathologist will classify the disease better if the whole organ is available.

Getting a biopsy from the base of the tongue is difficult. Many of these tumours are submucosal and certainly a punch biopsy from the surface will be valueless. Deep incisional biopsy is sometimes rewarding but even this yields a poor harvest. Many of these cases will present with a hardness at the base of the tongue but also with a metastatic neck node. A fine-needle aspiration or even an excisional biopsy of the neck node may be done to establish a diagnosis.

At the end of examination and biopsy under anaesthesia, the surgeon should know what the treatment modality will be. If it is to be surgery, then it may be useful to tattoo the lines of intended excision at this time, although this could wait until the time of the planned operation.

Treatment policy

Squamous carcinoma

It is intuitively attractive to split the oropharynx into its four anatomical sites and to lay down the treatment at each site. The way the tumours present, however, is not like this. They arise from a common mucosal covering that has had a wide-field change from exposure to alcohol and tobacco, and the tumours frequently extend from one area to the next without restrictions. Frequently it is impossible to say whether the tumour has arisen from the palate, the lateral wall, the tongue or the tonsil.

Another problem is that many patients present late and in poor biological status. There is a high incidence of alcoholism, liver cirrhosis and oesophagitis with varices. Taken in conjunction with poor nutritional status and the physiological defects of the surgery, decision-making is not easy.

Not only is there a high incidence of second malignancies in oropharyngeal tumours, but there is a high incidence of early and bilateral metastatic neck disease. Generally speaking, bilateral metastatic neck disease renders the patient almost incurable and, at best, the chances of survival from any modality are 10%.

In many of these poor subjects, the surgical resection will interfere greatly with the patient's ability to swallow and to handle secretions, so consideration has to be given as to how the patient is going to manage the upper airway if he or she does have a surgical resection and reconstruction.

The final point that creates a problem is in base-of-tongue tumours. To do a glossectomy for these is not an oncological operation. It is too near the pre-epiglottic space and it has to be combined either with a supraglottic laryngectomy or, more realistically, with a total laryngectomy. This often is taken as too much of a resection by both the surgeon and the

patient; thus some potentially curable patients are denied a chance of a cure on emotional grounds.

Given these strictures, however, we will set out our treatment policy in the traditional manner, hoping that the reader has taken to heart the preceding warnings about oversimplification.

Lateral wall tumours

Radiation would be expected to give an over 70% chance of 5-year survival in T_1 and T_2 tumours but would be fortunate to result in a 30–40% survival in a T_3 or a T_4 tumour. The results are very much worse if there are cervical node metastases. Some authors have suggested that if there are nodal metastases then radiotherapy has no place to play in management and that surgery should be the prime modality. Combined preoperative irradiation followed by surgery was in vogue for 15 years but it has now been replaced by primary surgery and postoperative irradiation.

The surgical resection for a lateral wall tumour is the commando operation. This consists of a radical neck dissection, and resection of the ascending process and part of the horizontal process of the mandible, the lateral oropharyngeal wall, part of the tongue base and part of the palate. If resection is small, the soft tissue defect can be closed with a lingual flap and, on rare occasions, primarily. More usually, tissue needs to be brought in from elsewhere, and the most satisfactory tissue to provide bulk as well as cover is the pectoralis major myocutaneous flap.

Base-of-tongue tumours

These present so late that radiotherapy is of little value. It is rare for the base of tongue to be resectable while leaving any useful anterior tongue and so total glossectomy is the minimal operation available, together with a unilateral or bilateral neck dissection. Access to the mouth can be from a lateral, commando-type approach, a midline jaw-splitting incision or a release of the oral cavity contents into the neck by a marginal incision round the floor of the mouth. As stated previously, a glossectomy is not an oncological operation and usually has to be combined with a total laryngectomy. The larynx can be sewn up in the usual way, and a pectoralis major myocutaneous flap provides adequate bulk for replacement of the tongue.

Posterior wall tumours

See Chapter 12.

Soft palate tumours

These are treated with radiotherapy primarily and, if there is recurrence, then a palatectomy is performed.

The best approach for this operation, which usually encompasses the superior part of the lateral wall, is a lateral one through an angular mandibulotomy. The best repair is to replace the soft palate with a dental prosthesis.

Inoperability

Finally, account must be taken of the patients who are inoperable. Inoperability occurs when the tumour extends too high in the nasopharynx or if the patient is in a poor biological condition, has distant metastases, or refuses treatment.

Lymphoma

Once a diagnosis of lymphoma has been established, the patient is usually taken over by the lymphoma treatment group. The disease must be classified and staged. Treatment will be by radiation alone if it is confined to the head and neck, or with adjuvant chemotherapy if it is generalized.

Most recurrences will take place within the first 18 months. If a recurrence does take place, the patient then only has a 10% chance of a long-term survival.

Minor salivary gland tumours

On the soft palate, benign pleomorphic adenoma is probably the commonest tumour. Once the diagnosis has been established, the adenomas are excised and the defect can be closed primarily, usually without any functional problems.

Minor salivary gland tumours occurring elsewhere in the oropharynx, however, are almost certain to be malignant. Adenoid cystic carcinoma should be treated as a squamous carcinoma with a wide-field excision and reconstruction. If it is treated primarily, no special attention needs to be given to extensive resection of nerves but if the patient has had previous treatment, then the resection needs to be wider than that applied to a squamous carcinoma.

Mucoepidermoid carcinoma presents much the same problem without the perineural spread. Although its biological behaviour is unpredictable, in the oropharynx it is better treated as a squamous carcinoma. Radiotherapy has little place in the management, either pre- or postoperatively, of these minor salivary gland tumours.

Failure of treatment

One in 5 will die of recurrence of the primary tumour. It is difficult to tell if a primary tumour has recurred once a myocutaneous flap has been put in place, but recurrence is often heralded by an increase in the amount of pain and trismus. An alteration of the swallowing pattern is also ominous. It is difficult to establish the diagnosis because tissue biopsy is often impossible and the anatomy is so distorted that the CT scan is usually unhelpful.

One in 10 will die of neck recurrence. The policy ought to be to do a radical neck dissection if nodes are palpable and a bilateral neck dissection if there are bilateral nodes. If there are no nodes and the patient is treated with radiation, then the neck should be electively irradiated, including the posterior triangle, because the incidence of occult nodes is so high.

One in 10 will die of distant metastases, 4% will die as a direct result of the primary treatment, and 6% will die of conditions unrelated to the tumour.

Thirty per cent of the 5-year survivors will get a second primary, of whom 66% will die.

Dysphagia

Dysphagia complicates many head and neck tumours and can follow a variety of head and neck surgical procedures. The symptom is considered here in the context of oropharyngeal tumours, however, as it constitutes the main problem after excision of part of the oropharynx. Deglutition is a uniquely semivoluntary reflex. It is impossible to swallow more than three or four times in the absence of oral bolus – a well-known physiological phenomenon which the reader can easily test. The decision to propel a bolus to the reflex trigger area in the posterior oropharynx is normally voluntary but once the reflex is triggered the bolus is propelled quickly past the vulnerable laryngeal inlet. Recent reconstructions of digitized barium X-rays suggest that the primary propulsive force is generated at the base of the tongue. Although there is a pharyngeal pressure wave, this probably has a clearing function and acts on the tail of the bolus (particularly when liquid) to reduce the risk of laryngeal aspiration. Following oropharyngeal surgery patients can have restriction of movement of the base of the tongue and impaired bolus propulsion. Also the bulk of the flap and the loss of sensory information from the hemipharynx can cause aspiration. In the initial postoperative phase swallowing is further impeded by the presence of a nasogastric tube. The temporary tracheostomy compounds the problem by altering subglottic pressure generation and tethering the trachea. The latter impedes the normal laryngeal ascent during the pharyngeal phase of swallowing which ensures that the laryngeal skeleton is tucked up under the base of the tongue and the epiglottis flipped over as the bolus passes the epilarynx.

Patients with advanced head and neck cancer are frequently nutritionally depleted at initial presentation. Postoperative nutritional support is an important consideration and in one study 85% of head and neck cancer patients required postoperative enteral feeding. Patients with preoperative weight loss greater than 4.5 kg (10 lbs) and those with pharyngeal tumours are more likely to require prolonged postoperative nutritional support. In one study 40% of patients required enteral supplementation for more than 1 month. While nasogastric feeding is adequate in the short term, it is associated with mechanical problems such as local irritation and erosion, aspiration and tube obstruction as well as being a socially inhibiting process.

The technique of percutaneous endoscopic gastrostomy (PEG) has in recent years been applied to head and neck patients. While the endoscopist carries out the initial gastroscopy the operator infiltrates the anterior abdominal wall with local anaesthetic. A needle and cannula are then inserted through the skin vertically and advanced until they can be seen by the endoscopist. The needle is withdrawn and a continuous-loop guidewire is pushed through the cannula and grasped by the endoscopist who draws it, together with the endoscope, through the patient's mouth. The mouth end of the wire is attached to the PEG tube. The abdominal end of the wire is then pulled until the tube has passed down the gullet and into the stomach. The compressible balloon passes easily, even through tight strictures. The tube is pulled out of the anterior abdominal wall until the balloon abuts the gastric mucosa.

Opponents to the routine placement of PEGs are concerned that the procedure may have an unacceptably high complication rate – reported to be as high as 16% in patients receiving concurrent chemotherapy. Specific complications include inability to place the tube because of pharyngeal or oesophageal obstruction. Review of over 120 carcinoma patients with attempted PEG replacement indicated that in fact postoperative complications were less frequently encountered than in patients having gastroscopy tube placement for other indications such as neurological disease.

One of the most frequently encountered causes of dysphagia in head and neck surgical patients is aspiration of ingested material or saliva into the upper respiratory tract. Modern techniques of video-recorded barium examination allow the observer to relate the occurrence of aspiration to the phase of the swallow cycle. Very small amounts of food should be given at each swallow, firstly to reduce the amount of aspirated material and secondly, to prevent the obscuring of laryngopharyngeal function by a large pool of contrast.

Aspiration can occur *before* the swallow reflex is initiated due to poor tongue control which causes some of the bolus to be lost into the pharynx. This problem is particularly encountered in patients who have resection of the anterior oral cavity. Patients who have had composite resection of the oropharynx suffer a variety of problems including delayed onset of the swallow reflex because of the damage to the afferent limb by resection of the anterior faucial pillar. Tongue mobility is also restricted in these patients who seem also to suffer from reduced pharyngeal peristalsis which results in aspiration *after* the swallow reflex because of reduced bolus clearance. Supraglottic laryngectomy causes a comparatively small reduction in oral and pharyngeal transit speed but there is severe impairment of the patient's laryngeal airway protection and elevation, together with base-of-tongue movement which contributes to the triggering of the swallow reflex. Aspiration is most likely to occur *during* the reflex after this procedure.

A comparison of oral cavity reconstruction with skin grafts, lingual flaps or myocutaneous flaps indicated that for comparable lesions of the mobile tongue, split-thickness skin grafts resulted in persistently better tongue mobility, speech and swallowing scores. The patients who had the highest score on tongue mobility also had the highest scores on the other tests. Tongue flaps in fact gave the worst results in this situation, perhaps because of the tethering of the disease-free side. Now the radial free forearm flaps are being increasingly used in oral and oropharyngeal reconstruction there is clearly a need for prospective studies to compare the rehabilitation of patients reconstructed by each method.

Technique of operations on the oropharynx

The commando operation

As outlined in Treatment policy, above, this operation is required for squamous carcinoma of the tonsil with a metastatic neck node, recurrent carcinoma of the lateral wall after radiotherapy, and for malignant salivary gland tumours of the lateral wall and soft palate. It is called a commando operation as an abbreviation for combined mandibular and oral cavity resection. The term does not relate to the extent of the operation or the bravery of the surgeon or patient.

A part of the mandible is removed, not because it is involved by tumour but because it is necessary to obtain access, and to make it possible to close the soft tissues. From time to time, people think it worthwhile to preserve the mandible in this condition but our experience shows that attempts to do so lead to an unsatisfactory soft tissue repair, trismus due to fibrosis of the pterygoid muscles, and often osteoradionecrosis of the mandible if it has been previously irradiated.

Preparation

Attention must be given to the teeth. All carious teeth must be removed and, if the patient has had previous radiotherapy, then it must be established that the remaining teeth are in good enough condition not to warrant complete extraction. When the mandible is cut, you must make sure that there is not a tooth root left near the cut edge of an irradiated mandible.

Start the operation with a tracheostomy and continue the anaesthesia through this route. Once the tracheostomy has been done, open the mouth and tattoo the excision line with methylene blue. It is also useful at this stage to fulgurate the tumour with diathermy in the hope of reducing possible later implantation. Once the mouth is entered and the tissue distorted, it is quite easy to get too close to the tumour, especially on the deep margin.

Next, prepare the skin in the usual fashion, put a Betadine swab in the mouth and towel the area.

Incision

Use a T-shaped incision and take the horizontal part of the incision round to the other side of the neck. This usually allows the upper skin flap to be taken over the mandible. It is not usually necessary to bring the horizontal incision up to split the lip, although it is very much easier if this is done (Fig. 17.4).

Carry out the radical neck dissection, making sure you clear the pre- and postvascular nodes around the facial artery, and making sure there is good clearance of the posterior triangle and the subdigastric area. Leave the neck dissection specimen pedicled on the posterior part of the submandibular gland at the angle of the mandible.

Excision

Incise the periosteum of the mandible with a knife and cut the insertion of the masseter. Elevate the periosteum on the lateral and medial side of the bone up to the coronoid process, the sigmoid notch and the neck of the mandible. Pass a Gigli saw around the neck of the mandible, divide it, and free the coronoid process from the temporalis insertion with Mayo scissors. Next, divide the mandible at an appropriate place on the horizontal portion with a Stryker saw (Fig. 17.1). If you do this cut before doing upper cuts, as it makes it very much more difficult to divide the coronoid process.

Enter the oral cavity and pull the tongue forward with a towel clip. Identify the tattoo marks and do the excision with cutting diathermy. It is almost certain that the external carotid artery will have to be ligated and the assistants should not retract too hard because occasionally the facial nerve can be traumatized.

At the end of the excision, wash out the wound, change gowns and gloves.

Reconstruction

There are three choices in reconstruction: a lingual flap; a pectoralis myocutaneous flap; and a deltopectoral flap.

The lingual flap

If the defect is relatively small, for example just the lateral wall without any palate or tongue excision, then measure the size of the flap that is required and cut a lingual flap, based posteriorly, just anterior to the circumvallate line. Make sure it includes the lingual artery at the base and the base of the flap should probably be the width of half of the tongue. Cut well down to the substance of the tongue and

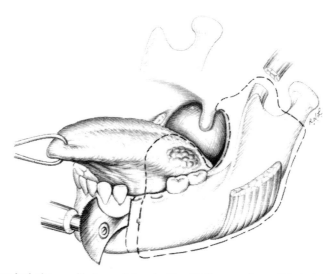

Fig. 17.1 Temporalis is detached, the mandibular neck is cut with a Gigli saw and mandible is divided with a Stryker saw at the mental foramen.

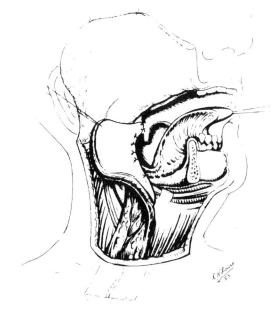

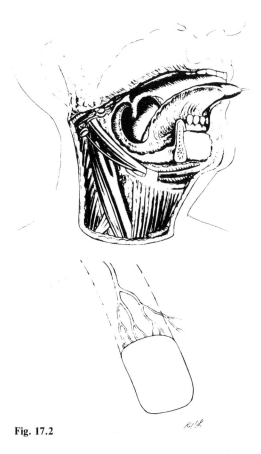

Fig. 17.3

Fig. 17.2

rotate the flap into the defect. Sew it into place in two layers with 3/0 chromic catgut and 3/0 Ethilon. Close the defect on the lateral side of the tongue by primary suture.

At a later date, a small freeing procedure may well be necessary as the tongue is often tethered.

The pectoralis myocutaneous flap

A description of the creation of this flap is given in Chapter 4. The flap is brought up through the neck and stitched into place and shaped as well as possible. The bulk of this flap disguises the loss of the ascending process of the mandible and is very good for cosmesis. If it goes too far down the pharynx, then it tends to be bulky and leads to aspiration due to the abolition of a lateral food channel (Figs 17.2–17.4).

The deltopectoral flap

This, of course, has the disadvantage of requiring two stages. Its advantage, however, is that it is thinner than the myocutaneous flaps and the patient often rehabilitates better. In an attempt to get away from the bulk of myocutaneous flaps, some surgeons

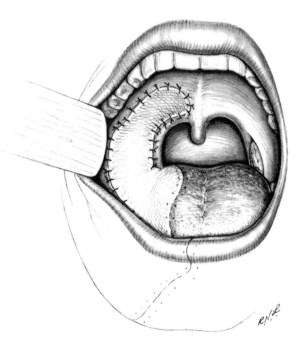

Fig. 17.4

use a free forearm flap for reconstruction. The forehead flap was used for many years because it had the advantage of being the correct thickness but this has largely fallen out of favour because of the bad scarring of the forehead.

Total glossolaryngectomy

Preparation

It is best to perform the tracheostomy as an initial step and to continue anaesthesia via this route. There is usually no problem about the lower margin in the laryngectomy and violation of tumour planes will not occur.

There is usually no need to carry out any tattooing. Place a Betadine swab in the mouth and carry out the neck dissection as required.

Excision

This can be done three ways: via a commando lateral approach; by doing a midline mandibulotomy; and by incising the mylohyoid and delivering the oral cavity into the neck.

We will describe the midline mandibulotomy approach.

The skin flap is raised from one angle of the mandible to the other and lifted up over the mandible. The periosteum of the mandible is divided in the midline and, if there are incisor teeth, the two central ones are removed. The mandible is marked in a V-shaped fashion and holes are drilled to take the wires (Fig. 17.5). The mandible is then cut in the V with a Stryker saw and the ends pulled apart. This then allows you to cut the mucosa of the floor of the mouth near the anterior part of the tongue, and the dissection is continued posteriorly, taking the lateral wall as necessary (Fig 17.6).

The laryngectomy is done in the usual fashion and the specimen removed. The wound is then washed, and gowns and gloves changed. An alternative to glossolaryngectomy is total glossectomy with clearance of the pre-epiglottic space (Fig. 17.7). All the tissues contained in this space, and the upper part of the thyroid cartilage are removed.

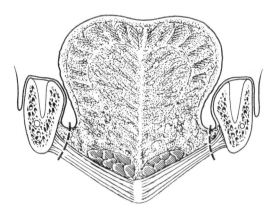

Fig. 17.6 Lateral limits of recection in total glossectomy.

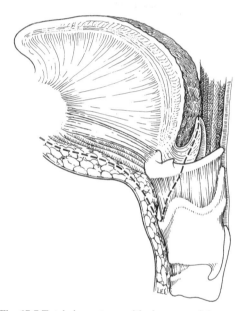

Fig. 17.7 Total glossectomy with clearance of the pre-epiglottic space.

Closure

The pharyngeal remnant is closed in the usual fashion using a Connel suture in two layers. At the upper end a defect will then remain where the pharynx meets the oral cavity.

A myocutaneous flap is cut and put in place, suturing it posteriorly to the pharyngeal remnant and laterally and anteriorly to the mucosa of the floor of the mouth (Fig. 17.8). The suturing is done from posterior to anterior; when the anterior part is reached, the mandibular ends are brought together and wired as shown in Figure 17.9.

Suturing the pectoralis muscle centrally over the pharyngeal remnant helps healing.

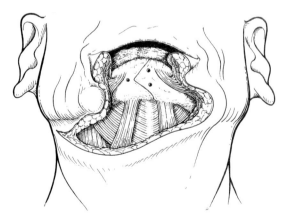

Fig. 17.5 Midline mandibulotomy cut after wiring holes drilled.

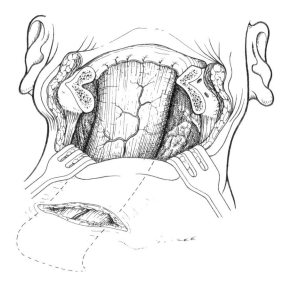

Fig. 17.8 Pectoralis major myocutaneous flap repair.

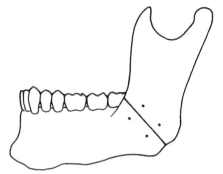

Fig. 17.10 Angular oblique mandibulotomy for access to the lateral oropharynx and palate.

penetrated with a fissure burr. With a Stryker saw, the bone is then cut obliquely, allowing the two ends to be lifted apart (Fig. 17.10). This gives access to the lateral wall of the oropharynx and direct access to the soft palate. The lateral wall and soft palate can then be removed (Fig. 17.11) and the wound washed. Gowns and gloves are changed.

Closure

The problem is that usually the whole lateral pharyngeal wall and the whole of the soft palate are removed. It is impossible to close this defect with a pectoralis major myocutaneous flap on its own. The defect is a curved base of skull and an oronasopharyngeal fistula. While it can be filled with a dental

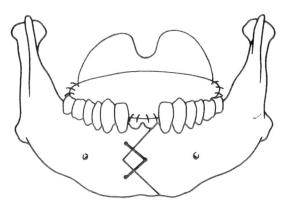

Fig. 17.9 Mandible wired in place and myocutaneous flap put in place and sutured to the mucosal remnant in the floor of the mouth.

Palatectomy

Preparation

A tracheostomy is made and the area to be removed from the oropharynx tattooed. A neck dissection is performed the pedicled at the angle of the mandible.

Excision

The mandibular periosteum is divided and the periosteum elevated off the ascending process of the mandible on both sides. At the angle, an oblique line is drawn. Work between the angle and the retromolar area. Sites of drill holes are marked and

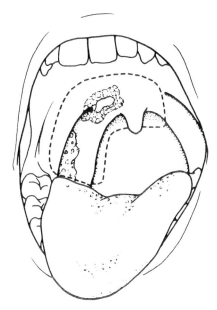

Fig. 17.11 Area of excision usually required for removal of a palatal tumour recurrence.

prosthesis and a pectoralis myocutaneous flap laterally, getting a good fit of prosthesis is difficult.

An alternative is to use a free jejunal flap to close
both defects. The flap, turned back on itself, mucosal
surface outwards, can form a new soft palate, and
laterally it can be laid open to close the lateral
pharyngeal wall. Getting an attachment to the hard
palate, however, may be difficult. Furthermore,
opening a short segment of jejunum compromises
the vascular supply.

Radiotherapy techniques

The radiotherapeutic technique chosen depends
upon whether or not the tumour is well-lateralized. If
there is a central tumour, or a large, lateral one
which either crosses or even encroaches on the
midline, there is a high probability of bilateral nodal
involvement. In such cases, the whole width of the
neck must be irradiated, whereas for small, laterally
placed tumours, treatment of a limited volume can
be effective. Such a set-up enables the contralateral
mucosa and parotid gland to be spared, and therefore it causes much less morbidity.

Carcinomas of the tonsil or lateral wall

Small tumours without nodes

Before considering small-volume treatment for a
lateral oropharyngeal tumour, it is essential that its
limits have been precisely identified at examination
under anaesthesia, and that any clinically occult
extension has been excluded by a CT scan. As in the
case of oral cavity tumours, it can be helpful for
treatment planning if the tumour margins are
marked by the insertion of inert metal seeds which
are used to indicate the position of the tumour on
radiographs. For T_1 or T_2 squamous carcinoma of the
tonsil or fauces which do not extend significantly into
the base of tongue or parapharyngeal area, and
where there is no lymphatic spread, small-volume
treatment is appropriate. Two ipsilateral fields are
used (Fig. 17.12), a posterior oblique and an anterior
oblique. Wedges are used to ensure that a homogeneous dose distribution is achieved (Fig. 17.13).
The fields extend from the level of the hard palate
superiorly down to the hyoid. Their anterior border
is through the central part of the tongue, and their
posterior limit is through the vertebral bodies. The
volume encompassed therefore includes the primary
tumour with an adequate margin and the jugulodigastric and parapharyngeal nodes, and extends to the
midline. For T_{1-2} N_0 tumours it is not necessary to
irradiate the lower neck prophylactically. The
patient is planned lying supine in a shell with the
mouth closed. A simulator check film is taken as a
permanent record of the intended treatment, and

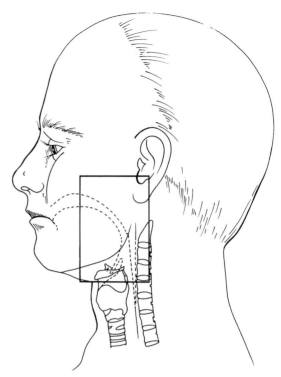

Fig. 17.12 Volume to be irradiated in the patient with a
small carcinoma of the lateral oropharynx without nodal
involvement.

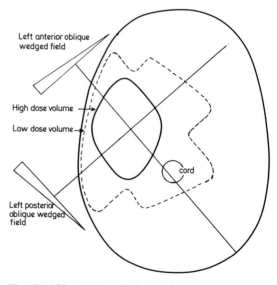

Fig. 17.13 Plan of the radiotherapy field arrangement for
a small lateral oropharyngeal tumour without nodal
metastasis.

portal verification films are taken to ensure that treatment is executed as planned. A dose of 55 Gy in 20 fractions over 4 weeks or its equivalent is given, using 4–6 MV X-rays from a linear accelerator.

Extensive lateral tumours and small ones with nodes

To embrace the primary tumour adequately and upper deep cervical nodes bilaterally a pair of lateral parallel opposed fields is used. Their margins are essentially the same as described for more limited tumours. Care is taken to ensure that these are extended if necessary to cover any direct tumour extension or nodal involvement. Although in most circumstances radiotherapists attach great importance to achieving a homogeneous dose distribution, the oropharynx provides an exception. If the tumour is confined to the tonsillar region and does not infiltrate the base of tongue or extend on to the palate, it is possible to weight the treatment, giving a greater dose to the affected side, and an adequate prophylactic dose to the contralateral nodes. If there is palpable nodal enlargement, the lower neck also is treated. An anterior field is used, the upper border of which matches the lower border of the parallel opposed fields. If the lymphadenopathy is bilateral, then obviously both sides of the lower neck are treated. A single anterior field covering the width of the neck is used, and a midline block is required to shield the cervical cord. If there is extensive or bulky nodal disease it may not be possible to achieve adequate coverage without including the spinal cord in the high-dose volume. A two-phase technique, similar to that described for pyriform fossa carcinoma, enables the dose to the cord to be kept within safe limits. In such circumstances the likelihood of cure is slim, but radical treatment may be attempted as it is sometimes successful. A dose of 55 Gy in 20 fractions over 4 weeks is often given, but for the reasons set out in the section on supraglottic carcinoma, many radiotherapists prefer a more protracted fractionation schedule.

Carcinoma of the base of tongue

The technique here is similar to that described above for bulky lateral wall tumours, or those with nodes. The inferior margin of the lateral fields should however be lower to cover actual or potential spread into the supraglottis. Also, if the tumour is confined to the tongue base, the upper margin is placed below the level of the hard palate and the patient is treated with the mouth open and the tongue depressed. This enables the mucosa of the roof of the mouth to be spared to some extent. Treatment of nodal disease, and selection of a fractionation schedule are as indicated above.

Carcinoma of the soft palate

In most cases this is treated by evenly weighted parallel opposed lateral fields, as described for extensive lateral wall tumours. In the rare event of finding a small T_1 squamous carcinoma, interstitial therapy alone may be chosen. The soft palate is an ideal site for a gold grain implant. The principal advantage of this approach is that because the treatment volume is small, the reaction will be minimized. Implantation is a particularly valuable treatment method when irradiation of a previous primary tumour has limited the scope for further external beam radiotherapy.

Lymphoma

For stage IE tonsillar lymphoma, it is routine to treat not only the involved site, but also the whole of Waldeyer's ring and the cervical lymph nodes. Large parallel opposed fields, similar to those needed for nasopharyngeal carcinoma, are used to cover the lingual and palatine tonsils, the adenoid area and the upper cervical lymph nodes. An anterior field with midline shielding is used to treat the lower neck. Lymphoma requires a lower radiation dose than that used for carcinoma. A 4 week course giving 40 Gy in 20 fractions is usually prescribed.

Controversies in management

How hard do you look for the second primary?

With an over 30% rate of second primary occurrence, every effort should be made to establish whether or not this is present before submitting the patient to the sort of surgery that is involved in the treatment of oropharyngeal cancer. It is the authors' custom to carry out bronchial cytology on all of these patients because the bronchus is the most likely other site. It is also wise to do as many biopsies as possible of the nasopharyngeal area because if there is going to be a nasty surprise, it will be at the upper level of the excision.

What do you do if you cannot get a positive biopsy from the base of the tongue?

Mention has been made of the common presentation of base-of-tongue tumours, i.e. with a node in the neck and a hard base of tongue but no positive biopsy. The authors have mentioned the use of a deep incisional biopsy in the base of the tongue and this is the method that is advocated. It is completely unjustifiable to do a glossolaryngectomy without a positive biopsy. In its absence, a wait-and-see policy, or removal of the neck node and irradiation to the area, should be adopted.

How do you manage a small adenoid cystic carcinoma that has been completely removed with the excision biopsy?

It is for this reason that the authors recommend incisional biopsy of tumours in this area. Very often tertiary referrals are see where there has been an apparently successful excision of a small adenoid cystic carcinoma. If this occurs, no notice should be taken of the clear margins described by the pathologist, and the operation appropriate for a squamous carcinoma should be performed, whether the tumour is in the base of the tongue or the lateral wall.

Is anything less than a total glossolaryngectomy allowable for base-of-tongue tumours?

It has been said several times that a total glossectomy is not an oncological operation for base-of-tongue tumours. The pre-epiglottic space is so close to the tumour-bearing area that this, at least, must be removed. The minimum operation would be removal of the hyoid, the epiglottis and the pre-epiglottic space, which would be a modified supraglottic laryngectomy. The authors have seen the occasional patient who has not aspirated after this procedure but, on the whole, the safe oncological procedure is a total glossolaryngectomy.

Which is the best reconstructive procedure?

The best reconstructive procedure is one that does not take too long, that is not too bulky and that preferably allows the patient as quick a rehabilitation as possible with a good chance of a complete take.

The forehead flap satisfied most of these criteria but, due to the scarring of the forehead, it has fallen into disrepute. The deltopectoral flap is the next best in this area but gravity works against it and there is often loss of the distal end of this flap. The free forearm flap is adequate for thickness but a beginner takes a long time to do the necessary vascular anastomosis.

The pectoralis myocutaneous flap or the latissimus dorsi flap are bulky but they have the advantages of being one-stage and also take is almost certain. If they are too bulky, they can be debulked at a later stage.

References and further reading

Surgical anatomy and pathology

Candela F C, Shah J, Jaques D P, Shah J P (1990) Patterns of cervical node metastases from squamous carcinoma of the oropharynx and hypopharynx. *Head Neck* 12:197–203.
Close L G, Brown P M, Vuitch M F, Reisch J, Sonaefer S D (1989) Microvascular invasion and survival in cancer of the oral cavity and oropharynx. *Arch Otolaryngol Head Neck Surg* 115:1304–9.
Danes B S, De Angelis P, Traganos F *et al*. (1990) Comparison of anatomical location of squamous cell carcinoma within the oral cavity and oropharynx with the incidence of in vitro hyperdiploidy. *Clin Genet* 37:188–93.
Hampal S, Hawthorne M (1990) Hypopharyngeal inverted papilloma. *J Laryngol Otol* 104:432–4.
Luna M A, Naggar A, Parichatikanond P, Weber R S, Batsakis J G (1990) Basaloid squamous carcinoma of the upper aerodigestive tract. Clinicopathologic and DNA flow cytometry analysis. *Cancer* 66:537–42.
Rasgon B M, Cruz R M, Hilsinger R L, Sawicki J E (1989) Relation of lymph-node metastasis to histopathologic appearance in oral cavity and oropharyngeal carcinoma: a case series and literature review. *Laryngoscope* 99:1103–10.

Investigations and treatment policy

Aspestrand F, Kolbenstvedt A, Boysen M (1990) Carcinoma of the hypopharynx: CT staging. *J Comput Assist Tomogr* 14:72–6.
Bataini J P, Jaulerry C, Brunin F, Ponvert D, Ghossein N A (1990) Significance and therapeutic implications of tumor regression following radiotherapy in patients treated for squamous cell carcinoma of the oropharynx and pharyngolarynx. *Head Neck* 12:41–9.
Calamel P M, Hoffmeister F S (1967) Carcinoma of the tonsil: comparison of surgical and radiation therapy. *Am J Surg* 114:582.
Conley J (1970) *Concepts in Head and Neck Surgery*. Stuttgart, Georg Thieme Verlag.
Fletcher G H, Lindberg R D (1966) Squamous cell carcinomas of the tonsillar area and palatine arch. *Am J Roentgenol* 96:574.
Fletcher G H, Jesse R H, Healey J E Jr, Thomas G W (1967) Oropharynx. In: *Cancer of the Head and Neck* MacComb W S, Fletcher G H (eds), Baltimore, Williams & Wilkins, pp. 179–212.
Johansen LV, Overgaard J, Overgaard M, Birkler N, Fisker A (1990) Squamous cell carcinoma of the oropharynx: an analysis of 213 consecutive patients scheduled for primary radiotherapy. *Laryngoscope* 100:985–90.
Ketcham A S, Hoyle R C, Chretien P B, Brace K C (1969) Irradiation twenty-four hours preoperatively. *Am J Surg* 118:691.
Kramer S, Gelber R D, Snow J B *et al*. (1987) Combined radiation therapy and surgery in the management of advanced head and neck cancer: final report of study 73–03 of the radiation therapy oncology group. *Head Neck Surg* 10:19–30.
Lederman M (1967) Cancer of the pharynx. *J Laryngol Otol* 81:151–72.
Leonard J R, Litton W B, Latourette H B, McCabe B F (1968) Combined radiation and surgical therapy: tongue, tonsils, floor of mouth. *Ann Otol Rhinol* 77:374.
Maciejewski B, Withers H R, Taylor J M, Hliniak A (1990) Dose fractionation and regeneration in radiotherapy for cancer of the oral cavity and oropharynx. Part 2. Normal tissue responses: acute and late effects. *Int J Radiat Oncol Biol Phys* 18:101–11.
Marcial V A, Hanley J A, Ydrach A, Vallecillo L A (1980)

Tolerance of surgery after radical radiotherapy of carcinoma of the oropharynx. *Cancer* **46**:1910–12.

Ogawa Y, Maeda T, Seguchi H *et al.* (1990) Application of the immunohistochemical method as a predictive assay in radiotherapy of squamous cell carcinoma of the oropharynx and hypopharynx. *Oncology* **47**:155–9.

Perez C A, Mill W B, Ogura J H, Powers W E (1970) Carcinoma of the tonsil: sequential comparison of four treatment modalities. *Radiology* **94**:649.

Powers W E, Palmer L A (1968) Biologic base of pre-operative radiation treatment. *Am J Roentgenol* **102**:176.

Powers W E, Tolmach L J (1964) Pre-operative radiation therapy: biological basis and experimental investigation. *Nature* **201**:272.

Rolander T L, Everts E L, Shumrick D A (1971) Carcinoma of the tonsil: a combined therapy approach. *Laryngoscope* **81**:1199.

Sagerman R H, Chung T, Cummings C W, King G A, Rabuzzi D D, Reed G F (1978) Surgical salvage after failure of radiation therapy in patients with advanced cancer of the oral cavity and oropharynx. *J Laryngol Otol* **92**:51–6.

Ricci S B, Grandi C, Salvatori P (1986) On the problem of radiotherapy in the treatment of oropharyngeal carcinoma; salvage surgery. *Rays (Roma)* **11**:127–31.

Rubin P (1971) Cancer of the head and neck: oropharynx. *JAMA* **217**:940–2.

Swallowing

Forgacs I, MacPherson A, Tibbs C (1992) Percutaneous endoscopic gastrostomy: the end of the line for naso-gastric feeding? *Br Med J* **304**:1395–6.

Gardine R L, Kokal W A, Beatty J D *et al.* (1988) Predicting the need for prolonged enteral supplementation in the patient with head and neck cancer. *Am J Surg* **156**:63–5.

Gibson S E, Wenig B L, Watkins J L (1992) Complications of percutaneous endoscopic gastrostomy in head and neck cancer patients. *Ann Otol Rhinol Laryngol* **101**:46–9.

Logemann J A (1985) Aspiration in head and neck surgical patients. *Ann Otol Rhinol Laryngol* **94**:373–6.

Logemann J A, Bytell D E (1979) Swallowing disorders in three types of head and neck surgical patients. *Cancer* **44**:1095–105.

Nash M (1988) Swallowing problems in the tracheotomized patient. *Otolaryngol Clin North Am* **21**:701–10.

Roukema J A, Werken C V D, Juttmann J R (1990) Percutaneous endoscopic gastrostomy as a standard procedure in head and neck surgery. *Arch Otolaryngol Head Neck Surg* **116**:730–1.

Surgical procedures

Ariyan S (1980) Pectoralis major, sternomastoid, and other musculocutaneous flaps for head and neck reconstruction. *Clin Plast Surg* **7**:89.

Babin R, Calcatera T C (1976) The lip-splitting approach to resection of oropharyngeal cancer. *J Surg Oncol* **8**:433.

Bakamjian V (1971) Experience with the medially based delto-pectoral flap in reconstructive surgery of the head and neck. *B J of Plast Surg* **24**:174.

Bakamjian V, Littlewood M (1964) Cervical skin flaps for intra-oral and pharyngeal repair following cancer surgery. *B J Plast Surg* **17**:191.

Biller H, Lawson W (1983) Total glossectomy. *Arch Otolaryngol* **109**:69.

Butlin T H (1900) *The Operative Surgery of Malignant Disease*, 2nd edn. London, J. and A. Churchill, pp. 175–86.

Conley J J (1962) The crippled oral cavity. *Plast Reconstr Surg* **30**:469.

DeSanto L W, Whicker J H, Devine K D (1975) Mandibular osteotomy and lingual flaps: use in patients with cancer of the tonsil area and tongue base. *Arch Otolaryngol* **101**:652.

Dubernick R C, Antoni J E (1974) Deglutition after resection of oral, laryngeal, and pharyngeal cancer. *Surgery* **75**:87.

Effron M Z *et al.* (1981) Advanced carcinoma of the tongue: management of total glossectomy with laryngectomy. *Arch Otolaryngol* **107**:694.

Figi F A, Masson J K (1953) Free skin grafting within the mouth. *Plast Reconstr Surg* **12**:176.

Givene C D, Johns M E, Cantrell R W (1981) Carcinoma of the tonsil. *Arch Otolaryngol* **107**:730.

Goepfert H, Jesse R H, Ballantyne A J (1980) Posterolateral neck bissection. *Arch Otolaryngol* **106**:618.

Jesse R H, Lindberg R D (1975) The efficacy of combining radiation therapy with a surgical procedure in patients with cervical metastasis from squamous cancer of the oropharynx and hypopharynx. *Cancer* **35**:1163.

Kaplan R, Million R R, Cassisi N J (1977) Carcinoma of the tonsil: results of radical irradiation with surgery reserved for radiation failure. *Laryngoscope* **87**:600.

Krause C J (1973) Carcinoma of the oral cavity – a comparison of therapeutic modalities. *Arch Otolaryngol* **97**:354.

Lindberg R D (1972) Distribution of cervical lymph node metastases from squamous cell carcinoma of the upper respiratory and digestive tract. *Cancer* **29**:1446.

McGregor I A (1963) The temporal flap in intra-oral cancer. *B J Plast Surg* **16**:318.

Martin H E (1957) *Surgery of Head and Neck Tumours*. New York, Hoeber Harper, pp. 12–13.

Martin H E, Sugarbaker E L (1941) Cancer of the tonsil. *Am J Surg* **52**:158.

Martin H E, Tollefsen H R, Gerold F P (1961) Median labiomandibular glossotomy. *Am J Surg* **102**:753.

Mantravadi R V P, Liebner E J, Ginde J V (1978) An analysis of factors in the successful management of cancer of tonsillar region. *Cancer* **41**:1054.

Marchetta F C, Sako K, Murphy J B (1971) The periosteum of the mandible and intraoral carcinoma. *Am J Surg* **122**:711.

McGuirt W F (1982) Panendoscopy as a screening examination for simultaneous primary tumours in head and neck cancer: a prospective sequential study and review of the literature. *Laryngoscope* **92**:569.

Mendenhall W M, Million R R, Cassisi N J (1980) Elective neck irradiation in squamous cell carcinoma of the head and neck. *Head Neck Surg* **3**:25.

Meyza J W, Towpik E (1991) Surgical and cryosurgical salvage of oral and oropharyngeal cancer recurring after radical radiotherapy. *Eur J Surg Oncol* **17**:567–70.

Million R R (1974) Elective neck irradiation for T_x N_0 squamous carcinoma of the oral tongue and floor of the mouth. *Cancer* **34**:149.

Million R R, Cassisi N J (1984) Oropharynx. In: Million R R, Cassisi N J (eds) *Management of Head and Neck Cancer*. Philadelphia, J B. Lippincott.

Million R R, Fletcher G H, Jesse R H (1963) Evaluation of elective irradiation of the neck for squamous cell carcinoma of the nasopharynx, tonsillar fossa, and base of tongue. *Radiology* **80**:973.

Parsons J T, Million R R, Cassisi N J (1982) Carcinoma of the base of the tongue: results of radical irradiation with surgery reserved for irradiation failure. *Layrngoscope* **92**:689.

Rollo J, Rozenbaum C V, Thawley S E (1981) Squamous carcinoma of the base of the tongue: a clinical pathologic study of 81 cases. *Cancer* **47**:333.

Sardi A, Walters P J (1991) Modified mandibular swing procedure for resection of carcinoma of the oropharynx. *Head Neck* **13**:394–7.

Schaefer S O, Muerkel M (1982) Computed tomographic assessment of squamous cell carcinoma of oral and pharyngeal cavities. *Arch Otolaryngol* **108**:688.

Schuller D (1984) Myocutaneous flaps in reconstructive surgery of the head and neck. In: Wolf G (ed) *Head and Neck Oncology*. Boston, Martinus Nijhoff.

Sessions D G (1983) Surgical resection and reconstruction for cancer of the base of the tongue. *Otolaryngol Clin North Am* **16**:309.

Sessions D G, Dedo D D, Ogura J H (1975) Tongue flap reconstruction following resection for cancer of the oral cavity. *Arch Otolaryngol* **101**:166.

Silver C E, Nadler B, Croft C B (1978) Oral and oropharyngeal carcinoma. *Arch Otolaryngol* **104**:278–81.

Smith P G, Collins S I (1984) Repair of head and neck defects with thin and double-lined pectoralis flaps. *Arch Otolaryngol* **110**:468.

Thawley S E (1986) Malignant neoplasms of the oropharynx. In: Cummings C W (ed) *Otolaryngology – Head and Neck Surgery*. St Louis, C. V. Mosby, pp. 1345–98.

Trotter W (1920) A method of lateral pharyngotomy for the exposure of large growths in the epilaryngeal region. *J Laryngol Rhinol Otol* **35**:289.

Trotter W (1928) Operations for malignant disease of the pharynx. *Br J Surg* **16**:485.

Weller S A *et al.* (1976) Carcinoma of the oropharynx: results of megavoltage radiation therapy in 305 patients. *Am J Radiol* **126**:236.

Wetmore S J, Swen J W (1984) Clinical management of regional metastases. In: Wolf G (ed) *Head and Neck Oncology*, Boston, Martinus Nijhoff.

18

Tumours of the nasopharynx

Surgical anatomy

The nasopharynx is a large space with rigid walls, 4 cm high, 4 cm wide and 2 cm deep. The anterior wall is formed by the choana and nasal septum, the floor by the soft palate, and the lateral wall by the eustachian tubes and the fossae of Rosenmüller. The roof lies inferior to the body of the sphenoid and is occupied by the adenoids in the adolescent; it merges with the posterior wall of the pharynx. The eustachian tubes are triangular in shape, the anterior wall joining the soft palate and the posterior wall being large and prominent. As the posterior wall is mobile, it requires space and this is provided by the fossa of Rosenmüller. This is a lateral extension of the nasopharynx lying above and behind the medial end of the eustachian tube. By adult life it may be as deep as 1.5 cm and is cleft-like. Its apex reaches the anterior margin of the carotid canal and its base opens into the nasopharynx at a point below the foramen lacerum medially. The inferior wall of the fossa is formed by a delicate mucosa covering the eustachian tube and levator palati muscle; the posterior wall is formed by the mucosa covering the dense pharyngobasilar fascia. The mandibular division of the fifth nerve lying in the parapharyngeal space is anterolateral to the apex of the fossa and is separated from it by fascia of the eustachian tube and the tensor palati muscle.

If a nasopharyngeal tumour penetrates the pharyngobasilar fascia, it invades the parapharyngeal space and can involve the foramen ovale, the foramen spinosum, the greater wing of the sphenoid and the retrostyloid compartment, which contains the carotid sheath, the last four cranial nerves and the cervical sympathetic trunk. This results in paralysis of the mandibular division of the trigeminal, trismus, vocal cord paralysis, tongue paralysis, Horner's syndrome and, occasionally, pharyngeal and palatal paralysis. Anterior spread of tumour from the fossa of Rosenmüller blocks the eustachian tube, resulting in conductive deafness, but spread up the tube to the middle ear is extremely rare. Spread through the foramen lacerum and along the internal carotid artery causes paralysis of the motor nerves to the eye and the upper two divisions of the trigeminal nerve. The intimate relationship of the carotid artery in the fossa of Rosenmüller also explains the relatively frequent finding of radiological destruction of the greater wing of the sphenoid without invasion of the eustachian tube.

In infancy the nasopharyngeal epithelium is columnar ciliated but in adults most of the epithelium has undergone squamous metaplasia, leaving only areas of columnar epithelium in relation to the fossa of Rosenmüller.

There is abundant lymphoid stroma in the submucosa of the nasopharynx. The ease of access to rich lymphatic channels is probably responsible for the high incidence of cervical node metastasis in nasopharyngeal carcinoma. The first echelon of nodes is the lateral retropharyngeal group. The uppermost one is known as the node of Rouviere. These nodes lie deep in the upper neck and cannot be palpated. The nasopharynx is a midline structure and, therefore, it is not surprising to find a high rate of bilateral neck node metastases.

Surgical pathology

Epidemiology

Nasopharyngeal cancer accounts for 18% of all malignant neoplasms in the Cantonese. It has a predilection for the Chinese who are natives of the Kwang Tung province. In Europe it forms less than 6% of all head and neck cancers but, in the Cantonese, it forms over 80%. In Singapore it is the second most common tumour: the normal Singaporean population distribution is 40% Chinese, 30% Malay, 28% Indian and 2% European, but the incidence of nasopharyngeal cancer is 87% Chinese, 10% Malay, 3% European and nil in the Indian population. In the

Japanese, Korean and North Chinese the incidence is as low as in the UK or USA, but in Kenyans, Tunisians, and Alaskans, it is much higher than in non-mongoloid races. American-born, second-generation Chinese have a lower risk of nasopharyngeal cancer than those born in China, but the risk is still eight times that of the resident non-Chinese population. In Hong Kong the rate is 124 per million, which is 25 times that found in Western Europe.

The aetiology of induction of nasopharyngeal cancer has been well explained as follows. The three important factors are:

1 The Epstein–Barr virus (EBV), which acts as a carcinogen;
2 a genetically determined susceptibility in the Cantonese;
3 an environmental factor, which is thought to be the eating of salted preserved fish and a deficiency of vitamin C in young Southern Chinese people.

In the Chinese the highest incidence is in the fourth decade of life; in the non-Chinese it is in the sixth decade. In the Chinese the male : female ratio is 3 : 1 and in the non-Chinese 2 : 1.

Environmental risk factors

In susceptible Chinese populations salted fish is one of the cheapest foods used to supplement rice and is probably eaten more often by the poorer segments of the population, in whom the disease is common. Studies from Hong Kong have confirmed that feeding salted fish to babies during weaning was a major risk factor and experimental studies have shown that 4 out of 20 Wistar rats fed salted fish developed carcinoma in the nose and paranasal region. A specific carcinogen has not yet been identified but it has been suggested that over 90% of nasopharyngeal carcinomas occurring in young Hong Kong Chinese could be attributed to the consumption of Cantonese-style salted fish during childhood. More recent studies have shown that other preserved foods also function as independent risk factors – dried fish, salted duck eggs, salted mustard green and fermented soya bean paste. The significance of environmental factors is supported by the epidemiological data, the observation of a plateau in the age incidence rate curve after the age of 40 and the observation that, while the high risks for the indigenous Chinese population in the Far East have remained static for the last 50 years, the incidence for the disease in the second and third generations of Chinese people born in North America has shown a relative decline.

Immunology

Although nasopharyngeal carcinoma is an epithelial tumour which arises many years after the peak incidence of EBV infection, the lesion appears to be related to the virus as the patients have an antibody response to the viral capsid antigen (VCA), the early antigen (EA) and the nuclear antigen (EBNA). Furthermore, Epstein-Barr viral markers have been found in nasopharyngeal carcinoma cell lines (but not yet in biopsy specimens). Only the undifferentiated forms consistently express EBNA. The fourth group of important Epstein–Barr-related antibody is antibody-dependent cellular cytotoxicity which is known to be effective in the destruction of viral-infected cells where the virus has induced the expression of membrane antigens. The titres of immunoglobulin G (IgG) and IgA to VCA and EA are useful diagnostic markers related to the tumour burden and thus also helpful in follow-up. The prognosis and survival are inversely related to VCA and EA antibodies, while high levels of antibody-dependent cellular cytotoxicity antibody are associated with a good prognosis.

The IgA antibody to VCA can also be used to screen for the tumour in high-risk (Chinese) populations. Although patients in Northern Ireland are reported to show elevated antibody levels to VCA and EA, a North American study found no relationship between post-treatment antibody titres and disease outcome. Conversely the antibody-dependent cellular cytotoxicity titre at the time of diagnosis is prognostic in patients in the USA. A direct relationship has been shown between IgA levels and circulating immune complexes whose immunosuppressive properties may account in part for the observed immunosuppression in nasopharyngeal carcinoma patients.

Studies of peripheral blood lymphocytes from nasopharyngeal carcinoma patients have been shown to have a normal proliferative response to phytohaemagglutinin but a low natural killer activity and no lytic activity against EBV-transformed B cells. This lack of cytotoxicity against an EBV-transformed B cell line is probably the result of the presence of a large number of suppressor T cells (OKT8 cells). In contrast, studies of the lymphocyte populations infiltrating a nasopharyngeal carcinoma show that some tumours have a predominance of helper (T$_4$) cells while in others suppressor cells predominate. Certainly the majority of the infiltrating lymphocytes are T cells. It is not clear from the literature which cell type predominates in nasopharyngeal lymphomas. One series from Hong Kong suggested that the majority of nasopharyngeal lymphomas were peripheral T cell neoplasms while a Japanese study showed a mixture of T cell and B cell origin. T cell lymphomas had a 5-year survival of only 12.5% while

B cell lymphoma had a 75% 5-year survival but the numbers of patients were very small.

Genetic factors

The major histocompatibility gene complex on the short arm of chromosome 6 has 6 loci: human leukocyte antigen (HLA) A, B, C, DR, DQ and DS. There are many alleles for each locus, and each determines a different antigen. Frequency of occurrence of these alleles varies among different ethnic groups. Different HLA types are associated with different patterns of clinical behaviour in nasopharyngeal carcinoma – for example, HLA AW19–B17 is associated with short-term survival while A2-BW46 is associated with intermediate-term survival. The occurrence of A2 without BW46 or B17 is associated with long-term survival, i.e. 5-year survival greater than 40%. (In British series the long-term survival from nasopharyngeal carcinoma in fact is considerably lower than this, probably because most patients tend to present late.) The interpretation of these findings is not clear because there is a different distribution of HLA in different age groups but a relative risk from a particular HLA type can be calculated. Despite the occurrence of more than 50 alleles at the HLA A and B loci only a few are associated with nasopharyngeal carcinoma.

A numerical alteration in chromosome complement in human dermal fibroblast cultures – hyperdiploidy with a normal occurrence of tetraploidy – was found in almost half of a series of 39 cases of carcinoma of the nasopharynx. The same pattern has been reported to be associated with the *in vivo* expression of certain heritable tumours and the average age of diagnosis was earlier in the group exhibiting the chromosomal abnormality. This has been taken to show a genetic predisposition for certain nasopharyngeal cancers.

Tumour types

Squamous cell carcinoma

Squamous cell carcinoma of the nasopharynx is divided into three types – keratinizing, non-keratinizing and undifferentiated. The squamous cell carcinoma constitutes 85% of all malignant tumours of the nasopharynx. A fourth variant is sometimes added, namely lymphoepithelioma, which is an undifferentiated tumour with lymphocytic infiltration among the tumour cells. Carcinomas may show marked structural variations, even in the same tumour, and this possibly explains the variety of tumours that are sometimes described in series of nasopharyngeal neoplasms. Although most classification systems divide the nasopharynx into the vault and lateral walls, it is usually impossible to say from where tumours arise. It is thought that most arise from the fossa of Rosenmüller but many will present with metastatic nodes before even declaring themselves in the nasopharynx. Almost half the patients will have metastatic nodes on first presentation. About 1 in 3 will have unilateral nodes and 1 in 5 bilateral nodes. The tumour spreads by direct infiltration into the basiocciput and the middle cranial fossa, paralysing all cranial nerves eventually from the third to the 12th. It can leave the nasopharynx by entering the orbit, the infratemporal fossa and the parapharyngeal space.

Other malignant tumours

In the adult, adenocarcinoma, adenoid cystic carcinoma and melanoma have been described but the second most common adult tumour is probably lymphoma. This is very rarely a Hodgkin's lymphoma; in 95% of cases it is non-Hodgkin's. It may be a plasmacytoma, either solitary or part of a generalized multiple myelomatosis. In children, rhabdomyosarcoma is the most commonly encountered malignancy in the nasopharynx and accounts for 30% of all malignancies in this site in children. These are classified as pleomorphic, embryonal, alveolar and botryoid. Histologically, the most common variety of rhabdomyosarcoma in the head and neck is the embryonal or botryoid embryonal form. Lymph node involvement occurs frequently (50%), and 12% will have distant metastases when first seen.

Nasopharyngeal angiofibroma

This is a rare condition and very few clinicians have experience of it in depth. It seems to be more common in the Middle East and the Indian subcontinent than it is in Europe or the USA. Girls are very seldom affected and the mean age at diagnosis is around 14 years. It arises from the base of the medial pterygoid plate and the sphenopalatine foramen and thus is not truly nasopharyngeal. Secondary involvement of the nasopharynx occurs because of accessability of the site to additional vascular attachments, following pressure ulceration of the lining epithelium. The lesion consists of angiomatous tissue and a fibrous stroma; both the maturity and quantity of these components may vary within individual tumours. Some are thus angiofibromas and others are fibroangiomas. It is thought that spontaneous regression occurs with age but this is entirely unproven and open to much doubt. The tumours are histologically benign but expand to involve the ethmoids, the orbit and the skull base. The majority are operable but, with the passage of time and several recurrences, they can pass beyond the field of the surgeon, when treatment becomes very difficult.

Investigations

History

One in 3 patients with a carcinoma presents with nasal symptoms such as epistaxis or nasal obstruction; 1 in 5 with conductive deafness; 1 in 5 with lymph node metastases; and 1 in 10 with pain. The remainder present with headache, diplopia, facial numbness, hypoaesthesia, trismus, ptosis and hoarseness. The average time between the appearance of the first symptom and first consultation is about 6 months. The patient's race is obviously very important and a Chinese person complaining of any of the above symptoms should be considered to have nasopharyngeal cancer until proved otherwise. A Caucasian over the age of 40 complaining of unilateral conductive deafness, or with an enlarged cervical lymph node, should be regarded with a similarly high degree of suspicion. In patients with advanced nasopharyngeal tumours, endocrine changes such as Cushing's syndrome, dermatomyositis, and pseudomyaesthenia gravis, also known as the Eaton–Lambert syndrome, have been reported.

Examination

Exophytic tumours are easily seen with a nasopharyngoscope or a postnasal mirror, but many tumours remain submucosal and may be missed. In large tumours the palate may be pushed down or may be paralysed, as may the vocal cords. The tympanic membrane on one side may be indrawn or there may be evidence of serous otitis media. There may be paralysis of one side of the tongue, and eye tests may display diplopia or a Horner's syndrome. If the tumour has spread into the parapharyngeal space, there may be trismus. With fifth nerve involvement there may be loss of facial, palatal or pharyngeal sensation. Seventy per cent of patients will have some degree of neck node involvement, whether it is unilateral bilateral enlargement or fixation, and this is very often the presenting feature.

A rhabdomyosarcoma presents in very much the same way as carcinoma and must, of course, be suspected if the patient is under the age of 12.

Similarly, angiofibroma occurs almost exclusively in boys around the age of puberty and should be suspected with someone presenting with nasal symptoms at this age. Angiofibromas are soft on palpation; fibroangiomas are often hard, tough and rubbery. There will not be any metastatic involvement, even though there is a big mass in the nasopharynx, and the patient will present with nasal symptoms or facial swelling.

Laboratory studies

Do a full blood count and erythrocyte sedimentation rate (ESR) in all patients, as repeated epistaxis may have caused an anaemia and a high ESR may raise the possibility of a lymphoma.

Do audiometry, including impedance tests to test for eustachian tube function; field tests and other specialized ophthalmic tests will also be required.

Titres for EBV-related antigens may be ordered. Patients with nasopharyngeal carcinoma have high titres of antibodies to Epstein–Barr viral capsid antigen and this increases with advancing clinical stage of the disease. Antibodies to the diffuse component of the EBV-induced early antigen are not usually demonstrable in stage 1 of the disease but, from stage 2 onwards, there is an increasingly high titre. Viral capsid antigen-specific IgA antibodies are invariably present in high-titre patients with nasopharyngeal cancer, and it has been suggested that the absence of these antibodies in a patient with clinical features suggestive of nasopharyngeal cancer may be used to exclude the diagnosis.

Radiology

The extent of a nasopharyngeal tumour is assessed by plain X-rays of the skull base, tomograms of the skull base, and computed tomography (CT) scan. With the ability to reconstruct coronal and axial views, the CT scan is the investigation of choice. This will define any evidence of destruction of pterygoid plates, foramen lacerum, foramen ovale, foramen spinosum or jugular foramen. Scans will give information about tumour extension into the ethmoid and sphenoid sinuses. They will also give further information about the presence of enlarged deep impalpable nodes in the retropharyngeal area.

Distant metastases to bone, lung and liver are searched for with the use of plain X-rays and scans.

Angiography used to be the test of choice in the assessment of an angiofibroma. This is now only used when embolization is considered as a treatment modality. A CT scan will show erosion of the medial pterygoid plate, lateral extension into the infratemporal fossa and invasion of the middle fossa by way of orbit or superior orbital fissure. It may show involvement of the sphenoid sinus in up to 70% of patients, of the infratemporal fossa in 60%, of the orbit in 30% and of the middle cranial fossa in 20%.

Magnetic resonance imaging, with its superior density resolution, shows the tumour edge more clearly, and its vascular nature is demonstrated by negative signals from vessels within the tumour.

Biopsy

This should be done under general anaesthesia. If a mass is seen, then the palate can be held forward with two catheters, visualized with a postnasal mirror and biopsy done transnasally with Tilley forceps. The biopsy may also be done under direct vision with a Yankauer's speculum.

If no tumour is seen and the nasopharynx is being harvested by biopsy for the investigation of a metastatic node with no obvious primary, then it is probably best to use an adenoid curette to obtain as big a sample as possible from the nasopharynx. Isolated blind biopsies have a much lower harvest rate. If a nasopharyngeal angiofibroma is suspected, then a great deal of thought should go into whether or not to do a biopsy. It is usually preferable not to do a punch biopsy because of the uncontrollable bleeding that may result. Diagnosis in these cases is very often possible without a biopsy because of the clinical and radiological findings.

Treatment policy

Radiation therapy is the primary treatment modality for nasopharyngeal carcinoma. The radiation field must be large, encompassing the nasopharynx, the base of the skull including the cranial foramina, the sphenoid sinus, the posterior ethmoid sinus, posterior orbit, posterior maxillary antrum and the posterior nasal cavity and, perhaps, the oropharynx and retropharyngeal nodes. It has been shown that elective irradiation of the uninvolved neck reduces the probablity of neck node metastases at a later date and so both sides of the neck are routinely irradiated.

Because of the large fields required, patients usually have bad side-effects from the irradiation, including anorexia, fatigue, mucositis and a persistent xerostomia. They may get trismus secondary to irradiation of the mandibular joint, and perhaps keratoconjunctivitis. The most severe complication was transverse myelitis, but modern techniques now avoid this. The 5-year survival depends on the node stage: in stage 1 disease the survival rates are between 70 and 80%; in stage 2 50–70% in stage 3 between 20 and 40%, and at stage 4, between 0 and 20%.

Surgery has almost no place in the management of a patient with nasopharyngeal carcinoma. Occasionally, where there is certain control of the primary and there is persistent or recurrent neck disease, then a radical neck dissection may be performed. Recurrence of tumour in the nasopharynx is treated with further radiotherapy but laser excision has been described. As recurrence will certainly indicate bone destruction, it is, however, difficult to see what this modality can offer. Various combined craniofacial procedures have been described for approach to the midline compartment of the skull. The original description was by Derome, and involved a transbasal approach combined with a transoral approach. These approaches, however, are more useful for the excision of benign tumours such as chordoma than for the carcinomas, which spread laterally and thus invalidate these procedures.

Nasopharyngeal lymphoma requires individual assessment, grading and combined therapy with radiation and chemotherapy.

Nasopharyngeal rhabdomyosarcoma now does very much better with the advent of triple therapy. The tumours do better when the bulk is excised and adjuvant chemotherapy and radiation therapy are used. The 2- or 3-year survival rate has gone up in the last decade from around 30% to around 80%.

Nasopharyngeal angiofibromas should be treated surgically because if they are left alone, they expand into neighbouring cavities, notably the orbit, causing blindness. Radiotherapy has been used as a curative modality and also to reduce the vascularity of tumours before surgery. Its use as a curative modality, however, should be limited to inoperable cases because the patient is almost always a young boy and radiotherapy will, at best, produce retardation of growth of the face and, at worse, tumour induction in later life.

Embolization is also enjoying increasing popularity as the skills of the radiologists improve. It requires considerable time and expertise to perform and, as well as being curative and preferable to the ligation of feeding vessels, it may actually produce an involution of the tumour.

If the tumours are confined to the nasopharynx with a small pedicle, then they are best approached and removed with a transpalatal approach. However, tumours that extend out of the nasopharynx into the posterior ethmoids and the infratemporal fossa should be removed via a lateral rhinotomy and a medial maxillectomy. This can be performed with a Moure's incision, and this is extended into a Fergusson incision or a Weber–Fergusson incision if infratemporal extension requires to be accessed. An alternative approach can be achieved by a Le Fort I osteotomy.

Radiotherapy technique

Nasopharyngeal carcinoma

The treatment volume includes the primary tumour, areas of actual or potential local spread, and the cervical lymph node areas. Both sides of the neck are treated, even if enlarged nodes are palpable only on one side, because the nasopharynx is a midline structure with bilateral drainage. The neck nodes are always treated, even in those few patients without lymphadenopathy at presentation, because of the high incidence of subclinical disease. This large treatment volume of necessity includes the spinal cord, which is a dose-limiting structure. A two-phase technique is therefore used, enabling the dose to the cord to be kept within tolerance but still allowing adequate treatment of overt disease.

The patient is treated lying supine in an individually prepared Perspex shell, which extends from the level of the eyebrows to the clavicles. The neck is extended to keep the anterior part of the oral cavity out of the field. The shell holds the patient immobile during treatment, and carries the marks indicating correct beam alignment and the position of the blocks used to shield critical structures.

For the first phase of treatment, large parallel opposed lateral fields are used. These extend from the level of the supraorbital ridge down to the clavicles. The anterior border is placed to include the entire neck, the oropharynx and the posterior parts of the nasal cavity and orbit within the treated volume. The posterior border encompasses the suboccipital area. The upper posterior corner is blocked to shield the brain, brainstem and optic chiasm. Care is taken, however, to ensure that this block does not impinge on the skull base which needs to be treated. An additional block shields the eye and anterior orbit (Fig. 18.1). A simulator check film is retained as a permanent record of the intended treatment. At the start of treatment, verification films are taken on the radiotherapy machine to ensure that the actual set-up matches the intended.

First-phase treatment is with 4–6 MV X-rays, giving 40 Gy in 20 fractions over 4 weeks. The patient is then replanned for the second phase, which follows on immediately after the first. Two smaller lateral fields now cover the primary tumour in the nasopharynx, base of skull, parapharyngeal space, sphenoid and posterior ethmoid sinuses and any extension into the nasal cavity or oropharynx (Fig. 18.2). If there is gross disease in the nasal cavity or ethmoid sinuses, an anterior field may be added to give adequate coverage of this area without compromising the eyes or optic nerves. The neck is treated by a single anterior field which matches on to the lower side of the lateral fields. This field has a central block to shield the vulnerable cervical cord (Fig. 18.3). The phase 2 volume receives a dose of 25 Gy in 12 fractions over $2\frac{1}{2}$ weeks, using 4–6 MV X-rays. The total dose is thus 65 Gy in 32 fractions over $6\frac{1}{2}$ weeks. If there is doubt about adequate coverage of any posterior lymph node masses, these may be boosted with small electron beam fields. The limited penetration of electrons enables sparing of the spinal cord.

As with other tumours such as supraglottic or pyriform fossa carcinoma with extensive nodal disease, where irradiation of most of the neck is required, the principal side-effect is mucositis. As the parotid glands are included in the irradiated volume, xerostomia exacerbates this. As it is easy for patients to stop eating and drinking almost com-

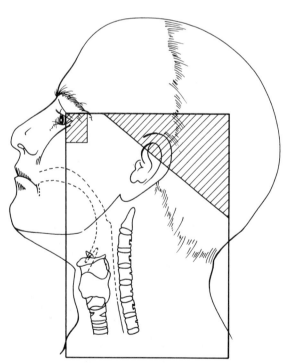

Fig. 18.1 Radiotherapy field for the first phase of treatment of nasopharyngeal carcinoma.

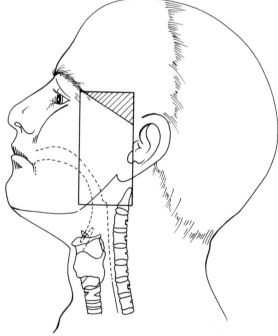

Fig. 18.2 Smaller field covering only the nasopharynx for the second phase of treatment.

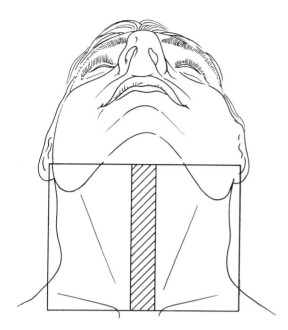

Fig. 18.3 Split anterior neck field for nodal irradiation.

pletely, they must be kept under close surveillance, especially during the latter half of treatment. Usually adequate oral intake can be maintained, but occasionally it may be necessary to resort to nasogastric feeding. It is important, however, to continue with the treatment as planned as interruptions in, or premature discontinuation of, treatment reduce substantially the likelihood of cure.

Juvenile angiofibroma

As indicated above, surgery is the treatment of choice, but for recurrent or inoperable cases, irradiation is a reasonable alternative, despite the slight risk of a subsequent radiation-induced malignancy. The tumour extent requires accurate delineation by CT scanning to enable the treated volume to be kept to a minimum. Lateral opposed portals or a three-field technique including an anterior field are suitable. A low dose of 30 Gy in 15 fractions over 3 weeks is adequate, but regression may be slow.

Surgical technique for nasopharyngeal angiofibroma

Approaches to the nasopharynx

There are four approaches to the nasopharynx:

1 *Transoral*. This is the approach used for nasopharyngeal biopsy, removal of adenoids and removal of nasopharyngeal cysts. The access is eased by anterior retraction of the palate and this is best done by passing rubber catheters through the nose and out of the mouth. This approach is of no value in the removal of angiofibroma.

2 *Transpalatal*. This is an approach that was formerly used for the removal of nasopharyngeal angiofibromas but it is not as popular now as it once was. It gives better access to the anterior nasopharynx than the transoral route but it gives inadequate access for the removal of an angiofibroma because there is poor access to the lateral nasopharynx, which is from where angiofibroma arises.

If it is done then the best incision is one that is placed just inside the upper alveolus to provide a large palatal flap. The incision is made down to the bone with a knife and the soft tissues are elevated from the bone backwards to the posterior edge of the hard palate. The exposure is increased by extending the incision backwards into the soft palate and if necessary dividing the greater palatine vessels on one side. The bony hard palate is then removed as necessary, using a cutting burr and bone-nibbling forceps.

The closure of the palatal flap is with 2/0 silk. It is important that there is always bone underneath the incision line or else an oronasal fistula occurs. Since removal of the bony hard palate is always necessary in this approach, it is important to make the incision as far forward as possible.

3 *Transmaxillary*. The maxilla is approached with an alveolar degloving incision which runs from tuberosity to tuberosity. Once the maxilla is exposed then osteotomies are done and the alveolus is fractured downwards. Occasionally there can be troublesome bleeding from a torn maxillary artery which may be difficult to deal with via this approach. While it gives adequate access it may need intramaxillary fixation in the postoperative period and as such probably more tissue damage than necessary is caused by the procedure for the removal of an angiofibroma. Nowadays it is more usual to repair with mini plates.

4 *Transnasoantral*. This is the preferred option now and there are two approaches to this.

The first is a degloving incision which is similar to the incision used for the transmaxillary approach, together with intercartilaginous and nasal transfixing incisions. The facial tissues can be elevated from both maxillas up to the frontoethmoid suture line. The inferior orbital limbs can be easily identified on both sides and although there is quite a lot of facial swelling in the postoperative period it avoids the creation of a facial scar.

The alternative approach is to use a Moure's incision and a lateral rhinotomy approach. This is more direct and gives slightly easier access but it does carry the complication of facial scarring.

All of the above approaches except the transoral approach are best accompanied by a temporary tracheostomy. It is not essential but it is safer, especially if any postoperative bleeding is expected, and it also gives better access because it removes the anaesthetic tubes from the operative field.

Removal of angiofibroma

Most angiofibromas are firm, and few are as vascular as expected. The vascularity of these tumours is now decreased by pre-operative embolization 48 h before surgery. They extend into the nasal cavity, the infratemporal fossa, the ethmoids and the sphenoids. The approach to the tumour is done by removing the medial wall of the maxilla and the ethmoids and using blunt finger dissection round the side of the maxillary antrum into the infratemporal fossa. The tumour is freed from the nasopharynx and infratemporal fossa and pedicled on the pterygomaxillary fossa which is where it arises from. With blunt dissection the two areas are joined and the tumour is removed. Any bleeding is controlled either directly or with a postnasal pack.

If a postnasal pack is inserted then the patient needs to be covered with antibiotics. The incisions are closed with Vicryl to mucosa and Nurolon to skin if a skin incision is used. The postnasal pack is removed after 48 h and it would be rare to have any complications after this period of time. In the degloving approach the facial swelling takes about a week to settle.

Controversies

Is nasopharyngeal carcinoma two different diseases?

This concept was first put forward by Scanlon and colleagues in 1967; these authors classified nasopharyngeal carcinoma into keratinizing squamous cell carcinoma and combined grade 4 undifferentiated carcinomas (lymphoepitheliomas, anaplastic carcinomas and transitional cell carcinomas). The EBV serological findings are different in the two groups. With the latter group, onset is at an earlier age, disease-free periods after treatment are longer, survival after treatment is greater, and the early and advanced neck metastases are more common. They are often small, submucosal and difficult to detect, and may be clinically occult. They are more radiosensitive than keratinizing squamous cell tumours, which are more likely to recur or persist in the nasopharynx after treatment. The keratinizing squamous cell carcinomas are more like the other carcinomas seen in the upper air and food passages.

It may also be a different tumour in Chinese and Caucasian people. There is a definite association between nasopharyngeal carcinoma and class 2 antigens in the Chinese, notably antigens A2, BW46 and B17. BW46 is a very uncommon antigen amongst whites and no significant associations have been found in Caucasians.

Why is there no good staging system?

The standard staging systems as set down by the American Joint Committee (AJC) and the International Union against Cancer (UICC) are artificial in that they divide the nasopharynx into often unidentifiable sites, and they do not take sufficient account of bony destruction of the base of the skull. The classification of cervical node metastases is done from a surgical point of view and not a radiotherapeutic one.

Separation of tumours confined to the nasopharynx and to T_1 (one subsite) and T_2 (two subsites) is not practical. Furthermore, a tumour may occur submucosally, making it difficult to evaluate its extent. The difference between T_3 and T_4 in the UICC classification is the presence or absence of bone involvement, but no mention is made of the involvement of cranial nerves, which may occur without demonstrable bone involvement.

Ho's classification is more acceptable (Table 18.1).

Similarly, the node classification is for the surgeon, whereas this is a radiotherapy disease. Ho's neck classification (Table 18.2) is more appropriate for the radiotherapist.

Table 18.1 Classification of tumours of the nasopharynx, according to Ho

T_1	Tumour confined to the nasopharynx
T_2	Tumour extended to nasal fossa, oropharynx or adjacent muscles
T_3	Tumour extended beyond T_2 limits and subclassified as:
T_{3a}	Bone involvement below the base of the skull
T_{3b}	Involvement with the base of the skull
T_{3c}	Involvement of cranial nerves
T_{3d}	Involvement of orbits, laryngopharynx or infratemporal fossa

Table 18.2 Classification of nodes in the neck; acording to Ho

N_0	No palpable nodes
N_1	Nodes in the upper cervical level above the thyroid notch
N_2	Nodes between the thyroid notch and supraclavicular fossa
N_3	Nodes palpable in the supraclavicular fossa

The management of recurrent nasopharyngeal carcinoma

When tumours recur only in the nasopharynx, re-irradiation, utilizing an implant with a radiation source to another 50 Gy or more, may be helpful and occasionally curative. Sometimes a palatal fenestration is performed to give access for intracavitary irradiation. The risk of further irradiation is, of course, transverse myelitis but this risk is usually worth taking. There are reports of 21% 2-year and 5% 5-year survival after reirradiation.

The use of chemotherapy for recurrent cancer of the nasopharynx has been disappointing and those cases that respond do so for only brief periods.

Recurrent angiofibroma

This can present a desperately difficult problem if it is after initial surgical removal. It is not so much of a problem after failed irradiation or embolization. It is said that fibroangiomas are more likely to recur than angiofibromas. These tumours do not have capsules and surgical removal may well leave tumour that it is hoped will involute. If it does not, and if it regrows, then further surgery with lateral rhinotomy and extensions of the medial maxillectomy must be used. If it goes into the sphenoid and its lateral walls, however, it becomes inaccessible to the surgeon. The treatment of 5 patients with recurrent angiofibroma using doxorubicin and decarbazine has been described.

References and further reading

Anatomy, pathology and investigation

Chan J K C, Ng C S, Lau W H, Lo S T H (1987) Most nasal/nasopharyngeal lymphomas are peripheral T-cell neoplasms. *Am J Surg Pathol* 11:418–29.

Fearon B, Forte, Brama I (1990) Malignant nasopharyngeal tumours in children. *Laryngoscope* 100:470–2.

Jacobs C, Hoppe R T (1985) Non Hodgkin's lymphomas of head and neck extranodal sites. *Int J Radiat Oncol Biol Phys* 11:357–64.

Sato H, Kurata K, Yen Y-H, Honjo T, Young Y-H, Hsieh T (1988) Extension of nasopharyngeal carcinoma and otitis media with effusion. *Arch Otolaryngol Head Neck Surg* 114:866–7.

Silver A J, Sane P, Hilal S K (1984) CT of the nasopharyngeal region. Normal and pathologic anatomy. *Radiol Clin North Am* 22:161–76.

Yanagisawa E, Isaacson G, Kmucha S T, Hirokawa R (1989) Videonasopharyngoscopy: a comparison of fiberscopic, telescopic and microscopic documentation. *Ann Otol Rhinol Laryngol* 98:15–20.

Genetic and immunological aspects of NPC

Anonymous (1989) Salted fish and nasopharyngeal carcinoma. *Lancet* 2:840–2.

Coyle P V, Wyatt D, Connolly J H (1987) Antibodies to Epstein–Barr virus in patients with nasopharyngeal carcinoma in Northern Ireland. *Irish J Med Sci* 156:182–4.

Danes B S, Boyle P D, Traganos F, Ringborg U, Melamed M R (1987) Evidence for genetic predisposition for some nasopharyngeal cancers by in vitro hyperdiploidy in human dermal fibroblasts. *Cancer Genet Cytogenet* 26:261–70.

Ho J H (1978) An epidemiologic and clinical study of nasopharyngeal carcinoma. *Int J Radiat Oncol Biol Phys* 4:182–98.

Lakhdar M, Ellouz R, Kammoun H et al. (1987) Presence of in vivo-activated T-cells expressing HLA-DR molecules and Il-2 receptors in peripheral blood of patients with nasopharyngeal carcinoma. *Int J Cancer* 39:663–9.

Neel H B, Taylor W F (1990) Epstein–Barr Virus-related antibody: changes in titers after therapy for nasopharyngeal carcinoma. *Arch Otolaryngol Head Neck Surg* 116:1287–90.

Sam C K, Prasad U, Pathmanathan R (1989) Serological markers in the diagnosis of histopathological types of nasopharyngeal carcinoma. *Eur J Surg Oncol* 15:357–60.

Shu M-M, Huang S-C (1988) Prognostic factors of patients with nasopharyngeal carcinoma. *Acta Otolaryngol* 458:34–40.

Sugimoto T, Hashimoto H, Enjoji M (1990) Nasopharyngeal carcinomas and malignant lymphomas: an immunohistochemical analysis of 74 cases. *Laryngoscope* 100:742–8.

Wolf G T, Wolfe R A (1990) Circulating immune complexes in patients with nasopharyngeal carcinoma. *Laryngoscope* 100:302–8.

Yan L, Xi Z, Drettner B (1989) Epidemiological studies of nasopharyngeal cancer in the Guangzhou area, China. *Acta Otolaryngol* 107:424–7.

Yu M C, Ho J H C, Lai S-H, Henderson B E (1986) Cantonese-style salted fish as a cause of nasopharyngeal carcinoma: report of a case-control study in Hong Kong. *Cancer Res* 46:956–61.

Radiotherapy of the nasopharynx

Budihna M, Furlan L, Smid L (1987) Carcinoma of the nasopharynx: results of radiation treatment and some prognostic factors. *Radiother Oncol* 8:25–32.

Chu A M, Flynn M B, Achino E, Mendoza E F, Scott R M, Jose B (1984) Irradiation of nasopharyngeal carcinoma: correlations with treatment factors and stage. *Int J Radiat Oncol Biol Phys* 10:2241–9.

Stillwagon G B, Lee D-J, Moses H, Kashima H, Harris A, Johns M (1986) Response of cranial nerve abnormalities in nasopharyngeal carcinoma to radiation therapy. *Cancer* 57:2272–4.

Vikram B, Strong E W, Manolatos S, Mishra U B (1984) Improved survival in carcinoma of the nasopharynx. *Head Neck Surg* 7:123–8.

Vikram B, Mishra U B, Strong E W, Manolatos S (1985) Patterns of failure in carcinoma of the nasopharynx. I Failure at the primary site. *Int J Radiat Oncol Biol Phys* 11:1455–9.

Vikram B, Mishra U B, Strong E W, Manolatos S (1986) Patterns of failure in carcinoma of the nasopharynx: failure at distant sites. *Head Neck Surg* 8:276–9.

Wang C C (1987) Re-irradiation of recurrent nasopharyngeal carcinoma – treatment techniques and results. *Int J Radiat Oncol Biol Phys* **13**:953–6.

Wazer D E, Schmidt-Ullrich R, Chasin W, Wu A, Buscher M (1989) High-dose boost irradiation techniques for carcinoma of the nasopharynx. *Am J Otolaryngol* **10**:173–80.

Yamashita S, Kondo M, Inuyama Y, Hashimoto S (1986) Improved survival of patients with nasopharyngeal squamous cell carcinoma. *Int J Radiat Oncol Biol Phys* **12**:307–12.

Surgery of the nasopharynx/juvenile nasopharyngeal angiofibroma

Andrews J C, Fisch U, Valavanis A, Aeppli U, Makek M S (1989) The surgical management of extensive nasopharyngeal angiofibromas with the infratemporal fossa approach. *Laryngoscope* **99**:429–37.

Bremer J W, Neel H B, DeSanto L W, Jones G C (1986) Angiofibroma: treatment trends in 150 patients during 40 years. *Laryngoscope* **96**:1321–9.

Cummings B J, Blend R, Keane T (1984) Primary radiation therapy for juvenile nasopharyngeal angiofibroma. *Laryngoscope* **94**:1599–1605.

Davis K R (1987) Embolization of epistaxis and juvenile nasopharyngeal angiofibromas. *Am J Radiol* **148**:209–18.

Farag M M, Ghanimah S E, Ragaie A, Saleem T H (1987) Hormonal receptors in juvenile nasopharyngeal angiofibroma. *Laryngoscope* **97**:208–11.

Harrison D F N (1987) The natural history, pathogenesis and treatment of juvenile angiofibroma. *Arch Otolaryngol Head Neck Surg* **113**:936–42.

Lee D A, Rao B R, Meyer J S, Prioleau P G, Bauer W C (1980) Hormonal receptor determination in juvenile nasopharyngeal angiofibromas. *Cancer* **46**:547–51.

Sasaki C T, Lowlicht R A, Astrachan D I, Friedman C D, Goodwin W J, Movales M (1990) Le Fort I osteotomy approach to the skull base. *Laryngoscope* **100**:1073–6.

Witt T R, Shah J P, Sternberg S S (1983) Juvenile nasopharyngeal angiofibroma: a 30 year clinical review. *Am J Surg* **146**:521–5.

19

Tumours of major salivary glands

Surgical anatomy

There are four main salivary glands – two submandibular glands and two parotids. There are 300–400 minor salivary glands occurring elsewhere in the upper respiratory tract, especially in the hard palate and lateral pharyngeal wall.

The removal of the major salivary glands is basically an anatomical dissection, so it is essential that any surgeon should know the anatomy of these regions intimately.

The *parotid gland* is described as having a superficial and a deep lobe with an isthmus in between; these lobes are separated by the facial nerve, which runs through the gland. This is the case in the cadaver, where the gland has been shrunk by formalin, but *in vivo* the gland should be regarded as a lump of bread dough poured over an egg whisk, the dough being the glandular tissue and the whisk the facial nerve. The facial nerve is surrounded by parotid tissue and intimately attached on all sides to glandular tissue.

The parotid gland extends from the zygoma superiorly to the oblique line of the sternomastoid inferiorly, and anteriorly to the midpoint of the masseter muscle. The duct runs over the anterior border of the masseter muscle to enter the mouth opposite the second molar tooth in the interdental line. The gland is covered by the investing fascia of the neck and there are six to eight lymph nodes outside this fascia and 10–12 lymph nodes embedded in the glandular tissue within the fascia.

The deep lobe of the parotid gland or the retromandibular portion lies in the parapharyngeal space anterior to the carotid sheath and styloid process and posterior to the infratemporal fossa. Medially is the superior constrictor muscle separating it from the tonsil and oropharynx (Fig. 19.1).

The *facial nerve* emerges from the stylomastoid foramen to enter the substance of the gland at its posteromedial surface. As the nerve exits from the stylomastoid foramen, it is surrounded by a thick layer of fascia, which is continuous with the periosteum of the skull base. It is, thus, very difficult to find the nerve at this point unless it is identified either distally or proximally within the mastoid process.

The standard landmarks to find the facial nerve within the parotid gland are as follows.

1 The tragal cartilage pointer: the tragal cartilage ends on a point that identifies the facial nerve 1 cm inferior and 1 cm medial to the pointer, under the temporomasseteric fascia.
2 If the posterior belly of the digastric muscle is followed up to the mastoid process, it will be found that the facial nerve bisects the angle formed by the bony tympanic plate and the muscle (Fig. 19.2).
3 If a finger tip is placed on the mastoid process with one edge of the finger on the tip of the mastoid and the end of the nail over the anterior border of the mastoid, the facial nerve lies halfway up the finger nail. This, however, gives no idea of the depth of the nerve, only an idea of the position.

Shortly after entering the substance of the parotid gland, the nerve divides into the two major trunks, the temporozygomatic and the cervicofacial. The branching of these nerves is rarely abnormal. On occasion the nerve will divide within the mastoid and will exit as separate branches but, in over 99% of cases, the standard single major trunk dividing into two is the expected pattern.

Many variations have been described thereafter, based on the peripheral branching patterns. These may be summarized into five types, varying from no anastomoses between the five branches to multiple vertical anastomotic connections (Fig. 19.3) The usual pattern is for terminal branches to go to the forehead, the eyebrow, the corner of the eye and lower eyelid from the temporozygomatic branch. The buccal branch can arise from either the upper division or the lower division of the nerve. This can give off vertical anastomotic branches to the temporozygomatic branch or the cervicofacial branch. It

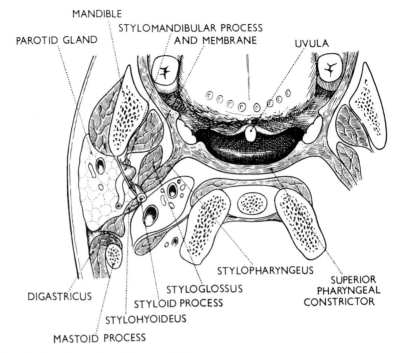

MANDIBLE

STYLOMANDIBULAR PROCESS
AND MEMBRANE

PAROTID GLAND

UVULA

DIGASTRICUS

STYLOID PROCESS

STYLOGLOSSUS

STYLOPHARYNGEUS

SUPERIOR
PHARYNGEAL
CONSTRICTOR

STYLOHYOIDEUS

MASTOID PROCESS

Fig. 19.1 Cross-section showing the relations of the parotid gland.

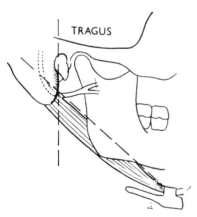

TRAGUS

Fig. 19.2 The facial nerve bisects the angle formed by the digastric and tympanic plate. It lies 1 cm inferior to the tragal cartilage.

supplies the lower eyelid, the centre portion of the face, the ala of the nose and the upper lip. The cervicofacial division divides into a branch to the upper lip, the corner of the mouth and the lower lip. The cervical branch goes to the platysma and is invariably divided during a parotidectomy.

It is essential to know the surface markings of the peripheral divisions of the nerve, in case they have to be used to find the facial nerve in a retrograde manner. The temporozygomatic branch crosses the

zygoma halfway between the intertragal notch and the lateral canthus. The buccal branch runs parallel to the parotid duct, 1 cm above it, and can be found on the masseter. The mandibular branch crosses the facial artery, 1 cm below the horizontal ramus of the mandible, one finger's breadth in front of the angle.

The other safe way to find the nerve is to carry out a facial nerve decompression within the mastoid. The oft-portrayed step of knocking the tip off the mastoid in order to find the facial nerve has more relationship to medical illustration than reality because the nerve is surrounded by a mixture of fascia and periosteum and it is virtually impossible to find it safely with this manoeuvre.

The *submandibular gland* fills the major portion of the submandibular triangle. It has a superficial portion that lies on the mylohyoid muscle, bounded anteriorly by the belly of the digastric, and this curves around the posterior part of the mylohyoid muscle to lie on the hyoglossus muscle and thus terminate in a duct entering the floor of the mouth. On the fascia, superficial to the gland, runs the mandibular branch of the facial nerve; deep to the gland is the lingual nerve superiorly and the hypoglossal nerve inferiorly, both lying in the hyoglossus muscle. There are several lymph nodes on the surface of the submandibular gland: the two most important ones lie in front of and behind the facial artery at the edge of the mandible and must be

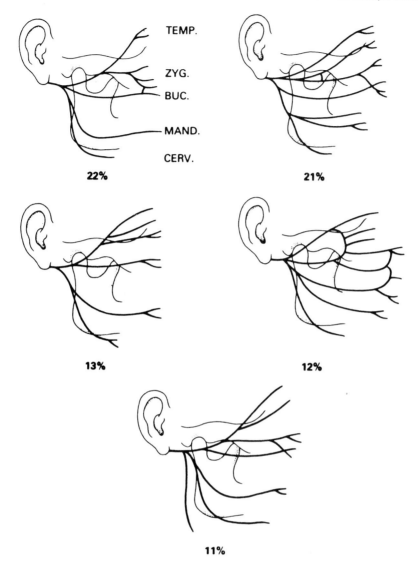

Fig. 19.3 Five types of division of the facial nerve.

recognized and sampled during the treatment of mouth cancer.

The *minor salivary glands* are mucus-secreting glands, situated throughout the upper respiratory tract. There are about 250 glands on the hard palate, 100 on the soft palate and 10 on the uvula. Palatal glands are not found in the midline nor anterior to a line between the first molar teeth, nor on the gingiva. Other glands are found in the submucosa of the inner surface of the lips, around the opening of the parotid duct, in the mucous membrane of the cheek, in the floor of the mouth, in the palatoglossal folds, on the inferior surface of the tongue, near the frenulum and within the palatine tonsil.

Other glands are found in the nose, the nasal sinuses, the larynx, the trachea and bronchi.

Surgical pathology

Salivary gland tumours are different from other head and neck tumours in several aspects. Firstly, some types of tumour in salivary glands are seen nowhere else in the body; secondly, squamous cell carcinoma, the commonest head and neck tumour, is extremely rare in these glands; and thirdly, there is a significant number of tumours of variable malignancy.

Major salivary glands are a mixture of serous and

mucous cells, drained by a series of ducts. The acinar structure is lined by an intercalated duct that drains into a striated duct and finally into an excretory duct. The cell structure of each of these areas is different and constitutes the cells of origin of various tumours.

Pleomorphic adenomas arise from intercalated duct cells and myoepithelial cells; striated duct cells give rise to oncocytomas; and excretory duct cells are the sites of origin for mucoepidermoid and squamous cell carcinomas.

Minor salivary glands are simple mucus-secreting structures and are the site of origin of adenoid cystic carcinoma. The lymph nodes that are within the parotid gland are the site of origin of adeno-lymphoma.

Benign tumours

Pleomorphic adenoma

This is also known as a mixed cell tumour; it arises from intercalated duct cells and myoepithelial cells. It is the commonest tumour of major salivary glands and, in the parotid gland, it forms 90% of all benign tumours and, in the submandibular gland, 50%. Although one pleomorphic adenoma has been recorded at birth, the average age at presentation is 40 years. It is usually unilateral but a few bilateral tumours have been described. The sex incidence is roughly equal.

The tumour grows slowly with long quiescent periods and short periods of rapid growth. About one-quarter of patients with this tumour have vague local discomfort, but it is usually symptomless apart from the lump, and the facial nerve is never para-lysed if the tumour is benign. Nearly all of these tumours occur in the tail of the parotid gland, just anterior to the lobe of the ear. They can also occur in the retromandibular portion of the parotid gland, either as solitary deep-lobe tumours or dumb-bell tumours. They are very rare elswhere in the parotid gland. On palpation, the tumour is usually smooth, superficial, round and mobile. The capsule of com-pressed normal parotid tissue varies in thickness and is lobulated because the tumour grows with pseudo-podial extensions through this capsule.

The cut surface is usually greyish white but it may have blue tinges; there also may be secondary cyst formation and haemorrhage. One tumour in 10 is highly cellular and, although showing no sign of malignancy, such a tumour is more prone to recur.

These tumours were orginally called mixed tumours because they were thought to contain epi-thelium and cartilaginous elements and were hence thought to be of mixed cell origin. This is no longer believed.

The tumour is highly implantable and the recur-rence rate after primary surgery is about 5%. If simple enucleation is performed, however, the recur-rence rate is between 20 and 30%.

Warthin's tumour

This is also known as a papillary cystadenoma lymphomatosum or adenolymphoma. It is a neoplas-tic proliferation of parotid tissue heterotopic within the lymph nodes that are normally present within the parotid gland. In essence, it is a monomorphic adenoma. It is commoner in men, the male : female rato being 7 : 1. It is seldom seen under the age of 30 and the average age at presentation is around 70 years. One in 10 tumours are bilateral; they are usually fluctuant, slow-growing and seldom show any spurts of rapid growth. The lump is not bosselated and it is usually situated in the tail of the gland. This tumour is never malignant. Even relatively solid tumours are soft and compressible, and the cystic ones have brown mucoid fluid inside them. Areas of solid whiteness are sometimes seen and these are due to lymphoid tissue.

Warthin's tumour accounts for 6–8% of all salivary gland tumours.

Oncocytoma

This is also known as an oxyphil cell adenoma and is another monomorphic adenoma. It accounts for less than 1% of all salivary gland tumours. Oncocytoma occurs in older patients and is seldom seen under the age of 50 years. The sex incidence is equal, and it presents as a painless, slow-growing lump. These neoplasms arise from the striated duct cells. Benign oncocytomas are usually cystic rather than solid; malignant variants have been reported but they are exceedingly rare.

Vascular tumours

These are the most common salivary tumours in children and are soft, painless masses.

Haemangioma accounts for more than half of the salivary gland lesions in children. They are much more common in females than males, and are usually diagnosed during the first year of life. The glandular parenchyma is replaced by vasoformative elements but normal glandular lobulation is maintained. The haemangioma may be capillary, cavernous, mixed or hypertrophic. In about 50% of patients, a cutaneous haemangioma coexists somewhere on the head and neck area.

Spontaneous regression definitely occurs in some vascular tumours so that no treatment should be offered until the age of 10 or 12 years. Surgery should only be performed if the tumour is enlarging.

Lymphangiomas are usually present at birth and again are commoner in girls than boys. The three types are simple lymphangioma, cavernous lymphangioma and cystic hygroma. The thin-walled lymph spaces invade the parotid and adjacent tissues and do not replace the glandular parenchyma like haemangiomas. The tumours are soft and fluctuant and usually transilluminate. If they cause disfigurement, they should be removed.

Granulomatous diseases

Sarcoidosis is usually bilateral and diffuse. A common presentation is, along with swelling of the parotid and lacrimal glands, chorioretinitis and progressive cranial nerve involvement, also known as Heerfordt's disease.

Tuberculosis is rare but is a possible infection of the lymph nodes on or within the parotid gland.

Actinomycosis can follow dental extraction or other oral trauma.

Cat-scratch disease is passed from wild or domestic animals to humans by a scratch and is due to a Gram-negative bacillus.

Cysts

Simple *retention cysts* within the parotid tissue are rare. If the patient has lived in the tropics and presents with a cystic lesion then suspect *Echinococcus* or a *hydatid cyst* (see also HIV-related cysts, p. 76).

The commonest cystic lesion is a Warthin's tumour, and areas of pleomorphic adenoma may also be cystic (see above).

Branchial cysts can occur within the lymph nodes in the gland and on the surface of the gland.

Lipomas can feel cystic. They usually lie lateral to the parotid gland but can extend anteriorly into the anterior compartment of the face. They must be differentiated from fatty infiltration, which is usually bilateral.

Tumours of variable malignancy

In this section we shall consider four tumours. The mucoepidermoid tumour is more likely than not to behave in a malignant manner and it carries more than a 50% mortality. Not all mucoepidermoid tumours however will behave aggressively. A significant portion will behave like indolent pleomorphic adenomas and the patient will present with a lump, have it excised and have no further problems.

For many years the acinic cell tumour was thought to be of very low-grade malignancy. Recent series however have shown that this tumour has probably been underestimated. It carries a significant mortality and, like adenoid cystic carcinoma, the survival must be measured in 20-year units rather than 5-year units.

Benign lymphoepithelial lesion is an enigma. It is not known whether it is part of a malignant process or whether it has only a propensity to move towards lymphoma. Finally, Sjögren's disease has to be included in this group because there is a small but significant number that will undergo lymphomatous change.

Mucoepidermoid tumour

This accounts for 4–9% of salivary tumours. Eighty-nine per cent are in the parotid gland, 8% in the submandibular gland and 1% in the sublingual gland. It is more common in minor salivary glands (41% palate, 14% buccal, 9% tongue, 5% lip). This is the commonest salivary gland tumour in children. There is an equal sex incidence; the tumour usually presents in the fifth decade. It may or may not be encapsulated and may be solid or cystic. Several cell types are seen – maternal, intermediate, epidermoid, columnar, clear and mucous. Pathologists divide these tumours into low-grade (well-differentiated) and high-grade (poorly differentiated). High-grade tumours comprise 10% of the total group and occur in older patients. They are commonly misdiagnosed as squamous carcinomas. A small proportion of the commoner low-grade tumours will behave in the same aggressive manner but the majority behave like pleomorphic adenomas. The tumours are usually unencapsulated and show a reactive stroma. Four out of 10 will have associated neck node metastases and the high-grade tumours have a 40% 5-year survival rate.

Acinic cell tumour

This accounts for 2.5–4% of all parotid tumours, and arises from the terminal tubular intercalated duct cells. It is sometimes bilateral and often encapsulated. The acinic cell tumour occurs in the fifth decade with a roughly equal sex incidence, but it is also the second most common salivary tumour in children. The majority behave like pleomorphic adenomas but some have an aggressive malignant course. There is a propensity for late recurrence, even 30 years after excision. Those that recur have a 10% regional node metastatic rate and a 15% distant metastatic rate. The 5-year survival is 90% and the 20-year survival rate between 50 and 60%.

Benign lymphoepithelial lesion

This was described in 1952 by Godwin. It is a pathological process that arises in the intralobular ducts like a punctate parotitis. As the ducts dilate, their cells disrupt and epidermoid metaplasia begins. Lymphocytes aggregate around the ducts and the lumen becomes obliterated. It is probably part of a lymphoreticular proliferative disease; it is not yet clear whether benign lymphoepithelial lesion evolves into malignancy or whether it is part of an immunological disorder that is going to become lymphoproliferative disease anyway.

It is a lesion isolated to the parotid gland and shows none of the systemic manifestations of Sjögren's disease.

Sjögren's syndrome

This was first described in 1933 by Henrik Sjögren, a Stockholm ophthalmologist. It is a multisystem disease, involving almost every system in the body. It is classified into two forms. Primary Sjögren's disease (the sicca syndrome) consists of xerostomia and xerophthalmia without an associated connective tissue disease. These patients are often extremely upset by the dryness of the mouth and frequently show psychiatric disturbances. They seldom have salivary gland involvement and 1 in 6 will progress to lymphoma.

Secondary Sjögren's syndrome shows the triad of xerophthalmia, xerostomia and a connective tissue disorder, which in 48% of cases will be rheumatoid arthritis. It may also be accompanied by systemic lupus erythematosus, scleroderma, polymyositis, primary biliary cirrhosis, autoimmune liver disease, chronic graft-versus-host disease and a number of other rarer autoimmune disorders. Thirty per cent will have involvement of the parotid in the form of recurrent bouts of parotitis, and a much smaller proportion go on to develop lymphoma.

Malignant tumours

There is no good staging system for major salivary gland cancer. Perhaps the best is offered by the American Joint Committee (AJC; Table 19.1).

One in 6 parotid tumours is malignant, as are 1 in 3 submandibular tumours and 1 in 2 minor salivary gland tumours.

Malignant tumours invade parotid tissue locally and usually extend into the retromandibular area of the parotid and the parapharyngeal space. They drain to the lymph nodes within the parapharyngeal space and to the deep jugular chain. They also metastasize to lymph nodes on the surface of the gland and to the pre- and postfacial nodes. They will ultimately involve the temporomandibular joint and the external auditory meatus, and perhaps the petrous bone.

The incidence is 12 per million of population and they form 3% of head and neck malignant tumours. The sex ratio is equal and they usually present in the fifth decade. They are commoner in blacks, Eskimos, Scots and survivors from radioactive exposure.

Forty-three per cent will involve the lateral lobe only and 27% will involve both lobes. Ten per cent will involve the deep lobe only and 20% extend beyond the glandular tissue.

Obviously facial nerve paralysis is the most striking sign of external invasion. The rates vary but Table 19.2 is the published consensus as to presentation with facial nerve paralysis.

Adenoid cystic carcinoma

This arises in major and minor glands: 25% occur in the parotid gland, 15% in the submandibular gland, 1% in the sublingual gland and the remainder (60%) in the minor glands. Seventy per cent of the minor gland tumours arise within the mouth. It forms roughly 40% of malignant tumours at all salivary sites.

Adenoid cystic carcinoma is commonly monolobular and usually measures 2–4 cm in diameter at the time of diagnosis. It is unencapsulated but appears circumscribed. On cut sections the neoplasm is moist and grey-pink in appearance and the growth pattern is infiltrative. One of its features is a marked tendency to invade nerves and this accounts for the high frequency of pain.

Only 15% will metastasize to lymph nodes – 8% at the time of presentation and 7% later. The hallmark, however, is the incidence of distant metastases in the lungs (40%), the brain (20%) and in the bones (20%). Approximately 40% of patients will ultimately manifest distant metastases but the incidence of such metastases in patients dying of the disease approaches 70%.

Adenoid cystic carcinoma can be imperfectly divided into four main patterns – cribriform, tubuloglandular, solid cellular and cylindromatous. The most probable source of the tumour is the intercalcated ducts.

It is slightly more common in women than men and

Table 19.1 American Joint Committee staging system for salivary gland cancer

T_0	No clinical evidence of primary tumour.
T_1	Tumour of 0.1–2 cm in diameter without significant local extension
T_2	Tumour of 2.1–4 cm in diameter without significant local extension
T_3	Tumour of 4.1–6 cm in diameter without significant local extension
T_{4a}	Tumour greater than 6 cm in diameter without significant local extension
T_{4b}	Tumour of any size with significant local extension

Table 19.2 Presentation of facial nerve paralysis in malignant tumours

Poorly differentiated carcinoma	23–26%
Adenoid cystic carcinoma	23–26%
Carcinoma ex pleomorphic adenoma	9–14%
Mucoepidermoid carcinoma	8%
Acinic cell carcinoma	3%

diagnosis under the age of 30 is unusual, the median age at presentation being in the sixth decade.

Carcinoma ex pleomorphic adenoma

One per cent of these tumours arises *ab initio*. The vast majority, however, arise from a pre-existing benign pleomorphic adenoma. The benign tumour should have been present for at least 10–15 years before malignant change occurs. About 1–5% of pleomorphic adenomas lasting this length of time are at risk of changing their biological character. When they become malignant they may still be grossly encapsulated; suspicious features are the occurrence of pain, a rapid growth spurt and excessive bosselation and infiltration at the periphery.

Regional lymph node metastases will occur in 25% and distant metastases in 30%. The 5-year survival is around 40% and the 15-year survival 19%.

Adenocarcinoma

This tumour forms about 3% of parotid tumours and 10% of submandibular minor salivary gland tumours. The sex incidence is equal and it can occur at any age. It is one of the commoner malignant salivary gland tumours seen in children. It may present as an asymptomatic mass or with typical malignant features. In the parotid, most occur in the deep lobe or extend beyond the gland when first seen. They are highly malignant with a high metastatic rate and the 5-year survival is only about 10%.

Squamous cell carcinoma

This is extremely rare (1%) in the parotid and is only slightly more common (5%) in the submandibular gland. Before arriving at a diagnosis of squamous cell carcinoma, the pathologist must rule out any possibility of this being a mucoepidermoid tumour or a malignant pleomorphic adenoma. You must also rule out the possibility of it being a metastasis in the lymph nodes in the parotid from a neighbouring skin tumour or from another head and neck primary site.

Two-thirds of the patients are men and the average age at presentation is in the seventh decade. It is an aggressive tumour and shows no tendency to encapsulation. It grows rapidly, causing pain, facial nerve paralysis, skin fixation and ulceration. About half will have metastatic neck nodes when first seen. It has a very bad prognosis from any method of treatment.

Sarcomas

These are extremely rare but neurofibrosarcoma, rhabdomyosarcoma, histiocytoma and Kaposi's sarcoma have all been described.

Metastatic tumours

The parotid gland has nodes within it and on the surface, so these can be the site of metastatic deposits. Eighty per cent of these are from skin of the face, temple or scalp, and they are usually melanoma or squamous carcinoma. The node metastases can be on the surface of the gland or in the deep portion of the stroma. They can also occur from infraclavicular sites.

Recurrent pleomorphic adenoma

This problem can be split into two categories. The first is where the recurrence can be expected after an inadequate lumpectomy for a pleomorphic adenoma. The second group is where the recurrence is unexpected after a superficial parotidectomy for pleomorphic adenoma. The possible causes of recurrence in this instance are bursting the capsule, carrying out an enucleation with no postoperative radiotherapy, and opening the tumour to carry out a frozen section. These tumours are highly implantable and after a superficial parotidectomy they may implant themselves on the retromandibular portion that lies under the facial nerve and the skin. There is, therefore, a sandwich effect, with the bread of the sandwich being the skin and the retromandibular portion of the parotid, and the filling being the tumour recurrence and the facial nerve. As many of the pseudopodia are infringed during the inadequate lumpectomy or the bursting of the capsule during manipulation, the recurrence is almost always multiple.

The problem of assessment, therefore, lies in knowing how far the tumour recurrence extends, its relationship to facial nerve and skin, and being able to do a total parotidectomy preserving as much facial nerve function as possible.

Investigations

History

Parotid tumours are usually unilateral, although Warthin's tumour can be bilateral. Pleomorphic adenomas almost always occur in the tail of the gland; if a tumour occurs in the body of the gland, suspect that it is not a pleomorphic adenoma. Neuromas of the facial nerve, myxomas of the masseter and lipomas occurring in the body of the gland may masquerade as pleomorphic adenomas. Benign tumours grow slowly over a period of years but malignant ones usually grow rapidly from the outset and the cardinal sign of malignancy is pain. They may also involve skin and/or the facial nerve. In inflammatory or calculus disease there is often marked fluctuation in the size of the glands, together with pain and tenderness. In these conditions, eating almost always causes an increase in pain and swelling.

Parotomegaly can occur with various endocrinopathies and systemic illnesses, so ask about other conditions such as myxoedema, diabetes, Cushing's disease, cirrhosis, gout and alcoholism. Young girls with parotid enlargement should be suspected of being bulimics until proven otherwise. Certain drugs such as the contraceptive pill, Thiouracil and Distalgesic can also cause parotomegaly. One in three patients with Sjögren's syndrome will present with parotomegaly, and it is also seen in granulomas.

Examination

Decide first whether the mass is in the parotid or outside it. Conditions outside the parotid that mimic parotomegaly are:

hypertrophy of the masseter
dental cysts
branchial cysts
myxoma of the masseter
neuroma of the facial nerve
temporal artery aneurysm
mandibular tumours
mastoiditis
lymphadenitis of parotid nodes
sebaceous cysts.

The next thing to establish is if only one gland is affected or not. Most tumours involve a single gland but sialectasis, benign lymphoepithelial lesion, Sjögren's disease, calculus disease and the endocrine conditions mentioned above usually affect more than one gland.

Decide if the lump is likely to be benign or malignant. The cardinal sign of malignancy is pain, and involvement of skin or facial nerve is absolutely diagnostic of malignancy.

Find out if the tumour is firm or cystic. Pleomorphic adenomas may present in either way but a cystic feeling should make you consider a Warthin's tumour or a mucoepidermoid tumour or a parotid cyst.

Always palpate salivary glands bimanually. This is particularly important in the submandibular gland or if calculus disease is suspected.

Always look inside the pharynx to see if there is a pharyngeal extension of a deep-lobe tumour.

In inflammatory disease, see if any pus can be expressed from the duct.

Laboratory tests

The appropriate endocrine tests should be done to exclude diabetes, myxoedema or Cushing's disease. In Sjögren's syndrome, do the erythrocyte sedimentation rate, protein electrophoresis, antinuclear factor and rheumatoid factor. In sarcoid involvement, do a Kviem test. Collection and examination of saliva have roused a great deal of research interest in the past but, to date, no useful practical clinical help has evolved from this investigation.

Radiology

Plain films

Parotid stones are almost always radiolucent while submandibular stones are nearly always radiopaque. Intraoral films are especially useful in this latter condition. Plain films may also be useful in differentiating some of the extraparotid causes of parotomegaly.

Sialography

This is the most useful radiological investigation in non-neoplastic salivary gland disease but it has only a limited place to play in the investigation of tumours.

Radiosialography

Scanning of the major salivary glands with technetium pertechnetate is not helpful. It used to be thought that Warthin's tumours were 'hot' whereas other tumours were 'cold', but time has not borne out this initial assessment.

Ultrasonography

This is useful in assessing the cystic nature of tumours. Retention cysts and true cysts of the parotid are sonolucent. Neoplasms appear as solid masses – except for Warthin's tumour. Malignant tumours have a low reflectivity whereas mixed tumours show variable reflectivity.

CT scanning

This is the gold standard for investigation of parotid tumours. The important thing to assess in the work-up of a parotid tumour is its extension in the deep lobe and its relation to the facial nerve. Computed tomography (CT) scanning, combined with sialography, usually allows this differentiation.

Magnetic resonance imaging

Magnetic resonance imaging has no significant advantage over CT scanning at the moment but its overall advantage is the lack of ionizing radiation. For salivary glands, the contrast between tumour and the surrounding tissue is greater than with CT scanning but tissue detail is less well-defined.

Biopsy

On no account should a discrete salivary gland mass be subjected to incisional biopsy. As there is a 9 out of 10 chance that a single parotid mass is a pleomorphic adenoma, incising it is not only unnecessary but will lead to an unacceptably high incidence of recurrence. The only acceptable biopsy in such cases is a superficial parotidectomy.

In recent years, fine-needle aspiration biopsy has become more acceptable as a means of diagnosing the pathology and nature of salivary gland masses without the complication of implantation. The use of this technique, however, depends on the presence of a pathologist who is both skilled and interested in the method.

If a tumour is obviously malignant, involving skin, then an incisional biopsy may be done to establish the tumour type before removing it together with the area of the biopsy.

If a diffuse enlargement of the salivary gland is probably not due to the tumour, then an incisional biopsy may be necessary, but this should usually be accompanied by a sublabial biopsy, which is the investigation of choice for the diagnosis of some of the granulomatous conditions and especially Sjögren's syndrome.

Treatment policy

The main problem of simple parotid masses is that a fairly major operation is done without a diagnosis being known. In 90% of cases, the clinical diagnosis is correct and a suspected simple tumour turns out to be a simple tumour. Occasionally, however, a malignant tumour may present as an isolated mass without pain, facial nerve involvement or skin involvement. The diagnosis may be suspected during surgery but usually becomes apparent only when the pathology report is returned to the unit.

In the case of a simple mass suspected of being a pleomorphic adenoma, a superficial parotid lobectomy is performed. Enucleation must never be performed. Even though it could be done quite safely for a Warthin's tumour or an oncocytoma, you do not know the diagnosis at this point in the operation, and a frozen section is not acceptable because of the danger of implanting a pleomorphic adenoma and because of the unreliability of frozen-section pathological diagnosis.

When some authors write about enucleation, they mean that they find the nerve and dissect the lower division, thus carrying out a lumpectomy with a cuff of healthy tissue around it. This is a very acceptable method of treating small pleomorphic adenomas and does not need to be followed with irradiation.

If you embark on a superficial lobectomy, you must be prepared to carry out a total parotidectomy if it is indicated, and thus you must be able to complete a total parotidectomy, preserving the facial nerve.

If, during the operation, the appearance of tumour is such as to suggest malignancy, then a frozen section must be performed. If, at this point, there is a high likelihood of the patient losing the facial nerve, then you must close the wound and discuss the changed situation with the patient. Although in the UK the consent form suggests that the surgeon can go on to perform any other operation that he or she sees fit to do, this cannot be taken literally. This item on the consent form is meant to relate to emergencies, not what is convenient for the surgeon or even for the patient. As alternative modes of therapy are available for a malignant tumour, including no treatment if the patient so wishes, then the patient must make up his or her mind whether or not he or she is willing to have the facial nerve sacrificed.

If, after the operation, the pathologist reports an intermediate grade of tumour or even a small adenoid cystic or malignant mixed-cell tumour, then you should reopen the wound and carry out a total parotidectomy, and consider postoperative irradiation.

If you suspect malignancy on clinical grounds then the treatment policy is affected by the following considerations:

Age
Metastatic spread
Facial nerve involvement
Mandibular involvement
Temporal bone involvement
Skin involvement
Trismus

The treatment policy will obviously be affected by all of the above. The operation may vary from a total parotidectomy with preservation of part of the nerve to a total parotidectomy, hemimandibulectomy, facial nerve sacrifice, petrosectomy, radical neck dissection and excision of skin in the area with subsequent reconstruction. While radical surgery if possible is the treatment of choice, a significant proportion of patients have disease which is inoperable either by virtue of disease extent, or by their age and general condition. In such cases primary radical irradiation after biopsy should be considered.

With recurrent pleomorphic adenoma, the aim of treatment is to carry out a total parotidectomy with preservation of as much facial nerve function as possible. Identification of the facial nerve is difficult in this instance because of scar tissue and the use of a stimulator is to be recommended. Finding the facial nerve using the peripheral branches is also very useful in this situation. Once the facial nerve is identified, a total parotidectomy may be attempted but a pleomorphic adenoma that is *on* a nerve is considered to be *in* the nerve and that portion should be sacrificed. It is usually possible, however, to keep a large number of the branches of the facial nerve intact, thus leaving the patient with useful nerve function.

Tumours in the submandibular gland are less common and are relatively simple to deal with. Those that are considered benign can be removed with a wide-field submandibular gland resection. Those that are considered to be malignant must be taken as floor-of-the-mouth tumours and the gland removed together with a radical neck dissection, and adjacent floor of mouth and perhaps mandible.

Technique of salivary gland operations

Superficial parotidectomy

Preparation and anaesthetic

Shave the hair for 2.5 cm behind the mastoid process, and remove all sideburns. Prepare the skin of one side of the face and neck from the midline to the clavicle, and from 2.5 cm behind the mastoid process down to the shoulder. It is important to see the whole of the side of the face during the operation, so place towels over the head at the hairline, down the back of the neck, and along the midline of the face. Towels in this position tend to slip, so stitch them in place. Tape the eyelids on the unoperated side to keep the eye closed, but not on the side of operation. It is important that the preparation includes the external meatus and that the external meatus is blocked during the operation with a piece of sterile cotton wool to stop it filling with blood clot.

The anaesthetic tube is taped to the opposite corner of the mouth, taking care not to distort the outline of the mouth. Also ask the anaesthetist before the operation not to use relaxant drugs. If he or she gives the patient curare the facial nerve is stimulated with difficulty.

Incision

The ideal incision begins near the upper part of the auricle, curves downwards into the tragal notch to avoid a scar contracture, continues downwards to the lobe of the ear, then curves backwards at almost a right angle to the tip of the mastoid process, and finally curves gently downwards towards the hyoid bone in a skin crease (Fig. 19.4).

Extend this incision down to the parotid fascia and to the fascia covering the sternomastoid muscle. It is often difficult to find the right plane because there is no platysma muscle to act as a guide, but once the plane immediately above the parotid gland has been found, elevate the skin flaps forwards to the edge of the masseter muscle. The great auricular nerve runs obliquely upwards and forwards at the junction of

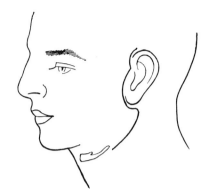

Fig. 19.4 Incision for parotidectomy.

the upper and middle thirds of the sternomastoid muscle. Do not divide it indiscriminately as it is a useful graft if the facial nerve must be resected. It is, however, impossible to remove the gland without dividing the great auricular nerve and this should be done as near the gland as possible, preserving the two terminal branches of the nerve.

Elevate the flap, turn it forwards, and place moist swabs on top of it. Very little posterior dissection is necessary, but free the lobe of the ear and stitch it to the upper drape.

Mobilization of the posterior surface

The key to this part of the operation is the cartilaginous external auditory meatus. Separate the gland from this until the whole of the cartilaginous meatus is quite free. It is best to start at the upper end of the parotid gland and separate this with scissors – this is quite safe as the facial nerve lies very much deeper than the cartilaginous meatus. Keep directly on the perichondrium; this avoids shredding the gland and injuring the nerve. Cotton wool balls soaked in adrenaline and held on the end of artery forceps are also helpful in creating relatively bloodless dissection. Continue elevating the gland off the cartilage right down to its lower border where it lies on the sternomastoid. With a knife elevate the gland off the sternomastoid until the anterior border of the sternomastoid is seen. Retract this and identify the posterior belly of the digastric muscle and the stylohyoid muscle, and trace them back to the mastoid process. Try to preserve the posterior facial vein as long as possible in order to minimize passive congestive bleeding.

Exposure of the facial nerve

The most important point about this step of the operation is that a nerve stimulator ought to be used to ensure the preservation of the facial nerve.

There are several ways described of finding the

facial nerve (see also Surgical anatomy, above), but the first method is probably the best.

1 Find the point on the end of the tragal cartilage. The nerve is 1 cm deep and inferior to this, surrounded by a small aggregation of fat and overlain by a small blood vessel.
2 Find the anterior border of the mastoid process and trace it up to where it meets the vaginal process of the tympanic bone. The facial nerve bisects the angle between the two pieces of bone.
3 It is also possible to find the nerve by following the posterior belly of the digastric muscle to where it meets the tympanic plate; the nerve bisects the angle between the two.
4 If the tumour is very large and overlies the previous approaches, or if the gland has been operated on before, then it is better to approach the nerve by finding the buccal branch (which goes to the upper lip). This branch runs parallel to and 1 cm below the arch of the zygoma going towards the corner part of the mouth; it is possible to find it at the anterior part of the gland and trace it backwards to the main trunk.
5 A method of tracing back the mandibular branch has been described, but it is not recommended because paralysis of this nerve leads to an ugly cosmetic deformity.

Hold the gland forwards with a malleable retractor, and find the nerve by opening up an artery forceps parallel to the nerve using the above landmarks, preferably the first (Fig. 19.5). During the early stages of the dissection numerous fine strands appear running in the direction of the facial nerve. Most beginners are worried that these are the nerve, but they do not respond to stimulation and when the nerve is finally seen deep in the wound it is instantly recognizable as a thick white cord, 2 or 3 mm wide. Final identification of the nerve is made by stimulating it.

Anyone operating on a parotid gland should be throughly conversant with all possible anomalies of the facial nerve. It may be pushed deep, inferiorly, or superiorly by a tumour. It may also divide in the stylomastoid foramen, thus appearing as five separate branches immediately anterior to the mastoid process.

Dissection of the nerve and removal of the superficial lobe

Once the nerve is found, trace it forward to its bifurcation, remembering that as soon as the nerve enters the gland it courses laterally in the gland substance. If attempts are made to follow the nerve in the horizontal plane then it will be damaged. It is best to dissect out the upper branch first; this is the more important of the two divisions as it supplies the eye. Always use very fine artery forceps (Fig. 19.6), run them along the nerve sheath and open them; this makes a tunnel. Cut along this with scissors, grasping the cut ends of the gland with artery forceps to retract them and stop the bleeding (Fig. 19.7). Tunnel along each branch consecutively, starting at the top and working downwards, and, by cutting the piece of parotid that lies between two branches (Fig. 19.8), peel the parotid out from above downwards. Try, if possible, to preserve the vertically disposed anastomotic filaments that join the nerves. Always test each piece of tissue with the stimulator before cutting it.

As the gland is dissected and lifted downwards, find the duct about its mid-portion, divide, and ligate it with 3/0 silk. When the gland is finally removed the facial nerve should be seen fully dissected out. All the terminal branches, the major bifurcations and

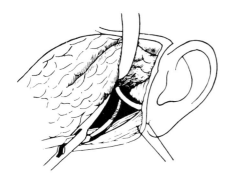

Fig. 19.5 With the gland retracted anteriorly, the facial nerve is seen 1 cm inferior and medial to the tragal 'pointer'. Note that artery forceps are opened parallel to the nerve and not at right angles.

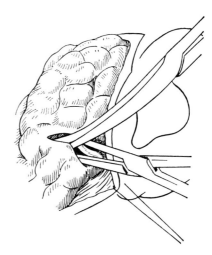

Fig. 19.6 Fine artery forceps make a tunnel along the nerve and hold up the parotid tissue, which is cut by scissors.

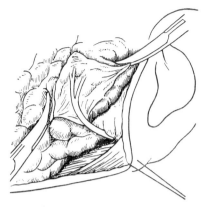

Fig. 19.7 The cut edges of the tunnel are held apart with artery forceps, thus enabling a further tunnel to be created.

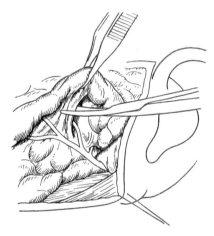

Fig. 19.8 When tunnels are made along two adjacent nerve branches, the bridge between the two is divided.

the main trunk should be stimulated. If one part of the nerve does not respond to stimulation, then close examination of that part should be made to make sure there is no break in continuity of the nerve. Occasionally interruption of conduction of a nerve may be caused by a haematoma in the medial surface of the perineural sheath. The only way to recognize this is with a stimulator – another important reason to use this instrument.

Closure

When the parotid gland is removed, wash the wound with saline and secure all bleeding points. Put one suction drain in place and bring it out posteriorly under the hairline. If it is brought out in the neck an

ugly puncture mark will be visible, which is undesirable, especially in women. Close the skin in two layers with 3/0 chromic catgut and 5/0 Prolene. When putting in the chromic catgut sutures it is easy to pucker the skin underneath the ear lobe as it is so thin; therefore, take great care at this point.

Complications

1   *General complications.*
2   *Nerve injury.* The steps to avoid nerve injury have been pointed out in the description of the operative technique. If any part of the nerve is transected, then repair it with 6/0 ophthalmic silk after trimming the ends square with a knife. The operating microscope is essential in this technique. When stitching the nerve it is important to stitch nerve sheath edge to nerve sheath edge, and not to evert the nerve or buckle it, as shown in Figure 19.14. It is possible to put two stitches in the sheath of each branch, and four to five sutures may be placed in the main trunk. If a haematoma is found in the perineural sheath, slit it open with a sickle knife and evacuate the haematoma.

   If the main trunk of the nerve is transected and reanastomosed, then there is no point in looking for any recovery of movement in under 6 months. The maximum improvement will occur at about 10–12 months.

   If the nerve could be stimulated at the end of the operation as described but weakness of part of the face is seen the day after operation, then the patient can be reassured that movement will always return. The quickest part of the face to recover normal function is the middle portion as there is a rich neural anastomosis to this area.

   Further mention will be made of permanent facial nerve damage later.
3   *Frey's syndrome.* This syndrome consists of painful sweating around the ear when the patient eats. It occurs in 25% of parotidectomies, usually within 3 months of the operation. Only about 1 in 5 of this group requires further treatment.

   It is due to regrowth of the secretomotor parasympathetic fibres into the space formerly occupied by the gland. As there is no gland present they grow into the skin. Whenever the patient eats, the reflex for salivation occurs and the skin blood vessels dilate and the sweat glands pour out sweat.

   The treatment is directed at interrupting this reflex arc and it can be done most easily by doing a tympanic neurectomy. This is done via a tympanotomy; the fibres of Jacobsen's nerve on the promontory are identified and divided. If a sufficient segment is excised, regrowth does not occur.
4   *Numbness of the ear.* This always happens after parotidectomy because the great auricular nerve is

always cut. Recovery of sensation slowly takes place over the next year.

5 *Salivary fistula*. It is surprising that this does not occur after every superficial parotidectomy as the bare surface of the deep lobe is left exposed. This happens rarely after a superficial parotidectomy, however, and if it does occur it always ceases spontaneously with time and pressure dressings.

6 *Xerostomia*. Removal of a superficial lobe only removes 30% of the saliva-producing tissue, so xerostomia is almost unknown after superficial parotidectomy.

Removal of a submandibular gland

The patient lies supine on the table, with the head turned to the opposite side and slightly extended. Prepare an area bounded by the mouth, the mastoid process, the clavicle and the midline in the usual fashion.

Place towels in position so that the angle of the mouth can be seen; it is helpful to use a steridrape to cover the field.

Make an incision 10 cm long, 2.5 cm below the mandible, in a skin crease and curve it slightly upwards anteriorly. Take the incision through the platysma and elevate flaps superiorly to the rim of the mandible and inferiorly to just below the hyoid bone, keeping the platysma in the skin flap. this plane may be obscured after sialadenitis.

The mandibular branch of the facial nerve comes into the neck one finger's breadth in front of the angle of the mandible and crosses the facial vessels. It then loops upwards after a variable distance towards the corner of the mouth. The usual technique of preserving the nerve is to transect and ligate the facial vessels and deflect them upwards; this may lead to damage to the nerve because it may be at, or slightly lower than, the point where the vessels are identifiable. It is better, therefore, to incise through the fascia of the gland at the level of the hyoid bone and reflect a flap upwards in the plane between the fascia and the actual surface of the gland. In this way the nerve need never be identified but will never be transected. If a facial nerve stimulator is available, then identification of the nerve is very much easier and it can be dissected upwards with accuracy. When the fascial cuff is developed and dissected upwards it is stitched to the upper flap, taking care not to include the nerve in the tie (Fig. 19.9).

The next step is mobilization of the gland. Start by identifying the facial vessels as they cross the mandible, one finger's breadth in front of the angle of the jaw. Identify and tie them separately with 3/0 silk. Because the fascial cuff has been elevated off the gland the dissection of the upper border of the gland from the mandible is an easy matter and only a few small vessels need be cauterized.

Separating the anterior part of the gland from the fat in the submental region can be tedious due to multiple small vessels, but a good plane is easily obtained with a knife.

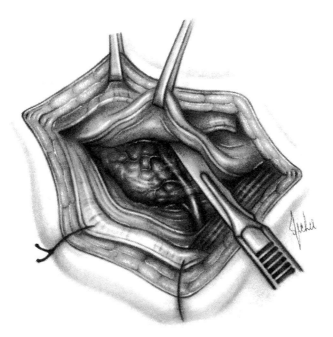

Fig. 19.9 The mandibular branch of the facial nerve can be protected either by dividing the artery and vein below the nerve, or by making a fascial cuff, as described in the text.

Follow the hyoid bone posteriorly and elevate the lower part of the gland.

The next step is to free the part of the gland that curves back over the mylohyoid muscle. This part of the gland can usually be pushed backwards off the mylohyoid muscle but this manoeuvre often has to be aided with the use of a knife until the free edge of the mylohyoid muscle is seen. Grasp the anterior part of the gland with Allis forceps, hold it upwards and outwards, and identify the facial artery and vein entering the lower part of the gland; transect and ligate them separately. It is often advisable to stitch the facial artery.

Next retract the posterior border of the mylohyoid muscle anteriorly to show the submandibular duct. This pulls the lingual nerve down in a U-shaped curve (Fig. 19.10), free it with a knife. This often causes troublesome bleeding from small veins in the area. Identify these accurately and on no account make blind attempts to secure haemostasis as this will almost invariably result in damage to the lingual nerve. Very often, pressure will stop the bleeding in this area. Before tying the submandibular duct, identify the hypoglossal nerve as it lies below the duct; then clamp the duct, cut and ligate it. The gland can then be removed and final haemostasis secured.

Put one suction drain in place and close the skin with 3/0 chromic catgut and 4/0 Prolene. No dressings are necessary.

Complications

1 *General complications.*
2 *Nerve injury.* The most usual injury is to the mandibular branch but steps to avoid this have been mentioned previously. If it occurs it gives rather an ugly cosmetic deformity and is not really an acceptable complication for a benign condition. One way of solving the cosmetic deformity is to cut the nerve on the opposite side, which will straighten up the mouth, but it will leave the lower lip immobile. This is not always successful, however, because the nerve supply to the lower lip can be shared between the mandibular and cervical branches.
3 *Lingual nerve injury* can also be avoided but it may occur if blind attempts at haemostasis are made after freeing the lingual nerve. There is little that can be done if this occurs. The same applies to any injury to the hypoglossal nerve. Unilateral anaesthesia or paralysis of the tongue, however, is a tedious rather than serious complication.

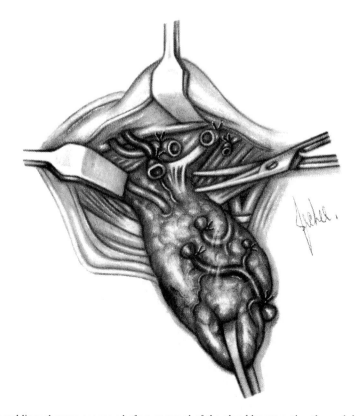

Fig. 19.10 The duct and lingual nerve are seen before removal of the gland by retracting the mylohyoid anteriorly.

Total parotidectomy

A total parotidectomy is usually performed for malignant tumours, recurrent pleomorphic adenoma or deep-lobe tumours. We shall describe here the total parotidectomy performed for a deep-lobe tumour.

Begin by carrying out a superficial lobectomy and peeling the gland off the facial nerve from above down. Pedicle the superficial lobe on the inferior pole or in the mid-zone, depending on the site of the tumour.

Using blunt-pointed iris scissors, dissect the whole length of the lower division of the facial nerve from its distal branches to the main trunk of the nerve. Also dissect the buccal division if it is coming off the lower main division. Do not lift the dissected nerve up but merely push it upwards. Even though the nerve is intact, it can be irreparably damaged by a severe axonotmesis if it is overstretched.

Dissect into the deep lobe to find the external carotid artery; clamp, cut and suture ligature it. Carry out a finger dissection of the parapharyngeal space and remove the retromandibular portion (Fig. 19.11). If the tumour of the deep lobe is large, then dislocate the mandible forwards to double the available space for removal (Fig. 19.12). An alternative is to direct the dissection downwards and to pull the mass below the mandible and extract it from behind the submandibular gland.

The finger dissection of the parapharyngeal space has been likened to enucleation but it is subtly different. An enucleation of a tumour of the superficial lobe of the parotid gland means going close to the tumour and probably violating its margins. In the parapharyngeal space, however, there is a lot of loose areolar tissue and the enucleation performed in the deep lobe is quite different from that which would be performed in the superficial lobe. At the end of the operation, the facial nerve and its branches should be stimulated so that the patient can be given some assessment of prognosis of facial nerve function, because it is almost certain that there will be at least a weakness of the lower part of the face after this manoeuvre.

Extended total parotidectomy

It is impossible to describe any one operation that will suffice for all large malignant tumours of the parotid gland, but in this section we describe a commonly performed procedure for a tumour in the body of the gland overlying the facial nerve.

The usual incision is made but, if neck nodes are palpable or if a radical neck dissection is required, then it is either done by making a parallel incision lower in the neck, thus creating a McFee procedure, or by dropping a perpendicular from the horizontal and then, with the parotid incision, creating a Fraser incision (Fig. 19.13).

If a cable graft is anticipated the great auricular nerve is carefully identified and dissected as close to the parotid as is safe and as far down the sternomastoid muscle as is possible (perhaps 6 cm). If this is not possible, then a sural nerve will have to be harvested from the patient's calf.

Once skin flaps have been elevated, the external meatus is transected and the skin lifted off the mastoid. Using a cutting burr, the mastoid antrum is

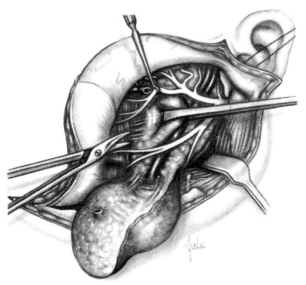

Fig. 19.11 Removal of deep lobe tumour between the upper and lower divisions of the nerve. The superficial lobe should be left attached to the deep lobe.

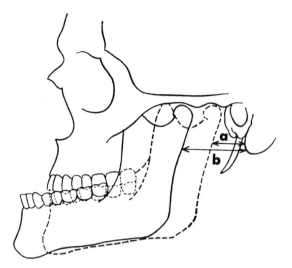

Fig. 19.12 Anterior displacement of the mandible to increase fossa space.

found and a simple mastoidectomy is done. The facial nerve is found at the genu and is decompressed down to its exit from the stylomastoid foramen. Having identified the exit point, the tip of the mastoid is then drilled off.

You then identify the peripheral branches of the facial nerve, namely the temporozygomatic, the buccal branch and the mandibular branch, as described in Surgical anatomy, above. These are followed into the gland as far as possible. You then try to find the main trunk of the facial nerve but this is sometimes impossible due to tumour spread. If it is, then the parotid is excised *en bloc*, carefully identifying the three peripheral branches. The parapharyngeal portion of the parotid is included in the resection

and the external carotid artery is ligated. The neck of the mandible is divided and the temporomandibular joint is freed. The zygoma is divided and, using a drill, this is joined on to the mastoidectomy and the external meatus and middle-ear contents are removed *en bloc* with the parotid and temporomandibular joint.

The facial nerve is grafted as described below.

The skin defect may be closed primarily if only a small amount of skin has been removed but usually, in an excision of this magnitude, skin overlying the tumour is also removed and perhaps a portion of the external ear. A pectoralis myocutaneous flap can be used to close the defect but it may be possible to use a trapezius island flap, based on the transverse cervical vessels.

Facial nerve grafting and facial nerve rehabilitation

Facial nerve grafting is an unsatisfactory surgical technique. Various eminent individuals have shown evidence of good results but by and large these are not replicated in the hands of the average surgeon. The reasons are twofold. Firstly, nerve grafting lies within the province of orthopaedic, plastic, general, otolaryngological and neurosurgery. The result is inevitably a dilution of expertise and experience. The facial nerve probably fares somewhat better than most, being restricted for the most part to the attentions of otolaryngologists and plastic surgeons. The second reason is that the intrinsic understanding of nerve growth and repair is imperfect. In fact the only significant advance in knowledge in the last 35 years has been the proof that a method of repair is only satisfactory if no tension exists at the suture line. Ignoring this important principle has perhaps been

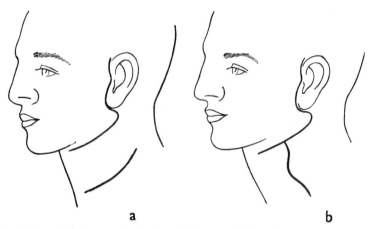

a   b

Fig. 19.13 Incision for total parotidectomy and radical neck dissection in (a) an irradiated patient, and (b) an unirradiated patient.

responsible for more failures of peripheral nerve repair than any other factor.

Peripheral nerve regeneration

The established view of peripheral nerve regeneration is that following transection of the nerve the axons and their myelin sheaths degenerate in the distal segment, leaving empty endoneurial tubes that are, in reality, the basement membrane of Schwann cells. Severed axons in the proximal stump undergo sprouting to form small unmyelinated pioneering axons, which enter the endoneurial tubes under the tropic and trophic influences of hypothetical surface and humoral agents, variously said to be produced by basement membrane, the Schwann cells themselves, or from end-organs. Many aspects of this theory derive from *in vitro* experiments and lack substantiations *in vivo* and undoubtedly represent an oversimplification. It is clear that endoneurial tubes are not essential for nerve regeneration. They may however affect the rate of regeneration early in its history.

Cable nerve grafts

A nerve graft is merely the vehicle along which new axons grow from the proximal stumps to the distal ends. The most important principles to be observed in the placing of these grafts are:

1 that the ends should be immobile;
2 that there should be no tension;
3 that the ends should make good contact with both proximal and distal ends of the nerve; and
4 that scar tissue should be prevented from growing between the nerve ends at the anastomosis.

A nerve graft can be taken without the aid of magnification but the nerve anastomosis should be performed using the operating microscope at 10 times power. Watchmaker's forceps should be used to hold the epineurium and crocodile scissors used to cut it. The ends of the nerve are best cut with a new no. 11 blade on a silicon block.

Sutures of 10/0 Prolene are used for the anastomosis (Fig. 19.14). They can either be applied to the endoneurium or to the facsicles. The question of whether epineurial or fascicular repair is better remains unresolved however. Although collagen tubes, vein grafts and adhesives were at one time popular, they have now been shown in animal experiments to reduce axonal regrowth.

If the main trunk (or one or both divisions) requires grafting, then the great auricular nerve autograft is the best choice. This is partly because of the proximity of the nerve to the operation site, which aids skin preparation and access, and also because the nerve is closer in size to the facial nerve

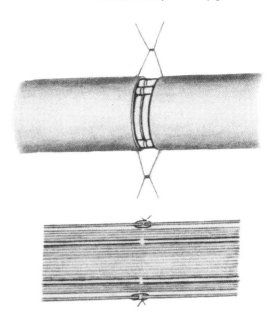

Fig. 19.14 Techniques of nerve anastomosis.

than the sural nerve. It should be noted however that this comparison of sizes relates to the nerve in its entirety and says nothing about the relative sizes of the contained fibres. Both the great auricular nerve and the sural nerve, being sensory, are likely to contain smaller nerve fibres conducting at slower speeds than the purely motor facial nerve.

If more than this requires to be grafted then the sural nerve autograft is the most frequent choice. For a large nerve several such strands are laid in parallel to form a cable graft. The harvesting of donor autograft has several disadvantages, including discrepancy in size between the graft and the damaged nerve and thus the need for additional donor nerve to make a cable graft. Cable grafts, not surprisingly, fare less well than single grafts of comparable thickness to the recipient nerve.

Freeze-thawed skeletal muscle grafts

Recently the idea of nerve repair using an autologous bioprosthesis has been reintroduced in the form of the coaxially aligned freeze-thawed skeletal muscle autograft. Although early results in digital nerves have been encouraging, adequate assessment in the laboratory and especially in clinical practice is lacking.

In the skeletal muscle where the fibres are longitudinally arranged the basement membrane of the myocytes consists of a parallel aligned matrix of tubes, each surrounding a single cell. It is thus similar in its cytoarchitecture and chemical composition to the matrix of Schwann cell basement membrane surrounding the neurons in a nerve. If the muscle can be made to degenerate, the result is structurally identical to that of a degenerating nerve, except that the tubes are larger in diameter. This is the basis of the concept of the freeze-thawed skeletal muscle graft. The sarcoplasm is disrupted by freezing in liquid nitrogen and hypo-osmotic thawing in distilled water provides an oriented matrix of parallel basement membrane tubes that function in a manner similar to a nerve graft.

Freeze-thawed skeletal muscle grafts are used in any situation where a nerve graft is required but they are especially useful where a large segment of the nerve has been removed. The best source of the skeletal muscle is either the sartorius muscle in the leg or, more realistically, the sternomastoid muscle in the neck.

Nerve crossover techniques

The facial–hypoglossal anastomosis is the most commonly used crossover technique. If the nerve trunk is sacrificed close to the stylomastoid foramen and if a peripheral part of the main trunk remains, then it is an easy matter to identify the hypoglossal nerve, divide it and join it on to the peripheral main trunk of the facial nerve. The hypoglossal nerve is larger than the main trunk of the facial nerve in many instances. The disadvantages of this technique is not the resulting paralysis of the tongue but rather when axonal growth occurs, associated movements and synkinesis can occur.

Cross-face anastomosis with the sural nerve is a time-consuming and tedious operation, and is seldom performed now.

Rehabilitation of the paralysed face when grafting fails

Lateral tarsorrhaphy

Inability to close an eye carries the risk of drying of the cornea and subsequent ulceration. To narrow the gap between the lids, a lateral tarsorrhaphy is performed by excising the mucosa over the lateral 1 cm of the upper and lower lids and stitching them together.

Lid implants

If the eye is closed but the aperture is an unsightly width, gold pellets can be implanted in the muscle of the upper eyelid to drag it downwards. Implants have to be specially made for the weight required. The incision in the upper lid is the same as for blepharoplasty except that no skin is excised.

Fascial sling

A strip of fascia lata is taken from the lateral side of the thigh with a fascia stripper. The strips are attached through drill holes in the zygomatic arch and run down through the subcutaneous tissue of the face to the orbicularis oris muscle, and from there they are taken back through the face and attached to the zygoma. Overcorrection is essential or the face falls within 3 weeks.

Muscle implants

Implants of pectoralis minor, along with its nerve supply, are placed around the angle of the mouth or eye in the hope that the muscle will become reinnervated.

Facelift

A standard facelift operation can improve a badly drooping and paralysed face but, even with creation of muscle hitches as in revision rhytidectomy, the skin stretches again and the procedure requires frequent revision.

Temporalis muscle swing

The temporalis muscle is useful in rehabilitating the paralysed face because, in addition to its attachment to the temporal bone, it is inserted into the coronoid process of the mandible and some dynamism is possible. Strips of muscle are freed from the temporal bone and overlying fascia; they are then attached to the orbicularis oris muscles of the midface region and the lateral end of the orbicularis oculi muscle.

Radiotherapy technique

Parotid gland

While radium needle implantation was once popular, especially for postenucleation treatment of pleomorphic adenomas, external beam therapy with 4–6 MV X-rays is now most often used. This enables the homogeneous treatment of the large block of tissue at risk. The technique is essentially the same for radical irradiation of an inoperable tumour as it is for postoperative radiotherapy. The wedge-shaped volume (Fig. 19.15) extends from the top of the zygoma superiorly, down to the hyoid bone, and from the anterior border of masseter to the mastoid. Medially it extends to the midline. It thus includes the entire parotid bed, the parotid duct, the parapharyngeal space and adjacent and upper deep cervical lymph nodes as well as covering the surgical scar. The upper limit may need to be extended if there is base of skull invasion, or any likelihood of spread of an adenoid cystic carcinoma along the

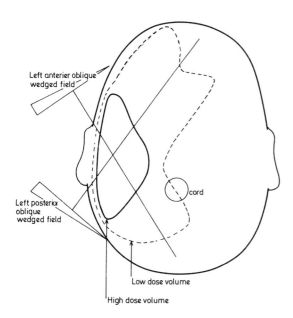

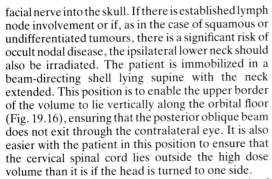

Fig. 19.15 Plan of radiotherapy field arrangement for irradiation of the parotid gland.

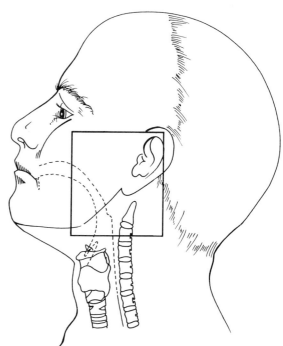

Fig. 19.16 Volume to be irradiated in parotid tumours.

facial nerve into the skull. If there is established lymph node involvement or if, as in the case of squamous or undifferentiated tumours, there is a significant risk of occult nodal disease, the ipsilateral lower neck should also be irradiated. The patient is immobilized in a beam-directing shell lying supine with the neck extended. This position is to enable the upper border of the volume to lie vertically along the orbital floor (Fig. 19.16), ensuring that the posterior oblique beam does not exit through the contralateral eye. It is also easier with the patient in this position to ensure that the cervical spinal cord lies outside the high dose volume than it is if the head is turned to one side.

The volume to be treated is covered with a pair of appropriately wedged lateral oblique fields, one anterior and one posterior. If the lower neck is to be treated, a single anterior field can be used, the upper border of which is carefully matched on to the lower border of the wedged pair. Where there is skin involvement by tumour, 0.5 cm of wax bolus is applied to the shell to circumvent the skin-sparing effect of megavoltage irradiation. A dose of 55 Gy in 20 fractions over 4 weeks or its equivalent should be used. For the postoperative treatment of pleomorphic adenomas, a direct electron field is a good alternative to a wedged pair arrangement of photon beams.

Submandibular gland

The radiotherapy technique used here is essentially the same as that used for floor of mouth tumours (Chapter 16).

Controversies in management

The management of tumour over the nerve

It may be possible to dissect directly on to the main trunk of the nerve, retracting the tumour out of the way and using the tragal pointer on the posterior belly of digastric as a landmark. To do this may run the risk of bursting the capsule of a pleomorphic adenoma or violating tumour planes in malignant tumours. Before attempting this, therefore, use must be made of the distal branch techniques as outlined above, and also of finding the facial nerve within the mastoid and dissecting it forwards. It is sometimes useful to carry out a radical neck dissection or an upper neck dissection in order to be able to come up to the nerve from below.

Management of adenoid cystic carcinoma that does not affect the nerve

Some years ago it was suggested that the facial nerve should be sacrificed in every case of adenoid cystic carcinoma. This is no longer accepted. If a small adenoid cystic carcinoma occurs in the tail or the body of the parotid gland, and if it is not lying on the facial nerve, then a total parotidectomy can be carried out with preservation of the facial nerve.

Management of recurrent pleomorphic adenoma

If a pleomorphic adenoma becomes implanted during a primary removal, then it is implanted in the deep lobe and is adjacent to the dissected facial nerve. Furthermore, the skin is placed directly on to the deep lobe and the tumour will grow into the skin. This means that not only should the deep lobe be removed but also the overlying skin, where it is contiguous with tumour.

The problem with recurrent pleomorphic adenoma is that the clinical assessment usually underestimates the spread.

The operation should begin by finding the facial nerve as in superficial parotidectomy; as there is a lot of scar tissue in the area, a stimulator is invaluable. All divisions of the nerve should be dissected and identified, and those that are contiguous with the recurrent pleomorphic adenoma should be sacrificed. It is usually possible, however, to preserve facial nerve function if there is careful preservation of the vertical anastomotic branches between the terminal divisions of the nerve. A total parotidectomy is performed, and small skin excisions are carried out and repaired as necessary.

Facial nerve reconstruction

There is no 'best buy' in methods of facial nerve grafting. Each method has its proponents but it can be said that the success of facial nerve reconstruction lies in the skill of the operator rather than the methods chosen. As long as the basic principles of nerve grafting are observed, as outlined above, then most patients should be able to regain facial tone at rest. Only the very successful grafts will allow of an equal smile and equal eye closure. The patient should be told not to expect any major return of function in under 6–12 months.

The choices available to the operator are epineural suturing, interfascicular suturing, and splinting with or without suturing.

A surprise diagnosis of a variable-grade tumour of the submandibular and parotid glands

This has been dealt with above. If the operator thought the tumour was benign at the first operation, then it is likely that he or she has not left any behind. In the parotid, a total parotidectomy should be done, but it is difficult to excise more in the submandibular region. If the tumour was contiguous with the floor of mouth, then perhaps a strip of tissue can be taken from this area for further pathological examination.

Each case should be seen at the combined surgery/radiotherapy clinic and a decision made with regard to postoperative irradiation.

Is a tumour on a nerve, in a nerve?

There can be no hard and fast guidance in this regard but it would be safe to assume that a tumour that is *on* a nerve, is *in* a nerve. The only exception to this is probably a pleomorphic adenoma or a monomorphic adenoma at first operation.

The patient wakes up with an unexpected facial paralysis

If a stimulator has been used and the nerve has reacted to electrical stimulation at reasonable levels, then the patient can be assured that the condition is temporary and will resolve within 3 months. It is important to use the stimulator at the end of the operation to get this information. The authors have seen interruption of facial nerve function with an intrasheath haematoma that would have been unrecognized had the stimulator not been used. An intact nerve at the end of the operation does not mean that the patient will regain facial nerve function. A grade 3 axonotmesis will often not recover and even though it may be better than a graft, the patient will have to wait 6–12 months to see both what recovery is going to take place and how much scarring has occurred, due to the intraneural bleeding that probably was produced with the tears in the axons.

Sjögren's syndrome and tumour formation

Sjögren's syndrome involves loss of suppressor T cell activity and decreased cell-mediated immunity. Patients with Sjögren's syndrome have a greatly increased chance of acquiring non-Hodgkin's lymphoma, Waldenström's macroglobulinaemia, immunoblastic sarcoma and carcinoma ex lymphoepithelial lesion. There is a 44 times greater than normal chance of developing lymphoma in Sjögren's syndrome and this can be compared with the 80 times greater than normal chance that transplant recipients have of developing lymphoma. The lymphoma is usually of histiocytic-predominant type.

Over 50 cases of carcinoma arising in benign lymphoepithelial lesion have been reported. Ninety-five per cent have been in the parotid and most have been in Eskimos or Orientals. It is an undifferentiated carcinoma of squamous origin and because of its proclivity to occur in Eskimos it has been described as an 'eskimoma'.

Are there any tests that tell you if a nerve is involved?

Although electroneurography has developed into a fairly sophisticated electrophysiological tool, it is seldom that information is gained from this investigation that is not obvious clinically. About three-quarters of any branch must be damaged by a tumour before there is loss of function of that branch. It is thus possible to have apparently good facial movement with tumour infiltration into the whole of the facial nerve. It is important to get informed consent from any patient undergoing parotid surgery. If there is little doubt that the tumour is benign then the patient can be told there is a less than 1% chance of facial nerve paralysis as a result of the operation, but they must also be told that such a paralysis might involve them in further surgery for facial nerve rehabilitation, both on the eye and the facial tissues, and that it will involve loss of oral competence.

If there is a suspicion that the tumour is malignant and the nerve is involved, then the patient must give informed consent for facial nerve sacrifice and grafting. If such consent is not obtained then the operation must be abandoned certainly within the legal framework of the UK, the patient woken up, and the problem rediscussed with him or her.

The capsule bursts during manipulation of a large pleomorphic adenoma

In this situation there is about a 10% chance of implantation recurrence. The chance of facial nerve damage in the removal of a recurrent pleomorphic adenoma is around 50%. It is thus important to minimize the effects of such spillage. All contaminated instruments should be removed from the scene of the operation and the gowns, gloves and drapes changed. The wound should be washed thoroughly for at least 5 min with sterile water.

The patient should then be seen by the radiotherapist and, depending on the patient's age, consideration given to the use of postoperative irradiation. The situation can be likened to the old-fashioned enucleation, which seemed to be a reasonably good operation provided it was accompanied by postoperative irradiation.

Is adenoid cystic carcinoma of the submandibular gland the same as adenoid cystic carcinoma of the floor of the mouth?

The submandibular gland is adjacent to the floor of the mouth and any tumour of it must be regarded as a tumour of the floor of the mouth. If it is an adenoid cystic tumour with its proclivity for growth along

nerve sheaths, then the lingual and hypoglossal nerves must be sacrificed along with the ramus mandibular nerve. Consideration also has to be given to the condition of the mandible and the proximity of the inferior dental nerve. Therefore, if an adenoid cystic tumour is diagnosed in the submandibular gland, then it should be treated as an oral cavity tumour.

Tumours of the parapharyngeal space

Surgical anatomy

The parapharyngeal space has been called the lateral pharyngeal space, the pharyngomaxillary space, the pterygomaxillary space and the pterygopharyngeal space. It is one of the peripharyngeal spaces and holds a key position by virtue of the vital structures passing through it, and because of its communication with other peripharyngeal spaces. Its anatomy has been well-described elsewhere. The contents of the compartments of the space are detailed in Table 19.3. The major consequence of the anatomy of the space is that tumours expanding within it can only grow medially and inferiorly.

The pharynx is surrounded by several spaces that form a complete ring around it. The spaces lie entirely deep to the superficial or anterior layer of the deep fascia and communicate more or less freely with each other around the muscles and vessels that pass through them. Posteriorly lies the retropharyngeal space and this is continuous laterally, both with the upper part of the carotid sheath and the lateral pharyngeal space; the latter passes anteriorly into the submandibular space where it communicates across the midline with the opposite side. The parapharyngeal space proper is bounded medially by the fascia of the pharynx, laterally by the pterygoid muscles and the sheath of the parotid gland. It extends upwards to the base of the skull but does not extend inferiorly below the level of the hyoid bone as it is limited here by the sheath of the submandibular gland. Posteriorly this space is directly continuous with the carotid sheath and its immediate lateral relation is the parotid space enclosing the parotid gland, the vessels which transverse the gland and the facial nerve. Anteriorly the parapharyngeal space communicates with the spaces about the floor of the

Table 19.3 Contents of the parapharyngeal space

Prestyloid space	Poststyloid space	Retropharyngeal space
Internal maxillary artery	Internal carotid artery	Lymph nodes,
Inferior alveolar nerve	Internal jugular vein	especially the
Lingual nerve	Cervical sympathetic chain	node of Rouviere
Auriculotemporal nerve	Glossopharyngeal nerve	
	Lymph nodes	
	Glomus system	

mouth; furthermore, it is adjacent to the submandibular gland so that infection can pass into it either from the pharynx, from the spaces around the mouth (dental infection), or from the submandibular gland.

Although strictly speaking the parapharyngeal space contains only the styloglossus and the stylopharyngeus muscles, we are concerned here with a clinical problem; that is the patient who presents with a mass lateral to but bulging into the pharynx; such a mass may arise either in the parapharyngeal space, in the deep part of the parotid space, or from the upper end of the carotid sheath.

Surgical pathology

The parapharyngeal space may harbour a wide variety of diseases. Tissues normally occurring in the space are shown in Table 19.4, along with the principal cell types. Acute inflammatory conditions in the nasopharynx and tonsillar regions may spread to the space and cause fatal carotid artery haemorrhage, false aneurysms of the carotid artery, or thrombosis of the internal jugular vein. Tuberculosis can also affect the lymph nodes in the space.

The commonest tumours are those arising in the deep lobe of the parotid gland, and they comprise 50% of parapharyngeal tumours. They may be dumb-bell-shaped because of constriction in the stylomandibular tunnel, and may present either as a pharyngeal or external swelling. The relative incidence of salivary tumours in this space is similar to that for the superficial lobe of the parotid. Malignant tumours tend to have a poorer prognosis than similar tumours of the superficial lobe.

Neurogenous tumours are the next commonest

Table 19.4 Tissues present either in or adjacent to the parapharyngeal space

	Tissue	Examples	Principal cell types
Digestive system	Salivary	Parotid gland	Acinar epithelial cells
		Minor salivary glands	Duct epithelial cell
			Myoepithelial cell
Nervous system	Peripheral nerves	Cranial nerves IX–XII	Schwann cell
		Lingual nerve	Fibroblast
		Auriculotemporal nerve	
	Autonomic ganglion	Superior cervical sympathetic ganglion	
	Sensory ganglion	Vagal ganglia	
Chemoreceptor system	Extra-adrenal paraganglion	Vagal body	Epithelioid cells
			Type I (glomus) cells
			Type II cells
Lymphatic system	Lymph nodes	Node of Rouviere	Lymphocytes
			Plasma cells
			Macrophages
			Reticulum cells
	Lymph vessels		Endothelial cells
Connective tissue	Dense		
	Irregular	Fascia and periosteum	Fibroblasts
	Regular	Stylomandibular ligament	
	Adipose	White and brown fat	Adipocytes
	Bone	Styloid process	Osteoblasts
Vascular system	Artery	Internal carotid, internal maxillary	Endothelial pericytes
	Vein	Internal jugular	Smooth muscle fibres
Muscle	Striated	Styloid muscles	Striated muscle fibres
	Smooth	Arterial wall	Smooth muscle fibres

type of tumour. These are schwannomas, neuro-fibromas, ganglioneuromas or neuroblastomas. Meningiomas may extend into the space though the jugular foramen.

Paragangliomas arise from extra-adrenal para-ganglia, most commonly from the carotid body, but also from the vagal body on the inferior ganglion of the vagus. Only 8% of carotid body tumours extend into the parapharyngeal space, and fewer than 10% of these are malignant.

Fibrosarcoma is the most common sarcoma des-cribed at this site. Lymphomas may arise in the parapharyngeal nodes. Other lesions include terato-mas, developmental cysts, lipomas, and, less com-monly, haemangiomas and rhabdomyosarcomas.

Malignant tumours may invade the space from the nasopharynx, oropharynx, mandible, maxilla or mouth. They may extend to the base of the skull because of the lack of anatomical barriers and thence through the foramina into the skull. The node of Rouviere is often the first site of metastasis of nasopharyngeal or antral carcinoma. Metastases to the node of Rouviere may cause palsies of the glossopharyngeal, vagus and hypoglossal nerves.

Salivary tumours may cause a parapharyngeal swelling in one of three ways: a minor salivary gland tumour; a parotid deep lobe tumour; or a parotid dumb-bell tumour.

Smooth swellings around or behind the tonsil displacing it medially or anteriorly may be due to a tumour arising from the mucous glands found out-side the capsule of the palatine tonsil. Three out of four of these tumours are benign pleomorphic ad-enomas and the vast majority of the rest are adenoid cystic carcinomas.

Tumours may arise from the deep lobe of the parotid gland, which is wedged between the mand-ible, the medial pterygoid muscle and the masseter anteriorly, and the sternomastoid and digastric mus-cles and the muscles arising from the styloid process posteriorly. The inner edge of the wedge protrudes into the parapharyngeal space. Between 2 and 4% of all parotid tumours develop primarily in the deep lobe. The pathology of tumours of the deep lobe is the same as that of tumours of the superficial lobe, most being benign pleomorphic adenomas.

Dumb-bell parotid tumours may cause swelling of the parapharyngeal space, though the most obvious clinical picture is the external swelling. The tumour passes into the para- and retropharyngeal spaces through the 'stylomandibular tunnel', which is bounded by the base of the skull above, the ascend-ing ramus of the jaw and the internal pterygoid muscles anteriorly, and the styloid process and the stylomandibular ligament posteriorly. Most of these tumours are pleomorphic adenomas, but one neur-oma has been recorded as presenting in this fashion, as has lymphatic leukaemia affecting the parotid lymph nodes.

Clinical features

A patient presenting with a mass pushing into the pharynx may have any of the diseases described above. Whatever the disease the history is usually a long one of many years. The tumours that arise from salivary tissue usually cause no other symptoms, other than that of a painless mass, though an adenoid cystic carcinoma may cause pain or numbness of immediately adjacent nerves, such as the inferior alveolar nerve.

Neurogenous tumours often paralyse the nerve from which they arise. The commonest schwannoma is that arising from the vagus which often presents with hoarseness due to paralysis of the vocal cord. Pain and rapid growth in schwannoma indicate malignant change, which almost always has a bad prognosis.

Paragangliomas of the carotid body seldom cause symptoms other than the presence of a mass, though as outlined above there may be a positive family history in which case the patient may have a phaeo-chromocytoma. About 30% of patients with a para-ganglioma present with a pharyngeal mass pushing the tonsil medially and anteriorly.

The glomus vagale tumour may present as an otherwise symptomless swelling, but much more commonly presents with the symptoms of paralysis of the vagus nerve and adjacent nerves, such as the hypoglossal and glossopharyngeal, or (as outlined above) with aural symptoms due to pressure of the tumour mass on the eustachian tube.

Examination

The tumour is examined to assess if it is mobile, if it is pulsatile and if possible to detect from which struc-ture it arises. The examination must be carried out by bimanual palpation with one finger in the mouth.

All the cranial nerves should be examined, but particularly the seventh, ninth, 10th, 11th and 12th. Paralysis of these nerves usually indicates origin from the nerve or invasion by a glomus vagale tumour. A paraganglioma of the carotid body rarely invades the adjacent nerves, and the salivary tumours only do so if they are malignant *ab initio* or if they undergo malignant degeneration, which is very uncommon.

Radiology

Plain soft tissue films are rarely helpful, apart from outlining the size of the mass.

The most useful radiological investigations are a CT scan and a carotid angiogram. The angiogram will show the characteristic picture of a carotid body tumour, or circulation through a glomus vagale tumour.

A sialogram of the parotid is rarely helpful although it may show displacement of the gland.

Biopsy

Biopsy should *never* be done of a swelling in the parapharyngeal space. It rarely gives the correct diagnosis; if the patient suffers from a salivary tumour it carries the danger of implanting tumour in the pharyngeal mucosa; and if the patient suffers from one of the vascular tumours the outcome is often fatal.

Diagnosis must therefore be made by a high index of clinical suspicion supported by radiology, particularly angiography.

Treatment

The same basic technique is used for all tumours. General anaesthesia with orotracheal intubation is induced. Position the patient with a sandbag under the shoulders, and turn the head to the side opposite the tumour. When the patient is draped perform a temporary tarsorrhaphy and leave the entire side of the face exposed to allow observation of facial nerve function.

Make a standard parotidectomy incision anterior to the pinna, curving under the lobule and then sweeping forward in a cervical skin crease to the level of the hyoid bone. Raise a flap of skin and platysma anterosuperiorly. Identify the anterior border of the sternomastoid muscle and the mastoid process posteriorly, and divide the great auricular nerve.

Separate the lower part of the superficial lobe of the parotid gland from the cartilaginous external meatus and mastoid process by blunt dissection. Then find the trunk of the facial nerve by one of the techniques described on page 279. Expose the lower division of the nerve with the aid of a nerve stimulator, as in a superficial parotidectomy (Fig. 19.17).

Divide the posterior facial vein, and remove the tail of the parotid gland and upper deep cervical lymph nodes. Identify the hypoglossal nerve curving anteriorly. Divide the posterior belly of the digastric muscle, which allows you to identify the internal and external carotid arteries, the internal jugular vein, the glossopharyngeal, vagus and accessory nerves and the sympathetic chain (Fig. 19.18). The external carotid artery gives off branches at this level and enters the deep lobe of the parotid gland superiorly. If necessary, ligate and divide the external carotid artery. Superiorly, follow the stylomandibular ligament, styloglossus muscle and the stylohyoid muscle to the styloid process with retraction of the angle of the mandible, parotid gland and external carotid artery. Divide the muscles and ligament close to the styloid process, which is then removed by bone-cutting forceps. This allows good access to the upper part of the parapharyngeal space and skull base. The tumour can now be removed by blunt and sharp dissection. Where there has been a previous intraoral incision or biopsy, remove pharyngeal mucosa in continuity with the primary tumour.

Small deep-lobe tumours may be removed between the divisions of the facial nerve, but with large tumours this may be technically impossible. This approach is used for neural sheath tumours, but the nerves of origin must be divided, as these tumours cannot be dissected from their nerve of origin.

Vagal body tumours are approached in the same way. They are generally close to the internal carotid artery and jugular vein at the skull base and are

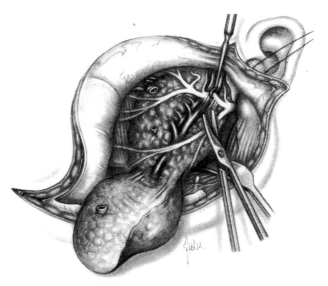

Fig. 19.17 Exposure of the facial nerve after partidectomy.

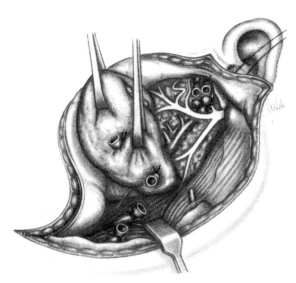

Fig. 19.18 Elevation of lower division of the nerve to access the deep lobe.

difficult to remove without damage to these structures. Sharp dissection is always required to remove these tumours.

References and further reading

American Cancer Society (1983) *Cancer Facts and Figures.* New York, American Cancer Society.

American Joint Committee for cancer staging and end results reporting (1980) *Manual for Staging of Cancer.* Chicago, AJC.

Armitstead P R, Smiddy H G, Frank H G (1979) Simple enucleation and radiotherapy in the treatment of the pleomorphic salivary adenoma of the parotid gland. *Br J Surg* **66**:716–17.

Bardwill J M (1967) Tumors of the parotid gland. *Am J Surg* **114**:498.

Batsakis J G (1982) *Tumours of the Head and Neck*, 2nd edn. Baltimore. Williams & Wilkins, pp 64, 194.

Batsakis J G, Regezi J A (1978) The pathology of head and neck tumors: salivary glands, part 1. *Head Neck Surg* **1**:59.

Batsakis J G, Regezi J A (1979) The pathology of head and neck tumors: salivary glands, part 4. *Head Neck Surg* **1**:340.

Batsakis J G *et al.* (1978) The pathology of head and neck tumors: salivary glands, part 2. *Head Neck Surg* **1**:167.

Batsakis J G, Chinn E K, Weimert T A (1979) Acinic cell carcinoma: a clinicopathologic study of thirty-five cases. *J Laryngol Otol* **93**:325.

Batsakis J G, Regezi J A, Bloch D (1979) The pathology of head and neck tumors: salivary glands, part 3. *Head Neck Surg* **1**:260.

Bjorkland A, Eneroth C M. (1980) Management of parotid gland neoplasms. *Am J Otolaryngol* **1**:55.

Buschke F, Galante M (1959) Radical preoperative roentgen therapy in primarily inoperable advanced cancers of the head and neck. *Radiology* **73**:845–7.

Byun Y S, Fayos J V, Kim Y H (1980) Management of malignant salivary gland tumours. *Laryngoscope* **90**:1052–60.

Chen K (1978) Metastasizing pleomorphic adenoma of the salivary gland. *Cancer* **42**:2407.

Chong G C, Beahrs O H, Woolner L B (1974) Surgical management of acinic cell carcinoma of the parotid gland. *Gynecol Obstet* **138**:65.

Christ T F, Crocker D (1972) Basal cell adenoma of minor salivary gland origin. *Cancer* **30**:214.

Clifford P P P (1979) Tumours of the nasopharynx. In: Maran A G D, Stell P M (eds.) *Clinical Otolaryngology.* London, Blackwell, pp. 315–27.

Conley J (1975) *Salivary Glands and the Facial Nerve.* New York, Grune & Stratton.

Conley J, Hamaker R C (1975) Prognosis of malignant tumors of the parotid gland with facial paralysis. *Arch Otolaryngol* **101**:39.

Conley J, Meyers E, Cole R (1972) Analysis of 115 patients with tumors of the submandibular gland. *Ann Otorhinolaryngol* **81**:323.

Corcoran M O, Cook H P, Hobsley M (1983) Radical surgery following radiotherapy for advanced parotid carcinoma. *Br J Surg* **70**: 261–3.

Corcoran M O, Webb R J, Hobsley M (1983) Recurrences after surgery for pleomorphic adenoma of the parotid gland. *Clin Oncol* **9**:181.

Cutchavaree A, Shuangshoti S, Kumut N (1984) Parapharyngeal neurogenic tumours: nine-year experience. *J Med Assoc Thai* **67**:350–5.

Davis R A *et al.* (1956) Surgical anatomy of the facial nerve and parotid gland based on a study of 350 cervicofacial halves. *Surg Gynecol Obstet* **102**:385.

DeCampora E, Camaioni A, Calabrese V, Corradini C, Crose A, D'Agnone N (1974) Conservative transmandibular approach in the surgical treatment of tumours of the parapharyngeal space. *J Laryngol Otol* **98**:1225–9.

Duncan W, Orr J A, Arnott S J, Jack W J (1987) Neutron therapy for malignant tumours of the salivary glands. A report of the Edinburgh experience. *Radiother Oncol* **8**:97–104.

Eby L S, Johnson D S, Baker H W (1972) Adenoid cystic carcinoma of the head and neck. *Cancer* **29**:1160.

Elkon D, Colman M, Hendrickson F R (1978) Radiation therapy in the treatment of malignant salivary gland tumors. *Cancer* **41**:502.

Eneroth C M (1964) Histological and clinical aspects of parotid tumors. *Acta Otolaryngol* **191**:(Suppl.):1.

Eneroth C M (1972) Facial nerve paralysis: a criterion of malignancy in parotid tumors. *Arch Otol* **95**:300.

Eneroth C M, Hjertman L, Moberger G (1967) Malignant tumors of the submandibular gland. *Acta Otolaryngol* **64**:514.

Eneroth C M, Hamberger C A (1974) Principles of treatment of different types of parotid tumors. *Laryngoscope* **84**:1732.

Evans J C (1966) Radiation therapy of salivary gland tumors. *Radiol Clin Biol* **35**:153.

Fee W E Jr, Goffinet D R, Calcaterra T C (1978) Recurrent mixed tumors of the parotid gland: results of surgical therapy. *Laryngoscope* **88**:265.

Ferrucci J T Jr, Wittenberg J, Margolies M N (1979) Malignant seeding of the tract after thin needle aspiration biopsy. *Radiology* **130**:345.

Fletcher G H, Jessee R H (1977) The place of irradiation in

the management of the primary lesion in head and neck cancers. *Cancer* **39**:862–7.

Fluur E (1964) Parapharyngeal tumours. *Arch Otolaryngol* **80**:557–65.

Foote F W Jr, Frazell E L (1953) Tumors of the major salivary glands. *Cancer* **6**:1065.

Foote F W Jr, Frazell E L (1954) Tumors of the major salivary glands. In: *Atlas of tumor pathology*, section 4, fascicle 11, Washington, DC, Armed Forces Institute of Pathology.

Frable W J (1983) *Thin Needle Aspiration Biopsy*. Philadelphia, W. B. Saunders.

Frable W J, Frable M A (1979) Thin needle aspiration biopsy: the diagnosis of head and neck tumors revisited. *Cancer* **43**:1451.

Gordon A B, Fiddian R V (1976) Frey's syndrome after parotid surgery. *Am J Surg* **132**:54.

Grage B G, Lober P H, Shahon D B (1961) Benign tumors of the major salivary glands. *Surgery* **50**:625.

Greyson N D, Noyek A M (1978) Nuclear medicine in otolaryngological diagnosis. *Otolaryngol Clin North Am* **2**:544.

Greyson N D, Noyek A M (1981) Oncocytoma radionuclide salivary scanning. *J Otolaryngol* **10**:15.

Guillamondegui O M, Byers R M, Luna M A, Chiminazzo H, Jesse R H, Fletcher G H (1975) Aggressive surgery in treatment for parotid cancer: the role of adjunctive postoperative radiotherapy. *Am J Radiol* **123**:49–54.

Hanna D C, Gaisford J C, Richardson G S, Bindra R N (1968) Tumours of the deep lobe of the parotid gland. *Am J Surg* **116**:524–7.

Hays L L, Novack A J, Worsham J C (1982) The Frey's syndrome: a simple, effective treatment. *Otolaryngol Head Neck Surg* **90**:419.

Hamperl H (1970) The myoepithelia-normal state: regressive changes, hyperplasia, tumors, *Curr Top Pathol* **53**:161.

Henry L W, Blasko J C, Griffin T W, Parker R G (1979) Evaluation of fast neutron teletherapy for advanced carcinomas of the major salivary glands. *Cancer* **44**:814–18.

Hillel A D, Fee W E Jr (1983) Evaluation of frozen section in parotid gland surgery. *Arch Otolaryngol* **104**:230.

Hobsley M (1981) Sir Gordon Gordon-Taylor: two themes illustrated by the surgery of the parotid salivary gland. *Ann R Coll Surg Engl* **63**:264–9.

Hodgkinson D J, Woods J E (1976) The influence of facial nerve sacrifice in surgery of malignant parotid tumors. *J Surg Oncol* **8**:425.

Hollander L, Cunningham M P (1973) Management of cancer of the parotid gland. *Surg Clin North Am* **53**:113.

Hugo N E, McKinney P, Griffith B H (1973) Management of tumors of the parotid gland. *Surg Clin North Am* **53**:105.

Isacsson G, Shear M (1983) Intraoral salivary gland tumors: a retrospective study of 201 cases. *J Oral Pathol* **12**:57.

Jackson G L, Luna M A, Byers R M (1983) Results of surgery alone and surgery combined with postoperative radiotherapy in the treatment of cancer of the parotid gland. *Am J Surg* **146**:497.

Johns M E, Coulthard S W (1977) Survival and follow-up in malignant tumors of the salivary glands. *Otolaryngol Clin North Am* **10**:455.

Johns M E, Regezi J A, Batsakis J C (1977) Oncocytic neoplasms of salivary glands: an ultrastructural study. *Laryngoscope* **87**:862.

Kagan A R, Nussbaum H, Handler S et al (1976) Recurrences from malignant parotid salivary gland tumours. *Cancer* **37**:2600–4.

Kahn L B (1979) Benign lymphoepithelial lesion (Mikulicz' disease) of the salivary gland: an ultrastructural study. *Hum Pathol* **10**:99.

King J J, Fletcher G H (1971) Malignant tumours of the major salivary glands. *Radiology* **100**:381–4.

Kumar P P, Good R R, Yonkers A L, Ogren F P (1989) High activity iodine-125 endocurietherapy for head and neck tumours. *Laryngoscope* **99**:174–8.

Lambert J A (1971) Parotid gland tumors. *Milit Med* **136**:484.

Lawrence W T, Lawrence W T Jr (1981) Malignant neoplasms of the major salivary glands. *J Surg Oncol* **17**:113.

Lawson V G, Leliever W C, Makerewich L A, Rubuzzi D D, Bell R (1979) Unusual parapharyngeal lesions. *J Otolaryngol* **8**:241–9.

Levitt S H, McHugh R B, Gomez-Marin O et al. (1981) Clinical staging system of cancer of the salivary gland. *Cancer* **47**:2712–24.

Lindberg L G, Ackerman, M (1976) Aspiration cytology of salivary gland tumors: diagnostic experience from six years of routine laboratory work. *Laryngoscope* **86**:584.

McCullough D T, Rye L, Redman R S (1981) Necrotizing sialometaplasia: a lesion of minor salivary glands that mimics malignancies. *Ann Plast Surg* **7**:480.

McEvedy B V, Ross W M (1976) The treatment of mixed parotid tumours by enucleation and radiotherapy. *Br J Surg* **63**:341–2.

McFarland J (1936) Three hundred mixed tumours of the salivary glands, of which sixty-nine recurred. *Surg Gynecol Obstet* **63**:457–68.

McIlrath D C, Remine W H, Devine K D, Dockerty M B (1963) Tumours of the parapharyngeal region. *Surg Gynecol Obstet* **116**:88–94.

Maran A G D (1979) Neck masses. In: Maran A G D, Stell P M (eds.) *Clinical Otolaryngology*, London, Blackwell, 288–305.

Maran A G D, Mackenzie I J, Murray J A M (1984) The parapharyngeal space. *J Laryngol Otol* **98**:371–80.

Marsh W L, Allen M S (1979) Adenoid cystic carcinoma: biologic behavior in 38 patients. *Cancer* **43**:1463.

Matsuba H M, Thawley S E, Devineni V, Levine L A, Smith P G (1985) High grade malignancies of the parotid gland: effective use of planned combined surgery and irradiation. *Laryngoscope* **95**:1059–63.

Mintz G A, Abrams A M, Melrose R J (1982) Monomorphic adenomas of the major and minor salivary glands. *Oral Surg* **53**:375.

Modan B, Baidatz D, Mart H et al. (1974) Radiation-induced head and neck tumours. *Lancet* **i**:277–9.

Mylius E (1960) The identification and the role of the myoepithelial cell in salivary gland tumors. *Acta Pathol* **50**:41.

Mustard R A, Anderson W (1964) Malignant tumors of the parotid. *Ann Surg* **159**:291.

Nigro M F Jr, Spiro R H (1977) Deep lobe parotid tumors. *Am J Surg* **134**:523.

Patey D H. Hand B H (1952) Diagnosis of mixed parotid tumours. *Lancet* **ii**:310–11.

Patey D H, Thackray A C (1975) The treatment of parotid

tumours in the light of a pathological study of parotidectomy material. *Br J Surg* **45**:477–87.

Perzik S L, Fisher B (1970) The place of neck dissection in the management of parotid tumours. *Am J Surg* **120**: 355–8.

Perzin K H, Gullane P, Clairmont A C (1978) Adenoid cystic carcinoma arising in salivary glands: a correlation of histologic features and clinical course. *Cancer* **42**:265.

Rafla, S (1977) Malignant parotid tumors natural history and treatment. *Cancer* **40**:136.

Rafla-Demetrious S R (1970) *Mucous and Salivary Gland Tumours* (1970) Springfield, Ill., Charles C Thomas.

Rampling R, Catterall M (1984) Facial nerve damage in the treatment of tumours of the parotid gland. *Clin Oncol* **10**:345–51.

Rice D H, Mancuso A A, Hanafee W N (1980) Computerised tomography with simultaneous sialography in evaluating parotid tumours. *Arch Otolaryngol* **106**:472–3.

Rossman K J (1975) The role of radiation therapy in the treatment of parotid carcinomas. *Am J Roentgenol* **123**:492.

Saksela E, Tarkkanen J, Kohonen A (1970) The malignancy of mixed tumours of the parotid gland. *Acta Otolaryngol* **70**:62–70.

Schantz S P, Potter J F (1983) Primary parotid cancer: factors influencing recurrence. *Ann Surg* **49**:477–82.

Schoss S M, Donovan D T, Alford B R (1985) Tumours of the parapharyngeal space. *Arch Otolaryngol* **111**:753–7.

Schuller D E, McCabe B F (1977) Salivary gland neoplasms in children. *Otolaryngol Clin North Am* **10**:399.

Shidnia H, Hornback N B, Hamaker R, Lingeman R (1980) Carcinoma of major salivary glands. *Cancer* **45**:693–7.

Sinner W N, Zajicek J (1976) Implantation metastasis after percutaneous transthoracic needle aspiration biopsy. *Acta Radiol Diagn* **17**:473.

Som P M, Biller H F (1979) The combined computerised tomography-sialogram. *Ann Otol Rhinol Laryngol* **88**:590–5.

Som P M, Biller H F, Lawson W (1981) Tumors of the parapharyngeal space: preoperative evaluation, diagnosis and surgical approaches. *Ann Otol Rhinol Laryngol* **90** (Suppl. 8):3–15.

Spiro R H, Huvos A G, Strong E W (1974) Adenoid cystic carcinoma of the salivary origin: a clinicopathologic study of 242 cases. *Am J Surg* **128**:512.

Spiro R H, Huvos A G, Strong E W (1975) Cancer of the parotid gland. *Am J Surg* **130**:452.

Spiro R H, Hajdn S I, Strong E W (1976) Tumors of the submaxillary gland. *Ann J Surg* **132**:463.

Spiro R H, Huvos A G, Strong E W (1978) Acinic cell carcinoma of salivary origin: a clinicopathologic study of 67 cases, *Cancer* **41**:924.

Spiro R H, Huvos A G, Strong E W (1982) Adenocarcinoma of salivary origin: clinicopathologic study of 204 patients. *Am J Surg* **44**:423.

Spitz M R, Batsakis J G (1984) Major salivary gland carcinoma. *Arch Otolaryngol* **110**:45.

Stell P M, Mansfield A O, Stoney P J (1985) Surgical approaches to tumours of the parapharyngeal space. *Am J Otolaryngol* **6**:92–7.

Stephens K L, Hobsley M (1982) The treatment of pleomorphic adenomas by formal parotidectomy. *Br J Surg* **69**:1–3.

Strong E W, Henschke U K, Nickson J J et al. (1966) Preoperative X-ray therapy as an adjunct to radical neck dissection. *Cancer* **19**:1509–16.

Suen J Y, Johns M E (1982) Chemotherapy for salivary gland cancer. *Laryngoscope* **92**:235.

Tannock I F, Sutherland D J (1980) Chemotherapy for adenocystic carcinoma. *Cancer* **46**:452.

Tapley N V (1977) Irradiation treatment of malignant tumors of the salivary glands, *Ear Nose Throat J* **56**:110.

Thackery A C, Lucas R B (1974) Armed Forces Institute of Pathology, *Tumours of the Major Salivary Glands*, Washington, DC, pp. 13–14.

Theriault C, Fitzpatrick P J (1986) Malignant parotid tumours. *Am J Clin Oncol* **9**:510–16.

Van Miert P J, Dawes J D K, Harkness D G (1968) The treatment of mixed parotid tumours. *J Laryngol Otol* **82**:459–68.

Vikram B, Strong E W, Shah J, Spiro R H (1980) Elective postoperative radiation therapy in stages III and IV epidermoid carcinoma of the head and neck. *Am J Surg* **140**:580–4.

Ward C M (1975) Injury of the facial nerve during surgery of the parotid gland. *Br J Surg* **62**:401–3.

Wheelis R F, Yarington C T Jr (1984) Tumors of the salivary glands: comparison of frozen-section diagnosis with final pathologic diagnosis. *Arch Otolaryngol* **110**:76.

Woods J E, Chong G C, Beahrs O H (1975) Experience with 1360 primary parotid tumors. *Am J Surg* **130**:460.

Work W P (1977) Parapharyngeal space and salivary gland neoplasms. *Otolaryngol Clin North Am* **10**:421–6.

Work N A, Hybels R L (1974) A study of tumours of the parapharyngeal space. *Laryngoscope* **84**:1748–55.

Work W P, Batsakis J G, Bailey D G (1976) Recurrent benign mixed tumor and the facial nerve. *Arch Otolaryngol* **102**:15.

20

Tumours of the thyroid gland

Surgical anatomy

The morbidity created by a poorly performed thyroid operation can be as great as or greater than the morbidity caused by leaving some thyroid lesions alone. Thus, it is vital to know the important points of surgical anatomy in relation to the thyroid gland, as well as the surgical pathology and behaviour of thyroid disease.

The superior thyroid artery runs down to the upper pole, in close proximity to the external branch of the superior laryngeal nerve; this nerve can be damaged if the vessel is ligated too high. The effect of section of this nerve is that the patient's vocal range is then limited but, unless he or she is a singer, it is unlikely to be noticed. The inferior thyroid artery arises from the thyrocervical trunk, pierces the prevertebral fascia medial to the carotid sheath, and enters the posterior part of the gland. Before any branch of the inferior thyroid artery is divided, it is necessary to identify the recurrent laryngeal nerve on each side.

The recurrent laryngeal nerves (Fig. 20.1) run in the tracheo-oesophageal groove and can be in front of, or behind, the inferior thyroid arteries. The nerves may occasionally lie lateral to the groove and even pass between the branches of the artery. At the level of the upper two or three tracheal rings they are closely applied to the posterior surface of the thyroid gland and may penetrate it. They usually divide into anterior and posterior branches before entering the larynx. On the right side it is important to remember that there are even more variations of the recurrent laryngeal nerve (Fig. 20.1). In some instances the recurrent nerve is not even recurrent. There may be extralaryngeal divisions as far as 3–4 cm below the inferior border of the cricoid.

The superior pair of parathyroid glands (Fig. 20.2) is usually in or near the capsule of the upper third of the thyroid gland, posteriorly at the level of the cricoid cartilage; the lower pair is much less posteriorly placed on the lower poles, close to the

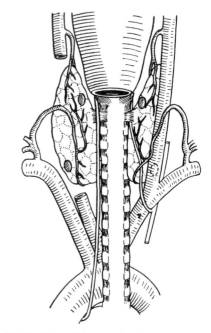

Fig. 20.1 Position of the parathyroid glands.

branches of the inferior thyroid artery. Parathyroid tissue can, however, occur anywhere in the neck.

The major lymphatic drainage is to the middle and lower deep jugular nodes, but some lymphatics drain to the pre- and paratracheal nodes and thus to the mediastinal nodes.

Surgical pathology

Incidence

Carcinoma of the thyroid gland is not common. The incidence is about 12 per million of the population in the UK; in the USA it is 36 per million per year. It is estimated, however, that only 6 people per million

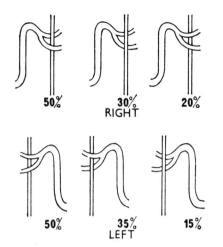

Fig. 20.2 Variations in the course of the recurrent laryngeal nerve.

die of thyroid carcinoma annually in the USA. Most deaths are from undifferentiated thyroid cancer. The otolaryngologist undertaking neck surgery must understand the pathology and the principles of treatment of thyroid cancer because a significant number of these patients will present with hoarseness due to invasion of the larynx, to recurrent laryngeal nerve paralysis, or with neck masses.

Aetiology

Four factors are now known to be of importance in the causation of thyroid cancer.

The first of these is an increased secretion of thyroid-stimulating hormone (TSH) by the anterior pituitary gland. It will be recalled that this thyroid secretion is controlled by a feedback mechanism between the pituitary and the thyroid. Thus, if the thyroid gland fails to secrete a sufficient amount of its hormones, thyroxine (T_4) and tri-iodothyronine (T_3), because of diminished uptake of iodine, then there is a rise in secretion of TSH by the pituitary gland. This can stimulate an abnormal gland to undergo malignant change.

Thus, in areas of the world such as Switzerland, where goitre is very common because of the diminished iodine intake, the incidence of thyroid cancer should be increased. This does in fact occur, the mortality rate in Switzerland from cancer of the thyroid being approximately 10 times that in England and Wales. Furthermore, the increased incidence is due to a higher number of follicular carcinomas occurring in nodular parenchymatous goitres. Conversely, in Iceland, where the intake of iodine is high, thyroid carcinoma is very uncommon and those that do occur are usually papillary in type.

It is hazardous to dismiss all thyroid enlargement

as benign adenomatous goitre. Up to 21% of patients who are found to have thyroid cancer have a history of 'goitre'. There is a 5% incidence of cancer in goitre patients. There is a 14% incidence of cancer in goitres that had a suspicion of malignancy and a 4% incidence in goitres removed for other reasons.

The second known aetiological factor in thyroid carcinoma is ionizing radiation. Between 1920 and 1940, young patients were treated by radiation to cause involution of the thymus, or of tonsils and adenoids, to treat adolescent acne, to treat tuberculous cervical adenitis, to control unwanted facial hair, and as a valid therapy for other malignancies. The association of irradiation with the subsequent development of thyroid cancer has been well documented over the past 30 years. One investigation found 8.3 cases of thyroid cancer per 1000 irradiation patients after a follow-up of 20 years. This exceeded the spontaneous rate by 100 times. The high-dose group had a rate 300 times that expected, and it was calculated that the mortality from thyroid cancer due to irradiation would be 38–52 cases per 10^6 persons exposed per rad of thyroid dose per year. The latent period before cancers occur is 10–15 years and the peak incidence is 20–30 years after exposure. It has also been found that 59% of the radiation-created tumours are multifocal, and 25% are node-positive.

The third factor, which is much less definite, is the genetic one. There does appear to be a definite tendency for hyperthyroidism, goitre and thyroid carcinoma to occur in members of the same family.

The fourth factor is the development of medullary carcinoma in patients with other endocrine neoplasias, in the context of the multiple endocrine neoplasia (MEN) syndrome.

Types of tumour

Tumours of the thyroid gland can originate from any of the cellular components of the gland – follicular and parafollicular cells, vascular endothelium, stromal fibroblasts and lymphocytes. The vast majority, however, arise from follicular cells, and other types are rare. The only known neoplasm of parafollicular cell origin is the medullary carcinoma. It is doubtful if fibrosarcoma and angiosarcoma occur, and malignant lymphomas are rare, usually arising within a lymphocytic thyroiditis.

Follicular cell neoplasms can be classified into three major categories – papillary, follicular and anaplastic (undifferentiated). The percentage distribution of these and medullary carcinoma is shown in Figure 20.3.

Papillary adenocarcinoma

This is the most differentiated tumour of all, and the most common (50%). It occurs in all age groups and is virtually the only thyroid cancer of children. Its

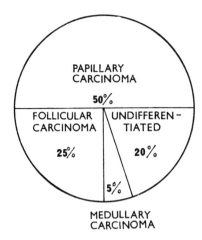

Fig. 20.3 Pathology of thyroid carcinoma.

most frequent age incidence, however, is from 40 to 49 years. Typically, papillary adenocarcinoma presents as a nodule in the thyroid; it is associated with a high incidence of enlarged cervical lymph nodes (60%). On occasion, the primary tumour in the thyroid may be so small as to be impalable and the patient then presents because of the neck node enlargement. The neoplasm is very often multifocal (80%) and found in both lobes. One in 10 patients with this disease has bony metastasis, and 1 in 5 pulmonary metastasis. The 10-year survival from occult or intrathyroid papillary carcinoma is over 90%, when it is extrathyroid, the 10-year survival falls to 60%.

In the older age groups the tumour tends to behave in a more aggressive fashion and may invade the larynx and trachea.

Follicular adenocarcinoma

This occurs in the older age groups, being commonest between 50 and 59 years, and seldom being seen under the age of 30. Twenty-five per cent of thyroid cancers are in this group. Typically it has a well-defined capsule and can be divided into two sub-groups depending on whether the capsule has or has not been breached.

Follicular carcinoma may present in one of two ways: either as obvious malignant change in a thyroid swelling that may have been present for many years; or, in an almost equal number of instances, because of the symptoms or signs of metastasis to the bones or lungs. As well as invading locally, therefore, these tumours commonly metastasize to bone. One patient in 3 will have a bone metastasis, especially to the flat bones and the ends of the long bones where red marrow is found. A high proportion (25%) will metastasize to the lungs and about 20% to lymph nodes. A typical feature is that many of these

tumours and their metastases readily take up radio-active iodine; they are the only thyroid tumours to do so.

Anaplastic neoplasms

These have no characteristic architecture and bear no resemblance to normal thyroid cells. They are aggressively malignant and have a high metastatic potential. They are subclassified into small cell, giant cell and spindle cell types, depending on the predominant cell morphology. The differential diagnosis includes metastatic malignancies and lymphoma. If metastatic neoplasms from other sites involve the thyroid, the commonest sources are the kidney and the breast.

Anaplastic tumours are common in the elderly and in women, and many of them are superimposed on a long-standing enlargement of the thyroid gland, which then begins to increase in size rapidly, associated with pain referred to the ear and hoarseness. They rapidly invade surrounding structures, such as the larynx, pharynx and oesophagus, and carry a uniformly bad prognosis. Ninety-two per cent of patients are dead within 1 year of treatment, and no therapy has any marked effect.

Medullary thyroid carcinoma

This occurs in the MEN syndrome (see above). It is frequently bilateral (90%), and cervical node metastasis varies from 25 to 50%. The tumours arise from the parafollicular or C cells, which secrete calcitonin, so that many patients with this tumour have large amounts of this hormone in their peripheral blood. Despite this, the serum calcium levels remain normal, which casts some doubt on the physiological importance of calcitonin in the regulation of calcium metabolism. Some of these patients also suffer from severe diarrhoea, which has now been shown to be caused by prostaglandin secreted by the tumour and its metastases. There may also be a cryptic phaeochromocytoma, which may be synchronous or may appear in symptomatic form as much as a decade before or after the medullary cancer.

Other neoplasms

Thyroid lymphomas are sometimes difficult to differentiate from the rare, small cell type of anaplastic carcinoma unless immunocytochemistry is used. These tumours are commoner in elderly women and may be related to pre-existing Hashimoto's disease.

The Hürthle cell adenoma is extremely uncommon. It should be regarded as a malignant tumour containing Askanazy cells. It arises from follicular cells containing abundant eosinophilic granular cytoplasm and the term 'oxyphil cell tumour' is sometimes used.

Investigations

History

A history of radiation in childhood and a family history of thyroid disease is important to establish.

The patient's age is the most critical factor. The likelihood of malignancy is high in young patients, lessens in middle age, and increases again after the age of 50–60 years. The incidence of anaplastic thyroid cancer increases after the age of 50–60 years. A thyroid nodule in a patient under 30 years old has a 15–35% chance of malignancy. Of these, over 80% have cervical lymph node metastases. In elderly males, the likelihood of a solitary thyroid mass being malignant is 6%.

Forty per cent of patients will present with neck node metastases. Hoarseness (13%), pressure on the airway or oesophagus (8%) and pain, often referred to the ear (5%) are other presenting features.

Pain, rapid growth of a mass, and unilateral vocal cord paralysis are ominous signs, and are seen in 70% of patients with anaplastic thyroid cancers.

Examination

Examine the thyroid gland, looking particularly for hardness. Note if any swelling goes up and down when the patient swallows, and try to get below the swelling in the midline. If there is a retrosternal prolongation of the tumour, extend the patient's neck and see if the tumour comes up into the neck. Cysts feel as if they are full of fluid, colloid nodules feel doughty, and papillary and medullary cancers frequently feel like hard rubber nodules. Anaplastic tumours are hard, fixed and craggy, and lymphomas are frequently diffuse.

Palpate the neck and axilla carefully for lymph nodes and finally, examine the larynx and pharynx for invasion by tumour or vocal cord paralysis.

Radiology

X-ray the chest and soft tissues of the neck, the former to show metastases, and the latter, deviation and compression of the trachea. Psammoma bodies are characteristic of papillary thyroid cancer and, when they are calcified in advanced tumours, they may appear as finely stippled areas on soft tissue films.

Ultrasonography can distinguish purely cystic nodules. Only rarely (less than 5%) is a cystic nodule associated with a thyroid cancer.

The computed tomography (CT) scan is of help in assessing the extent and relationship of larger thyroid tumours.

The 'gold standard' of investigation is the thyroid scan, using technetium (^{99m}Tc), which has a very short half-life. A dose of 37 MBq of technetium is injected intravenously and the neck is scanned within the next half-hour. Typically, a follicular carcinoma and its metastases take up radioactive iodine, whereas no other tumour does so in its natural state. A 'cold' area may thus be the site of a carcinoma but all nodules that are 'cold' on scan are far from being malignant, as this appearance may be due to haemorrhage or degeneration in a cystic goitre. The majority of malignant lesions (95%) are 'cold' but the incidence of malignancy in solitary 'cold' nodules is only 5–30%.

'Hot' nodules may be associated with general glandular hyperfunction and, in general, are not operated on for the suspicion of cancer.

Unless, the nodule is hyperfunctioning, clinical criteria rather than the appearance of a scan should contribute most to the decision of whether to treat surgically.

Laboratory investigations

Measure the T_3 and T_4 and serum calcium to provide baselines for the postoperative management of the patient. Measure the thyroid antibodies, as Hashimoto's disease may be difficult to distinguish clinically from carcinoma. If medullary carcinoma is suspected, measure the calcitonin in the peripheral blood before and after measures to provoke the stimulation of calcitonin.

Biopsy

A thyroid lobectomy, encompassing the lesion, will give the best material that can be evaluated for histological purposes. It is easier, however, to do a cutting needle-core biopsy or a fine-needle aspiration biopsy. The major difficulty with fine-needle aspiration comes in the assessment of whether or not a follicular neoplasm is benign or malignant.

Treatment policy

The treatment of thyroid malignancy is multidisciplinary in nature, involving five distinct and complementary modalities. These are surgery, radioiodine treatment, external beam radiotherapy, hormonal manipulation and chemotherapy. Selection of the most appropriate combination depends on both the tumour pathology and extent of disease.

In general, for operable differentiated carcinoma of follicular cell origin, the most important treatment is full surgery. This usually entails total thyroidectomy and removal of involved lymph nodes. Subsequently ablation of the inevitable remnant of thyroid tissue should be undertaken with radioiodine. Later, the patient is scanned to see if there is any residual focus of uptake in the neck or elsewhere, which would indicate active malignancy requiring radio-iodine therapy. Those patients with differentiated carcinoma of follicular cell origin which does not accumulate iodine, and patients with medullary carcinoma, should receive postoperative external beam therapy if surgery was incomplete or in the case of any extrathyroid spread. Meticulous long-term follow-up is mandatory, maintaining patients with differentiated carcinoma of follicular cell origin on doses of thyroid hormone adequate to suppress TSH production. Radical external beam radiotherapy is often indicated for patients with undifferentiated carcinoma, and those with inoperable differentiated or medullary carcinoma. Patients with thyroid lymphoma will require radiotherapy, and perhaps chemotherapy also.

Papillary adenocarcinoma

A patient with papillary adenocarcinoma will usually have a mass in one lobe of the thyroid, very often associated with enlarged lymph nodes in the neck. The most important part of treatment is surgery, a thyroidectomy and neck dissection. There is controversy, however, over how much thyroid to remove and what sort of neck dissection to carry out. For example, some consider that in a young woman with a solitary, very small tumour without nodal metastases, lobectomy alone is adequate. Similarly, if a partial thyroidectomy is performed for multinodular goitre, and histology reveals an unsuspected focus of microscopic malignancy, no further treatment is required.

Nevertheless there are several cogent reasons for advocating more radical surgery in the majority of patients. Firstly, the tumour is multifocal in the majority of patients. Secondly, patients treated with limited surgery are significantly more likely both to have a local recurrence and to die from their malignancy than those who have had complete excision. Similarly, transformation from an initially well-differentiated tumour to an anaplastic carcinoma is more common after minimal surgery. Finally, the use of thyroglobulin as a tumour marker, and the use of radioactive iodine for the imaging and treatment of differentiated carcinoma are both completely dependent on the absence of functioning normal thyroid tissue. In addition it should not be forgotten that to reoperate on the thyroid is technically more difficult than to do an adequate operation the first time around, when fewer complications are likely to result.

For these reasons, total thyroidectomy is the operation of choice. In reality, the morbidity resulting from a truly total thyroidectomy is unacceptable, and so a near-total thyroidectomy is performed, in which a sliver of the contralateral lobe, containing

one parathyroid, is preserved. The extent of nodal surgery depends on the extent of lymphatic involvement. The lymphatics of the thyroid gland drain to nodes in the tracheo-oesophageal groove, to mediastinal (particularly thymic) nodes, to the pre-laryngeal node, and to the jugular chain; some of the lymphatic trunks also pass through the wall of the trachea. From this it is obvious that a true radical neck dissection for a thyroid cancer, with all its draining nodes, would be a massive and mutilating bilateral procedure. What is therefore practised instead is removal of all enlarged nodes, including where necessary those in the mediastinum, without attempting a full clearance of uninvolved nodes, or sacrificing the sternomastoid, jugular vein or accessory nerve. The aim of the combined total thyroidectomy and limited lymphadenectomy is to remove all macroscopic malignancy.

Subsequently, in the immediate postoperative period, before thyroid hormone replacement has been started, remaining thyroid function should be ablated with a single dose of radioiodine. This is done whether or not the tumour itself concentrates iodine. In fact, most papillary carcinomas have a follicular component and about 80% of well-differentiated carcinomas of follicular cell origin – not just follicular carcinoma – accumulate iodine adequately for imaging and therapy. Scanning with radioiodine for functioning residual disease or metastases is undertaken at 3 months, by which time the initial treatment will have abolished residual normal tissue. Earlier assessment is not possible, as the avidity of tumour for iodine is always considerably less than that of normal thyroid tissue. If any uptake is demonstrated, a therapy dose is given. This is repeated every 3–6 months until all tumour is eradicated or the disease progresses. In the minority of patients whose tumours do not accumulate iodine, postoperative external beam radiotherapy should be considered if the operative clearance was dubious or macroscopically incomplete, or if there was extensive nodal involvement.

After this combined primary treatment with optimal surgery and radioiodine or external irradiation, the patient should be placed on a dose of T_4, usually 300 mg/day, adequate to suppress TSH levels fully. Thereafter patients should be followed up regularly. As the disease may recur after decades of inactivity, surveillance should probably be for life. Thyroglobulin assay has now replaced routine radioiodine scanning, although this is of course indicated if thyroglobulin levels rise. Patients with inoperable differentiated carcinoma which fails to accumulate iodine may benefit from radical radiotherapy.

Follicular adenocarcinoma

The management of follicular adenocarcinoma is very similar to that of papillary tumours. The mainstay of treatment is surgery. This entails a total thyroidectomy with removal of any masses in the neck or superior mediastinum. Subsequently ablation of the thyroid remnant is performed, followed in 3 months by screening for residual disease in the neck or metastases. Haematogenous spread is more common with follicular than with papillary carcinoma. The most frequently affected sites are lung and bone. In contrast to squamous carcinoma of the head and neck, and indeed most other solid tumours, distant dissemination is not a death sentence. About half of those receiving radio-iodine for pulmonary deposits alone will survive 10 or 15 years. The prognosis is, however, much worse for those with osseous disease, and in patients whose tumours fail to concentrate iodine. With follicular tumours, adequate iodine uptake is less likely in the elderly and in those with less well-differentiated tumours. Following initial treatment, suppressive T_4 replacement and regular surveillance with thyroglo-bulin measurement are indicated, as in the case of papillary carcinoma.

Medullary carcinoma

The principal treatment advised for the patient with medullary carcinoma is surgery. This should be radical and entails total thyroidectomy and removal of any enlarged lymph node masses, extending the operation into the superior mediastinum if necess-ary. If an unexpected diagnosis of medullary carci-noma is made following lobectomy, lymph node biopsy or other incomplete surgery, reoperation is required to remove remaining disease. As these tumours arise from the parafollicular cells, it is not surprising that they do not accumulate radioiodine.

Postoperative radiotherapy is indicated if there is any suggestion of residual disease in the neck, whether clinically, pathologically or because the tumour markers, calcitonin and carcinoembryonic antigen, fail to return to normal despite the absence of haematogenous spread. Patients with disease considered inoperable either due to the advanced nature of the primary tumour or nodal disease, or because of serious intercurrent illness, should be considered for radiotherapy. Although the aim of this is principally palliative, a full 'radical' treatment course is required, and cure may be anticipated in a proportion. Although medullary carcinoma is more chemoresponsive than carcinoma of follicular cell origin, and some patients have benefited from pallia-tive chemotherapy, there is no regimen that can be considered as routine for patients with this disease. Because of its significant toxicity and limited effi-cacy, cytotoxic drug treatment should only be con-sidered for patients with distressing symptoms refractory to other treatments.

Anaplastic tumours

A biopsy is mandatory to confirm that a patient suspected to have an anaplastic carcinoma does not have lymphoma which may be curable. Apart from this, surgery, and also radioiodine, has no part to play in the management of anaplastic carcinoma. Regression may, however, be produced by radical radiotherapy, but early recurrence is the rule, lead-ing almost inevitably to death within 6–12 months. Attempts to improve the dismal prognosis in this disease with chemotherapy have been disappointing, and none is recommended. In some patients the disease may be so advanced at presentation that, once the diagnosis is confirmed, no active treatment is the kindest policy.

Thyroid lymphoma

If the clinical condition at presentation permits, patients with thyroid lymphoma should be fully staged prior to treatment. The system is the same as for extranodal lymphoma at other sites. That is, patients with disease confined to the thyroid com-prise stage I, those also with nodal disease in the neck or mediastinum are in stage II and those with subdiaphragmatic nodal disease fall into stage III. Evidence of extranodal involvement in organs other than the thyroid, such as the liver, gut or bone marrow indicates stage IV disease.

Although no surgery other than biopsy is usually considered to be necessary for lymphoma at other sites, surgical removal of bulk disease has been shown to improve both local control and survival in patients with thyroid lymphoma. Thyroidectomy is therefore indicated if feasible, although radiother-apy remains the principal treatment for thyroid lymphoma. While radiotherapy may produce a very dramatic resolution of the tumour mass, treatment must continue until the end of the prescribed course to ensure sustained local control. Patients with high-grade histology and more advanced disease should in addition receive appropriate chemotherapy, if permitted by their general condition.

Thyroid nodule

For many years there has been controversy about how to manage the solitary thyroid nodule. There are two incontrovertible facts, however. Firstly, a proportion of them may be malignant and secondly, a nodule that appears to be solitary on palpation may merely be part of a multinodular cystic goitre.

If an apparently solitary nodule is found in a patient who is euthyroid, then ultrasound investi-gation and a technetium scan should be performed. If the ultrasound shows that it is a solitary cyst, then fine-needle aspiration is done together with cytology. If it is benign, then the patient may be observed on a regular basis or investigated for thyroiditis. If there is a suspicion of malignancy, a follicular pattern or a Hürthle cell pattern, then the patient should have the minimum biopsy, which is a lobectomy plus removal of the isthmus.

If the technetium scan shows a multinodular goitre, then the only reason to operate is for hyperfunction, obstruction or rapid increase in size. If it shows a cold nodule, then in those with a high cancer risk a lobectomy and removal of the isthmus should be performed. Those with a high cancer risk are under 30 years, have had prior head and neck irradiation, have a hard nodule that has shown some growth potential, have hoarseness, airway obstruction, palpable cervical nodes, a nodule bigger than 3 cm, fixation of nodule, and a family history of MEN 2.

If the patient is over 30 years, and has a soft nodule that is not fixed, then a fine-needle aspiration biopsy should be done, and surgery considered if it is malignant and has a follicular or a Hürthle cell pattern.

Technique of operations on the thyroid gland

Lobectomy

Incision

Position the patient with the neck extended, and prepare and drape the neck in the usual way. Mark out a collar incision with methylene blue in a skin crease over the middle of the thyroid gland. Never cut without making a mark as this easily leads to an asymmetrical scar.

Cut through skin and platysma, and with traction on the flaps elevate them down to the sternum and up to the upper edge of the thyroid cartilage. Then retract the flaps and exclude the skin from the wound by using a Joll's thyroid retractor.

Isolation of the recurrent laryngeal nerve

The essential step in a lobectomy is preservation of the recurrent laryngeal nerve; isolate it first and ensure its safety (Fig. 20.4).

Find the nerve low in the neck, where it lies in the groove between the trachea and the oesophagus. Approach this plane by separating the strap muscles vertically in the midline: then either retract the strap muscles laterally or divide them low in the neck. Dissect posteriorly next to the wall of the trachea, inferior to the thyroid isthmus as far as the groove between the trachea and the oesophagus, deep in the neck. The recurrent laryngeal nerve lies in this groove, although occasionally it may be a little lateral to this but still deep in the neck. It is readily recognizable as a fairly thick nerve about 2 mm wide.

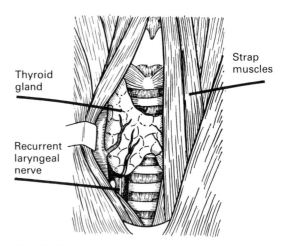

Fig. 20.4 Exposure of recurrent laryngeal nerve.

It is a good idea to practice recognition of this nerve during total laryngectomy, when it does not matter if it is cut.

During the course of this dissection, tie and divide the inferior thyroid veins.

Removal of the gland

After finding the recurrent laryngeal nerve trace it upwards, lifting the gland off it. Never lift up the nerve or squeeze it. Just dissect all tissues off it, leaving it undisturbed in its bed. Also never use diathermy near the nerve, and tie all bleeding points using small mosquito forceps and fine ties, being careful never to catch the nerve in a tie.

After elevating the lower part of the gland progress is held up because of the lateral attachments of the gland. Therefore, next retract the strap muscles, divide the middle thyroid vein (Fig. 20.5) and divide the loose fascia lateral and posterior to the middle part of the gland.

The whole of the lobe can now be easily swung medially and upwards, to allow dissection of the recurrent laryngeal nerve to proceed.

About this time the next thing to look for is the inferior thyroid artery. Divide it well lateral to the recurrent laryngeal nerve and transfix the proximal end.

Continue dissecting the recurrent laryngeal nerve until it divides and disappears into the larynx. Mobilize the upper lobe, transfixing the vascular pedicle and preserving the superior laryngeal nerve. Lastly remove the lobe (Fig. 20.6) including the isthmus, and a small slice of the opposite lobe to prevent an unsightly bump after healing has taken place.

Palpate the jugular lymphatic chain, remove individually any obviously enlarged nodes and send them for examination.

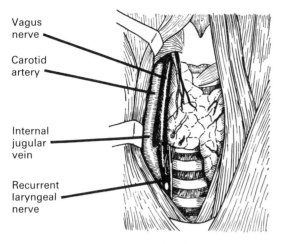

Vagus
nerve

Carotid
artery

Internal
jugular
vein

Recurrent
laryngeal
nerve

Fig. 20.5 Division of middle thyroid vein.

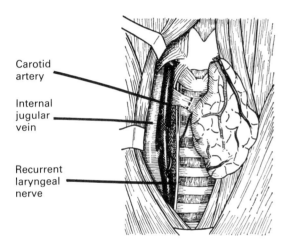

Carotid
artery

Internal
jugular
vein

Recurrent
laryngeal
nerve

Fig. 20.6 Division of superior thyroid pedicle.

Wash the wound in the usual way, and close it with suction drainage.

Total thyroidectomy

This operation is required for follicular adenocarcinoma and for medullary carcinoma, and for papillary adenocarcinoma where there is spread to lymph nodes.

Incision

A gland dissection will often be required, either at the time or later. Access for this can be gained by a collar incision with lateral limbs up to the mastoid process and down to the clavicle at the insertion of the trapezius.

Isolating the recurrent laryngeal nerve

Patients needing a total thyroidectomy may have spread of the tumour beyond the capsule of the thyroid gland. For this reason it may not be possible to preserve the recurrent laryngeal nerves and the parathyroid glands. This is unfortunate because division of the recurrent laryngeal nerve on one side, or unilateral loss of the parathyroid glands, can be compensated for, whereas the loss of both recurrent laryngeal nerves or all the parathyroid tissues leads to problems.

Begin dissection in the same way, by separating the strap muscles in the midline, and then either divide or retract them. Continue the dissection down the side of the trachea to the tracheo-oesophageal groove, and proceed to identify the recurrent laryngeal nerve in the same way as in a lobectomy. If the tumour has invaded outside the capsule in the region of the nerves, sacrifice them rather than the patient's chance of survival.

Removal of the gland

Continue the dissection in the same way as for a lobectomy, provided there is no spread beyond the gland. It may be necessary on occasion to include surrounding invaded structures in the dissection, particularly part of the tracheal wall. Once the lobe is free do not divide the isthmus but mobilize the opposite lobe in the same fashion and remove the gland in one piece.

In total thyroidectomy it is important to preserve at least two of the parathyroid glands if possible. As they are embedded in the substance of the thyroid gland, this means that a small sliver of thyroid tissue must be preserved. The glands are inconstant in position, the upper pair being the most constant, lying opposite the cricoid cartilage. Magnification helps in recognizing the glands, which are tan-coloured, and are most easily found by following the anastomotic branch between the superior and inferior thyroid arteries, near which they lie, on the back of the thyroid gland.

In a papillary adenocarcinoma, if glands are palpable, enlarge the incision by a lateral limb extending up to the mastoid process: if necessary, further access can be gained by a lower lateral limb running downwards to the clavicle at the point of insertion of the trapezius. Then remove individually any obviously enlarged glands. A formal radical neck dissection is not only unnecessary but is also illogical in this disease.

In medullary carcinoma it may be necessary very occasionally to split the sternum and dissect out glands in the superior mediastinum. Although this operation is not difficult, the help of a thoracic surgeon will usually be needed.

If part of the tracheal wall has been removed it

must now be repaired. There are two ways of doing this: either by Marlex mesh or by reanastomosis.

Marlex is a synthetic material supplied in a mesh. Cut a piece large enough to fit the defect and stitch it into place with sutures of Marlex. The mesh allows granulation tissue to grow through into the lumen of the trachea, so that ciliated epithelium can regenerate on its inside.

Reanastomosis of the trachea is described in Chapter 11. If less than four rings of the trachea are involved, they can be resected and continuity restored by end-to-end anastomosis (p. 157)

Closure

If for any reason the patient having a total thyroidectomy needs a tracheostomy, do it through a hole in the lower flap and not through the incision.

Wash the wound in the usual way and close it with suction drainage and clips.

Aftercare

1 General care.
2 Thyroid replacement. Replacement with T_4 is always needed. In patients with papillary carcinomas with no metastases, begin replacement a few days after operation, with 0.2 mg L-thyroxine daily. It is unnecessary to give this in a divided dose. Even if a lobectomy has been done, T_4 should still be given to prevent stimulation of the remaining thyroid tissue by TSH if the patient has a papillary carcinoma.
3 Follow-up. Patients with papillary carcinoma should be followed for many years at 3-monthly intervals to detect the appearance of enlarged lymph nodes. If these do appear, remove them individually – it is unnecessary to carry out a formal radical neck dissection.

Patients with follicular carcinoma should have a ^{123}I or ^{131}I scan and uptake every 6 months and should be treated with radioactive iodine if more than 10% of a tracer dose is retained. The technique is described on p. 000.

Complications

1 General complications.
2 Respiratory obstruction. This should not occur after a lobectomy, but may occur after a total thyroidectomy if there was tracheal compression before operation.
3 Bleeding. Two common sites of bleeding after thyroidectomy are the inferior thyroid veins and the branches of the inferior thyroid artery in the vicinity of the recurrent laryngeal nerve. The danger is pressure on the exposed trachea, resulting in respiratory obstruction. If this happens, open the wound in the ward and return the patient to theatre; look for the bleeding points carefully, and if they are in the vicinity of the recurrent laryngeal nerve, clamp and tie them carefully using mosquito forceps and fine ties – *never* use diathermy in this area.
4 Hypoparathyroidism – immediate or delayed. This should be looked for by serum calcium estimation, in the immediate period after operation and at 6 monthly intervals. If it occurs treat it by calcium and vitamin D supplements, as outlined on page 28.

Radiotherapy techniques

Radioiodine treatment

The procedure to be followed for both ablation of residual normal thyroid tissue and treatment of functioning residual disease or metastases is the same. The patient should be admitted to a hospital and accommodated in a single room equipped, for radiation protection purposes, with private toilet facilities or a commode. The patient should have been warned to avoid iodine-containing foods over the previous 3 weeks and should not have had any recent radiological investigations such as intravenous urography which use iodine-containing contrast media. As most patients with thyroid cancer are women, many of child-bearing age, the possibility of pregnancy must be excluded before radioiodine therapy is given. Lactating mothers must stop breast-feeding their infants. The patient must either not have commenced or should have stopped thyroid hormone replacement in time to allow endogenous TSH levels to rise and stimulate uptake of iodine. The TSH level should be measured before radioiodine therapy, if it is not greater than 33 mu/l exogenous TSH administration is required.

The isotope of iodine used for therapy is ^{131}I, given as a drink or capsule of sodium iodide. The dose prescribed is 3 GBq (80 mCi) for ablation of a small thyroid remnant, or 5.5 GBq (150 mCi) for treatment of tumour. The whole-body effective half-life of this radionuclide is considerably shorter than its physical half-life of 8 days, as the variable biological half-life is often less than a day. In contrast, such is the avidity of differentiated thyroid carcinoma for iodine, that the effective half-life in tumour, although again variable, is at least 3 days. The significance of this is that scanning 3 or 4 days after administration of a therapy dose allows imaging of the tumour after the whole-body radioiodine level has become negligible. Accumulation of radioiodine occurs not only in the thyroid gland and carcinoma, but also in the bladder and salivary glands. In order to minimize the radiation dose to pelvic organs and prevent sialitis or xerostomia, the patient should drink plenty to establish a diuresis, and suck lemon sweets to stimulate salivation. The patient is discharged home when the measured whole-body radio-activity has fallen to the permissible level of 30 MBq (about 1 mCi) if travelling home by private car or, if going by bus or train, to 15 MBq (less than 0.5 mCi).

When the need for further ^{131}I therapy or diagnostic scanning is anticipated, suppressive thyroid hormone replacement should be with T_3, 20 μg three times daily, rather than with T_4, as its half-life is considerably shorter, enabling a more rapid rise in TSH levels after its withdrawal. It is necessary to stop T_3 replacement about 10 days prior to radioiodine administration in order to allow TSH levels to rise adequately.

External beam radiotherapy

The planning of radiotherapy for thyroid carcinoma is complicated by various factors. Firstly, a large volume must be covered to encompass both the primary tumour and draining nodal areas. Secondly, the body contour changes rapidly in both the sagittal and coronal planes. In addition, the spinal cord lies just behind the target volume. Great care must be taken to ensure that the radiation dose received by this critical structure is kept within its tolerance, while an adequate radiation dose must be delivered to the tumour. For simulation and treatment the patient lies supine, with the cervical spine as straight as possible, immobilized in a shell. This covers the whole neck and upper chest, extending from the base of the skull, down to nipple level. The central axis of the treatment beam is angled so that it is perpendicular to the spinal cord. To enable accurate dosimetry,

at least three contours are taken (Fig. 20.7), parallel to the central axis, on which the position of the tumour, cord and air gaps can be marked. The advent of CT planning has made this process much easier and more accurate.

The volume to be treated depends on the tumour type and extent of disease. For treatment of differentiated carcinoma of follicular cell origin following optimal surgery without bulky nodal disease, the treatment volume can be limited to the tumour bed and adjacent nodal areas bilaterally. The upper and lower margins of the volume are the hyoid bone and the suprasternal notch. When there has been extensive nodal disease, the volume must be extended posteriorly to include all cervical nodes and also inferiorly to the carina to include the superior mediastinum. Similarly, in the case of anaplastic and medullary carcinoma, a large volume must also be treated. In addition, treatment of the medial supraclavicular fossa nodes is also recommended in these histological types if there was bulky central disease. In cases of lymphoma yet more generous fields are used, with the upper limit at the submentomastoid line, the lower limit at the carina and laterally including the supra- and infraclavicular nodes.

Several conceptually different techniques have been devised to overcome the difficulties outlined above. In centres where high-energy (20 MeV) electrons are available, a direct anterior electron field can be used. This has the advantage of delivering a fairly uniform dose to a particular depth of tissue, beyond which the dose falls off quite rapidly. A tissue-equivalent wax compensator is prepared which lies centrally and on the sides of the shell and, taking into account the increased transmission of

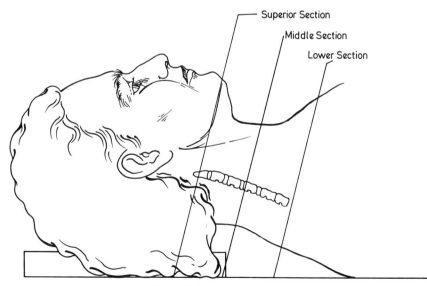

Fig. 20.7 Levels at which contours are taken for radiotherapy planning purposes.

electrons through the air in the trachea, limits the dose to the cord. Laterally in the neck there is less wax anteriorly to attenuate the electron beam, but there is wax at the sides to maintain the dose on the skin surface. With this arrangement the high dose volume is horseshoe-shaped, encompassing the nodes, yet sparing the cord (Fig. 20.8).

Many radiotherapy centres are, however not equipped with electron facilities of the appropriate energy, and conventional megavoltage photon therapy must be used instead. Here, a small, anterior volume may adequately be treated with two wedged anterior oblique fields (Fig. 20.9). Larger volumes are often treated with a two-phase technique. Initially an anterior and posterior parallel opposed pair of fields is used, with lead blocks to shield the lung apices and, in lymphoma, the oral mucosa. The dose to the spinal cord is limited by use of a central spine block on the posterior field. The dose given in the first phase should be adequate to sterilize microscopic disease, and the lower dose received by the cord is well-tolerated. The second phase treats a smaller volume. The site of previous or residual bulk disease is irradiated to a high dose by a more complex technique. Often a three-field technique with a direct anterior and two anterior oblique fields is used. Custom-made tissue compensators provide

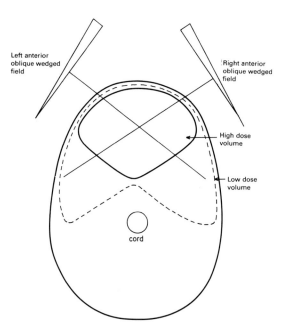

Fig. 20.9 Field arrangement for irradiation of a small anterior volume.

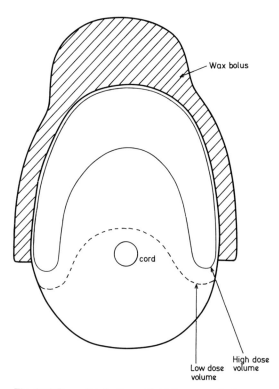

Fig. 20.8 Dose distribution with high-energy electron treatment of thyroid cancer.

the best way of ensuring dose homogeneity. Alternatively, careful use of wedges in both planes can compensate to some extent for the changing contour in both directions, if proper tissue compensator facilities are not available. In the case of thyroid lymphoma, where a lower total dose is necessary, the phase 1 technique alone is adequate.

The dose prescribed for localized treatment of well-differentiated tumours is 60 Gy in 30 fractions over 6 weeks. In the first phase of wide-field treatments for anaplastic, medullary, or extensive differentiated tumours, a dose of 50 Gy in 25 fractions over 5 weeks is given, with a phase 2 boost of a further 10–15 Gy in 10–12 additional daily fractions. Lymphoma requires a dose of 40 Gy in 20 fractions over 4 weeks.

Controversies

Fine-needle aspiration biopsy

Fine-needle aspiration biopsy of a thyroid mass is the diagnostic test of choice, provided there is a physician able to obtain a good sample by the technique, and provided there is a trained cytologist experienced in the analysis of these biopsy specimens. It is a simple test requiring inexpensive equipment, and it can give a same-day result.

The major limitation relates to the small amount

of tissue obtained. The main problem is with follicular neoplasms because their biological potential cannot be determined from cytological characteristics. In papillary carcinoma, papillary formations or psammoma bodies are found in the sample. The demonstration of amyloid establishes the diagnosis of medullary carcinoma; highly pleomorphic cells suggest anaplastic or metastatic tumours. Hürthle tumours can be recognized by their cytoplasmic texture.

A fine-needle aspirate will give information as to the fluid content of any mass. If a mass is cystic and after aspiration has a significant residual solid mass, then there should be a repeat biopsy and aspiration.

A skilled cytologist will be able to differentiate between the different types of thyroiditis, i.e. granulomatous thyroiditis (de Quervain's), subacute thyroiditis (Hashimoto's) or invasive thyroiditis (Riedel's).

The false-negative rate varies from 0 to 4% and the false-positive rate varies between 0 and 29%. These rates, of course, depend on the experience and skill of the cytologist.

Biological behaviour of follicular tumours

The biological behaviour of follicular tumours must be judged from the presence or absence of an invasive growth pattern. A completely encapsulated follicular tumour should be classified as benign, but any evidence of invasive growth classifies it as a carcinoma even though there is a lack of the cytological characteristics of malignancy. Sometimes invasion may be detected only after a careful examination of an apparently encapsulated nodule and the adjacent vessels. The diagnosis of follicular carcinoma, therefore, cannot be made from a needle aspirate.

The value of the thyroid scan

When used for scans, ^{131}I delivers significant irradiation to the thyroid. To avoid this irradiation, ^{99m}Tc or ^{123}I is used for diagnostic scans because of the short half-life which is measured in hours.

Clearly, 'cold' or 'hot' nodules do not present a major problem. The problem nodule shows normal or spotty uptake. The definition of a thyroid mass by scan depends on where it is. Smaller posterior nodules may be overlain by active thyroid tissue; multiple small nodules may give a relatively homogeneous appearance. The scan is of great value in the thick muscular neck, where it can confirm suspicious clinical findings. It can give information as to whether a mass is closely related to the thyroid or outside the thyroid. A scan cannot locate accurately the position of a cancer within the thyroid stroma.

Extent of the thyroidectomy

In follicular carcinoma and in medullary carcinoma there is little debate as to the operation. It ought to be a total thyroidectomy.

There is debate, however, as to the best option for papillary thyroid tumours. Papillary cancer is frequently multifocal and small lesions in the contralateral lobe will be missed if a simple lobectomy is done. The contralateral lobe contains minute foci of papillary cancer in 36% of specimens. Less than 10% of these, however, will declare as frank carcinomas in the ensuing years.

If ^{131}I therapy is to be used postoperatively, then all active thyroid tissue should be ablated and this is an argument also for a total thyroidectomy. Males, and all patients older than 40 years, have a higher chance of recurrence and so a total thyroidectomy may be considered in these subjects. The reason not to do a total thyroidectomy is probably based on the assumption that complications are less with a lobectomy. In skilled hands, this should not be the case.

Is it worth doing extended operations?

In view of the lethal nature of anaplastic carcinoma, it is never worthwhile operating on the larynx, pharynx and oesophagus in association with thyroid removal for these tumours.

Surgery is worth considering, however, in the management of invasive papillary follicular or medullary carcinoma. Very often a sternotomy is necessary to extirpate extensions of these tumours and the paratracheal nodes. They tend to have a pushing margin and so areas of thyroid and tracheal cartilage can be pared off, preserving these structures; if there is significant invasion, then a laryngectomy and also excision of part of the trachea can be done. If the tumour invades all of the trachea, then a segment of trachea should be excised and an end-to-end anastomosis performed. If the tumours invade posteriorly and involve the oesophagus, then a laryngopharyngecotmy is worth doing, reconstituting the pharynx either with a pectoralis major myocutaneous flap or a free jejunal transplant.

The dysphonic patient after thyroidectomy

If the patient has voice alteration immediately after a thyroid operation, then it may be due to a neuropraxia and axonotmesis, or to a division of the nerve.

The authors do not believe that the traditional way of assessing cord movement after a thyroidectomy, by having the anaesthetist look at the larynx during the recovery phase, is a valid test. It is almost impossible to see vocal cord movement as an isolated event during the recovery period and, very often, mass movement of the larynx is mistaken for movement of the cords.

Opinions vary as to whether reopening the neck in the event of vocal cord paralysis is worthwhile. The recurrent laryngeal nerve may be included in a suture involving the inferior thyroid artery but the harvest of the search for this factor is low. In spite of this, the authors feel that the operative site should be explored immediately in the event of any major nerve paralysis.

If the cord is in the midline, then the patient will recover sufficient voice but may retain some breathlessness on severe exertion such as tennis or jogging. If the cord is in the abducted position, then a later medialization procedure may be indicated.

If a patient has a reasonable voice after thyroidectomy and develops hoarseness some weeks later, then it is likely that the vocal cord damage relates to the operation. The recurrent laryngeal nerve will seldom, if ever, be paralysed by the formation of scar tissue. The voice may be normal after the operation due to oedema of the vocal cords from intubation or manipulation of the larynx during removal of the thyroid. This may disguise a cord paralysis, and the dysphonia may only come to light as the cordal oedema subsides, thus leaving a gap between the cords on phonation.

The stridulous patient after thyroidectomy

If a patient has stridor after a thyroidectomy, then both the vocal cords are in the mid-position. This should be confirmed by laryngoscopy and, if it is confirmed, the neck should be reopened. The patient should have a temporary tracheostomy and both recurrent laryngeal nerves should be explored. There may be involvement of the nerve with a suture but if a transected nerve is cut, then it is worthwhile performing a primary nerve anastomosis because the alternative is a permanent tracheostomy.

The patient who is left with a permanent tracheostomy in this instance has the choice of keeping the tracheostomy and thus having a good voice but an external deformity; or of having a Woodman's operation, which will close the tracheostomy but will result in a breathy voice.

References and further reading

Pathology

Bell R M (1986) Thyroid carcinoma. *Surg Clin North Am* **66**:13–30.

Davis N L, Gordon M, Germann E, Robins R E, McGregor G I (1991) Clinical parameters predictive of malignancy of thyroid follicular neoplasms. *Am J Surg* **161**:567–9.

Deftos L J, Bone H G, Parthemore J G (1980) Immunohistological studies of medullary thyroid carcinoma and C cell hyperplasia. *J Clin Endocrinol Metab* **51**:857–62.

Farbota L M, Calandra D B, Lawrence A M Paloyai E (1985) Thyroid carcinoma in Graves's disease. *Surgery* **98**:1148–52.

Favus M J, Schnieder A B, Stachura M F et al. (1976) Thyroid cancer occurring as a late consequence of head-and-neck irradiation: evaluation of 1056 patients. *N Engl J Med* **294**:1019–25.

Fernandes B J, Bedard Y C, Rosen I (1982) Mucous-producing medullary cell carcinoma of the thyroid gland. *Am J Clin Pathol* **78**:536–40.

Har-el G, Hadar T, Segal K, Levy R, Sidi J (1986) Hurthle cell carcinoma of the thyroid gland. *Cancer* **57**:1613–17.

Mahoney J P, Saffos R O, Rhatigan R M (1980) Follicular adenoacanthoma of the thyroid gland. *Histopathology* **4**:547–57.

Shimaoka K, Tsukada Y (1980) Squamous cell carcinomas and adenosquamous carcinoma originating from the thyroid gland. *Cancer* **8**:1833–42.

Shvero J, Gal R, Avidor I, Hadar T, Kessler E (1988) Anaplastic thyroid carcinoma; a clinical, histological and immunohistochemical study. *Cancer* **62**:319–25.

Sizemore G W (1987) Medullary carcinoma of the thyroid gland. *Semin Oncol* **14**:306–14.

Investigations

Bashist B, Ellis K, Gold R P (1982) Computed tomography of intrathoracic goiters. *Am J Radiol* **140**:455–60.

Black E G, Sheppard M C, Hoffenberg R (1987) Serial serum thyroglobulin measurements in the management of differentiated thyroid carcinoma. *Clin Endocrinol* **27**:115–20.

Brendel A J, Guyot M, Jeandot R, Lefort G, Manciet G (1988) Thallium-201 imaging in the follow-up of differentiated thyroid carcinoma. *J Nucl Med* **29**:1515–20.

Brunt L M, Wells S A (1987) Advances in the diagnosis and treatment of medullary thyroid carcinoma. *Surg Clin North Am* **67**:263–80.

Edmonds C J, Hayes S, Kermode J C, Thompson B D (1977) Measurement of serum TSH and thyroid hormones in the management of thyroid carcinoma with radioiodine. *Br J Radiol* **50**:799–807.

Friedman M, Toriumi D M, Maffee M F (1988) Diagnostic imaging techniques in thyroid cancer. *Am J Surg* **155**:215–23.

Hall T L, Layfield L J, Philippe A, Rosenthal D L (1989) Sources of diagnostic error in fine needle aspiration of the thyroid. *Cancer* **63**:718–25.

Harmer C (1991) Multidisciplinary management of thyroid neoplasms. In: Preece P E, Rosin R D, Maran A G D (eds) *Head and Neck Oncology for the General Surgeon*, London, W. B. Saunders, pp. 55–90.

Higgins C B, Auffermann W (1988) MR imaging of thyroid and parathyroid glands: a review of current status. *Am J Radiol* **151**:1095–106.

Lennquist S (1987) The thyroid nodule: diagnosis and surgical treatment. *Surg Clin North Am* **67**:213–32.

Miller J M, Kini S R, Hamburger J I (1985) The diagnosis of malignant follicular neoplasms of the thyroid by needle biopsy. *Cancer* **55**:2812–17.

Nathan A R, Raines K B, Lee Y M, Sakas E L, Ribbing J M (1988) Fine-needle aspiration biopsy of cold thyroid nodules. *Cancer* **62**:1337–42.

Sessions R B, Diehl W L (1989) Thyroid cancer and related nodularity. In: Myers E N, Suen J Y (eds) *Cancer of the*

Head and Neck, New York, Churchill Livingstone, pp. 735–89.

Surgery of the thyroid gland

Eisele D W, Goldstone A C (1991) Electrophysiologic identification and preservation of the superior laryngeal nerve during thyroid surgery. *Laryngoscope* **101**:313–15.

Harada T, Shimaoka K, Mimura T, Ito K (1987) Current treatment of Graves' disease. *Surg Clin North Am* **67**:299–314.

Kark A E, Kissin M W, Auerbach R, Meikle M (1984) Voice changes after thyroidectomy: role of the external laryngeal nerve. *Br Med J* **289**:1412–15.

Katz A D, Bronson D (1978) Total thyroidectomy: the indication and results of 630 cases. *Am J Surg* **136**:450–4.

Lipton R J, McCaffrey T V, Litchy W J (1988) Intraoperative electrophysiological monitoring of laryngeal muscle during thyroid surgery. *Laryngoscope* **98**:1292–6.

Noguchi S, Murakami N (1987) The value of lymph node dissection in patients with differentiated thyroid cancer. *Surg Clin North Am* **67**:251–61.

Rossi R L, Cady B, Silverman M L, Wool M S, Horner T A (1986) Current results of conservative surgery for differentiated thyroid carcinoma. *World J Surg* **10**:612–22.

Schroder D M, Chambors A, France C J (1986) Operative strategy for thyroid cancer: is total thyroidectomy worth the price? *Cancer* **58**:2320–8.

Sluis R F van der, Wobbes T (1985) Total thyroidectomy: the treatment of choice in differentiated thyroid carcinoma? *Eur J Surg Oncol* **11**:343–6.

Starnes H F, Brooks D C, Pinkus G S, Brooks J R (1985) Surgery for thyroid carcinoma. *Cancer* **55**:1376–81.

Thomas C G, Croom R G (1987) Current management of the patient with autonomously functioning nodular goiter. *Surg Clin North Am* **67**:315–28.

Wells S A, Dilley W G, Farndon J R, Leight G S, Baylin S B (1985) Early diagnosis and treatment of medullary thyroid carcinoma. *Arch Intern Med* **145**:1248–52.

Index